HULL ROYAL INFIRMARY
T24644

For Churchill Livingstone:

Commissioning Editor: Timothy Horne
Project Development Manager: Janice Urquhart
Project Manager: Frances Affleck
Design: Jim Farley

PREFACE

'We believe that communication by verbal and written methods is the fundamental basis for study and learning. Nevertheless, in the modern setting where knowledge is increasing so rapidly and in a subject such as pathology where morphological changes are a major component, we consider that the visual image has an important facilitating role.'

Since these comments were written in the preface to the first edition 18 years ago, medical education has changed considerably. There has been a recognition of the adverse effects of 'information overload' on medical students, separation of 'core' and 'special study topics' and an increasing emphasis on the understanding of basic mechanisms. The place of pathology in the curriculum has also altered, especially in those medical schools which have changed from a subject-based to a topic- or problem-based curriculum. Nevertheless, pathology remains one of the foundations of clinical medicine.

In this fifth edition the general layout and style and the division into general and systemic chapters have been retained. We have concentrated on 'core' topics and on what we feel to be clinically relevant pathology. We have attempted to accommodate, but also keep in perspective, the continuing rapid expansion in knowledge of cell and molecular pathology, but recognise that our attempts at simplification do not tell the whole story.

We are indebted to our colleagues, Drs Alan Mowat (Chapter 5, Immunity) and George Lindop (Chapter 7, Cardiovascular Diseases) for detailed advice and criticism and to Drs Wilhelmina Behan and Torquil MacLeod for helpful discussions in the preparation of this edition. Credit for any improvement is theirs; the shortcomings are our responsibility.

P. S. Macfarlane
R. Reid
R. Callander

MEDICAL LIBRARY
ERMEC
HULL ROYAL INFIRMARY
ANLABY ROAD
HULL HU3 2JZ

CONTENTS

Introduction	ix
1. Cell and Tissue Damage	1
2. Inflammation	31
3. Healing	47
4. Infection	61
5. Immunity	87
6. Neoplasia	113
7. Cardiovascular Diseases	155
8. Respiratory System	249
9. Gastrointestinal Tract	289
10. Liver, Gallbladder and Pancreas	341
11. Haemopoietic and Lympho-reticular tissues	383
12. Genitourinary System	463
13. Nervous System	543
14. Musculo-skeletal System	605
15. Endocrine System	645
Index	669

INTRODUCTION

Pathology is the study of disease. It describes the manifestations of the disease, its progress and sequelae and attempts to determine the cause (aetiology) and underlying mechanisms (pathogenesis). It forms a bridge between basic science and clinical practice.

Disease occurs when there are variations of structure outside the normal range.

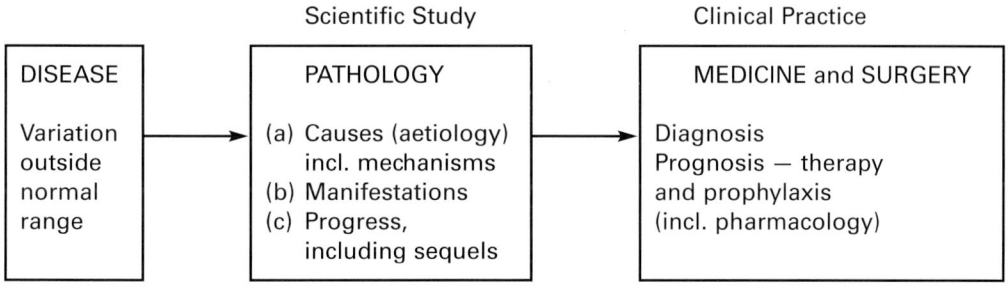

The manifestations of a disease are the sum of the damage done by a harmful agent and the body's response. The variation in these components accounts for the great diversity of disease, which can then be classified into four main groups:

DEVELOPMENTAL INFLAMMATORY NEOPLASTIC DEGENERATIVE

Causes of disease

The various factors involved are considered in 2 broad groups:
(1) Environmental factors and (2) Genetic factors.

ENVIRONMENTAL FACTORS are many and are classified under the following general headings:

Physical agents Among these are trauma, radiations, extremes of heat and cold, electrical power, i.e. the application to the body of an excess of physical energy in any form.

Chemical poisons These are increasing in number particularly with the advances in industrial processing. Some act in a general manner, such as cyanide which is toxic to all cells. Others act locally, for example strong acids and caustics. Another group exhibit a predilection for certain organs — paraquat affects the lungs, phosphorus and organic solvents cause damage especially in the liver and kidneys.

Iatrogenic disease is an important subgroup, not uncommon in present times due to the development of powerful drugs, many of which have undesirable side effects.

Nutritional deficiencies and excesses They may arise as a result of poor supply, interference with absorption, inefficient transport within the body or defective utilisation. In addition, the effects may be of a general nature as in starvation or lack of oxygen or they cause specific damage, for example, in vitamin deficiencies. Dietary excess plays an important role in diseases in Western countries.

Infections and infestations Viruses, bacteria, fungi, protozoa and metazoa all cause disease. They may do so by causing cell destruction directly as in certain virus infections, for example poliomyelitis, or protozoal infections, for example malaria. In many cases, however the damage is done by toxins elaborated by the infecting agent as in diphtheria and tetanus. As with poisons they may have a general effect or show a predilection for certain tissues.

Abnormal immunological reactions The immune process is normally protective but in certain circumstances the reaction may become deranged. Hypersensitivity to various substances can lead to alarming shock-like conditions — anaphylaxis or to more localised lesions such as asthma. In other circumstances the immune process may act against the body cells — autoimmunity. This can be seen in certain endocrine diseases such as thyroiditis.

Psychological factors cause and influence disease processes in several ways: (a) psychological stress may lead to mental illness; (b) their influence on the individual's symptoms and reaction to established somatic disease is apparent; (c) they are important components in disease caused by addiction, for example alcohol, tobacco; (d) finally it is thought that psychogenetic factors, by as yet ill-defined mechanisms, may be causally related to such diseases as hypertension, coronary arterial thrombosis and ulcerative colitis.

GENETIC FACTORS are the results of the actions of single genes and groups of genes. Research, such as the human genome project, has led to rapid expansion in knowledge. Both variations in 'normal' genes and mutations which radically affect the function of 'abnormal' genes influence the development of disease.

Normal genes

There is considerable genetic variation among individuals, both between and within races and even within families. These genetic polymorphisms strongly influence SUSCEPTIBILITY and RESISTANCE to disease. For example:

1. The susceptibility of fair skin to damage by ultra-violet light (and the development of skin cancer) is well known and the mechanism — lack of the protective pigment melanin — is obvious, and presumably determined on evolutionary grounds.
2. The human leucocyte antigen (HLA) system is a complex of genes on chromosome 6 in which there is a great allelic variation. An individual's HLA type strongly influences the development of many disorders especially autoimmune diseases.

Abnormal genes

The mutations which give rise to disease vary from point mutations affecting single base pairs (e.g. sickle cell anaemia) to chromosomal abnormalities affecting many genes (e.g. Down's syndrome). Many mutations appear to arise spontaneously, some follow exposure to radiation or chemicals and others are transmitted in the germline. There is even variation in the rate of mutation, often determined by variation in the genes responsible for DNA repair. INHERITED diseases, where the genetic abnormality directly determines the disease are relatively rare: in contrast there is a genetic component in many diseases.

Age and disease

Different diseases affect different age groups. Developmental disorders and degenerative diseases affect the opposite extremes of life, while tumours, in general, affect an ageing population.

Physiological ageing itself implies a gradual loss of cellular and body vitality usually associated with atrophy of tissues and organs. This process is accentuated and mimicked by the degenerative disease of old age so that physiological and pathological states tend to merge. Nevertheless the student should attempt to identify the distinctions between ageing and disease. Additionally, in old age multiple diseases coexist and also interact with one another. Drug induced disorders are also common in this age group.

METHODS IN PATHOLOGY

The traditional methods of careful naked eye and light microscopic examination of organs at autopsy have been supplemented by the much wider use in clinical practice of biopsy and cytology where tissue or cells are removed during life for diagnosis. Endoscopic and fine needle techniques allow biopsies to be obtained from most parts of the body. In addition, technological advances have allowed examination at more detailed levels:

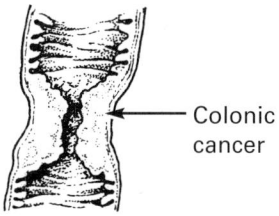

Naked eye examination.

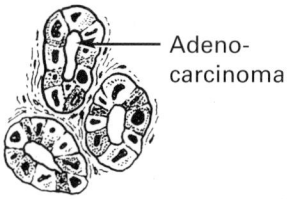

Light microscopy
– morphology.

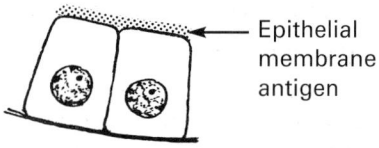

Immunocytochemistry
– demonstration of specific proteins.

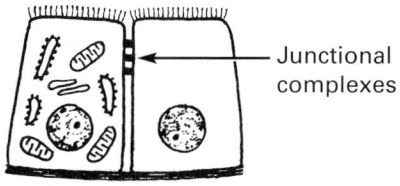

Electron microscopy
— organelles.

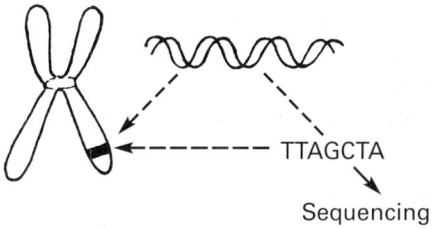

Molecular biology
— chromosomal analysis.

These increasingly sophisticated methods tend to influence the student to focus on detailed mechanisms at the molecular levels. It should not be forgotten that simple methods of gross examination and histological assessment are fundamental to the study of diseases. The following descriptions begin therefore with gross and microscopic pathology and proceed to the more detailed cellular changes when they are known. The student will find that such an approach is the basis of their learning in clinical practice.

CHAPTER 1

CELL AND TISSUE DAMAGE

Cellular Physiology and Pathology	2
Control of Cell Number	3
Apoptosis	4
Cell Damage	5
Necrosis	6–8
Necrosis — Autolysis	9
Cell Damage — Hydropic Swelling	10
Cell Damage — Fatty Change	11
Free Radicals	12
Cell Damage — Radiation	13
Atrophy	14
Ageing	15
Heredity, Genes and Disease	16, 17
Mitosis and Meiosis	18
Genetic Abnormalities and Associated Disorders	19–21
Amyloid Deposition	22, 23
Amyloid Classification	24
Calcification	25
Endogenous Pigmentation	26–28
Endogenous Pigmentation — Degenerations	29

CELLULAR PHYSIOLOGY and PATHOLOGY

To understand diseases of the body systems or individual organs, requires knowledge of the function and dysfunction of individual cells. This is a topic of great complexity and only the basic principles can be outlined.

Cellular physiology is characterised by:

(a) Close interdependence of the various cellular components and activities (though it is convenient to describe them separately).

(b) Balancing control mechanisms aimed at maintaining constant conditions (i.e. homeostasis).

(c) Very efficient compensatory and repair mechanisms to minimise damage.

PLASMA MEMBRANES

Main functions.

1. Maintain integrity of cell.
2. Contact with extracellular environment
   e.g. cell surface receptors.

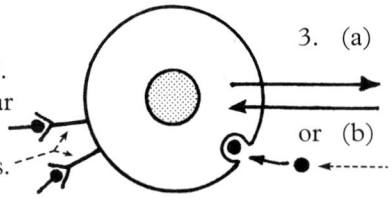

3. (a) Passage of ions through permeable channels e.g. Na^+, K^+

   or (b) Passage of complex molecules by pinocytosis or phagocytosis.

Any disorder may lead to dysfunction or cell death.

MITOCHONDRIA These are the main sites of ENERGY production.

Disorder of energy production affects all cellular functions.

Source	Production		Utilisation
O_2 + glucose →	ADP → ATP (oxidative phosphorylation) →	release of energy →	for all cellular activities

NUCLEUS

The nucleus controls all cellular activities through the action of at least 50, 000 genes, each of which encodes a protein with structural, enzymatic or control functions.

Damage to DNA (e.g. by ionising radiation) is particularly likely in dividing cells. There are effective repair mechanisms but severe damage usually leads to cell death by apoptosis (see page 4).

Germ cell DNA damage (i.e. to spermatogonia or oocytes)

1. Severe damage to chromosomal structure → Prevention of conception; Early abortion
2. Less severe damage to groups of genes or single genes → Developmental abnormalities; Hereditary disease; Susceptibility to diseases

Somatic cell DNA damage

This is acquired during life. Damage to **stem cells** is especially important.

The development of cancer (p. 151) through activation of oncogenes or loss of tumour suppressor genes is the most important example.

LYSOSOMES

These membrane bound organelles contain hydrolytic enzymes and are responsible for digestion and disposal of complex substances. → Disorder may lead to escape of enzymes or to cellular overloading (e.g. storage disorders).

CONTROL OF CELL NUMBER

In adult life the CELL NUMBER is fairly constant: this is achieved by complex control mechanisms which evenly balance the continuing formation of new cells with cell loss.

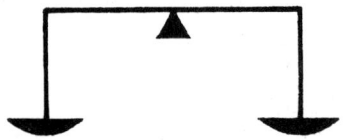

During SOMATIC GROWTH cell proliferation outweighs cell loss.

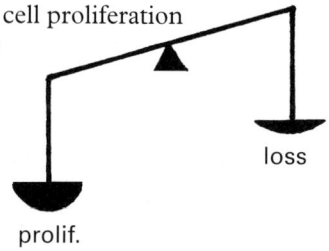

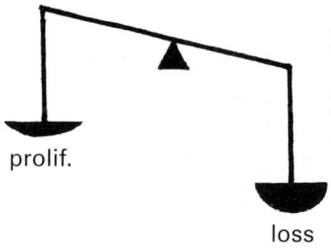

In the ATROPHY of old age, cell loss outweighs cell proliferation.

Also in many diseases the balance is lost.

Cell proliferation — the Cell cycle

In adult life, cells fall into 3 main groups in respect of their proliferation potential.

	Proliferation potential	**Examples**
1. LABILE CELLS	rapid proliferation and cell turnover	gut lining epithelial cells
2. STABLE CELLS	slow proliferation and cell turnover	hepatocytes
3. PERMANENT CELLS	NOT able to proliferate	neurones

In preparation for division, a cell passes through 4 consecutive phases (G_1, S, G_2, M) ending in **Mitosis** (M).

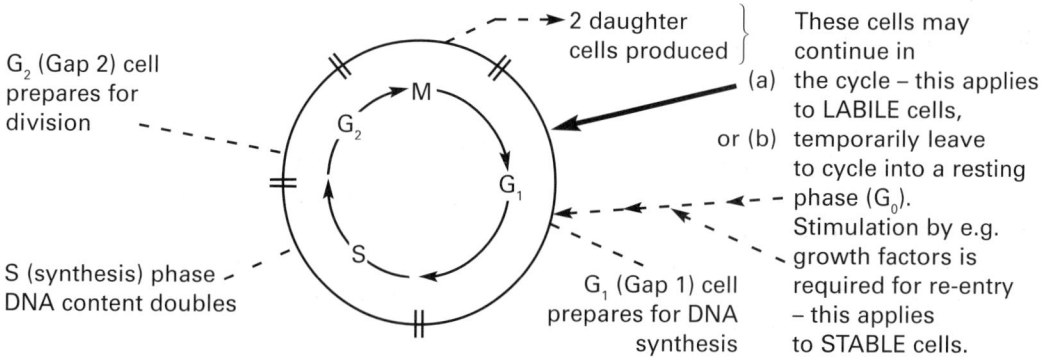

Various growth promotors, inhibitors and drugs influence the cycle at various stages.

Knowledge of the cycle underlies the understanding of mechanisms involved in HEALING and REPAIR and in CARCINOGENESIS.

APOPTOSIS

Apoptosis (programmed cell death) (Greek: apoptosis = falling off, like leaves from a tree) is an important process in health and disease by which effete, abnormal or unwanted cells are eliminated. It differs from necrosis (p. 5) and is an active process. A few examples are:

Apoptosis in health

In embryogenesis and development

(i) Metamorphosis of tadpole to frog.

(ii) Loss of autoreactive response of 'T' cells in the **thymus** preventing auto-immune attack.

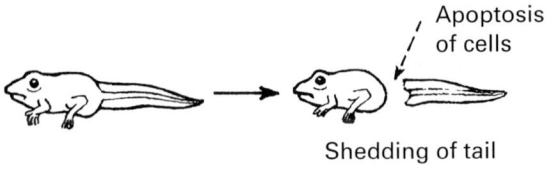

(iii) In atrophy and involution, often on withdrawal of hormones, e.g. menstrual breakdown of endometrium.

Apoptosis in disease

(i) Irradiation, (ii) Virus infection, (iii) Action of cytotoxic 'T' cells, e.g. in rejection of transplanted organs.

(iv) In tumours, apoptosis and proliferation rates together control the rate of tumour growth.

Apoptosis is a rapid process usually affecting single cells scattered in a population of healthy cells. It is considered in 2 stages:

Stage 1: **The dying process**

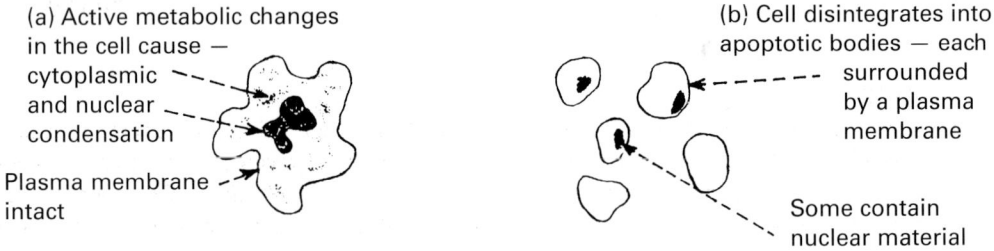

Stage 2: **The elimination process**

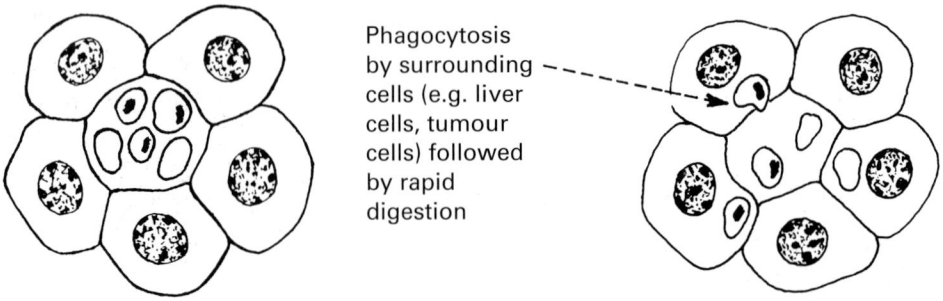

Note

1. The surrounding cells move together to fill the vacant space leaving virtually no evidence of the process.
2. The presence of intact plasma membranes around the apoptotic bodies explains the absence of inflammation.

CELL DAMAGE

A wide variety of noxious agents can damage cells. These can be grouped as follows (the individual diseases mentioned are illustrative examples):

1. **Reduced oxygen supply** — respiratory disease, cardiovascular disease, anaemia
2. **Physical agents** — mechanical trauma, excessive heat or cold, radiations
3. **Chemical agents** — these continue to increase enormously with the complexity of industrial processes
4. **Toxins** — bacteria, plants, animals e.g. snakes
5. **Viruses**
6. **Abnormal immunological reaction** — hypersensitivity states, glomerulonephritis
7. **Nutritional deficiencies** — vitamin deficiency and malabsorption syndromes
8. **Genetic abnormalities** —Down's syndrome

The severity of the injury determines the outcome:

(a) **Mild injury** can be reversed by

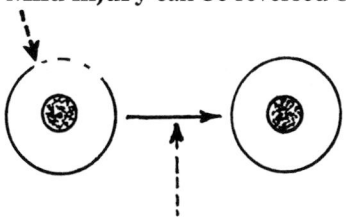

repair mechanisms

(b) **Severe injury** results in cell death by one of two mechanisms:

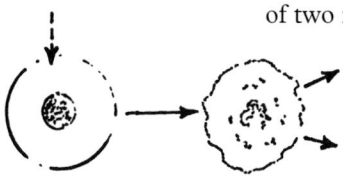

1. NECROSIS (cells simply die)
2. APOPTOSIS (an active process)

NECROSIS

This term describes death of a cell or group of cells, typically following severe hypoxia, physical or chemical injury. Death of the cell is associated with rapid depletion of intracellular energy systems. Initially there are no morphological changes, but within a few hours the cell membrane and intracellular organelles are disrupted. Electron microscopy demonstrates these changes earlier than light microscopy.

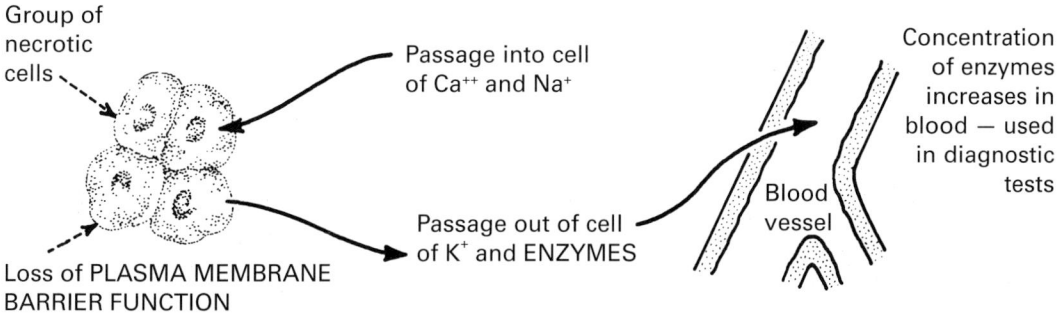

What we recognise as necrosis is due to denaturation and coagulation of protein and/or digestion of the cell by released enzymes. There are several naked eye appearances depending on which of these predominates.

1. Coagulative necrosis is the classical appearance.
2. In colliquative necrosis, the tissue is softened by enzymatic digestion.

NECROSIS

COAGULATIVE NECROSIS

This type of necrosis is frequently caused by lack of blood supply and is exemplified well in infarcts of solid organs, e.g. heart, spleen and kidney.

Naked eye appearance of kidney

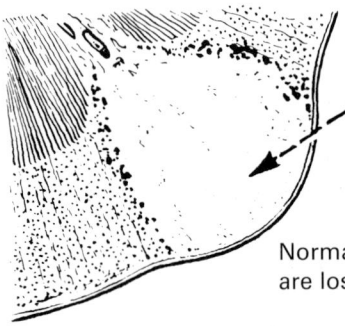

Microscopic appearance

Necrosis *Normal kidney*

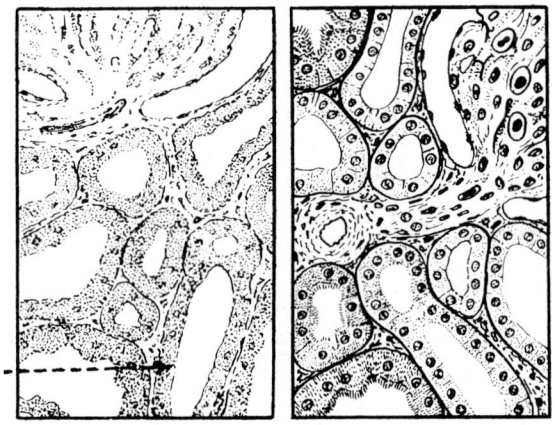

At *light microscopic level* the following changes in the cell are seen:

1. The nucleus shows one of two changes (a) Karyolysis (b) Karyorrhexis.
2. The cytoplasm becomes opaque and strongly eosinophilic (affinity for the red dye, eosin).

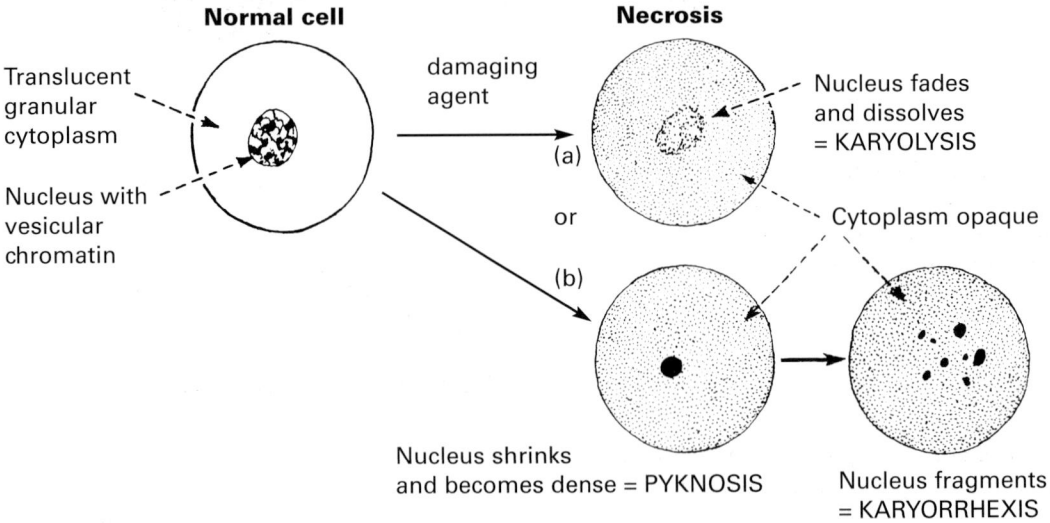

At *electron microscope (E.M.) level*, in addition to the above nuclear changes, disorganisation and disintegration of the cytoplasmic organelles and severe damage to the plasma membrane are seen.

NECROSIS

COLLIQUATIVE NECROSIS

In the brain consistently, and in other tissues when they contain a large amount of fluid and enzyme activity is marked, necrotic areas undergo softening and are filled with pigmented or turbid fluid, with complete loss of structure.

An **abscess** (see p. 40, 41) is an example of colliquative necrosis caused by the enzymatic action of polymorphonuclear leucocytes.

GANGRENE

This is a complication of necrosis. In certain circumstances necrotic tissue is liable to be invaded by putrefactive organisms which are both saccharolytic and proteolytic. Foul-smelling gases are produced and the tissue becomes green or black due to breakdown of haemoglobin. Obstruction of the blood supply to the bowel is almost inevitably followed by gangrene, e.g.:

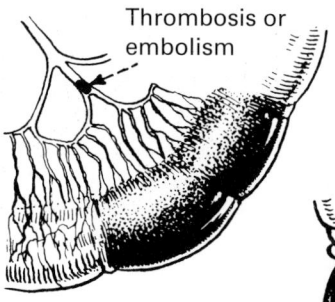

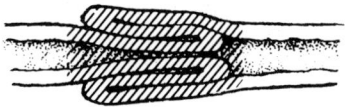

Intussusception

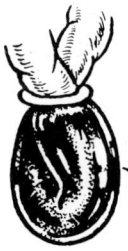

Strangulated
hernia

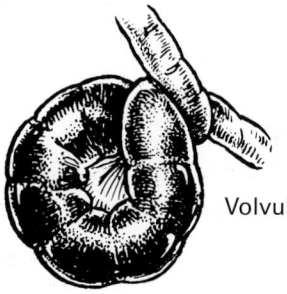

Volvulus

Gangrene also occurs on the skin surface following arterial obstruction. It is particularly liable to affect the limbs, especially the toes in diseases such as diabetes.

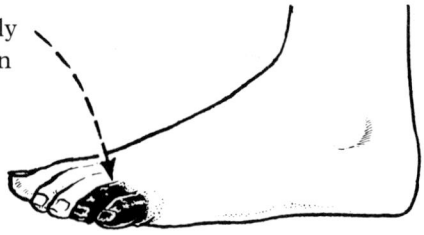

A special type of gangrene follows infection with clostridial organisms (gas gangrene; see p. 70).

NECROSIS

CASEOUS NECROSIS (CASEATION)

The necrotic tissue assumes a cream-cheesy appearance, slightly greasy to the touch. It is commonly seen in tuberculosis (see p. 72).

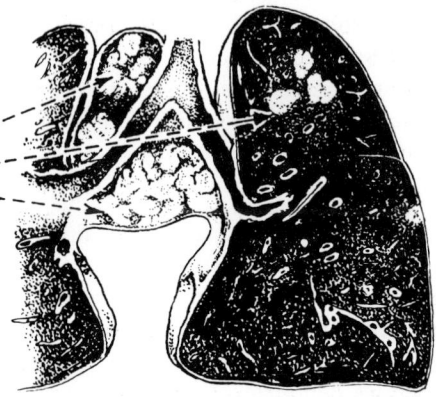

FAT NECROSIS

Adipose tissue is damaged in pancreatitis and occasionally due to trauma. The special appearances are due to the action of lipases on triglycerides as follows:

TRIGLYCERIDES (released from necrotic fat) → FATTY ACIDS + Ca^{++} → Insoluble SOAPS

↑ LIPASE usually pancreatic

E.g. Appearances in omentum and mesenteries.

Naked eye

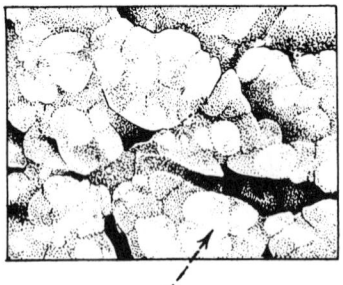

Opaque white patches

Microscopic

Normal fatty tissue

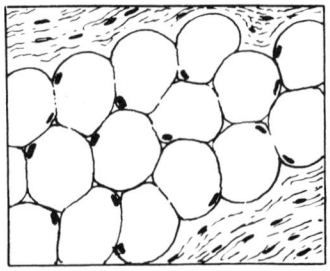

Necrotic

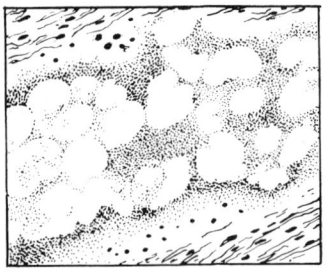

Note loss of nuclei and cell structure, and deposition of insoluble soaps.

FIBRINOID NECROSIS

This is a descriptive term in which connective tissues and especially arterial walls are infiltrated by a strongly eosinophilic hyaline material which shows some of the characteristics of fibrin. Any actual necrosis is usually inconspicuous.

NECROSIS – AUTOLYSIS

SEQUELS OF NECROSIS

1. When small numbers of cells are involved, the cellular debris is removed by PHAGOCYTOSIS (see p. 36).
2. With larger numbers of dead cells, there is an inflammatory response with **organisation** and fibrous repair (see p. 41).
3. When the necrotic tissue cannot be completely removed or organised, deposition of calcium may be an additional feature, for example in TUBERCULOUS CASEOUS NECROSIS. This feature is important in radiological diagnosis. It is sometimes described as 'dystrophic' (page 25).

AUTOLYSIS

The process of 'self-digestion' begins after the death of the cell (as described above) and proceeds at a rate dependent on the local enzyme content; it is an inevitable sequel of necrosis. However, the term is more commonly applied to the changes which take place in tissues removed from the body and in the whole body after death.

In practice, autolysis can be modified or inhibited as follows:

(1) by REFRIGERATION
↓
ENZYME activity slowed down
↓
Whole body 'preserved'
↓
AUTOPSY performed without undue haste

(2) by FIXATION
↓
CHEMICALS added (e.g. formalin) or HEAT
↓
ENZYMES and PROTEINS DENATURED
↓
AVAILABLE for PATHOLOGICAL PROCESSING

CELL DAMAGE – HYDROPIC SWELLING

The various agents which can cause cell necrosis may also cause lesser cell damage which is reversible when the injurious agent is removed.

The appearances and effects are considered under these headings: (1) **hydropic swelling**, (2) **fatty change**, (3) **radiation** and (4) **atrophy**.

HYDROPIC SWELLING

Hydropic swelling — formerly called Cloudy swelling — proceeds to hydropic vacuolation.

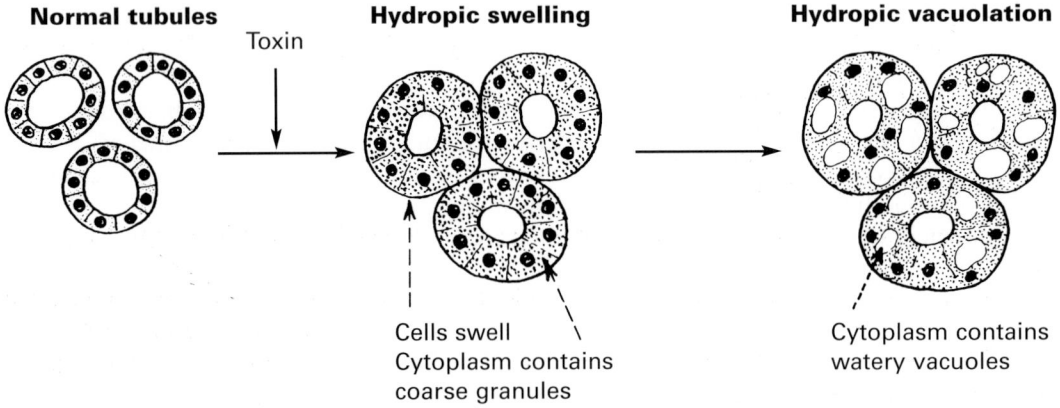

The damaged organs become swollen and on section have a pale and swollen appearance.

Electron microscopic (E.M.) appearances indicate the mechanisms:

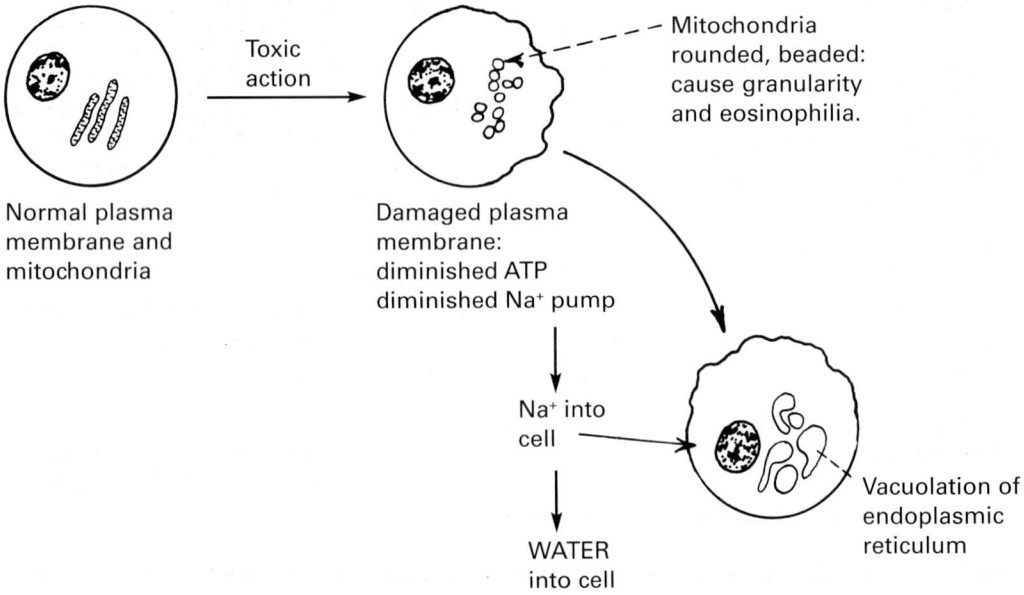

CELL DAMAGE – FATTY CHANGE

This is accumulation of fat in non-fatty tissues, especially the parenchymatous organs, skeletal muscles and the heart, which have a high metabolic rate.

The essential problem is the inability of the non-fatty tissues to metabolise the amount of lipid presented to them, resulting in its accumulation within the cells. The most important causes range from direct cell poisons through clinical conditions associated with reduced cellular energy.

CELL POISONS
Bacterial,
Chemical e.g. Chloroform, Alcohol.

CLINICAL DISORDERS
Anoxia due to anaemia,
cardiac failure, respiratory disease.
Diabetes mellitus, Chronic malnutrition.

→ REDUCED cellular ENZYME activity → Inability to metabolise fat → Accumulation of fat in cells

In normal non-fatty tissues the intracellular fat is not visible by light microscopy using conventional fat stains.

In fatty change, the accumulated fat is visualised using frozen sections and fat-soluble dyes: in routine paraffin sections the fat has been dissolved and is indicated by clear vacuoles.

For example, in the **LIVER**, the increase of deposited fat causes enlargement of the organ. Its distribution varies with the cause, e.g.—

(1) Lack of Oxygen – in anaemia and cardiac failure

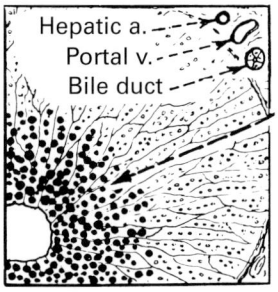

Fats tend to be deposited furthest from the arterial blood supply (hepatic arteriole) around the efferent vein (hepatic venule)

(2) Poison, Toxins etc – alcohol, infections, organic solvents

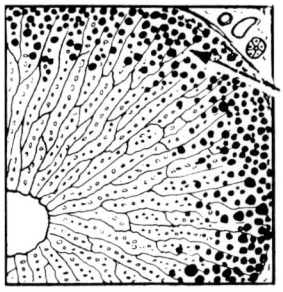

Fat is found nearest the afferent blood supply (portal venule and hepatic arteriole)

EFFECTS OF FATTY CHANGE

Impairment of cellular function is usually due to the pathological process causing the fatty change (e.g. anoxia in severe anaemia) and not to the physical presence of fat within the cell. In the liver, for example, very large accumulations of fat do not impair basic liver functions.

A possible exception is the myocardium in certain circumstances.

(a) **Rapid or large transfusion** + Fatty myocardium → Increased ventricular pressure; → Weak muscle fibres → Dilatation of heart → Cardiac failure

(b) **Sudden excessive exertion** + Fatty myocardium → Rise in blood pressure; → Weak muscle fibres → Temporary left sided cardiac embarrassment

FREE RADICALS

The formation of free radicals is now thought to be an important contributory factor in many disease processes.

Free radicals are molecules with a single unpaired electron in an outer orbital position: they react vigorously with and modify a wide range of molecules affecting particularly lipids (of cell membranes), DNA and proteins.

A dot above the chemical symbol indicates the presence of a free radical: e.g. $OH^{\bullet}$ = hydroxyl radical: $O_2^{\bullet}$ = superoxide radical.

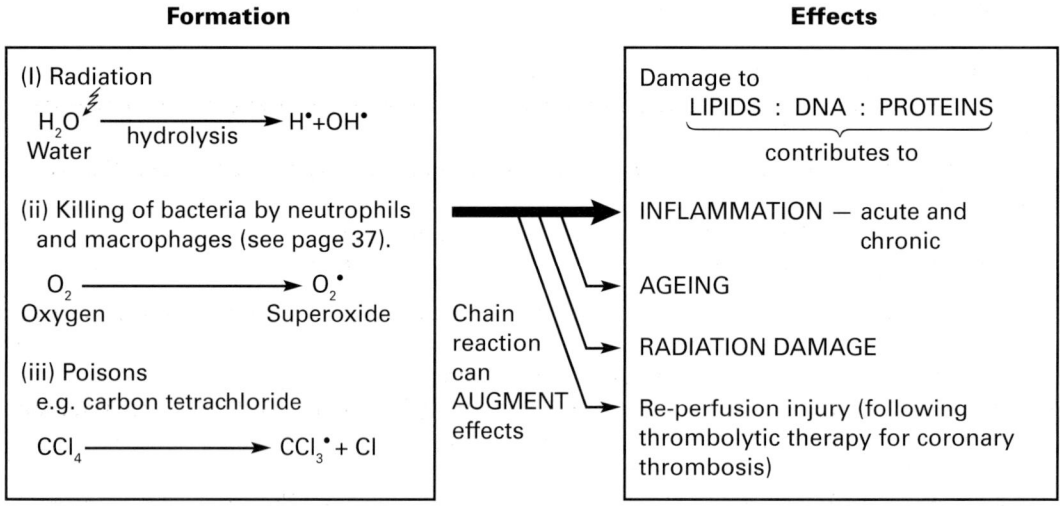

Defence mechanisms to free radicals

Some free radicals decay spontaneously (e.g. $O_2^{\bullet}$) but they can also be removed by ANTIOXIDANTS e.g. Vitamin E and also by the action of enzymes such as superoxide mutase and catalase.

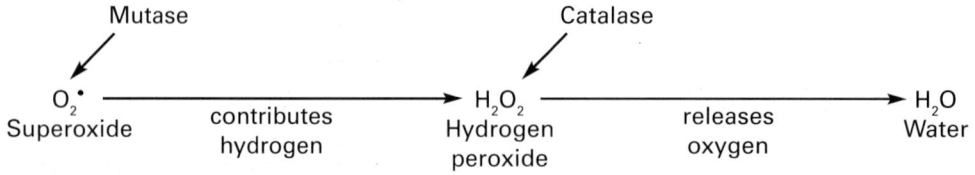

CELL DAMAGE – RADIATION

High energy (ionising) radiation, particularly in the form of gamma (γ) or X-rays can cause serious cellular and tissue damage.

At cellular level there are 2 mechanisms involving:

1. The cell **CYTOPLASM**

   A large dose of radiation hydrolyses water producing damaging **free hydroxyl** radicals: acute cell death follows

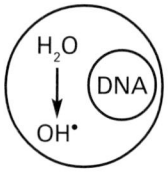

2. The cell **NUCLEUS**

   Lower doses damage DNA with 2 results:
   (a) failure to replicate
   (b) mutation with variable genetic abnormalities

These effects will be considered under 3 headings:

1. The **localised effects** complicating radiotherapy in the tissues adjacent to the therapeutic field.

   Following any reparable acute damage a latent period precedes persistent injury. This is caused by:

   (a) damage to blood vessels } leading to (a) *ischaemia*
   (b) damage to fibroblasts } leading to (b) *dense fibrosis*

   Injury to organs which are difficult to shield is seen, for example, in skin, eyes, alimentary tract, bladder, lungs, gonads and spinal cord.

   In surgical practice, wound healing is seriously impaired.

2. Some of the mutations may lead to cancer, particularly leukaemias and lymphomas. (About 2% of all malignancies are associated with radiation.)

   The mechanisms are described on page 148.

3. **Whole body radiation** is usually the result of atomic explosion. The acute effects which are related to large doses are summarised below.

Dose (Grays)	**Result**	**Mechanism**
above 50	Death in a few hours	All cells damaged but particularly **CNS:** CEREBRAL OEDEMA ↓ COMA
5–10	Death 3–7 days	Mucous lining of **intestine** destroyed: DIARRHOEA: SEPTICAEMIC SHOCK
2–5	Death 2–3 weeks	**Bone marrow** destroyed: LEUCOPENIA THROMBOCYTOPENIA ↓ INFECTION: HAEMORRHAGE
0.2-1	Damage to fetus in early pregnancy	Embryonal cell mutation

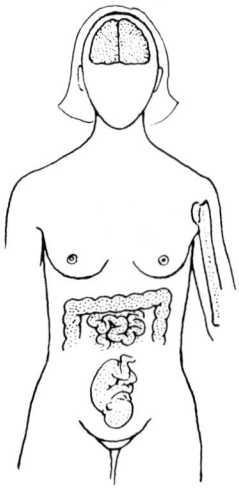

ATROPHY

This is a simple decrease in cell size or number, resulting in a shrinkage of affected tissues and organs. The most common example is atrophy of old age (see p. 15).

Causes

(1) **Gradual diminution in blood supply** ⟶ Reduction in oxygen supply and nutrients ⟶ General fall in cell activity and shrinkage, e.g. narrowing of coronary arteries → myocardial atrophy

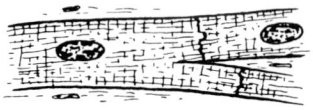

Normal

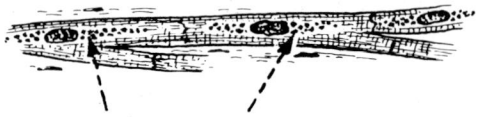

Accumulation of lipofuscin around nucleus

Lipofuscin ("wear and tear" pigment) is a golden yellow pigment representing undigested lipid material derived from cellular metabolism.

(2) **Reduced functional activity** (disuse atrophy) ⟶ Diminished demand for nutrition ⟶ Atrophy of cells

E.g. Lack of exercise ⟶ Atrophy of skeletal muscle
E.g. Obstruction of gland duct ⟶ Atrophy of gland (Apoptosis is important here)

(3) **Interrupted nerve supply** ⟶ Reduced reflex and metabolic activities, e.g. atrophy of skeletal muscles after destruction of motor nerves as in poliomyelitis.

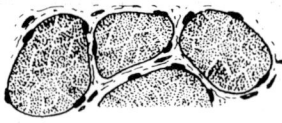

← Normal

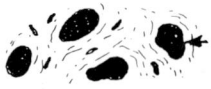

← Loss of structure and shrinkage

(4) **Endocrine deficiency** ⟶ Loss of trophic mechanism ⟶ Reduced metabolic activity in dependent tissues

E.g. Pituitary deficiency ⟶ Atrophy of ⟶ Thyroid
⟶ Adrenals
⟶ Gonads and genital organs

(5) **Pressure** ⟶ Interruption of blood supply and interference with function, e.g. neoplasm pressing on surrounding tissues.

Atrophy is reversible provided the cause is eliminated or deficiencies restored.

AGEING

The distinction between 'true' ageing and ageing complicated by disease processes may be difficult; since therapy can be directed at the latter the distinction is important in clinical practice.

The changes associated with *true* ageing would be seen in a theoretical 'ideal' environment (minimal stress).

The following diagram is illustrative. The main controlling factors are *intrinsic*, i.e.
genetic: ? associated with expression of ageing genes in mitochondria:
? loss of cells' ability to divide due to telomeric shortening (ends of chromosomes).

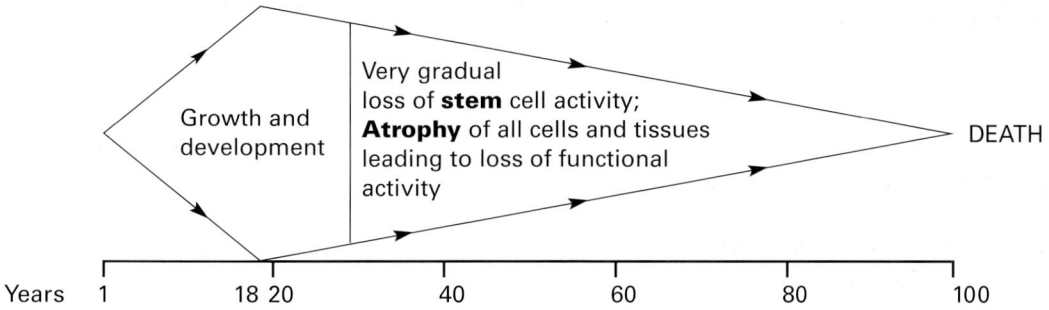

In the real environment this theoretical concept of ageing is accelerated and aggravated by two groups of *extrinsic* factors:

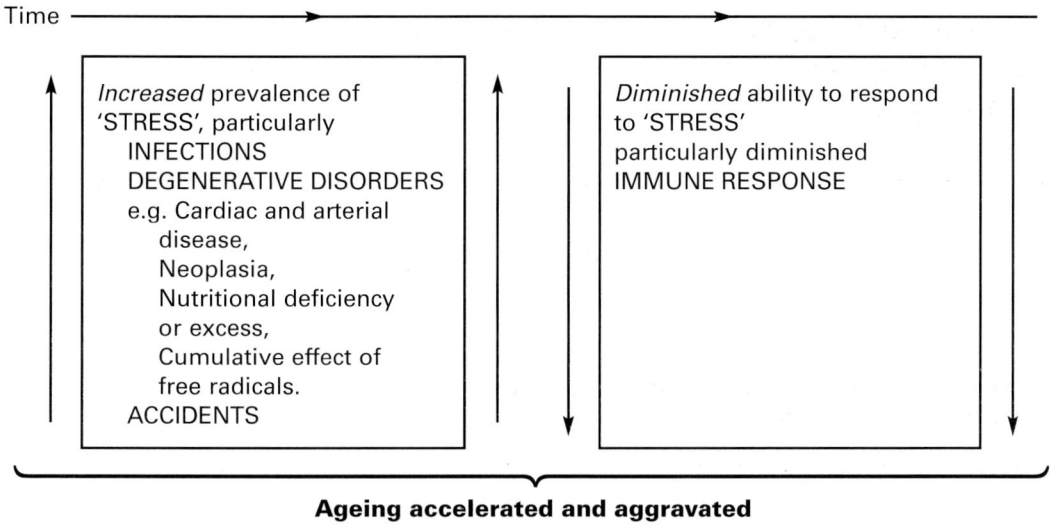

N.B. Death is only very rarely, if ever, due to 'pure' ageing. It is the result of disease — either a single process or, with increasing age, more often several causes.

HEREDITY, GENES AND DISEASE

CELL NUCLEUS AND CHROMOSOMES

Knowledge of the GENETIC influence on disease is expanding very rapidly. The following can only be a brief outline of basic facts:

The cell **NUCLEUS** contains structures, CHROMOSOMES, which transmit hereditary traits from one generation to the next and also control the synthesis of all the proteins in the body.

The 46 chromosomes which most human nuclei contain are not identifiable in differentiated cells or cells in the non-proliferating phase of the cell cycle (G_0).

The different morphological appearances of nuclei in histological sections indicate to some extent the amount of nuclear activity.

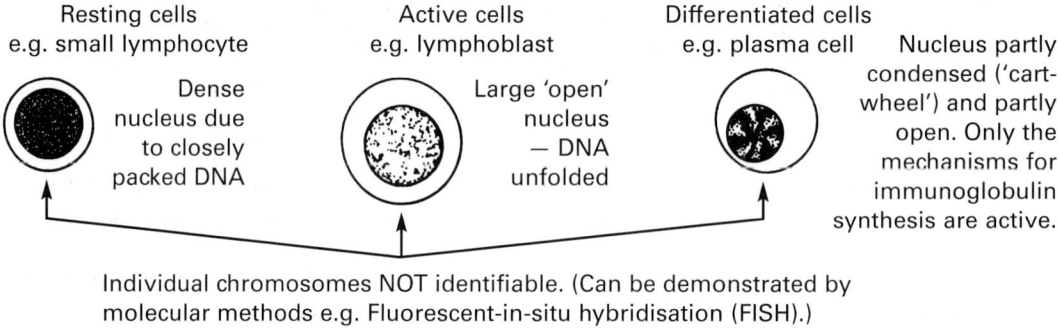

CHROMOSOMES

During MITOSIS the chromosomes condense into specific morphological forms which are identifiable by light microscopy: when colchicine is added to a cell culture, mitosis is arrested at the metaphase: chromosomes are then separable and can be studied.

Diagram of a typical chromosome

Banded appearance

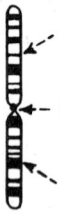

Note: This appearance represents a very condensed and coiled molecular arrangement i.e. inactive.

The following features are specific to each chromosome: (1) Overall length, (2) position of centromere (this dictates the length of each arm) and (3) the pattern of banding.

e.g.

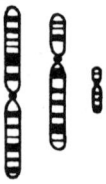

Using these morphological criteria each chromosome is identified and numbered 1 to 22.

The sex chromosomes are labelled

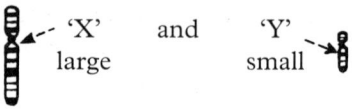

A typical normal chromosome map (karyotype) shows 22 pairs of different but identifiable chromosomes ..... plus 2 sex chromosomes,

Each pair is called an AUTOSOME and consists of a PATERNAL and MATERNAL chromosome.

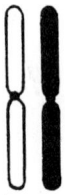

x22

either 2 large X = FEMALE

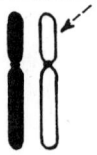

or 1 large X and 1 small Y = MALE

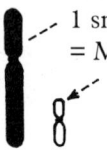

HEREDITY, GENES AND DISEASE

DEOXYRIBONUCLEIC ACID (DNA)

Since Watson and Crick defined the molecular structure of DNA in 1953, there has been a great increase in knowledge of the 'genetic code'. Each chromosome is a very long single molecule of deoxyribonucleic acid (DNA), condensed during mitosis.

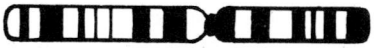

It is extended to its characteristic structure when active:

The **DOUBLE HELIX**

Diagram of a very small part of a very long molecule.

2 long spirals of nucleotides [consisting of a deoxyribose (sugar) + phosphate] around a central axis, complementary but running in opposite directions.

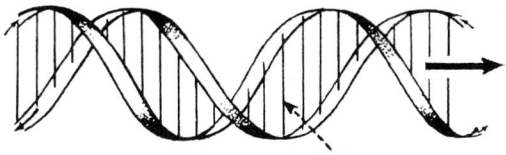

Extending to millions of base pairs

Joined by purine and pyrimidine base pairs

The essential function is to initiate and control the synthesis of proteins from amino-acids. All types of protein (structural proteins, hormones, receptors, intra-cellular messengers etc.) are ENCODED along the molecule.

A **GENE** is the unit of the chromosome responsible for the synthesis of a single SPECIFIC PROTEIN. Genes vary in length but on average occupy about 20,000 base pairs of the molecule.

There are about 50,000 genes in all the human chromosomes, not all are active: some are repetitive: some form clusters subserving related activities [e.g. MHC (HLA) locus, see page 92].

There is a complex REGULATION of gene activity involving stop and start signals, promotor and enhancer functions all within the DNA structure. Many genes have now been sequenced as part of the *'human gene project'*.

Gene expression and protein synthesis

A gene consists of coding regions (EXONS) interspersed with non-coding regions (INTRONS). In transcription the introns are eliminated and all the exons are transcribed to a ribonucleic acid form (mRNA) which is a copy of the DNA-code sequencing the amino-acids required for the production of a specific protein.

The simplified diagram illustrates:

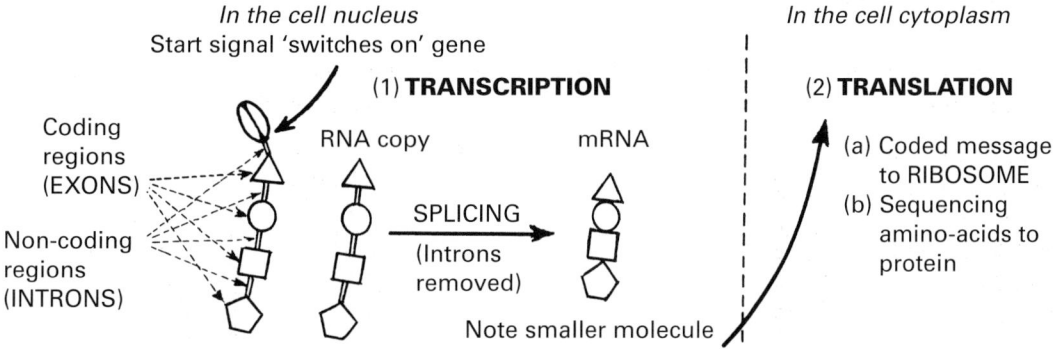

MITOSIS AND MEIOSIS

MITOSIS is the process by which SOMATIC cells proliferate ensuring *exact replication of the daughter cells*. Following the stimulus to proliferate, the chromosomes condense and replicate exactly.

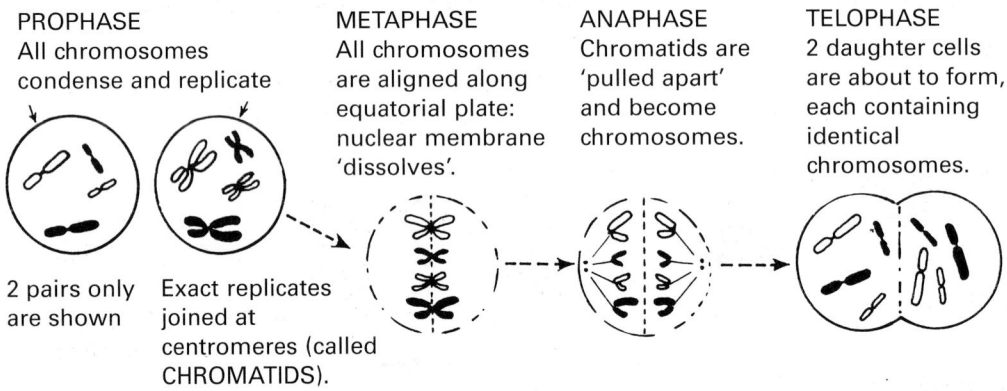

MEIOSIS is a complex process occurring during GAMETOGENESIS: it involves the reduction and division of chromosomes in such a way that (1) a random mixture of both parental genes is present in the gamete and that (2) the chances are equal for fertilisation to result in either sex.

This simple diagram shows the important results of meiosis.

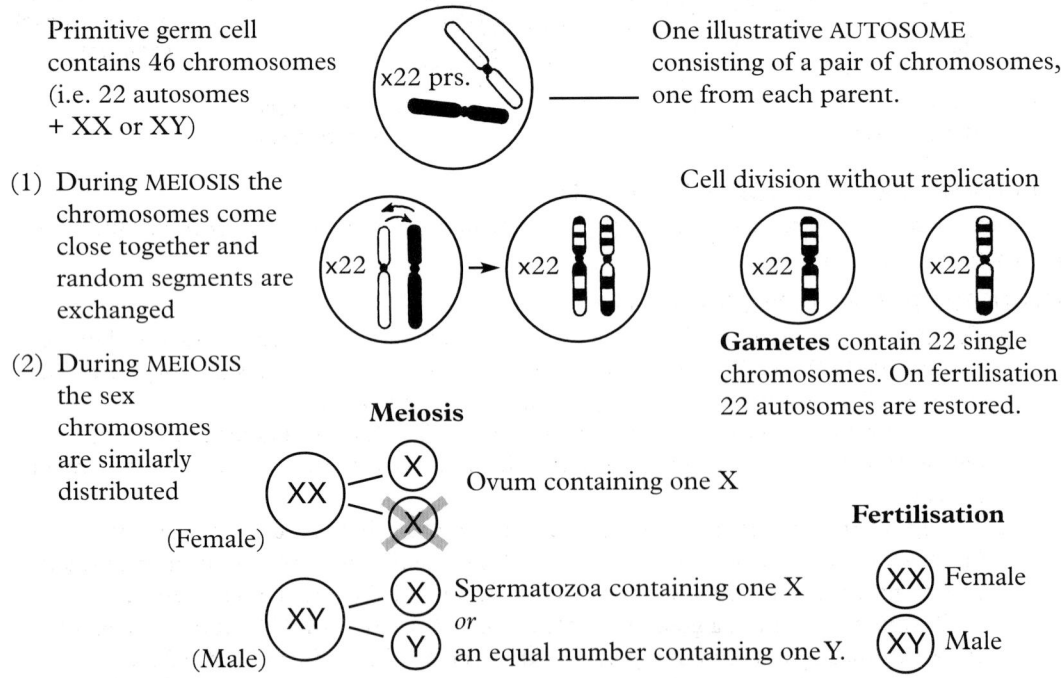

Note: In this simplified diagram a preliminary replication before meiosis and mitotic divisions after meiosis are omitted. The chances of error can be seen to be greatly increased.

GENETIC ABNORMALITIES AND ASSOCIATED DISORDERS

It is not surprising that errors arise during these complex genetic activities. GERM CELLS and proliferating SOMATIC CELLS (including STEM CELLS) are susceptible to such errors.

They may occur spontaneously or be potentiated by external influences.

It is important to distinguish between germ cell and somatic cell abnormalities.

GERM CELL ABNORMALITIES

Errors which have arisen during germ cell development are transferred to the fertilised ovum and thence to all cells including the germ cells of the new individual.

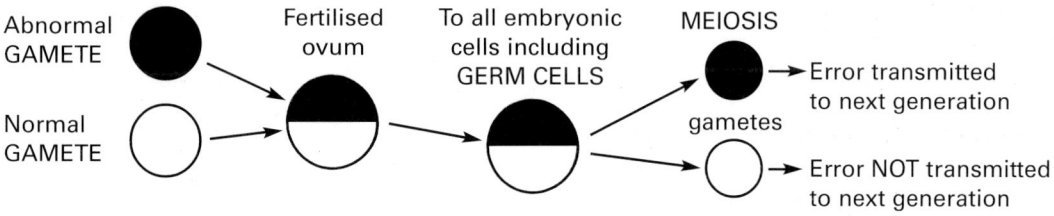

ABNORMALITIES arising in SOMATIC CELLS

These tend to cause restricted effects: they are not transmitted to next generation.

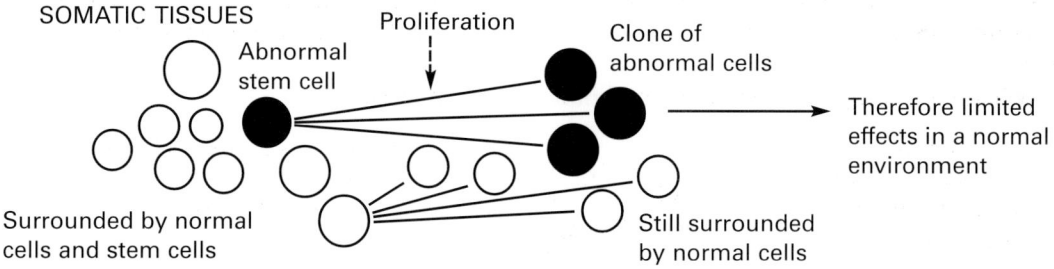

TYPES OF GENETIC ABNORMALITIES

They range from large, involving whole chromosomes, through parts of chromosomes, to gene clusters and single genes.

CHROMOSOMAL ABNORMALITIES

(1) ***Polyploidy*** — when the chromosomal numbers are increased by an exact multiple of the normal (23) e.g. 23 × 3 = 69 chromosomes. Such nuclei are seen in hypertrophied muscle cells and ageing liver cells (i.e. somatic cell polyploidy).

Such gross chromosomal abnormalities occurring during gametogenesis or at fertilisation are usually incompatible with life and are a common cause of spontaneous abortion.

(2) ***Aneuploidy*** — where the number of chromosomes is increased usually by one (TRISOMY) or decreased by one (MONOSOMY). Early spontaneous abortion is again common: survivors show mental retardation and varied physical abnormalities.

Down's syndrome is a good example of AUTOSOMAL TRISOMY and is due to an extra chromosome (i.e. Trisomy 21 — karyotype 47XX + 21 or 47XY + 21).

The abnormality occurs in utero after fertilisation of the ovum and is therefore autosomal. Increasing maternal age is a potentiating factor in Down's syndrome and many other genetic defects.

GENETIC ABNORMALITIES AND ASSOCIATED DISORDERS

CHROMOSOMAL ABNORMALITIES (continued)

(3) ***Structural abnormalities***

Despite the existence of efficient repair mechanisms structural errors do arise when the long DNA molecules are accidentally broken during the dramatic physical changes occurring at replication. They include, for example, duplication and deletion of gene clusters and single genes: and translocation of fragments of DNA between chromosomes.

SINGLE GENE DISORDERS

Factors regulating the production of the final specific protein are extremely complex and interacting:

1. *In the nucleus* — *In the cytoplasm*

Activity of other genes

↓

promotion
enhancement
start/stop signals → single gene activity (including the RNA transcription and movement) → ↑ or ↓ ← detailed control of each step in protein synthesis

↓

Therefore GENETIC EXPRESSION very VARIABLE

2. The corresponding genes on each parental chromosome exert important influences on each other. The inheritance of the Rhesus blood group D is illustrative: there are two possibilities at the D locus on the chromosome — 'D' or 'd'. The 3 possible combinations give rise to the actual blood group (phenotype) as follows:

	Homozygous		Heterozygous	
Genotype	DD	dd	Dd	
Blood group (phenotype)	D	d	D	→ The presence of one D confers the blood group D i.e. D is DOMINANT.

→ The presence of two d's is required to confer the blood group d, i.e. d is RECESSIVE.

This concept is important in *inherited single gene disorders*.

(1) In DOMINANT inheritance any HETEROZYGOUS offspring bearing the abnormal trait will be affected: mating with a normal partner statistically produces 50% of normal offspring and 50% affected.

(2) In RECESSIVE inheritance only HOMOZYGOTES for the trait are affected. Such cases usually arise from the mating of 2 heterozygous CARRIERS who, by definition, are themselves unaffected.

The results of mating are as follows: (A = affected gene, N = normal gene)

NN = normal individual: NA = carrier: AA = affected individual.

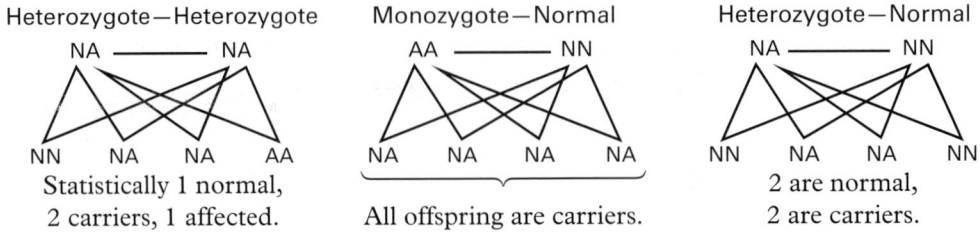

GENETIC ABNORMALITIES AND ASSOCIATED DISORDERS

The concept of dominant and recessive traits is useful in genetic counselling. Long lists of dominant and recessive disorders are available: only a few important examples are given.

Autosomal dominant — neurofibromatosis, Huntington's disease: polyposis coli: congenital spherocytosis.

Autosomal recessive — cystic fibrosis, congenital deafness, mucopolysaccharidoses.

Sex-linked disorders are usually recessive and are carried on the X-chromosome: males are affected and females are carriers. Important disorders are haemophilia and muscular dystrophy.

METABOLIC DISORDERS (inborn errors of metabolism)

These are inherited disorders of single genes which code for the enzymes concerned in many metabolic pathways. The clinical effects show considerable variation in severity.

Examples are: disorders of carbohydrate (including glycogen storage), lipid and amino-acid metabolism: lysosomal storage: and membrane transport (including cystic fibrosis).

Note: Not all single gene abnormalities cause, by themselves, significant pathological effects. As indicated above, the controlling factors are complex and include the important effects of 'modifying genes'. It seems likely that abnormal recessive genes exist in the normal population but only present as clinical disorders in rare special circumstances.

MULTIFACTORIAL DISORDERS

Most human diseases have a genetic component but environmental factors usually play a very important part in the pathogenesis.

COMBINED ACTIVITY of SEVERAL GENES (both normal and abnormal) + ENVIRONMENTAL FACTORS ⟶ DISEASE

Examples are: atopic (allergic) disorders: diabetes mellitus, hypertension, rheumatoid arthritis and various infections.

SOMATIC CELL GENETIC DISORDERS

When mutation occurs after fertilisation of the ovum and at any stage throughout life the effects are limited to the disordered cell(s) and progeny. The clinical effects tend to be localised.

NEOPLASMS and hamartomas are examples of somatic cell genetic disorders (see Carcinogenesis).

Note: In the systematic section of this book significant genetic contribution to the pathogenesis of diseases will be recorded.

AMYLOID DEPOSITION

Amyloid is a waxy substance deposited in the extracellular tissues, particularly around blood vessels and in basement membranes. Various forms of amyloid are seen and they have varying effects. Amyloid is resistant to degradation and its deposition tends to progress relentlessly.

Nature of Amyloid

Chemical: amyloid fibrils are made up of

(i) A major variable component >90%.

(ii) A minor constant component, AMYLOID P PROTEIN — a glycoprotein normally found in serum.

Physical: whatever its composition, amyloid fibrils are arranged in a β-pleated configuration: this accounts for its resistance to degradation and its staining properties.

Detection

At *post-mortem*, the affected organs are pale, enlarged and have a firm, waxy texture.

STAINING with LUGOL's IODINE
- AMYLOID — DEEP BROWN
- NORMAL — YELLOW

On *biopsy* material, specific stains and electronmicroscopy are needed.

(i) **Light microscopy**

CONGO RED STAIN
- AMYLOID — RED STAINING: APPLE GREEN BIREFRINGENCE in POLARISED LIGHT.
- NORMAL — PALE PINK: NO BIREFRINGENCE.

IMMUNOSTAINING — for specific constituents e.g. P protein.

(ii) **Electronmicroscopy** — specific appearance: closely packed interlacing fibrils 70 to 100 Å in diameter.

Pathological effects

AMYLOID DEPOSITION
- → Pressure on adjacent cells → ATROPHY
- → Blood vessels
  - → Narrowing
  - → Increased permeability → TRANSUDATION of PROTEIN out of vessels

AMYLOID DEPOSITION

Almost any tissue in the body may be affected by amyloid deposition, but the most important changes occur in the kidney, gastrointestinal tract and the heart. Other organs, such as the liver and spleen, may also be grossly affected without serious functional impairment.

KIDNEY

In severe cases the kidneys are pale, firm and waxy, and with the iodine test the glomeruli stand out as brown dots to the naked eye.

Renal biopsy is useful in the diagnosis of amyloidosis.

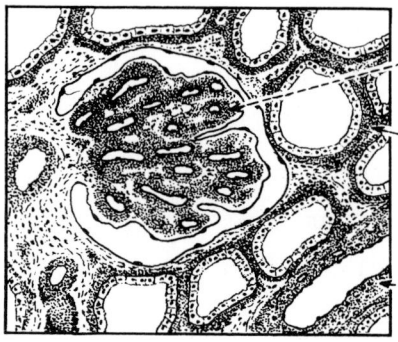

Effects: Glomerular capillary permeability altered

↓

GROSS PROTEINURIA → NEPHROTIC SYNDROME → late renal failure

GASTROINTESTINAL TRACT

Due to altered permeability of the capillaries, the patient suffers from diarrhoea and protein loss. There may also be malabsorption, nutritional deficiencies and electrolyte imbalance.

Rectal biopsy is useful in the diagnosis of amyloidosis.

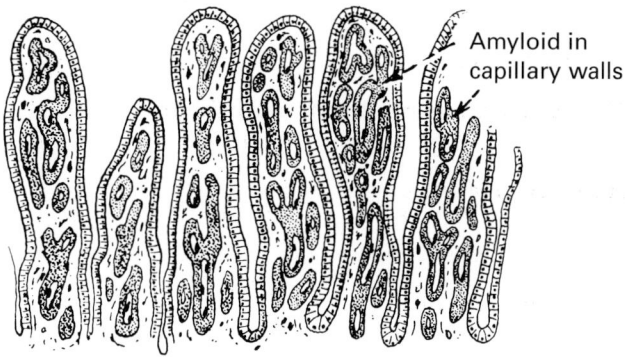

HEART

Amyloid deposition occurs around the cardiac muscle fibres and the capillary basement membranes. The heart is enlarged with apparently thick muscular walls but much of the thickness is due to amyloid deposition.

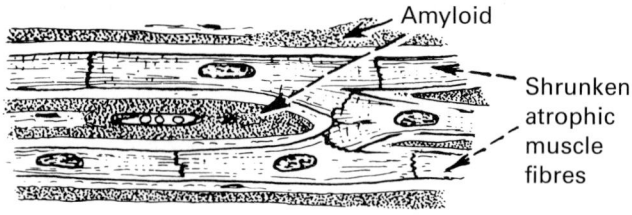

Effects: Cardiac failure develops mainly due to the mechanical effect of amyloid, making the heart muscle stiff and preventing cardiac filling (restrictive defect). The blood supply to the muscle fibres is also impaired.

AMYLOID CLASSIFICATION

Amyloid was previously classified into 2 main groups.

(i) Primary i.e. without known cause.

(ii) Secondary i.e. associated with chronic inflammatory disease.

Knowledge of the mechanisms of amyloid deposition has made this classification obsolete. Instead:-

1. SYSTEMIC AMYLOIDOSIS

(a) *Associated with monoclonal plasma cell proliferation*
(e.g. myeloma, monoclonal gammopathy, Waldenstrom's macroglobulinaemia).

Increased production of:
Variable protein — AL (Amyloid Light chain derived) — from fragments of immunoglobulin, especially lambda light chains.

(b) *Associated with chronic inflammation*
(e.g. tuberculosis, osteomyelitis, rheumatoid arthritis, bronchiectasis).

Increased production of:
Variable protein — AA (Amyloid A protein) — derived from serum AA protein, an acute phase reactant in many inflammatory conditions.

Summary of formation of amyloid

Abnormal (monoclonal) proliferation of plasma cells
↓
Abnormal immunoglobulins esp. lambda light chains
Proteolysis →
↓
AMYLOIDOGENIC PROTEIN > 90% (AL)
+ Amyloid P glycoprotein < 10%
↓
SYSTEMIC AMYLOID (AL)

Long continued active inflammation
↓
Acute phase reactant protein
↓ ← Proteolysis
AMYLOIDOGENIC PROTEIN > 90% (AA)
+ Amyloid P glycoprotein <10%
↓
SYSTEMIC AMYLOID (AA)

2. LOCALISED AMYLOIDOSIS

In ENDOCRINE TUMOURS — amyloid derived from polypeptide hormones e.g. medullary carcinoma of thyroid — calcitonin derived amyloid.

In OLD AGE — the amyloidogenic protein is related to pre-albumin. Deposits of amyloid occur in the heart, brain and joints. In Alzheimer's disease (p. 565) local amyloid deposition in the brain is important.

CALCIFICATION

Abnormal deposits of calcium salts occur in 2 circumstances: dystrophic calcification and metastatic calcification.

1. DYSTROPHIC CALCIFICATION

Local deposits of calcium may occur in:

(a) **Necrotic tissue which is not absorbed** e.g. old caseous lesions of tuberculosis; old infarcts; old collections of pus; dead parasites; in fat necrosis associated with pancreatitis.

(b) **Tissues undergoing slow degeneration** e.g. hyaline areas in benign tumours e.g. fibroids (p. 509); in arteries due to atheromatous degeneration or in old age; in old thrombi; diseased or abnormal heart valves.

The mechanism may be as follows:

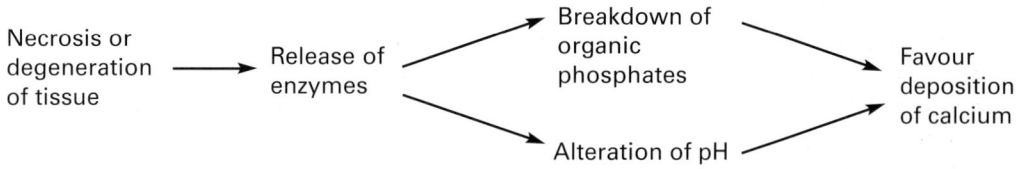

Note: The presence of radio-opaque Ca^{++} is of diagnostic use particularly in old healed disease (e.g. tuberculosis) and also in some tumours, e.g. breast cancer where very small deposits of calcium may be present.

2. METASTATIC CALCIFICATION

In this case the essential feature is an increase in the calcium X phosphate product in the blood (usually hypercalcaemia).

The mechanisms are complex: the 2 usual mechanisms are simplified as follows:

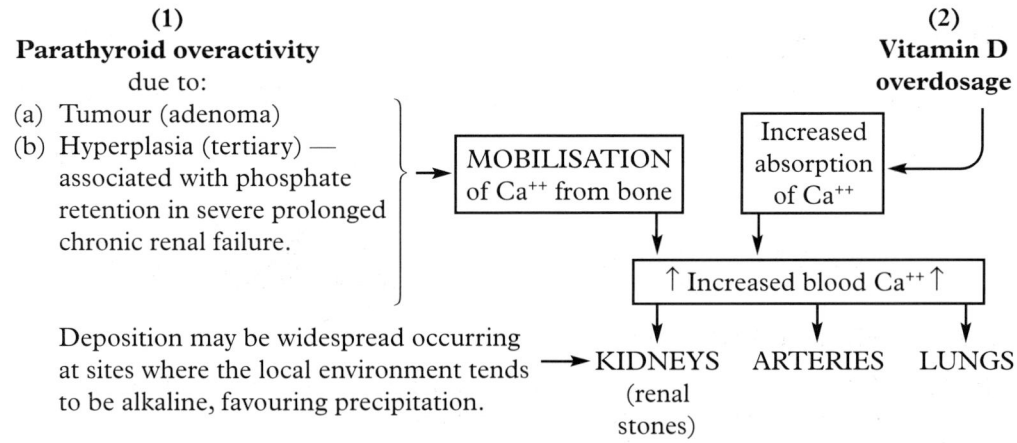

About 5% of MALIGNANCY cases — particularly with carcinoma of the breast and lung — have HYPERCALCAEMIA, although most do not live long enough to have significant systemic deposition.

The mechanisms are (1) secretion by the tumour of a protein [parathyroid hormone related peptide (PTHrP)] which mimics the action of parathormone and (2) of less importance, the local release of bone resorbing cytokines by tumour metastases in bones.

ENDOGENOUS PIGMENTATION

IRON-CONTAINING PIGMENT

Two main pigments are derived from the breakdown of red blood cells.
(1) HAEMOSIDERIN and (2) BILIRUBIN.

The detailed mechanism is described on page 346 in relation to JAUNDICE.

HAEMOSIDERIN

The iron derived from red cell breakdown is held in the spleen, liver and bone marrow, combined with apoferritin. In the plasma it is transported by transferrin. The two mechanisms maintain an equilibrium between the iron contents in these three sites. When the amount of iron within the cells becomes excessive and overloads the ferritin system, it is deposited in a brown granular form — haemosiderin. This occurs in 2 situations:

1. **Local breakdown of red cells in tissues e.g. in**

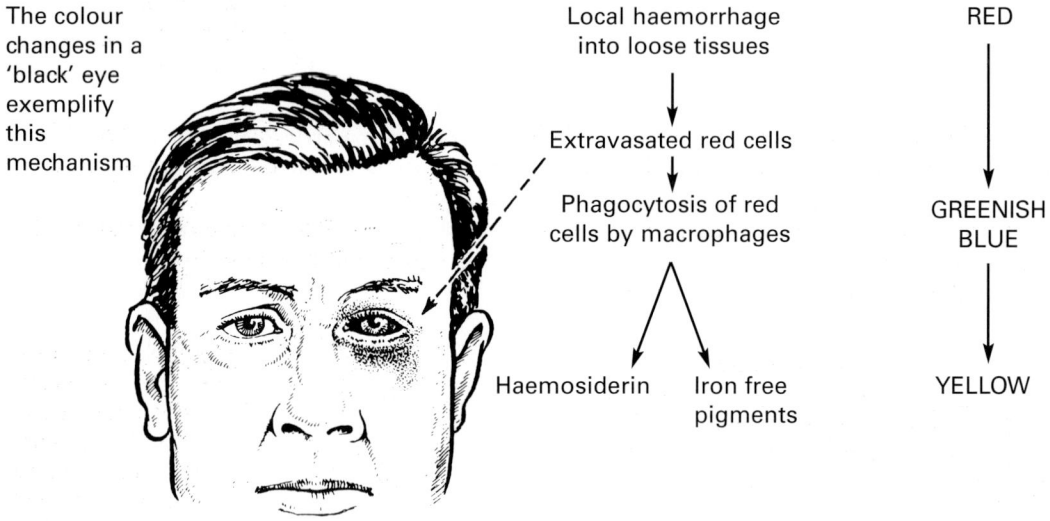

2. **Visceral siderosis**

(a) *Haemosiderosis*

This is seen in the liver, spleen and sometimes the kidneys in cases of haemolytic anaemia, and in patients requiring repeated blood transfusion. The change is most strikingly seen in the liver, which becomes deep brown. Iron is found in the Kupffer cells first and, later, in liver cells. Easily demonstrated by the Prussian blue reaction. These iron deposits very rarely cause organ damage, in contrast to haemochromatosis.

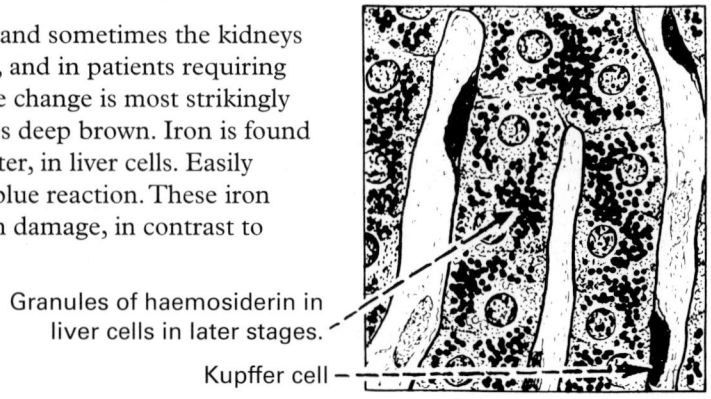

ENDOGENOUS PIGMENTATION

Haemosiderin (continued)

(b) *Haemochromatosis (Bronzed diabetes)*
The absorption of iron from the intestine is controlled by the ferritin-transferrin mechanism already mentioned.

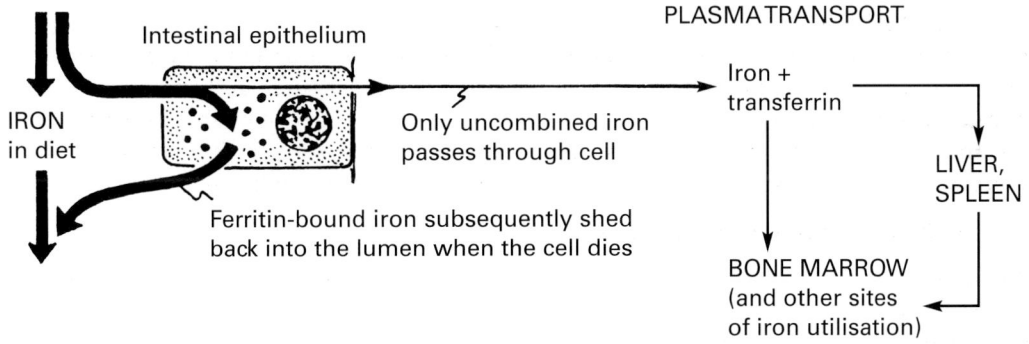

The ferritin content of the intestinal epithelium, iron saturation of the plasma, stores of iron in the liver and spleen and the demand for iron by the bone marrow form a balancing mechanism preventing overloading of any part of the system.

In haemochromatosis the absorption of iron is virtually uncontrolled, due to an inherited defect on chromosome 6. The system becomes overloaded and iron is deposited as haemosiderin in many sites, the main ones being:

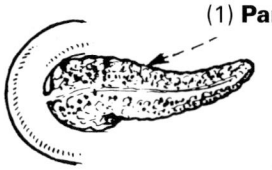

(1) **Pancreas** — associated with fibrosis which may destroy islet tissue ≡ DIABETES MELLITUS

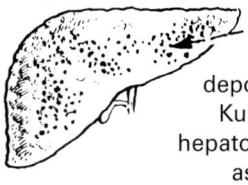

(2) **Liver** — massive iron deposition in both Kupffer cells and hepatocytes, usually associated with fibrosis (CIRRHOSIS)

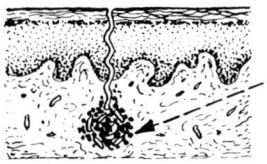

(3) **Skin** — mainly around sweat glands. Excessive melanin is also deposited, hence this condition is sometimes termed 'bronzed diabetes'

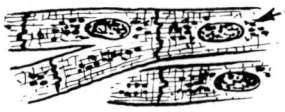

(4) **Heart muscle**

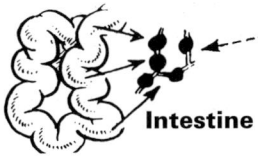

(5) **Mesenteric lymph nodes**

Intestine

Haemosiderin may be found in almost any site in the body.

ENDOGENOUS PIGMENTATION

Haemoglobin

Occasionally, intravascular haemolysis occurs. Haemoglobin appears in the urine, giving it a dull red colour — in the severe acute situation (e.g. incompatible blood transfusion) acute renal tubular necrosis occurs. If the condition is chronic, as in paroxysmal haemoglobinuria, some of the haemoglobin is reabsorbed and subsequently broken down so that iron, as haemosiderin, appears in the renal tubular epithelium.

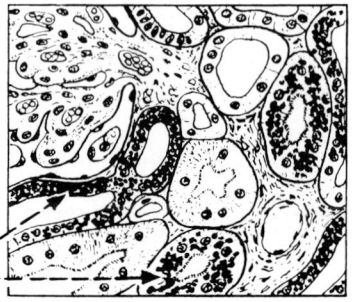

(Demonstrated by the Prussian blue reaction)

Haematin (or haemazoin)

This is a brown pigment produced by malarial parasites from haemoglobin. It is taken up by the monocytes in the blood and subsequently deposited in the liver and spleen.

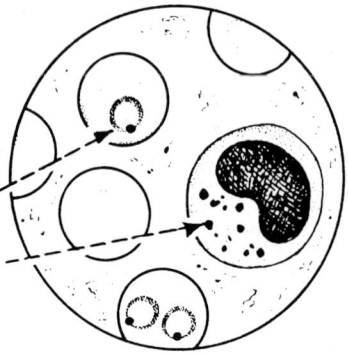

Lipofuscin

This is a yellowish brown pigment having a high lipid content, often found in the atrophied cells of old age — 'wear and tear' pigment. It is particularly common in the heart muscle, and the term 'brown atrophy' is often applied.

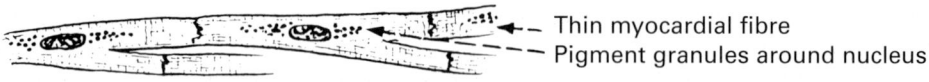

It is also found in liver cells, testes and nerve cells.

EXOGENOUS PIGMENTATION – DEGENERATIONS

EXOGENOUS PIGMENTATION

Pigments may be introduced by inhalation, ingestion or injection. The most important are those introduced by inhalation of dusts in industrial processes.

Inhalation

The commonest substances inhaled are COAL DUST (carbon) — black, and STONE DUST (silica) — grey.

The particles reach the alveoli especially if the bronchial ciliary action is disturbed by chronic bronchitis.

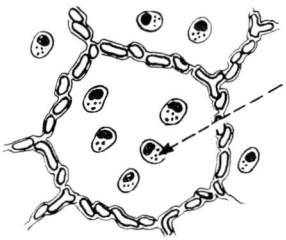

Particles taken up by macrophages in alveoli

Transported into lymph channels and deposited in small focal aggregates throughout lungs and hilar lymph nodes

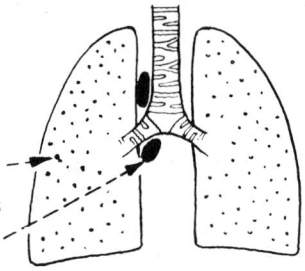

The effects are described in detail under PNEUMOCONIOSIS.

Ingestion

Pigmentation can be caused by chronic ingestion of metals such as silver or lead. In both, the skin has a metallic hue, and in the case of lead a blue line appears on the gums due to interaction between lead and hydrogen sulphide. Excessive intake of carrots can lead to yellowish red skin pigmentation caused by carotene.

Injection

Tattooing is the most striking example of pigmentation following injection.

DEGENERATIONS

(1) **Hyaline**

This is a descriptive term meaning a glossy, refractile appearance, seen in sections stained with haematoxylin and eosin. It is most commonly encountered in the form of dense collagen, particularly in benign tumours such as leiomyomas where the collagen has replaced muscle fibres, and in blood vessels in arteriosclerosis.

The term 'Mallory's hyaline' refers to an *intra*cellular accumulation of cytoskeletal proteins e.g. in alcoholic liver disease.

(2) **Mucoid**

This is a common change in epithelial tumours which secrete mucin. In these cases the epithelial cells undergo degeneration and appear to dissolve in the mucin.

Connective tissue may also accumulate mucin. Spaces filled with mucopolysaccharides (e.g. hyaluronic acid) appear between the fibres. The change is common in some tumours and the term 'myxomatous' may be used.

CHAPTER 2

INFLAMMATION

Inflammation	32
Acute Inflammation	33–38
Sequels of Acute Inflammation	39–41
Chronic Inflammation	42, 43
Ulceration — Simple	44
Ulceration — Malignant	45
Inflammation — Anatomical Varieties	46

INFLAMMATION

Inflammation is the dynamic process by which living tissues react to injury. They concern vascular and connective tissues particularly.

Causes:

Various agents may kill or damage cells:

PHYSICAL
- Trauma
- Heat or cold
- Radiation

CHEMICAL
- Simple chemical poisons, e.g. acids
- Organic poisons, e.g. paraquat

INFECTIVE
- Bacteria
- Viruses
- Parasites

IMMUNOLOGICAL
- Antigen-antibody
- Cell-mediated

... and any other circumstance leading to tissue damage, e.g. VASCULAR or HORMONAL DISTURBANCE.

The inflammatory reaction takes place in the surviving adjacent vascular and connective tissues; the specialised parenchymal cells do not directly participate.

The initial stages are known as the **acute** inflammatory reaction. Where the process is prolonged the inflammation may be **subacute** or **chronic**.

ACUTE INFLAMMATION

The classical signs are:

REDNESS (rubor)
HEAT (calor)
SWELLING (tumor)
PAIN (dolor)
LOSS OF FUNCTION (functiolaesa).

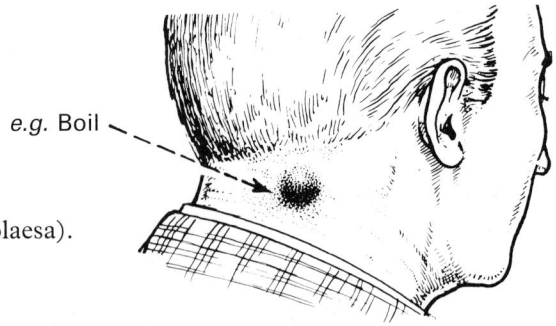

These gross signs are explained by changes occurring at microscopic level. Three essential features are:

1. **HYPERAEMIA**
2. **EXUDATION OF FLUID**
3. **EMIGRATION OF LEUCOCYTES**

ACUTE INFLAMMATION

HYPERAEMIA

The hyperaemia in inflammation is associated with the well known microvascular changes which occur in Lewis' triple response — a FLUSH, a FLARE and a WEAL. It occurs when a blunt instrument is drawn firmly across the skin and illustrates the vascular changes occurring in acute inflammation.

The stroke is marked momentarily by a white line due to VASOCONSTRICTION.

The flush, a dull red line, immediately follows and is due to CAPILLARY DILATATION.

The flare, a bright red irregular surrounding zone, is due to ARTERIOLAR DILATATION.

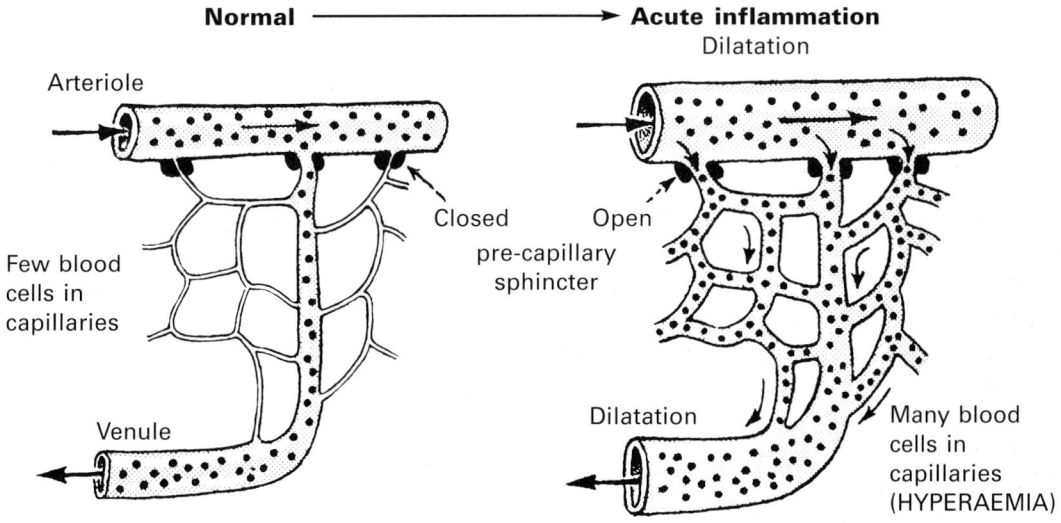

Mechanisms involved are:

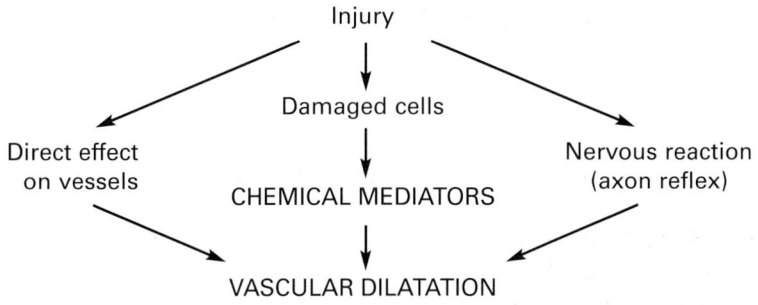

HYPERAEMIA explains the classical signs of REDNESS and HEAT.

ACUTE INFLAMMATION

EXUDATION

Exudation is the increased passage of protein-rich fluid through the vessel wall into the interstitial tissue. It explains the **weal** in Lewis' triple response.

Advantageous results

Fluid increase

↓

Dilution of toxins

Contents of fluid

(a) Globulins → protective antibodies

(b) Fibrin deposition → Helps to limit spread of bacteria

(c) Various factors promoting subsequent healing

Mechanism

(1) ***Protein passage***

Chemical mediators → Endothelial contraction — formation of gaps

↓

Chemical mediators → Increased permeability

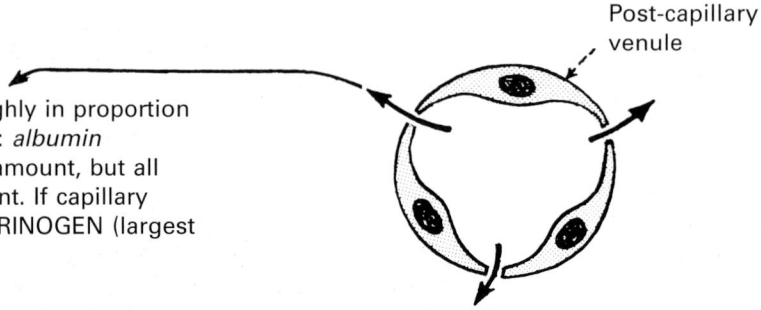

Leak of **proteins**, roughly in proportion to their molecular size: *albumin* (smallest) greatest in amount, but all plasma proteins present. If capillary damage is severe, FIBRINOGEN (largest molecule) escapes.

(2) ***Fluid movement***

Hyperaemia → Capillary blood pressure rises

Loss of protein from capillaries → Reduced plasma osmotic pressure

Interstitial tissue protein increase → Increased tissue osmotic pressure

→ INCREASED FILTRATION PRESSURE

↓

Local swelling (OEDEMA) — 3rd classical sign

↓

Increased lymph flow from area

ACUTE INFLAMMATION

EMIGRATION OF LEUCOCYTES

Neutrophils and mononuclears pass between the endothelial cell junctions by amoeboid movement through the venule wall into the tissue spaces. In this process both neutrophils and endothelial cells are activated and both express cell adhesion molecules initially SELECTINS and then INTEGRINS.

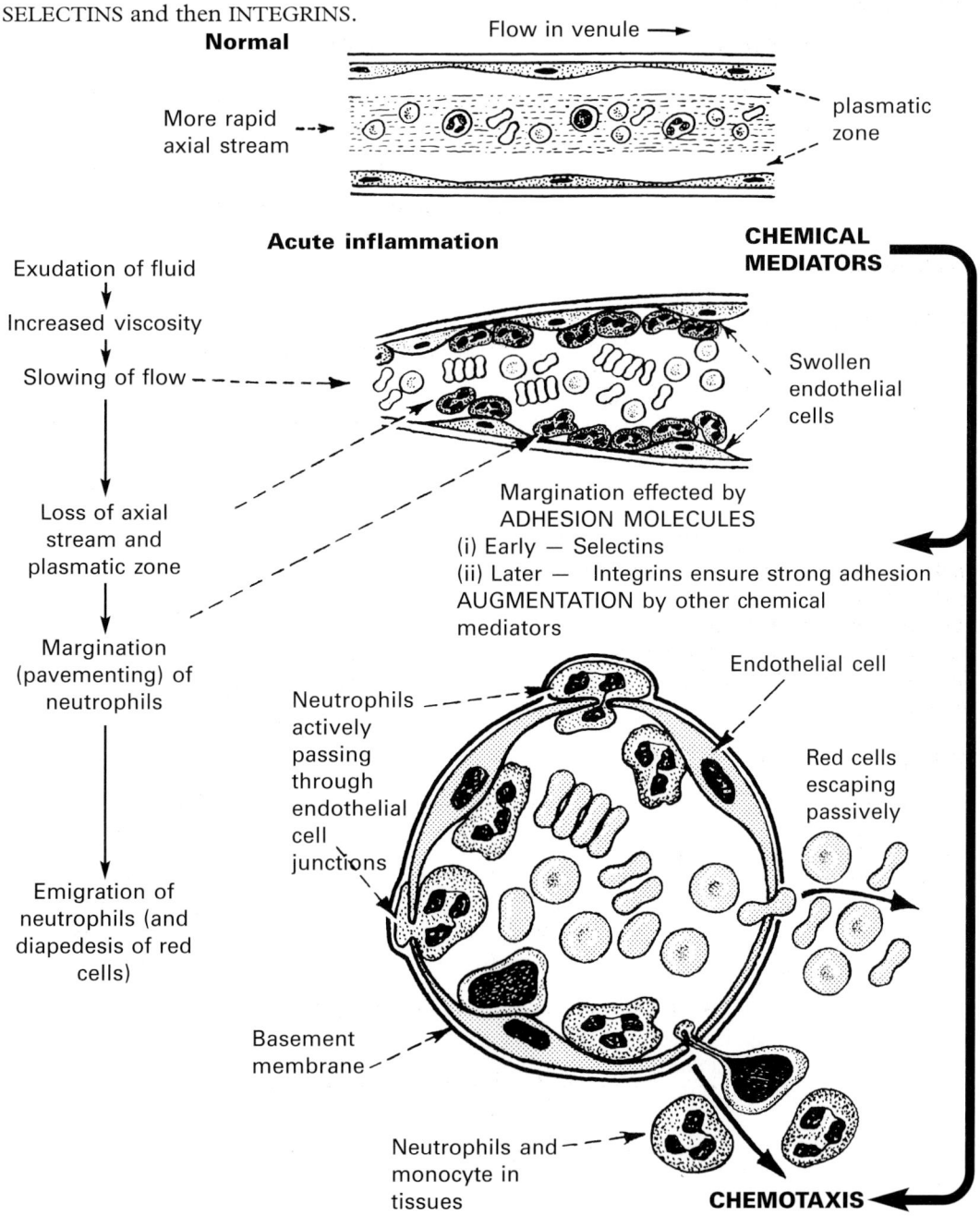

ACUTE INFLAMMATION

CHEMOTAXIS

The initial margination of neutrophils and mononuclears is potentiated by slowing of blood flow and by increased 'stickiness' of the endothelial surface.

After penetration of the vessel wall, the subsequent movement of the leucocytes is controlled by CHEMOTAXIS. The cell moves in response to an increasing concentration gradient of the particular chemotactic agent, usually a protein or polypeptide.

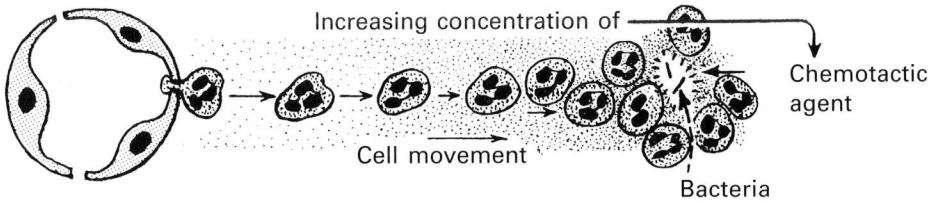

Important examples of chemotactic agents are:

Fractions of the COMPLEMENT SYSTEM (esp. C5a)
Factors derived from arachidonic acid by the neutrophils — LEUKOTRIENES
Factors derived from pathogenic BACTERIA
Factors derived from sensitised lymphocytes — CYTOKINES.

The process helps to explain the apparently purposeful movement of leucocytes and their aggregation in large numbers in inflammation.

PHAGOCYTOSIS

This is the process by which neutrophils and macrophages ingest debris and 'foreign' particles. It is similar to the feeding process of the amoeba.

It is an important defence mechanism in bacterial infections particularly.

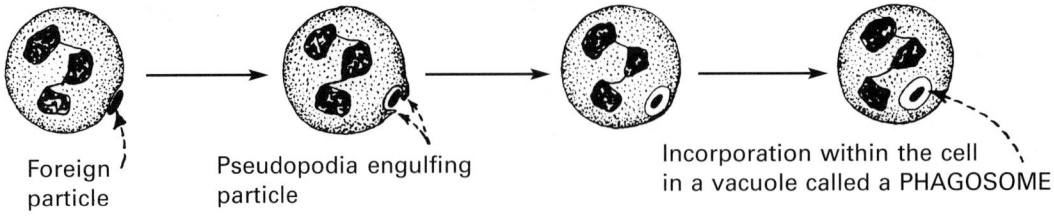

Factors influencing the efficiency of phagocytosis:

(1) OPSONINS — antibodies of both natural and specific immune type, especially antibodies of IgG class (page 96).
(2) Fractions of the COMPLEMENT system.
(3) The PHYSICAL STATE of the cellular environment.

The opsonic activity is enhanced when it is confined within a solid organ or rigid medium such as a fibrin network; where the conditions are looser and more fluid, activity is diminished.

ACUTE INFLAMMATION

Sequels of phagocytosis

NEUTROPHIL *(natural life span 1–3 days)*

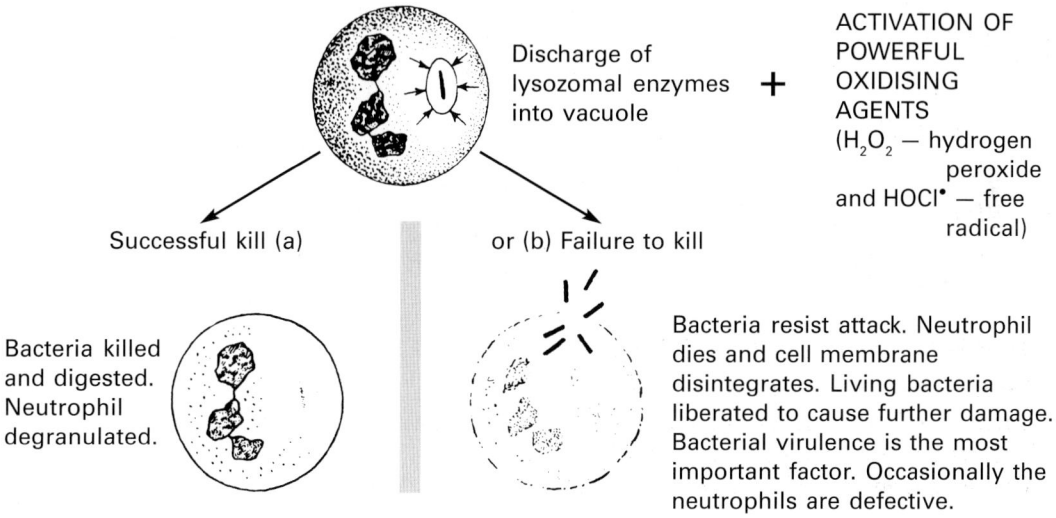

MACROPHAGE *(natural life span — months to several years)*

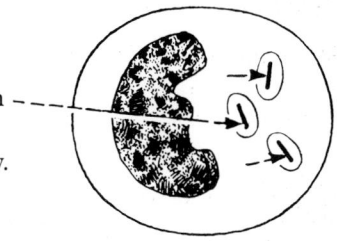

(a) Successful kill may be accomplished.
(b) Failure to kill may allow bacteria to continue to live within the cell which may move via lymphatics to adjacent parts. This partly explains the spread of tuberculosis in the body.
(c) All debris (including dead polymorphs) which has been ingested by macrophages is gradually removed from the site of the inflammation.
(d) Antigenic material from bacteria available for presentation to the immune system.

Side effects: The liberation of enzymes and oxidising agents into adjacent tissues contributes in varying degree to the tissue damage seen in several diseases, e.g. rheumatoid arthritis, progressive pulmonary emphysema.

ACUTE INFLAMMATION

THE ROLE OF CHEMICAL FACTORS

Various substances are credited with roles in the inflammatory process; they have complex overlapping actions, many of which are only imprecisely defined. Regulatory mechanisms prevent uncontrolled progression of the inflammatory process.

Agents associated with vascular dilatation and increased permeability include:

1. *Vaso-active* AMINES — these appear early and their action is short.

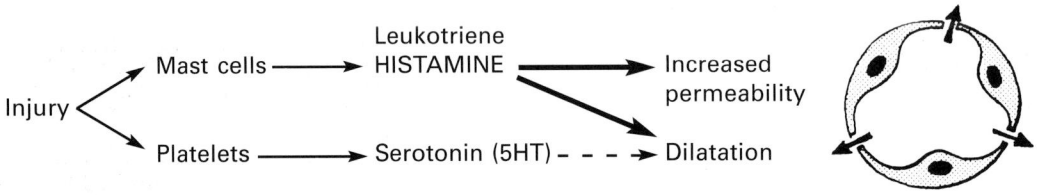

2. *Vaso-active* POLYPEPTIDES formed by specific enzyme action (breakdown products of proteins and tissues).

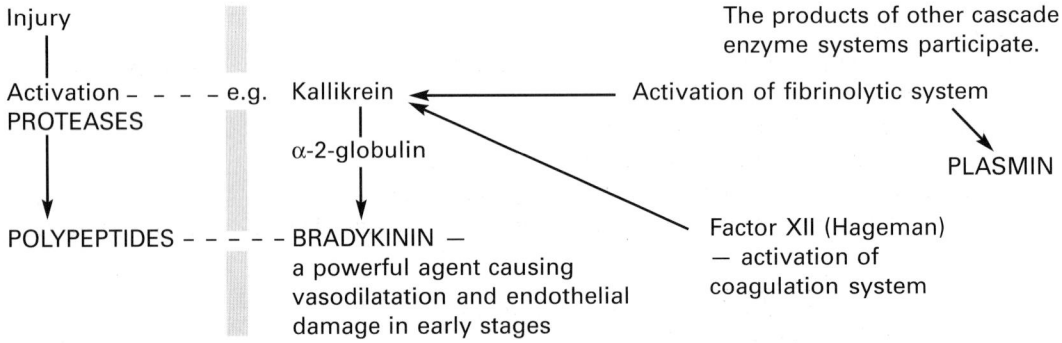

3. MISCELLANEOUS AGENTS influencing the inflammatory processes include:

- Toxins from bacteria
- Complement factors C3a and C5a
- Prostaglandins
- Leukotrienes } (from leucocytes)
- Lysosomal enzymes } (from leucocytes)
- Interleukins (macrophages)
- Globulin permeability factor
- Lymph node permeability factor
- Products of DNA and RNA breakdown
- Antigen-antibody complexes
- Tumour necrosis factor
- Nitric oxide (from endothelial cells)

SEQUELS OF ACUTE INFLAMMATION

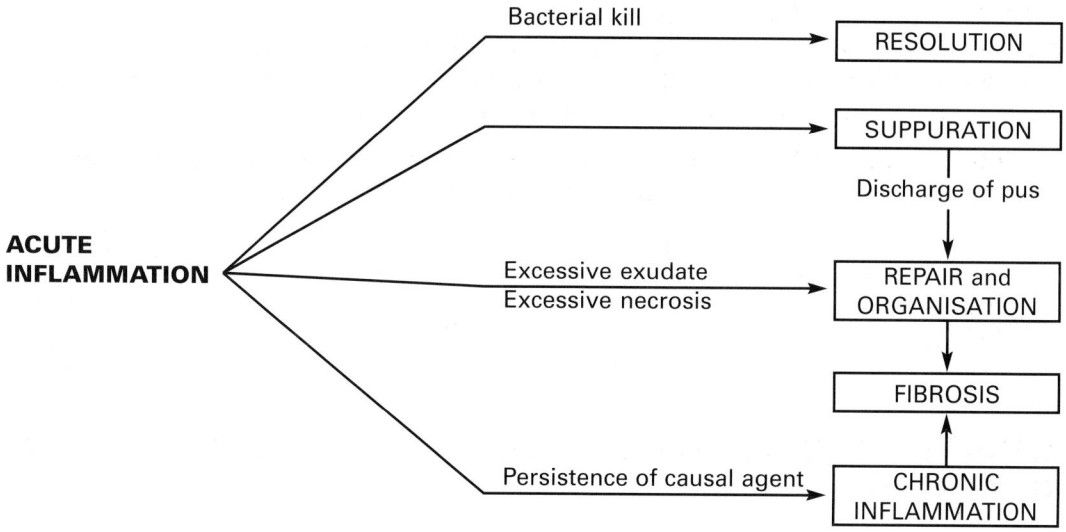

RESOLUTION

This means the complete restoration of normal conditions after the acute inflammation. The three main features which potentiate this sequel are:

1. minimal cell death and tissue damage
2. rapid elimination of the causal agent, e.g. bacteria
3. local conditions favouring removal of fluid and debris.

Resolution of lobar pneumonia (bacterial inflammation of lung alveoli) is a good example:

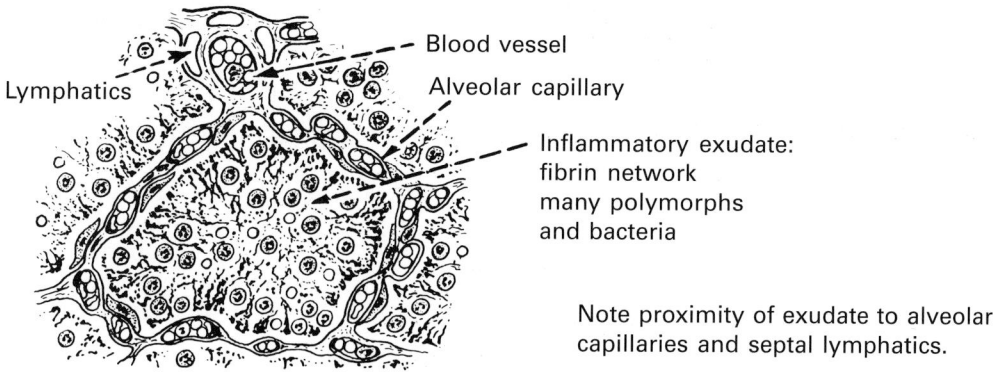

Following bacterial kill the mechanism is as follows:

1. Solution of fibrin by enzyme action (polymorphs and fibrinolysin)
2. Removal of fluid by blood vessels and lymphatics
3. Removal of all debris by phagocytes to hilar lymph nodes
4. The capillary hyperaemia diminishes and restoration to normal is complete

SEQUELS OF ACUTE INFLAMMATION

SUPPURATION

This means the formation of PUS; where pus accumulates an ABSCESS forms.

Infection by pyogenic (pus-forming) bacteria is the usual cause, e.g. staphylococcal abscess (or boil). The pus in this case is a thick, creamy yellow fluid which, on centrifugation, separates thus:

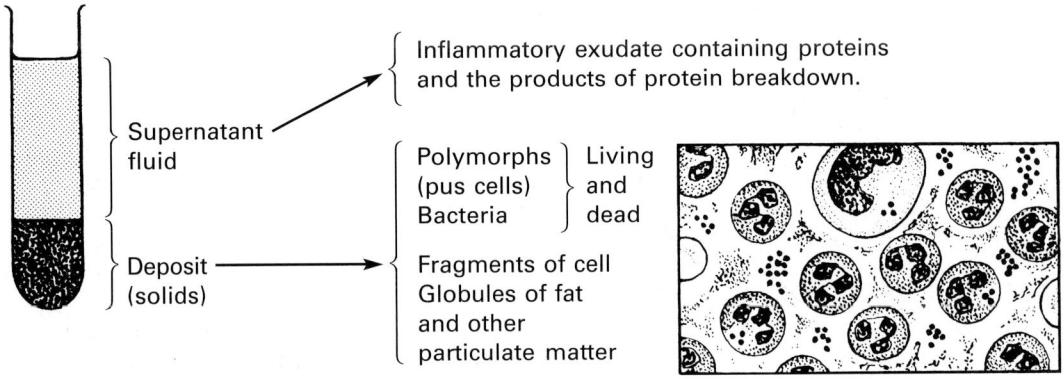

Evolution of an abscess

The usual evolution of an abscess is as follows:

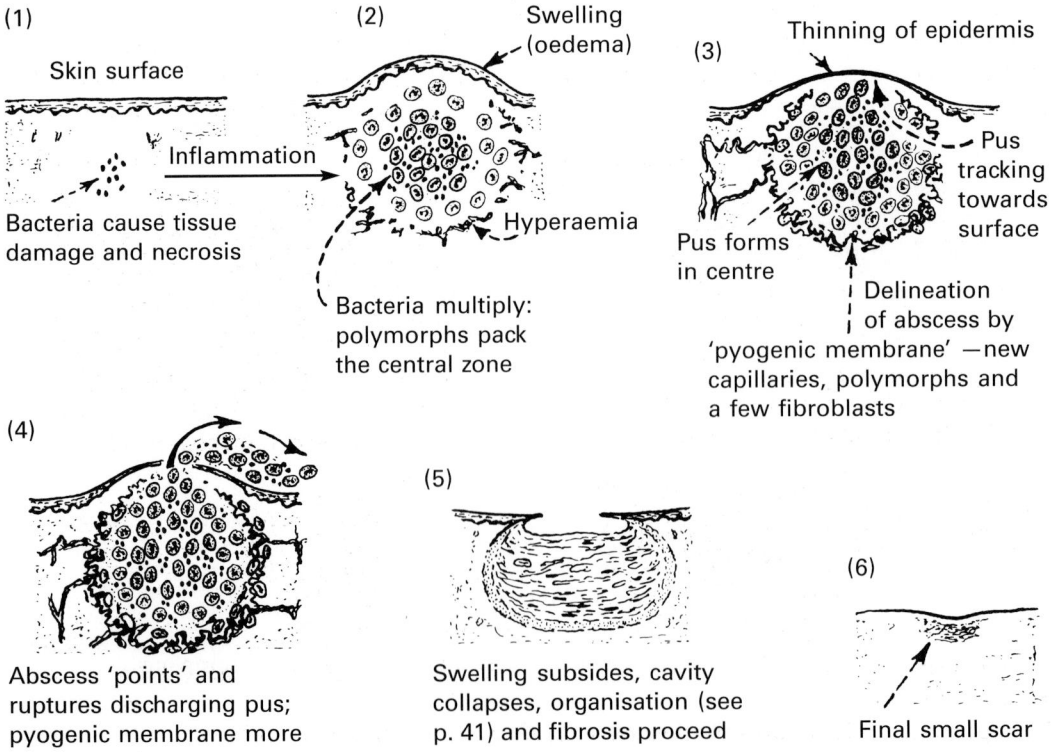

SEQUELS OF ACUTE INFLAMMATION

Evolution of an abscess (continued)

When the abscess is deep-seated, the process may be modified as follows:

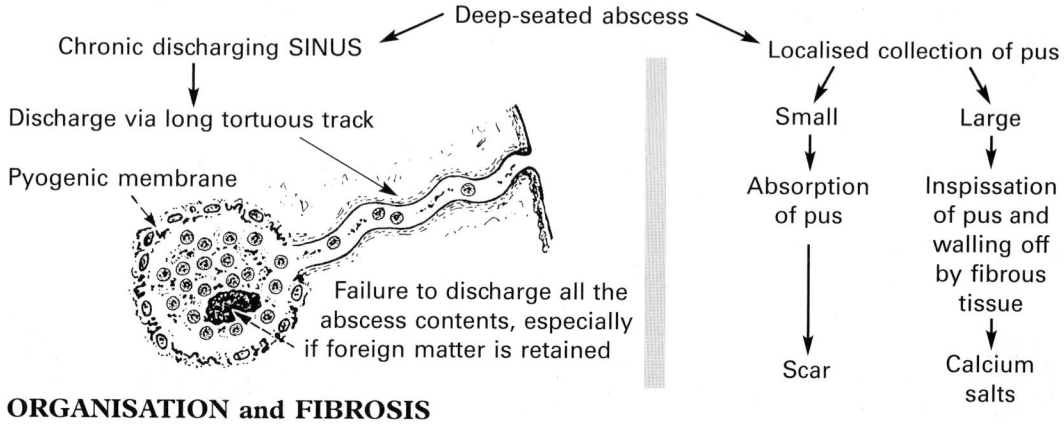

ORGANISATION and FIBROSIS

Organisation occurs when, during the acute inflammatory process, (a) there is excessive exudation or necrosis or (b) when local conditions are unfavourable for the removal of exudate and debris. The term also applies to the local reaction to the presence of thrombus and also the necrosis associated with infarction.

The changes are similar to those described in wound healing viz — the growth of new capillaries into the inert material (exudate or thrombus), the migration of macrophages and the proliferation of fibroblasts resulting in FIBROSIS.

A good example of organisation following acute inflammation is seen in the pleura overlying pneumonia. The inflammation of the lung tissue proper usually resolves completely (p.269); in contrast the pleural exudate is not easily removed and organisation takes place.

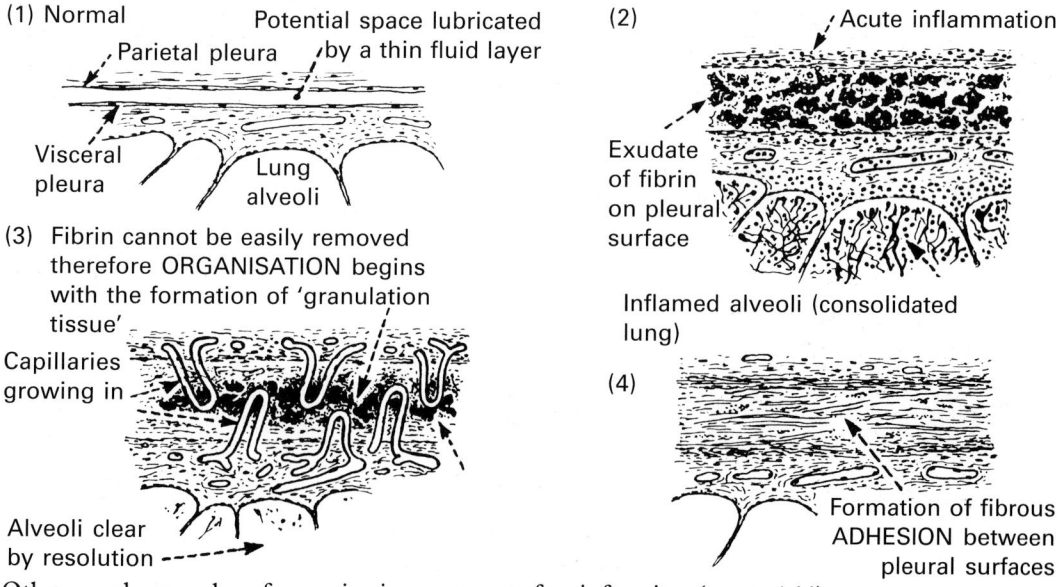

Other good examples of organisation are seen after infarction (see p. 164).

CHRONIC INFLAMMATION

Chronic Inflammation may (a) follow acute inflammation if the causal agent is not removed: or (b) be 'primary' i.e. there is no pre-existing acute stage.

The essential changes are

1. Absence of polymorphs; the appearance of lymphocytes and plasma cells. Macrophages play an increasingly important role (see Granulomas, p. 43). In some cases, giant cells form.
2. Proliferation of vascular endothelium by 'budding' — formation of new capillaries (angiogenesis).
3. Proliferation of fibroblasts with collagen production —
4. Fibrosis.

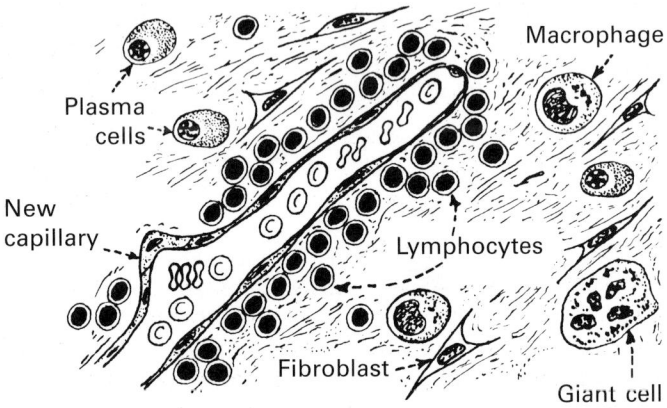

Common causes of 'primary' chronic inflammation include:

(a) Persistent infections e.g. tuberculosis, leprosy — where the organisms are resistant to neutrophil attack.
(b) Foreign material e.g. silicates, including asbestos.
(c) Auto-immune diseases e.g. auto-immune thyroiditis.
(d) Conditions of unknown aetiology e.g. sarcoidosis: Crohn's disease.

Cellular interactions

The various cells in chronic inflammation release messengers e.g. cytokines, which influence each other's behaviour.

In the illustrative diagram below, ↓ denotes one cell type changing to another: ⚡ denotes activity of a messenger.

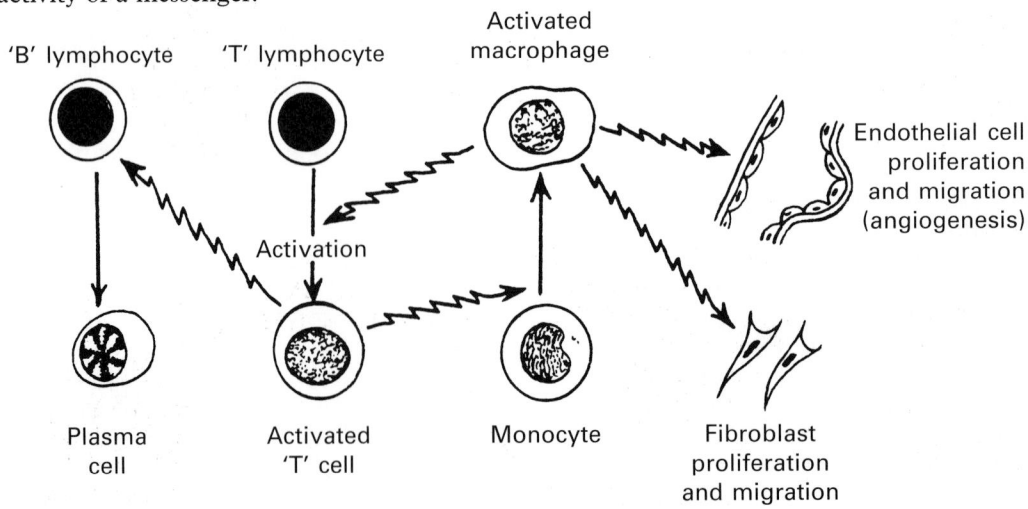

CHRONIC INFLAMMATION

GRANULOMATOUS INFLAMMATION

This is the term given to forms of chronic inflammation in which modified macrophages (epithelioid cells) accumulate in small clusters (follicles) surrounded by lymphocytes. The small clusters are called GRANULOMAS. The basic lesion in TUBERCULOSIS is a good example.

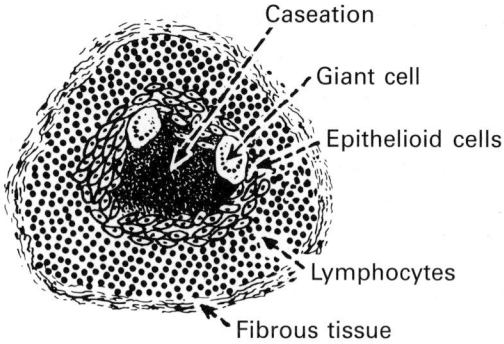

Similar follicles are seen in:

Sarcoidosis — a rare inflammatory disease of unknown aetiology affecting especially the lymph nodes and lungs, but also many other organs

'Talc' granuloma — where particular silicates introduced into the tissues evoke an inflammatory reaction after a latent period (usually years)

Crohn's disease — a chronic inflammatory disease affecting the terminal ileum and colon (see p. 311).

Lymph nodes draining ulcerated areas in which breakdown of lipid is occurring.

N.B. In all of these follicular granulomatous diseases the basic lesion may be identical, but CASEATION only occurs in tuberculosis.

The epithelioid cells of the follicular granulomas are modified macrophages, and giant cells are derived from macrophages usually by cell fusion but occasionally by nuclear division without cytoplasmic separation.

The Langhans' giant cell — seen in chronic granulomata, e.g. tuberculosis and sarcoidosis.

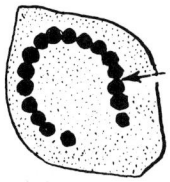

The foreign body giant cell — seen in association with particulate insoluble material.

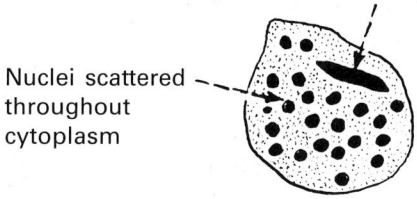

Mechanism of granuloma formation

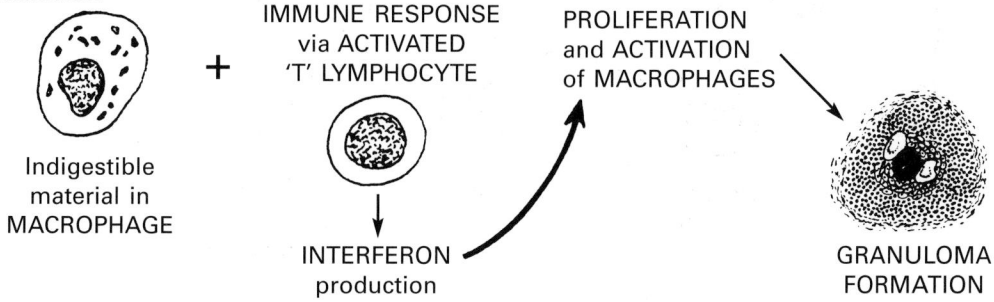

ULCERATION – SIMPLE

ULCERATION is a complication of many disease processes.

An **ulcer** is formed when the surface covering of an organ or tissue is lost due to necrosis and replaced by inflammatory tissue.

The most common sites are the alimentary tract and the skin.

Ulcers are divided into two main groups: (1) SIMPLE (inflammatory) and (2) MALIGNANT (cancerous).

The word 'simple' is used here in the limited sense of contrasting with 'malignant': 'simple' ulcers may have serious consequences.

Evolution of a simple ulcer

Acute ulcer

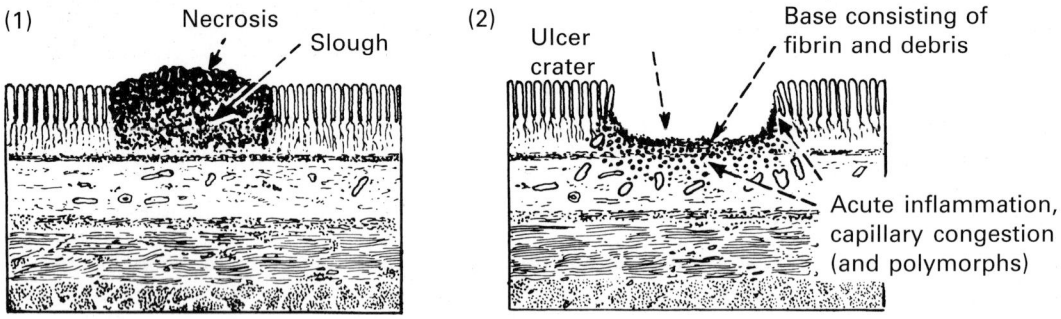

Healing can occur at this stage with restoration to normal, but if irritation (e.g. bacterial action, slight trauma, digestive juices and acid) continues, a CHRONIC ULCER forms.

Chronic ulcer

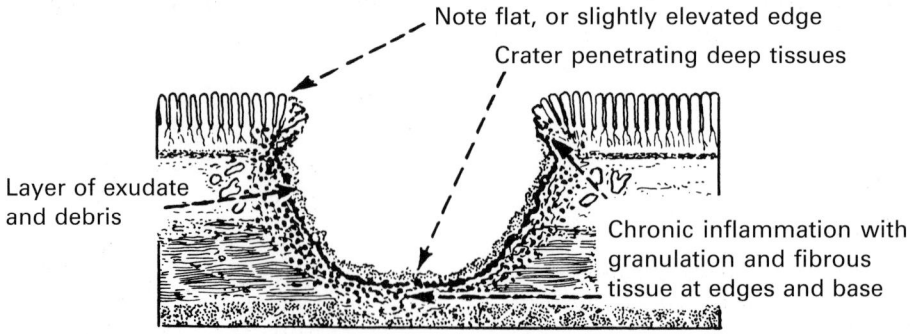

Healing of a chronic ulcer may be impeded by the secondary obliterative changes in the blood vessels due to the chronic inflammation, and it is inevitably associated with a variable amount of scarring.

ULCERATION – MALIGNANT

Evolution of a malignant ulcer (ulcerated tumour)

Such an ulcer is the result of the growth of a malignant tumour.

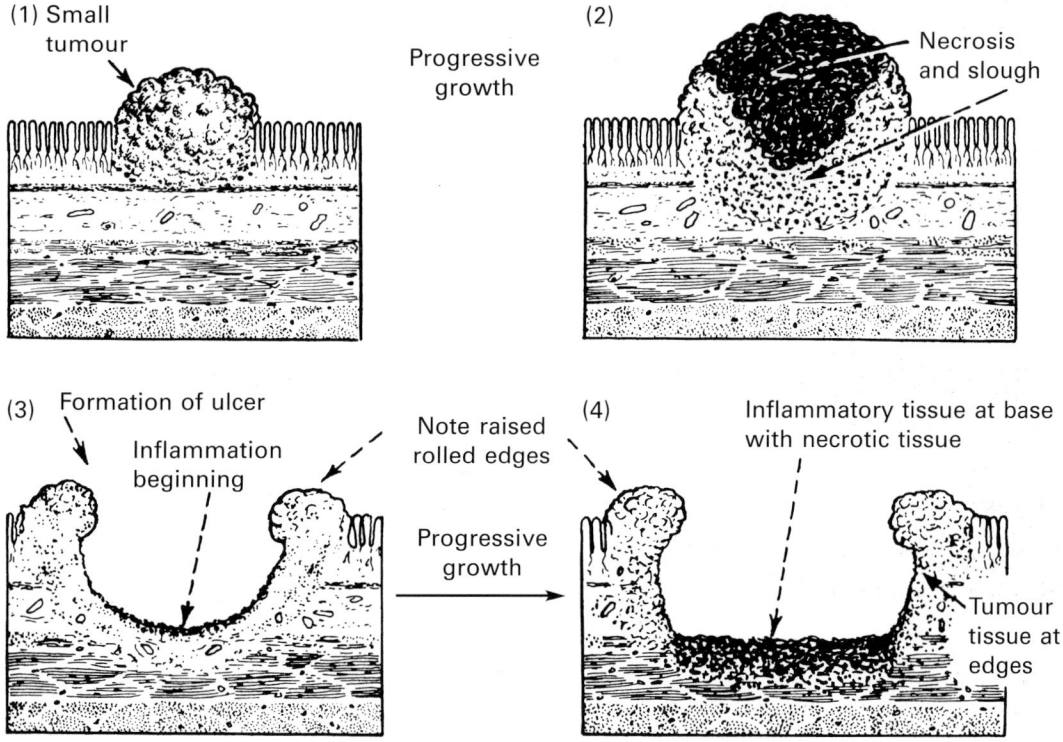

The differences between simple and malignant ulcers are most prominent at the edges — from which a diagnostic biopsy should be taken.

Simple ulcer

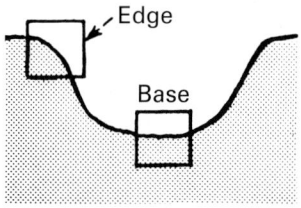

Biopsies from edge and base both show inflammation

Malignant ulcer

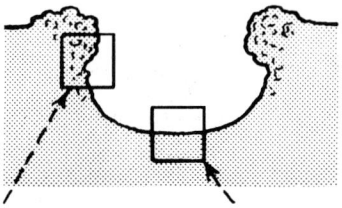

Biopsy from edge likely to show malignant tumour

Biopsy from base may miss malignant tumour

INFLAMMATION – ANATOMICAL VARIETIES

SINUS

A sinus is a tract lined usually by granulation tissue leading from a chronically inflamed cavity to a surface. In many cases the cause is the continuing presence of 'foreign' or necrotic material.

Examples include:

- **Sinuses associated with osteomyelitis** (inflammation of bone).
  Where necrosis of bone occurs, chronic sinuses form over it.
- **Pilonidal sinus** (pilonidal = nest of hairs).
  Seen in the mid-line over the sacrum (natal cleft) where hairs which have penetrated deeply under the skin are associated with chronic relapsing inflammation.

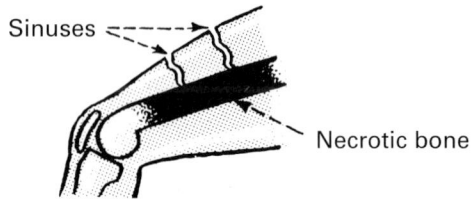

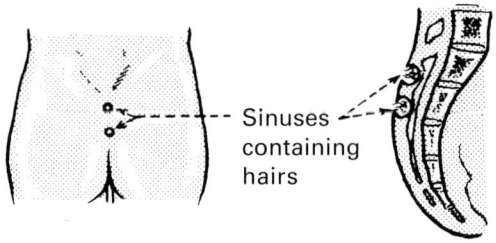

FISTULA

A fistula is a track open at both ends, through which abnormal communication between two surfaces is established.

There are two main types:

1. **Congenital** — due to developmental abnormality: any inflammation is superimposed.
2. **Acquired** — due to:

(a) Trauma

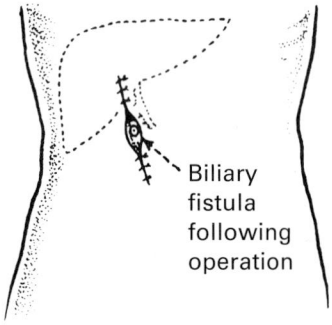

(b) Inflammation

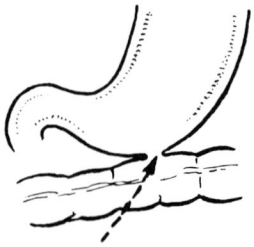

Gastrocolic fistula in Crohn's disease (p.311)

(c) Necrosis – particularly of tumour

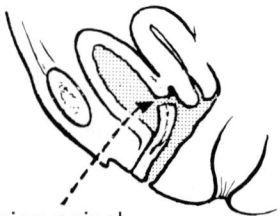

Vesicovaginal fistula following radionecrosis in treatment of cancer of cervix

An **EMPYEMA** is a collection of pus in a body cavity or hollow organ. The term refers usually to the pleural cavity or the gall bladder.

CELLULITIS occurs when inflammation spreads in the connective tissue planes.

CHAPTER 3

HEALING

Healing	48
Wound Healing	49–51
Healing — Fibrosis	52
Healing — Special Situations	53–60

HEALING

Healing is the final stage of the response of tissue to injury.

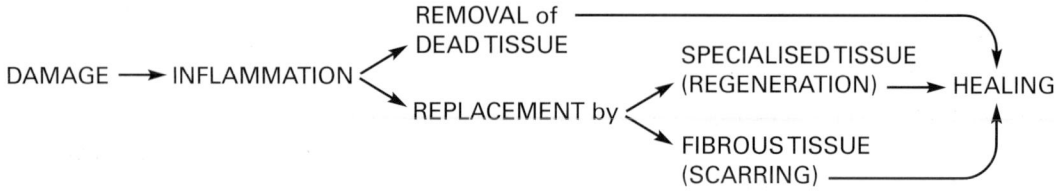

The capacity of a tissue for REGENERATION depends on its PROLIFERATIVE ABILITY and on the type and severity of the damage.

Three broad GROUPS of cells are considered in the context of the cell cycle (p. 3).

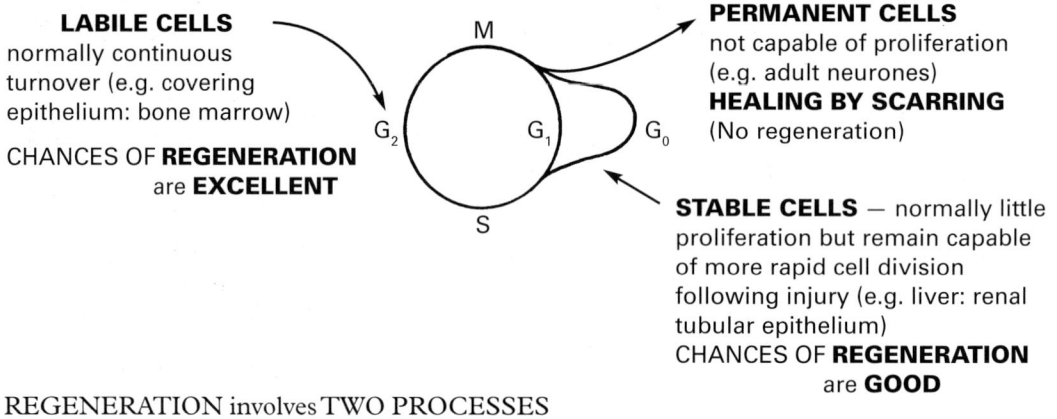

REGENERATION involves TWO PROCESSES

1. PROLIFERATION of SURVIVING CELLS to replace lost tissue.
2. MIGRATION of SURVIVING CELLS into the vacant space.

The FACTORS which CONTROL healing and repair are complex: they include the production of a variety of **growth factors**.

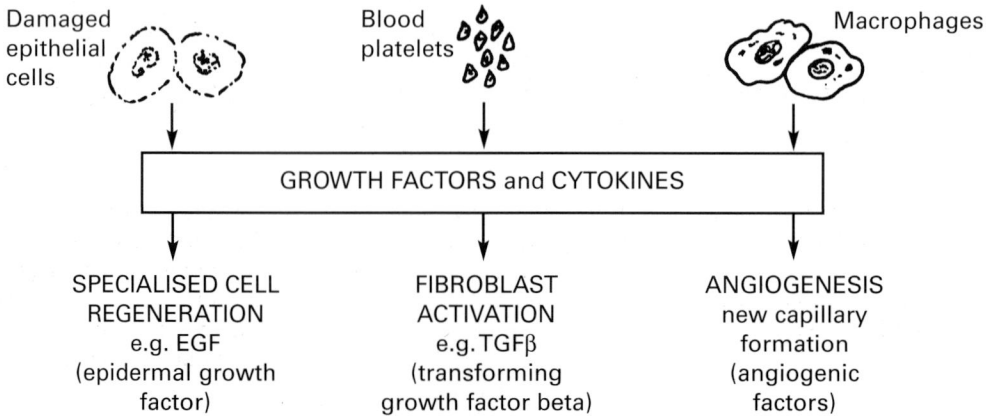

WOUND HEALING

Healing of a wound demonstrates both epithelial regeneration (healing of the epidermis) and repair by scarring (healing of the dermis).

Two patterns are described depending on the amount of tissue damage. These are essentially the same process varying only in amount.

1. Healing by first intention (primary union)
This occurs in clean, incised wounds with good apposition of the edges — particularly planned surgical incisions.

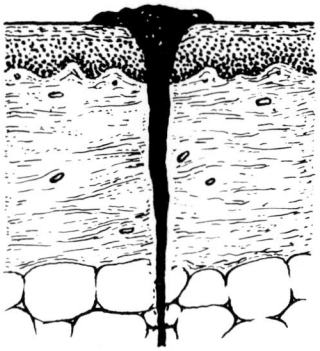

Immediately: Blood clot and debris fill the small cleft.

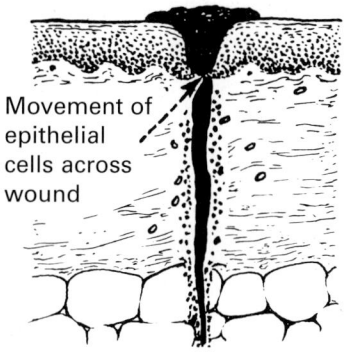

2–3 hours: Early inflammation close to edges.
Mild hyperaemia and a few polymorphs.

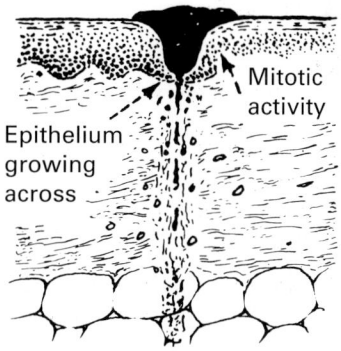

2–3 days: Macrophage activity removing clot.
Proliferation of blood vessels.
Fibroblastic activity.

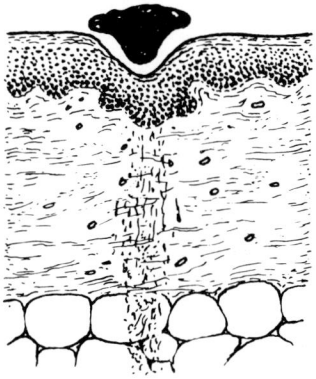

10–14 days: Scab loose and epithelial covering complete.
Fibrous union of edges, but wound is still weak.

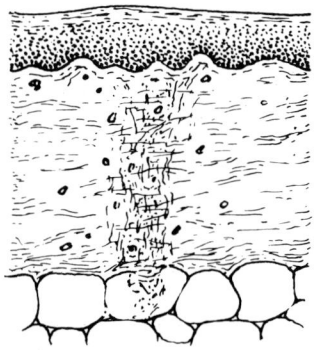

Weeks: Scar tissue still slightly hyperaemic.
Good fibrous union, but not full strength.

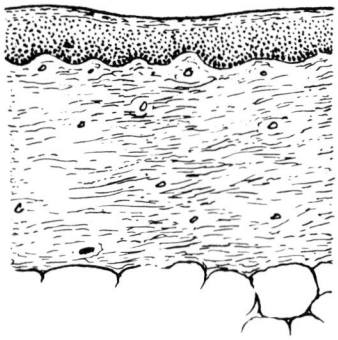

Months — years: Devascularisation.
Remodelling of collagen by enzyme action. Scar is now minimal and merges with surrounding tissues.

WOUND HEALING

WOUND HEALING (continued)

2. **Healing by second intention (secondary union)**
   This occurs in open wounds, particularly when there has been significant loss of tissue, necrosis or infection.

Early

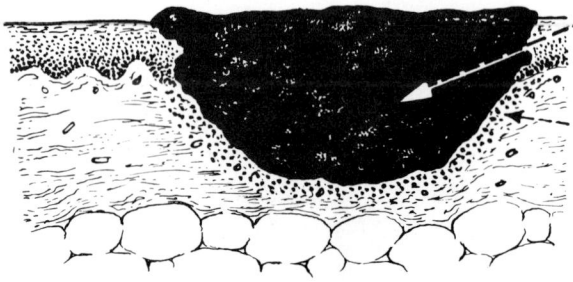

A few days

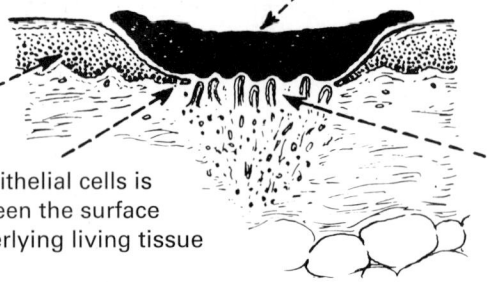

1 week approximately

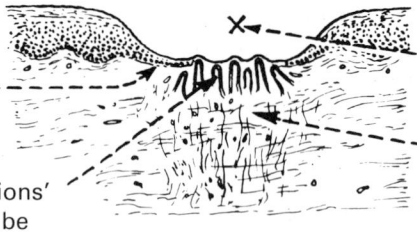

Capillary loops form small 'granulations' in the base of the wound. These can be seen by the naked eye and, historically, are the origin of the term 'granulation tissue'. This term is now used in a wider context to describe tissue consisting of newly formed capillaries with fibroblasts and macrophages and occurring in many circumstances in addition to wounds.

2 weeks onwards

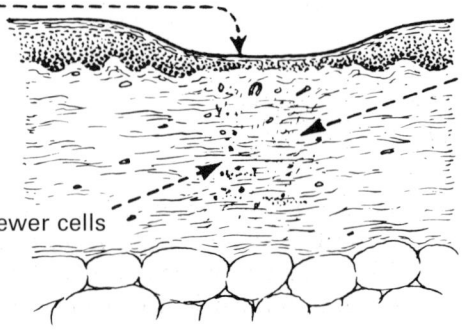

WOUND HEALING

Healing by second intention (continued)

Months

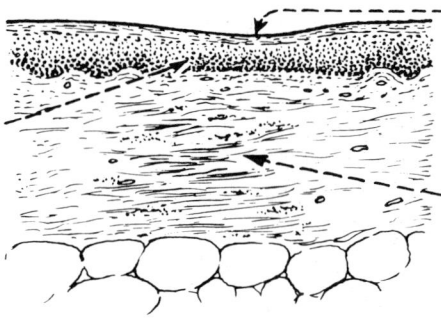

Note that the differences in the two types of wound healing are quantitative: the essential pathological processes are the same.

Wound contraction

Wound contraction which is beneficial and begins early, is due mainly to the young, specialised 'myofibroblasts' in the granulation tissue exerting a traction effect at the wound edges. The exposed surface is reduced by gradual regeneration of the surface epithelium. The remodelling of the collagen continues for many months.

COMPLICATIONS

Contracture

Later, CONTRACTURE with distortion due to thickening and shortening of collagen bundles may cause serious cosmetic and functional disability, particularly in deep and extensive skin burns and around joints if muscles are seriously damaged.

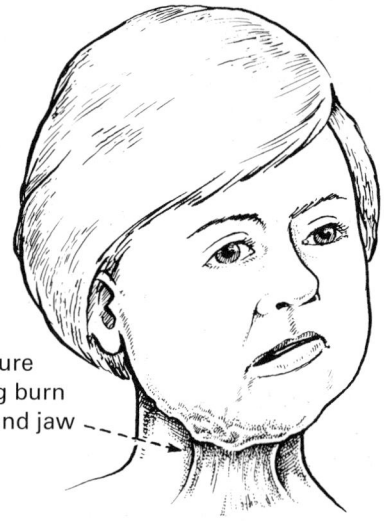

Occasional complications

1. At the edges and base of a wound granulation tissue may form in excess and prevent proper healing ('exuberant granulations': 'proud flesh').

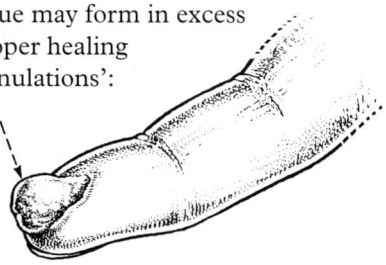

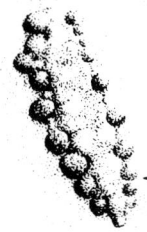

2. The formation of excess collagen in the form of thick interlacing bundles which causes marked swelling at the site of the wound is known as a KELOID. The essential cause is unknown. It is particularly common in blacks.

HEALING – FIBROSIS

FIBROSIS is the end result of WOUND HEALING, CHRONIC INFLAMMATION and ORGANISATION.

Formation of fibrous tissue

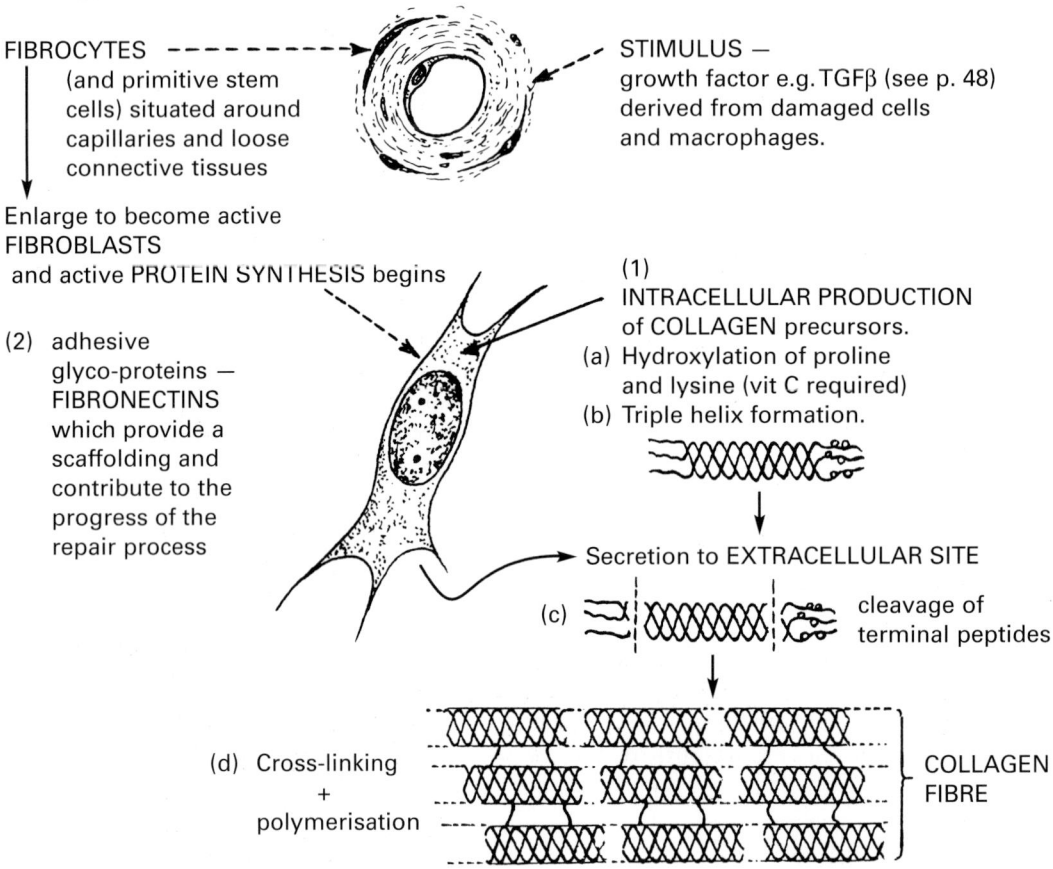

REMODELLING follows: Action of COLLAGENASE + secretion of COLLAGEN ⟶ SCAR TISSUE (reversion to FIBROCYTES)

Factors delaying wound healing

1. Local
   INFECTION, a POOR BLOOD SUPPLY, excessive movement and presence of foreign material DELAY HEALING.
2. General
   DEFICIENCY of VITAMIN C
   DEFICIENCY of AMINO ACIDS (in malnutrition)
   DEFICIENCY of ZINC
   EXCESS of ADRENAL GLUCOCORTICOIDS
   DEBILITATING CHRONIC DISEASE
   } Failure of proper collagen synthesis with delayed healing and weak scars.

HEALING – SPECIAL SITUATIONS

INTERNAL SURFACES

The regeneration of the covering epithelium is very similar to that of the skin, as seen for example in the alimentary tract.

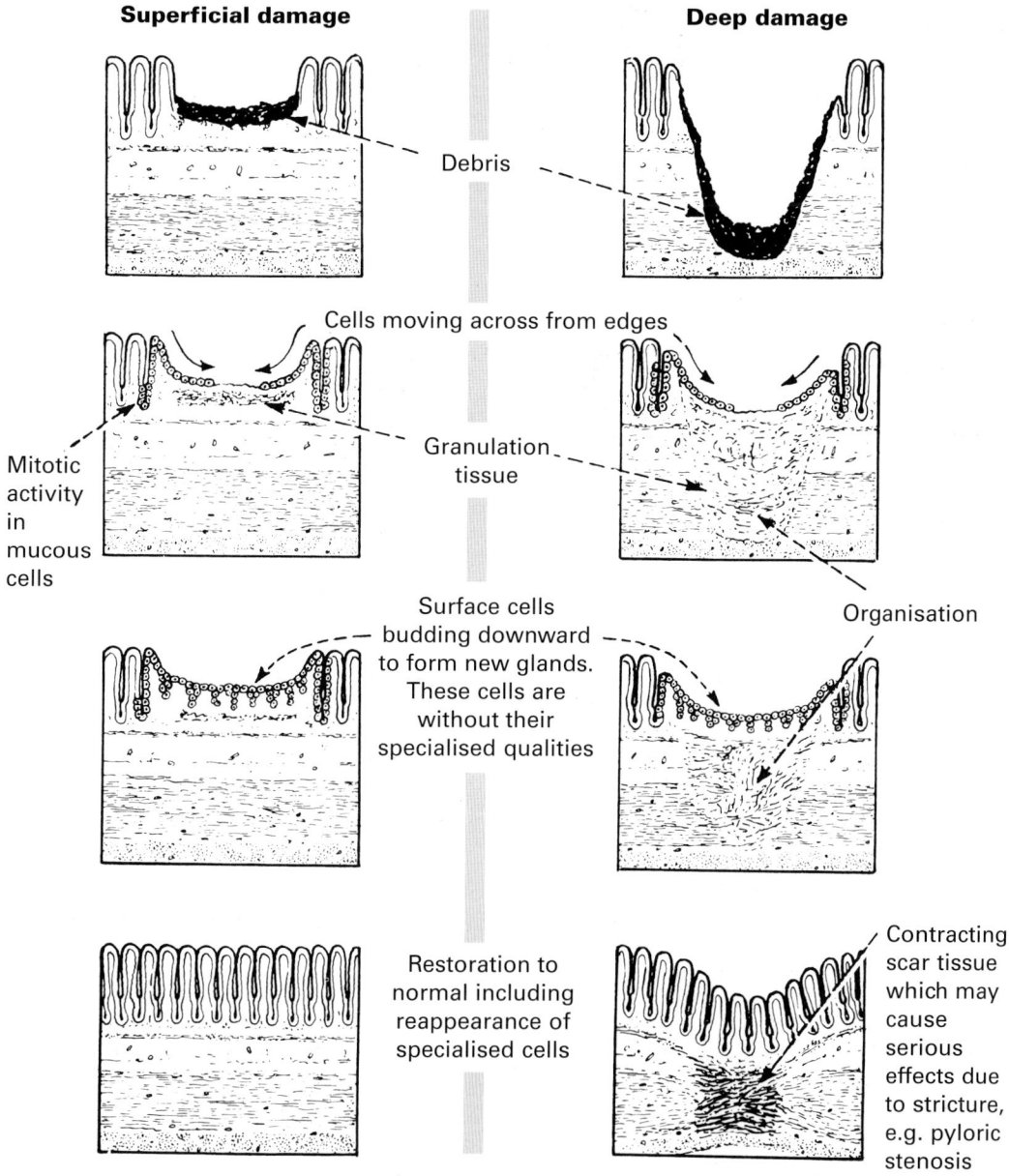

HEALING – SPECIAL SITUATIONS

SOLID EPITHELIAL ORGANS

1. **Following gross tissue damage — including supporting tissue** (post-necrotic scarring).

e.g. **Kidney** **Liver**

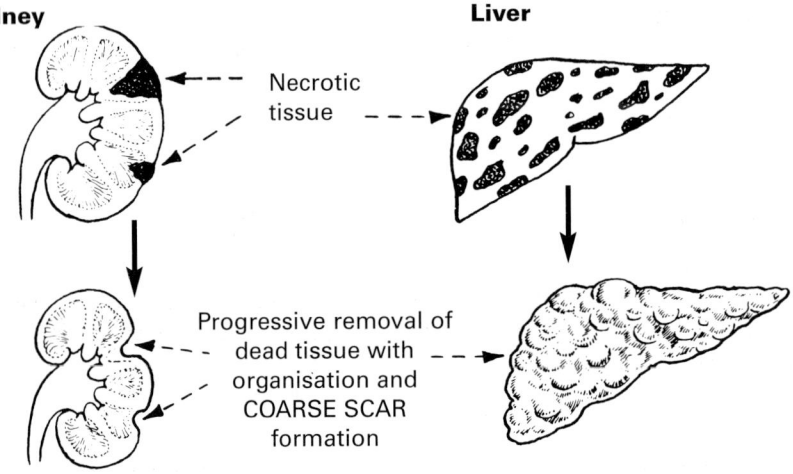

2. **Following cell damage with survival of the supporting (reticular) tissues**

e.g. **Tubular necrosis in kidney** **Perivenular hepatic cell necrosis**

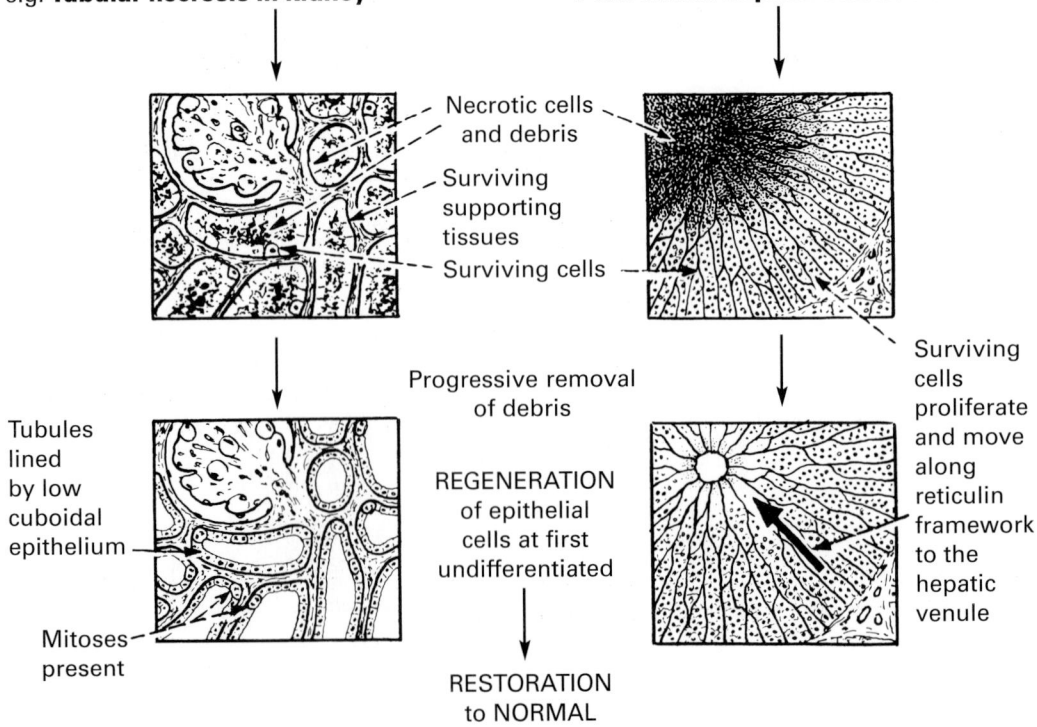

HEALING – SPECIAL SITUATIONS

MUSCLE

Muscle fibres of all 3 types — skeletal, cardiac and visceral — have only limited capacity to regenerate.

When a MASS of muscle tissue is damaged, repair by SCARRING occurs. This is particularly important in the HEART after infarction.

If the damage affects individual muscle fibres diffusely and with varying severity, then regeneration of the specialised fibres is possible (e.g. the myocardium may recover completely from the effects of diphtheria toxin and virus infection).

NERVOUS TISSUE

Central nervous system

Regeneration does not occur when a neurone is lost.

In cases of acute damage, the initial functional loss often exceeds the loss of actual nerve tissue because of the reactive changes in the surrounding tissue. As these changes diminish, functional restoration commences.

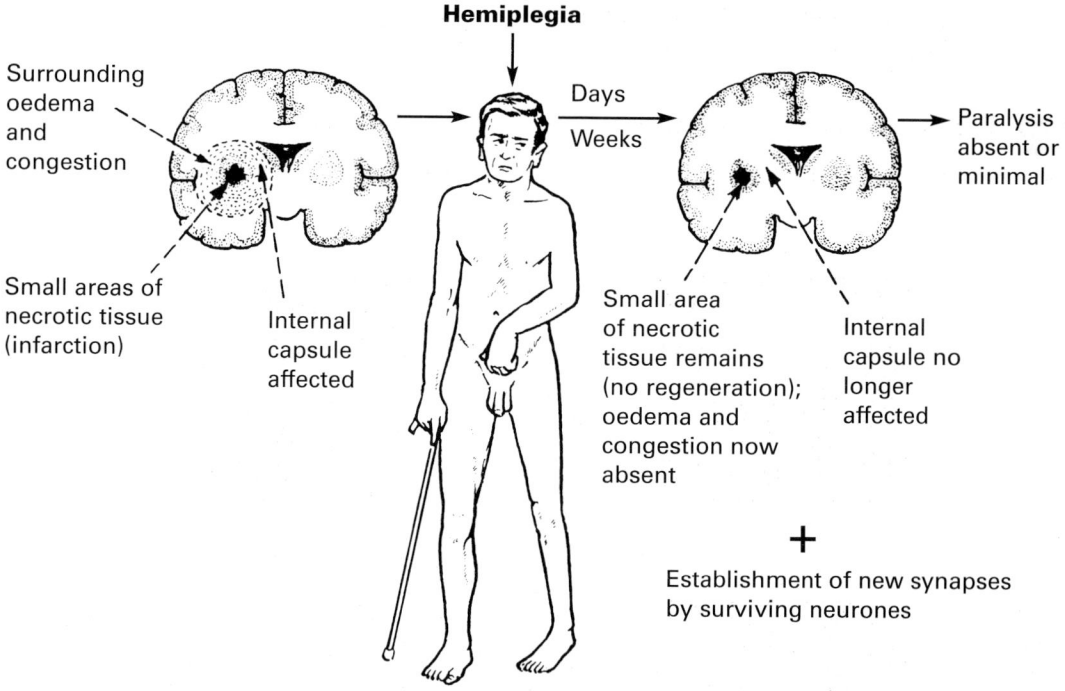

Scarring within the CNS is by proliferation of ASTROCYTES and the production of fibrillary glial protein — a process known as GLIOSIS.

HEALING – SPECIAL SITUATIONS

NERVOUS TISSUE (continued)

Peripheral Nerves

When a peripheral nerve is damaged, the axon and its myelin sheath rapidly degenerate distally. The supporting tissues of the nerve (neurilemma) degenerate slowly.

Regeneration can occur because the central neurone of which the axon is a peripheral extension is remote from the site of damage.

A spinal motor nerve is taken as an example.

Normal Spinal cord

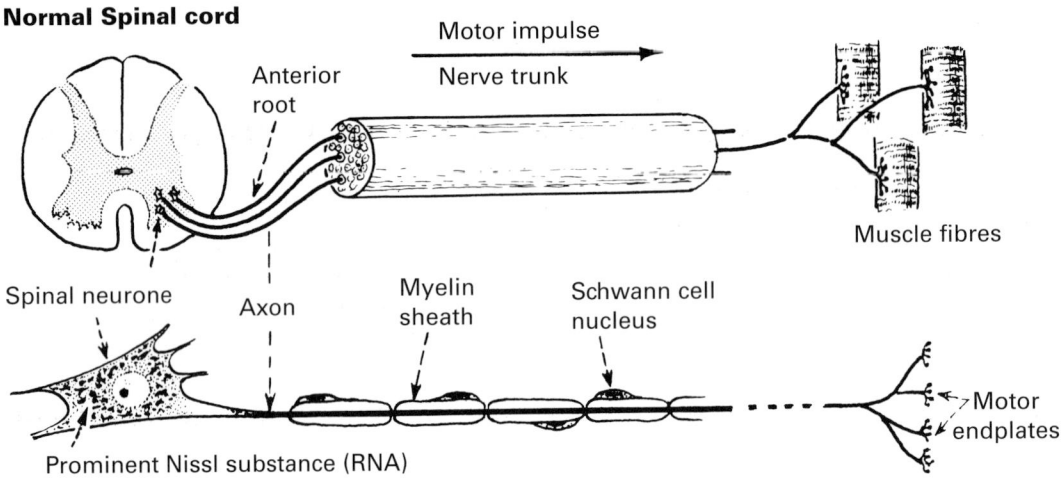

Results of damage

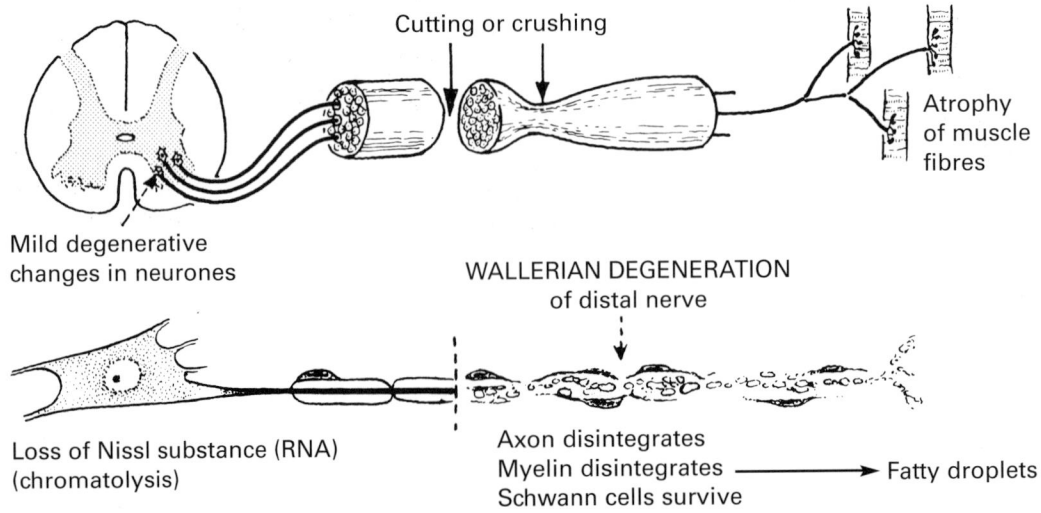

HEALING – SPECIAL SITUATIONS

PERIPHERAL NERVES (continued)

Regeneration takes the form of a sprouting of the cut ends of the axons.

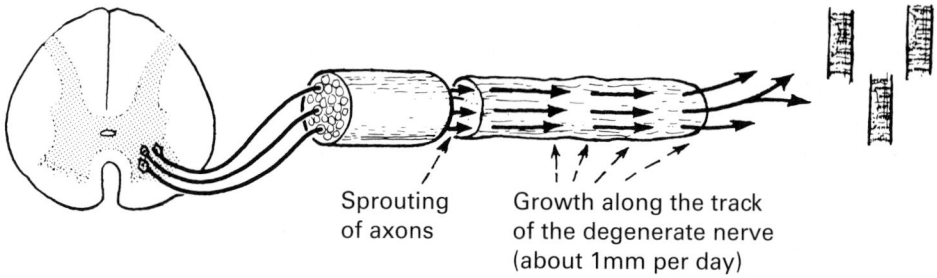

The results depend on the apposition of the distal remnant with the sprouting axons.

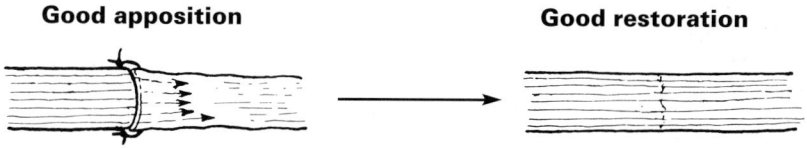

The best results are seen in crushing injuries where the sheaths remain in continuity.

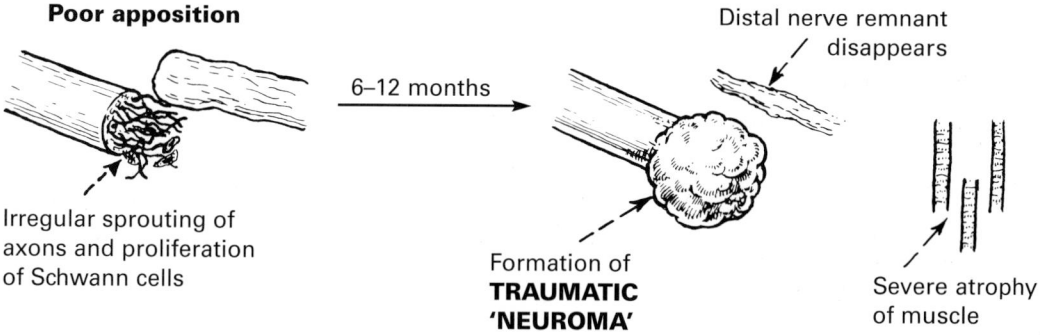

HEALING — SPECIAL SITUATIONS

BONE

A fracture is usually accompanied by damage to or haemorrhage into adjacent soft tissues which are repaired by the process of organisation (page 41), while the bone is repaired by regeneration.

Events following a fracture

(1) *Immediate effects*

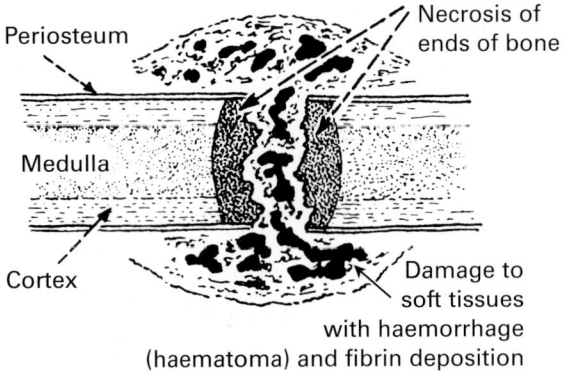

(2) *Early reaction-inflammatory*
First 4-5 days

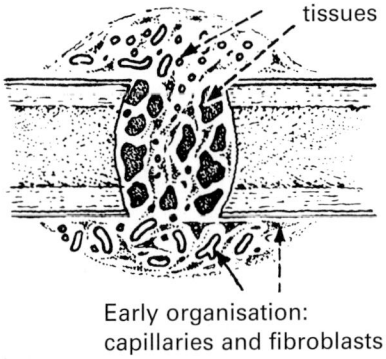

(3) *Formation of callus*
(early bone regeneration)
— after 1 week.

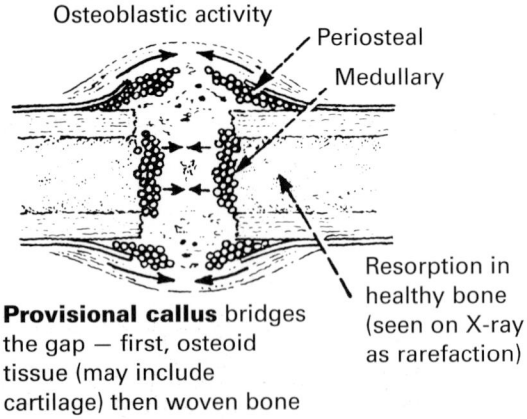

(4) *Mature callus*
— from 3 weeks onwards

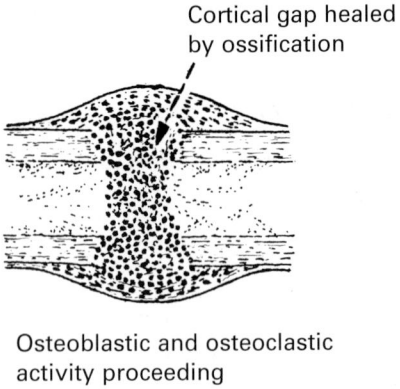

(5) *Remodelling of callus*
Definitive — weeks into months

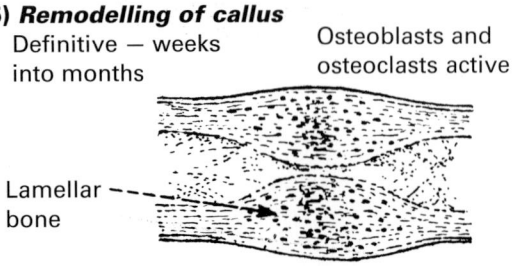

(6) *Final reconstruction*
Months later

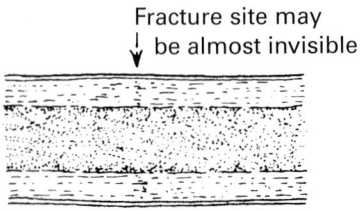

HEALING – SPECIAL SITUATIONS

EVENTS FOLLOWING A FRACTURE (continued)

Complications

1. *Fat embolism* may occur in fracture of long bones due to entry of fat from the marrow cavity into the torn ends of veins.

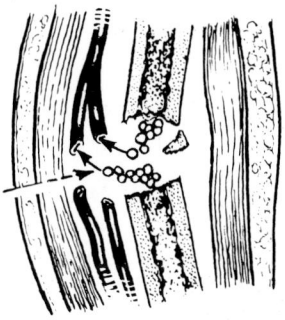

2. *Infection*
   If the overlying skin is breached in any way, i.e. the fracture is 'compound', the risk of infection is greatly increased; this is an important adverse factor in the healing process.

   E.g.

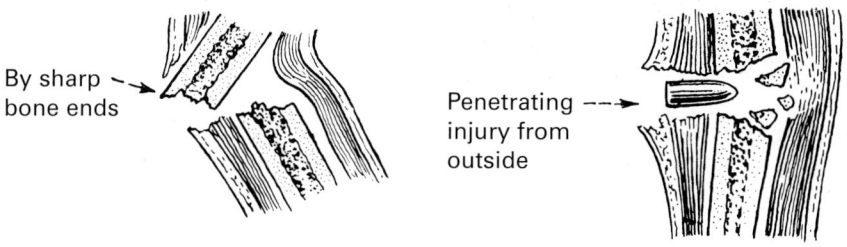

PATHOLOGICAL FRACTURE

When the break occurs at the site of pre-existing disease of the bone, the term 'pathological fracture' is applied.

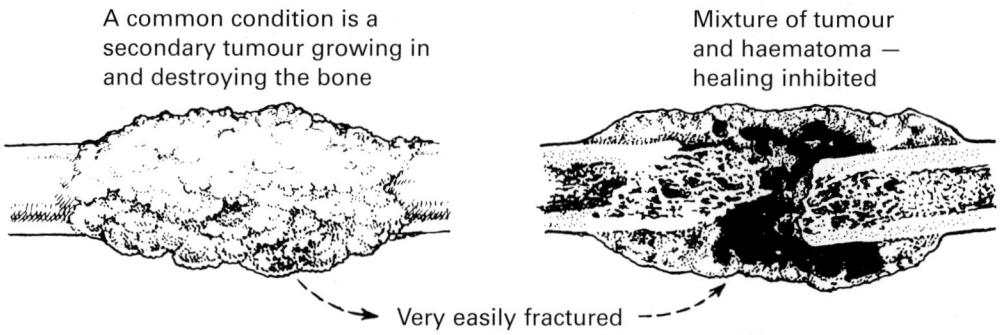

HEALING – SPECIAL SITUATIONS

FACTORS INFLUENCING HEALING OF FRACTURES

ADVERSE	FAVOURABLE
1. Local factors	
(a) *Infection* } See previous page (b) *Pathological fracture* } See previous page	
(c) *Poor apposition and alignment*	*Good apposition*
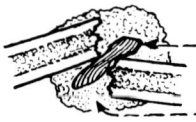 There may be interposition of soft tissue, e.g. muscle Large irregular callus: slow repair, permanent deformity of bone	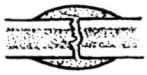 Small callus, quick repair
(d) *Continuing movement of bone ends*	*Good immobilisation*
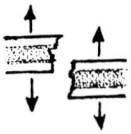 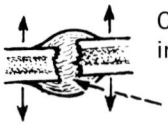 Callus formation inhibited Fibrous union In extreme cases, a rudimentary joint (pseudoarthrosis) may form 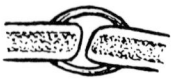	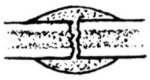 Small callus, good bone formation
(e) *Poor blood supply*	*Good blood supply*
This is largely influenced by the anatomical site of the fracture, for example: (a) Nutrient artery entering remote from the fracture or damaged by fracture (e.g. scaphoid, femoral head) (b) Fracture through area devoid of periosteum (*e.g.* neck of femur) (c) Minimal adjacent soft tissue (*e.g.* tibia).	In favourable conditions blood supply is derived from: (a) periosteal arteries (b) nutrient artery (c) adjacent soft tissues.
2. General factors	
(a) *Old age*	*Youth*
(b) *Poor nutrition* — e.g. famine conditions, malabsorption lead to lack of protein, calcium, vit D and vit C.	*Good nutrition* — especially protein, calcium, vit D and vit C.

CHAPTER 4

INFECTION

Infection 62–67
Acute Bacterial Infection 68–71
Chronic Bacterial Infection (Granulomas) 72–77
Virus Infections 78–81
Host/Virus Interaction 82, 83
Opportunistic Infections 84
Infection — General Effects 85, 86

INFECTION

There are very many infections: the chapter will deal only with principles and a few examples.

Infecting agents which cause disease are said to be PATHOGENIC.

Type of Infecting Agent	Example	Example of Disease
BACTERIA (a very wide range)	STAPHYLOCOCCUS	ABSCESS
VIRUSES (a wide range)	HERPES ZOSTER	CHICKENPOX and SHINGLES
FUNGI (a limited range)	CANDIDA	BUCCAL and VAGINAL THRUSH
PROTOZOA	PLASMODIUM	MALARIA
Infestation with PARASITES WORMS and FLUKES	ECHINOCOCCUS GRANULOSIS	HYDATID DISEASE

COLONISATION AND COMMENSAL GROWTH

Vast numbers of bacteria normally colonise the external body surfaces (skin, alimentary and upper respiratory tracts). Most are of low pathogenicity and some may actually be beneficial to the host, for example:

1. By producing nutrient chemicals, e.g. vit B12
2. By competing with and excluding pathogens.

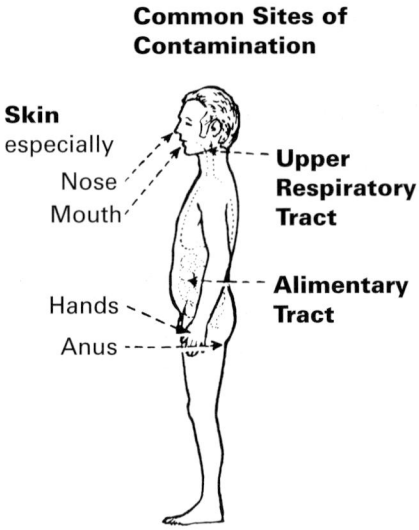

INFECTION AND INFECTIOUS DISEASE

INFECTION occurs when microorganisms invade the sterile internal body tissues. (Multiplication usually follows invasion.)

An INFECTIOUS DISEASE occurs when infection is associated with clinically manifest tissue damage.

Routes of entry of infecting organisms

1. Through the *skin* or *mucous membranes*
   (a) By direct close contact, e.g. venereal disease: HIV.
   (b) By contamination of abrasions and wounds, e.g. wound infections, rabies.
   (c) By inoculation, e.g. insect bite — yellow fever, syringe — hepatitis B and C, AIDS.

2. By *ingestion*
   Contaminated food and water, e.g. enteric fever, hepatitis A, poliomyelitis, cholera.

3. By *inhalation*
   Dust and droplets, e.g. influenza: tuberculosis.

INFECTION

Factors influencing the establishment of infection

1. *In the HOST*
In addition to a good state of general health and nutrition, the following mechanisms operate in preventing and limiting infection.

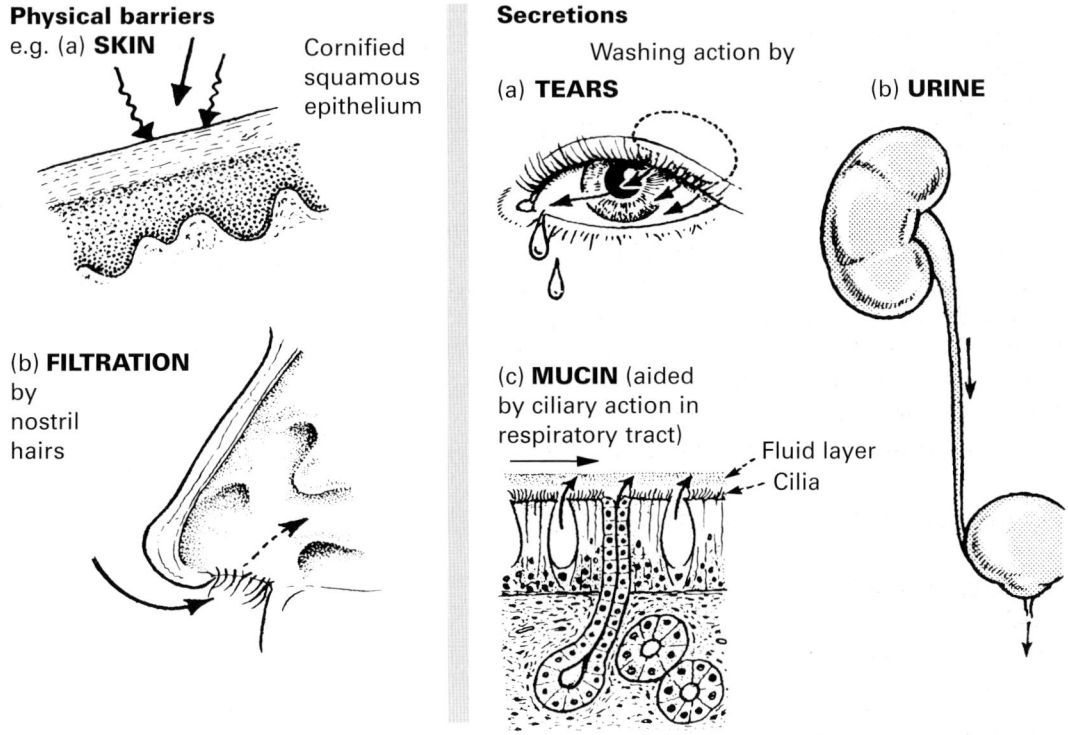

Chemical action

(1) Acid secretion in stomach and urinary tract.
(2) Lysozymes — enzymes capable of dissolving bacterial capsules, e.g. in tears and saliva.
(3) Immunoglobulin A (IgA) — a specialised immunoglobulin (see p. 97), — tears: intestinal secretions.
(4) Non-specific inhibitory substances — urine, sweat, sebum.

2. *In the MICRO-ORGANISM*

Factors potentiating invasive capacity include:
(1) **Quantity of dose** — the larger the dose the more likely that the defences are penetrated.
(2) **Virulence** — a variable factor, and often poorly defined, includes:
  (a) Capacity to resist phagocytosis and enzyme attack,
  (b) Adhesive properties,
  (c) Production of exoenzymes which act on host tissues, e.g. hyaluronidase (streptococci), coagulase (staphylococci) and of toxins, e.g. leucocidins, enterotoxins.

INFECTION

Factors influencing the course of infection

Once infection has occurred, important defence mechanisms operate:

1. **Inflammation** in the **acute** local reaction (see p. 33) tends to limit the spread of organisms. In some important diseases, there is no acute local inflammatory response at the site of entry, e.g. Brucellosis (undulant fever) and many virus infections.
   In the **chronic** inflammatory reaction (see p. 42), the formation of fibrous tissue also helps to localise infection.
2. **Phagocytosis** (see p. 36) *NB* some organisms may survive or multiply within phagocytes — usually associated with chronic infection. Good examples are tuberculosis, brucellosis, leprosy.
3. **The Immune Response** (a) *Humoral antibody* reactions e.g. agglutination, opsonisation, lysis via complement — especially important in *Bacterial* infections.
   (b) *Cell-mediated* reactions — especially in *Viral* infections.
4. **Interferons** — a group of non-specific anti-viral agents (see page 83).

Examples of failure of protective and defence mechanisms

1. **In skin** — direct breach by wounding and burns; softening of the surface by exposure to water and sweat or due to skin disorders.
2. **In the respiratory tract** — inhibition of ciliary movement by nicotine in smokers potentiates infection.
3. **In the stomach** — in achlorhydria (no hydrochloric acid) organisms flourish in the stomach.
4. **When secretions are prevented from flowing freely** by narrowing of natural passages, bacterial growth in the 'stagnant' fluid is potentiated (e.g. enlarged prostate urethral obstruction, urinary infection).
5. **When commensal growth is impaired** by antibiotic treatment, pathogenic bacteria may colonise the 'vacant site'.
6. **Deficiency of the immunological system:**
   (a) natural deficiency due to hereditary defect,
   (b) acquired due to administration of drugs in treatment of disease, e.g. steroids, cytotoxic drugs; specific virus infection, e.g. Human Immunodeficiency Virus (HIV) causing Acquired Immune Deficiency Syndrome (AIDS).
7. **Deficiency of phagocytosis** — especially polymorphs (either low numbers or deficient function — see page 37).
8. **In debilitating diseases** such as diabetes, chronic failure and nutritional deficiency.
9. **Genetic susceptibility** — may be a factor in some infections.

INFECTION

Mechanisms by which disease is produced
The local reaction to infections is usually INFLAMMATORY and is evoked by cellular damage and death. The detailed mechanisms are different in bacteria and viruses.

BACTERIA
1. Production of toxins (poisons)

Exotoxins	Endotoxins
Secreted by living bacteria	Integral part of bacterial cell wall Release on death of organism (usually Gram-negative)
Simple proteins	Lipid-polysaccharide complexes
Neutralised by specific antibody (antitoxin)	Do not stimulate antitoxin production
Often have specific enzyme activity and may act on specific organs or tissues	Cause fever and ENDOTOXIC SHOCK. Act by damaging capillaries and disturbing the coagulation system as well as causing necrosis. Activate fibrinolytic and complement cascades: facilitate release of chemical mediators of acute inflammation.

2. **Hypersensitivity reaction causing tissue injury**
This is a form of the immune response in which reaction between the bacterial protein and sensitised lymphocytes initiates the inflammatory reaction (see p. 108).

3. **Tissue invasion: lymphatic spread and invasion of blood stream**

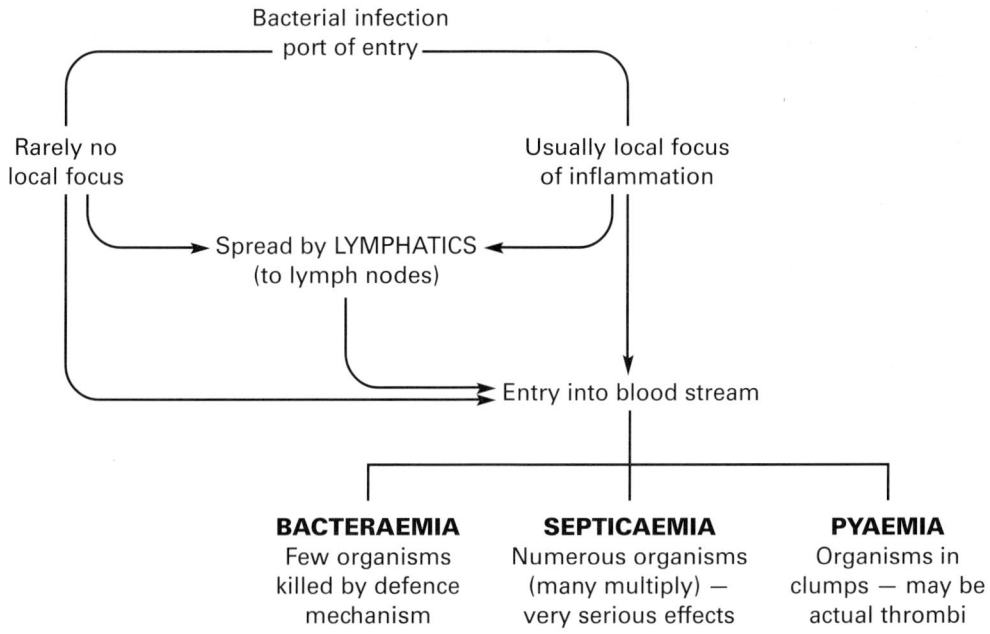

ACUTE BACTERIAL INFECTION

PYOGENIC BACTERIA

Staphylococcus aureus

Gram-positive spherical organism in clusters

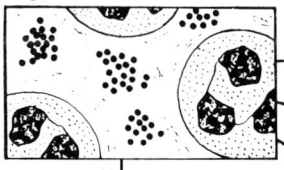

Produce an enzyme — coagulase — which deposits fibrin at the site and tends to localise the infection with production of an abscess containing pus

Common sites of carriage
(usually without symptoms)

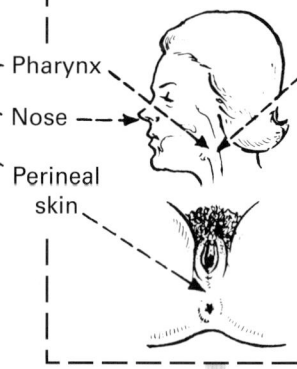

Streptococcus pyogenes

Gram-positive spherical organisms in chains

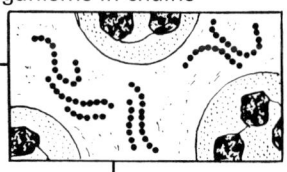

Produce numerous enzymes, e.g. hyaluronidase — liquifies ground substance; streptokinase — dissolves fibrin: and leucocidin, — kills polymorphs and tends to promote spreading inflammation.

Note: Staphylococci are becoming increasingly resistant to multiple antibiotics (MRSA = methicillin resistant staphylococcus aureus).

Lesions produced

Skin infections — pustules, boils, carbuncles
Wound infection
Staphylococcal broncho-pneumonia may be a serious complication in epidemic influenza
Exotoxin production → food poisoning: toxic shock syndrome.

Skin infections — impetigo, erysipelas, cellulitis
Wound infection
TONSILLITIS and pharyngitis
Exotoxin production
↓
The skin rash of scarlet fever

GENERAL BLOOD SPREAD

PYAEMIA (and septicaemia)
OSTEOMYELITIS — acute inflammation of long bones — particularly in children

SEPTICAEMIA

NB Rheumatic fever and acute glomerulonephritis are complications of streptococcal infection in which the heart and kidneys are damaged. This is caused by disturbance in the immune mechanisms and is not due to the actual presence of streptococci in the heart and kidneys.

ACUTE BACTERIAL INFECTION

PYOGENIC BACTERIA (continued)

NEISSERIA

Meningococcus

Both are **Gram-negative intracellular** diplococci

Carried in nasopharynx.
Causes **purulent** *meningitis* and, in children, occasionally a fatal septicaemia.

Skin rash

Massive adrenal haemorrhage

(Waterhouse-Friderichsen syndrome)

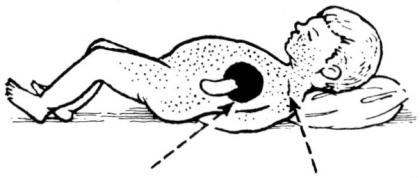

Massive adrenal haemorrhage

Purpuric skin rash

Gonococcus

Carried in genital mucous membrane.
Causes purulent inflammation of urethra in male and of uterine cervix in the female with spread to adjacent organs.

Male

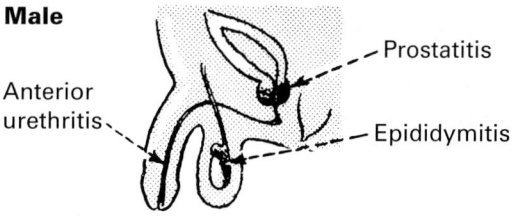

Female

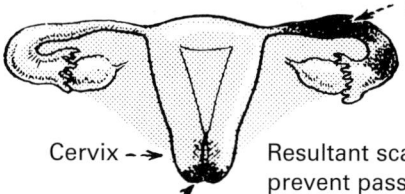

Gram-negative bacilli

These are usually commensals in the alimentary tract and include facultative and obligatory anaerobes.

'Coliform' organisms can cause local inflammation in the alimentary tract, the urinary tract and wound infections.

In addition, ENDOTOXINS liberated in the blood stream cause severe SHOCK (page 172).

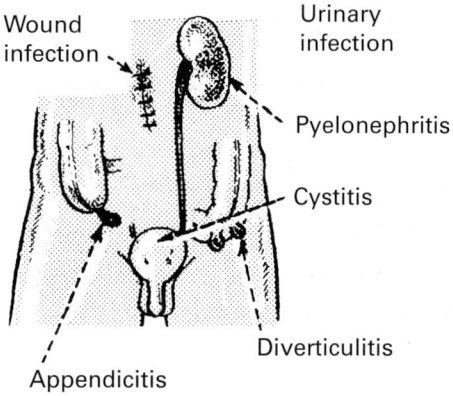

FOOD POISONING

E. Coli 0157 — a commensal in cattle is a human pathogen — production of a powerful **virocytotoxin** is associated with the **haemolytic uraemic syndrome** (see p. 491) and may cause death in the very young and elderly.

ACUTE BACTERIAL INFECTION

GANGRENE

Gangrene is a form of NECROSIS in which a special type of bacterial activity is superimposed. The bacteria proliferate in and digest the dead tissues often with the production of gases. There are two main types: PRIMARY and SECONDARY.

Primary (gas gangrene)

This occurs occasionally in civilian practice but is a serious complication of war wounds. It is due to infection of deep contaminated wounds by bacteria of the CLOSTRIDIA group — ANAEROBIC sporulating Gram-positive bacilli (the commonest organism is *Cl. perfringens*). The anaerobic conditions and the presence of necrotic tissue favour the multiplication of these anaerobes with the formation of GAS BUBBLES and further spreading necrosis. Spread is rapid and there is associated TOXAEMIA.

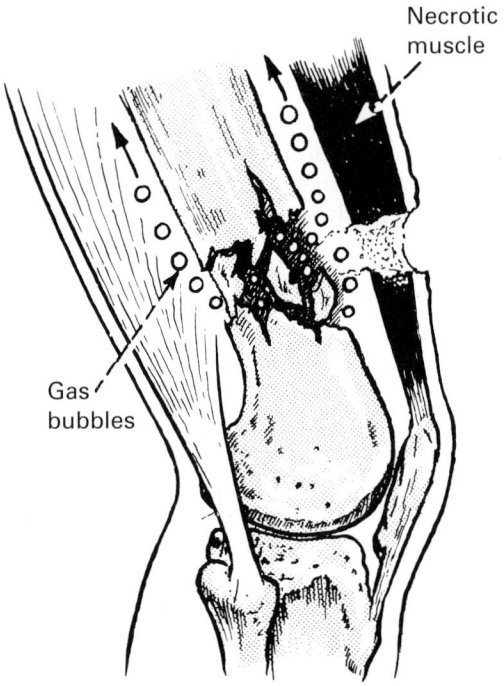

Secondary

This is due to invasion of necrotic tissue usually by a mixed bacterial flora including putrefactive organisms. It occurs in two forms: WET and DRY.

Wet gangrene. The tissues are moist at the start of the process either due to oedema or venous congestion. Examples are in strangulation of viscera and occlusion of leg arteries in obese diabetic patients.

Dry gangrene. Occurs especially in the toes and feet of elderly people suffering from gradual arterial occlusion. The putrefactive process is very slow and only small numbers of putrefactive organisms are present.

ACUTE BACTERIAL INFECTION

TETANUS

This is a toxigenic disease — the organism itself does not cause local tissue damage. The effects are due to a powerful EXOTOXIN secreted by the organism. This is in contrast to the usual bacterial diseases where tissue damage is important and is due to the local bacterial action.

The infecting organism, *Clostridium tetani*, a STRICT ANAEROBE, is a Gram-positive rod. Often the presence of a terminal spore gives a characteristic drum-stick appearance. The highly resistant spores are widespread in the environment due to contamination by animal faeces.

Method of Infection

Contamination of wounds in which there are anaerobic conditions, e.g. deep-penetrating wounds and wounds with severe soft tissue damage (road traffic accidents and battle casualties); only very occasionally trivial thorn punctures.

In developing communities the umbilical stump of the newborn may be infected by faecal material.

Effects:

The exotoxin is highly potent and causes paroxysmal muscular spasm which becomes progressively more severe and was fatal in many cases: modern therapy including muscle relaxation and ventilation has improved the prognosis dramatically.

Course

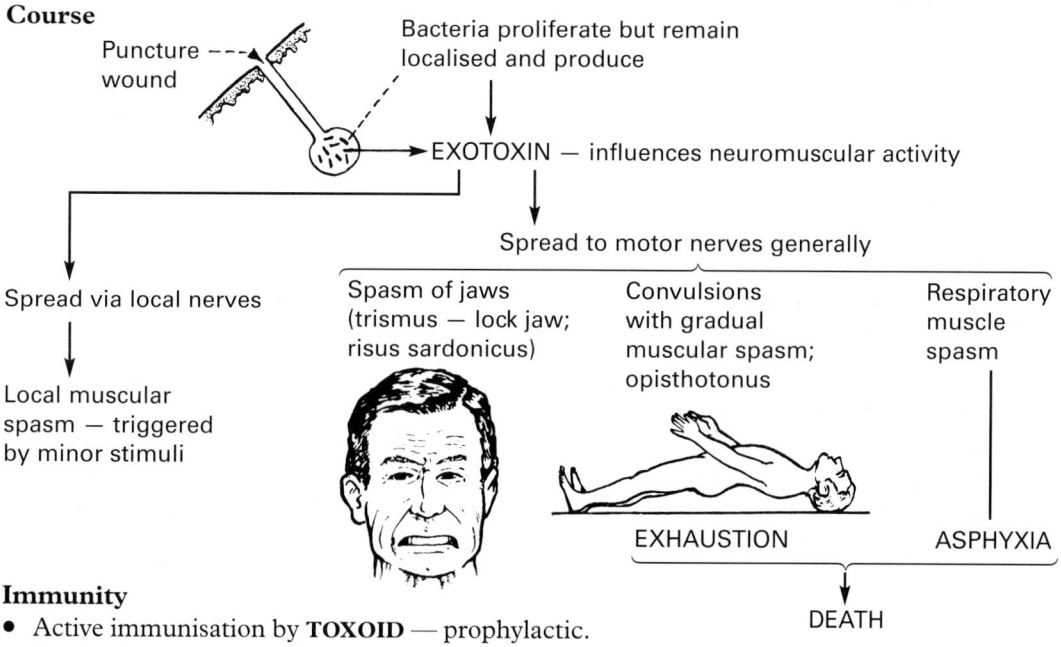

Immunity

- Active immunisation by **TOXOID** — prophylactic.
- Passive immunisation by **ANTITOXIN** — therapeutic (only effective before toxin is fixed to nerve tissues).

Note: Clostridium Difficile, another commensal in the alimentary tract, may cause serious disease in special circumstances (page 322).

CHRONIC BACTERIAL INFECTION (GRANULOMAS)

In these infections chronic inflammation is the basic mechanism (see p. 43). The detailed evolution of the inflammatory reaction is modified by several factors of which the immune response of the host is important (see p. 89).

TUBERCULOSIS

Tuberculosis is caused by the *Mycobacterium tuberculosis* (tubercle bacillus: TB) an organism which has a resistant waxy component in its structure and is acid and alcohol-fast (i.e. resists bleaching with strong acid and alcohol after being stained red with fuchsin). The disease rapidly declined in Western Europe and North America after World War II due to (a) improved nutrition and hygiene, (b) BCG immunisation and (c) chemotherapy (note: drug resistance is becoming an increasing problem). Patients with AIDS are at particular risk: other 'at risk' groups are the elderly, the immunosuppressed and alcoholics. The disease remains prevalent in developing countries.

The tuberculous follicle (tubercle)

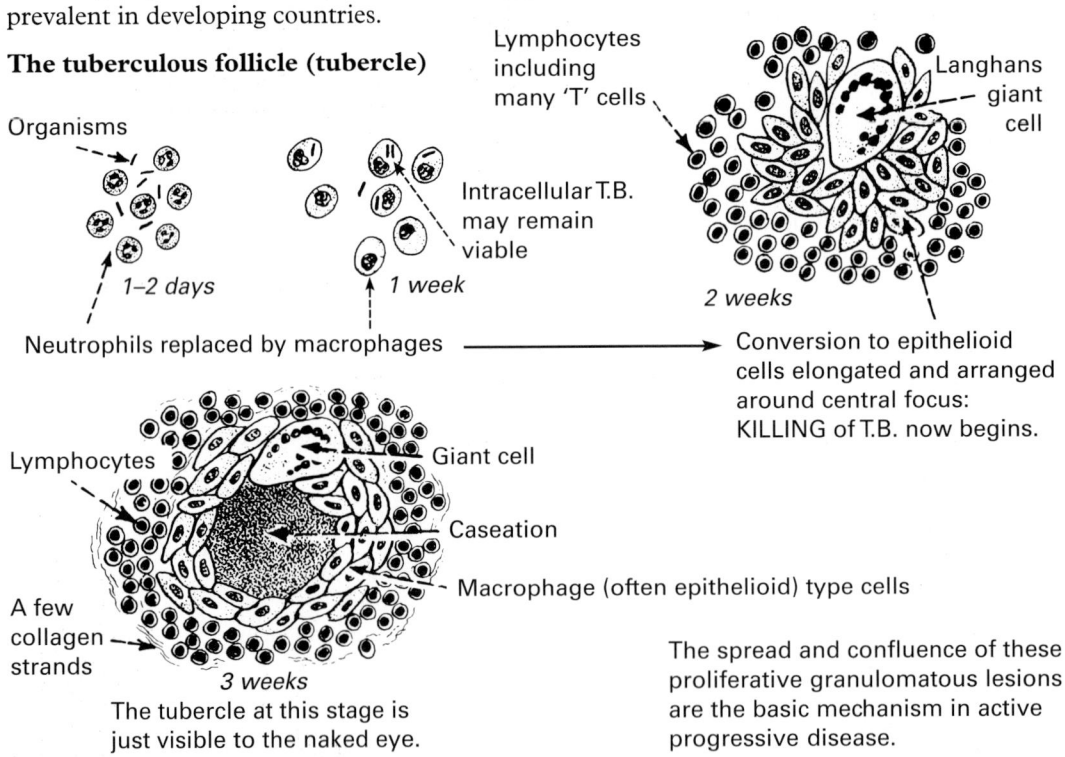

The role of **cell-mediated immunity** (see p. 93) in combating infection is well seen in the evolution of the tuberculous follicle.

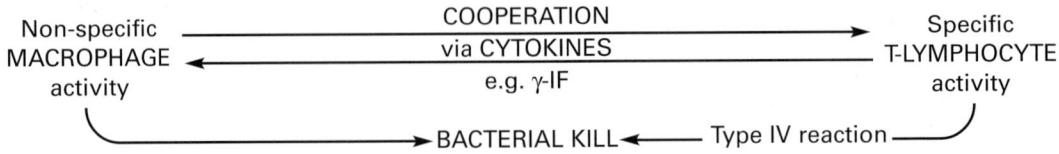

The caseation is the result of the combined effects of (a) the Type IV hypersensitivity reaction, (b) bacterial activity and (c) ischaemia.

CHRONIC BACTERIAL INFECTION (GRANULOMAS)

TUBERCULOSIS (continued)

Primary infection

Usually seen in non-immune children in first contact with tuberculosis. A few bacilli infect the PRIMARY SITE — usually at the periphery of the lung but also occasionally in the pharynx (tonsil) or small intestine.

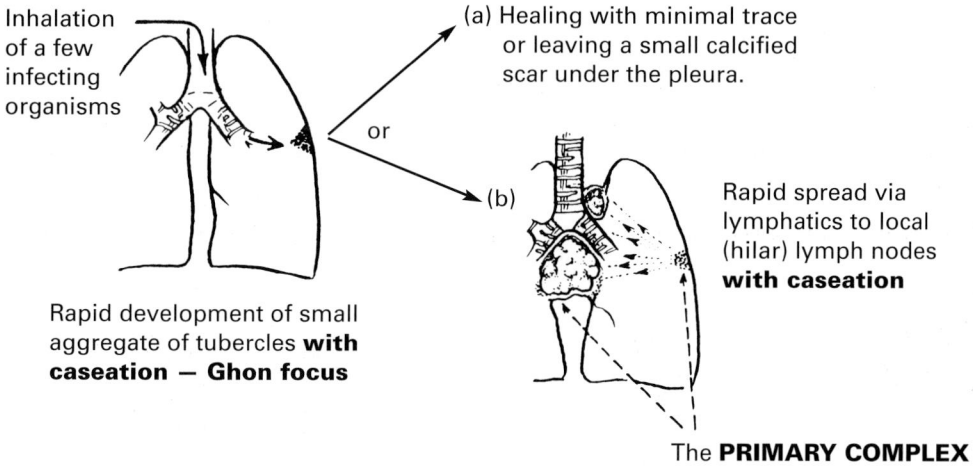

Healing can occur at this stage, leaving calcified lymph nodes, or occasionally the disease spreads via blood stream (a) generally or (b) to individual organs.

General spread

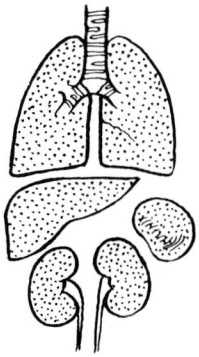

Miliary tuberculosis

Scattering of small pale tubercles throughout the body (milium = millet seed)

Spread to individual organs

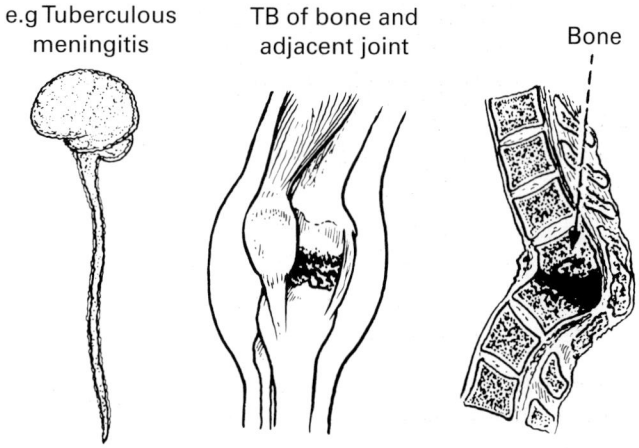

CHRONIC BACTERIAL INFECTION (GRANULOMAS)

TUBERCULOSIS (continued)

Re-infection tuberculosis

This occurs in older children and adults who have had a primary infection or have received BCG vaccination by which a variable degree of immunity to the tubercle bacillus has been established.

The evolution of the disease is much slower than in the primary infection and fibrosis tends to limit the spread, but in untreated cases gradual extension with destruction and scarring of tissues is usual.

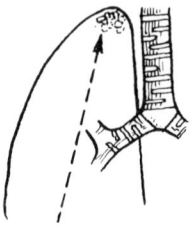

The usual site of reinfection is the lung apex

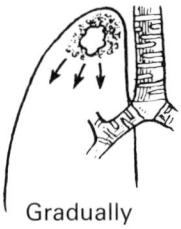

Gradually progressive disease destroying lung tissue: CAVITATION is common.

If the individual's immunity is impaired for any reason, the disease may spread locally more rapidly with increased caseation or in the miliary form.

NB In apparently well-healed tuberculosis, the tubercle bacilli can survive for many years in scarred and calcified tissues and are able to re-establish active disease — REACTIVATION of tuberculosis. This is the commonest form nowadays in Western countries, occurring in late middle and old age among people who were originally infected when tuberculosis was common.

Variations in the basic mechanism

1. *Exudative* inflammation occurs particularly in serous cavities.

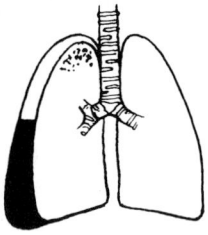

e.g. Pleurisy with effusion

Ascites in abdominal tuberculosis — with adherence of viscera

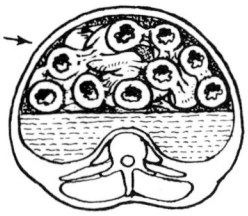

2. *Cold abscess* — where caseation is marked, the tuberculous pus may track to a surface as a 'cold' abscess and sinus.

3. *Fibrotic tuberculosis* — in this condition the body's reparative mechanism is dominant but not sufficient to ensure complete healing; a slow progressive fibrosis with scarring results. This is seen particularly in lung infections.

4. *Acute caseating 'non-reactive' tuberculosis* is seen when the individual's immunity is seriously impaired; massive caseation with little cellular reaction occurs: macrophages are packed with viable tubercle bacilli.

OTHER MYCOBACTERIAL INFECTIONS: human infections are rare: *M. bovis* - from cattle: *M. avis* from birds.

Note: Infection by *Avian tuberculosis* occurs as a complication of AIDS.

CHRONIC BACTERIAL INFECTION (GRANULOMAS)

ACTINOMYCOSIS

Actinomycosis is a localised but gradually spreading chronic suppuration affecting the lower jaw particularly; the ileocaecal region of the bowel and occasionally the lung.

The organism — *Actinomyces israelii* — widespread in nature, is a Gram-positive, branching, filamentous anaerobe found around the teeth and in the pharyngeal crypts. In the tissues, it forms yellow, densely felted together spherical colonies just visible to the naked eye: the pus is seen to contain 'sulphur granules'.

Sites of infection

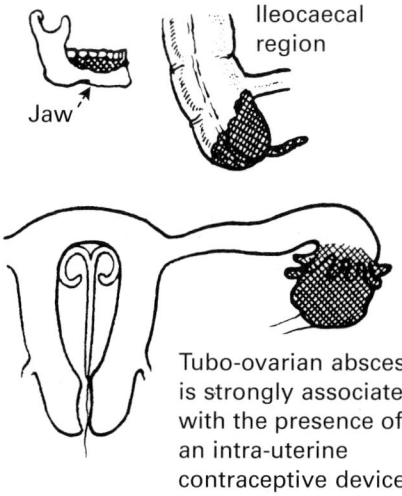

Abscess formation

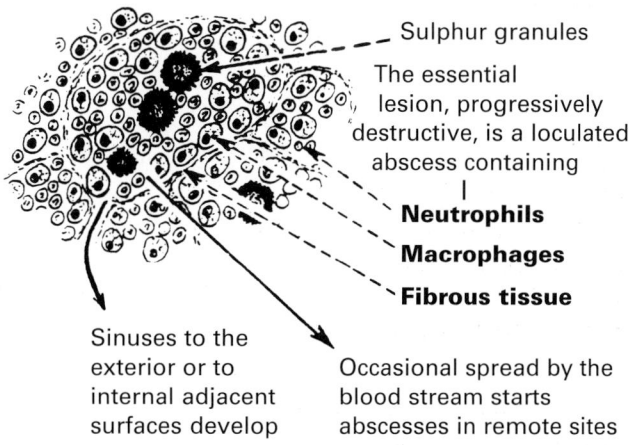

LEPROSY

This slowly progressive disease which causes serious effects by damage to peripheral nerves is still widespread in the tropics and subtropics. The infection is acquired by close, prolonged contact and is due to *Mycobacterium leprae*, a slender acid and alcohol-fast bacillus. The disease presents in two contrasting extreme forms and with cases of intermediate type.

1. Lepromatous leprosy

Disfiguring nodularity of the skin — 'leonine facies'.
Peripheral nerves affected late.
The lesions contain lymphocytes, plasma cells and macrophages — filled with organisms
Organisms + + + in tissues.

2. Tuberculoid leprosy

Focal areas of skin pallor and anaesthesia due to early involvement of nerves.
Basic lesion is a follicular granuloma (tubercle) not unlike the true tubercle follicle.
Organisms are scanty.

These differences are due in the main to differences in the immune reaction of the host.

Cell-mediated immunity is markedly diminished.

Cell-mediated immunity is well developed.

CHRONIC BACTERIAL INFECTION (GRANULOMAS)

SYPHILIS

Syphilis is a venereal infection; the usual sites of entry of the infection are the penis and the vulva or vagina. Extra-genital infection also occurs.

The organism is a spirochaete (*Treponema pallidum*) with a close set, regular spiral, demonstrated by dark ground illumination, silver staining or immuno-fluorescence. Although it very rapidly dies outside the body it has a highly invasive capacity on contact with mucous membranes.

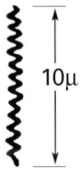

PRIMARY SYPHILIS

During the first three weeks after infection, the spirochaetes spread in the blood throughout the body without any noticeable effects. Then the primary lesion — hard chancre — appears at the original site of entry.

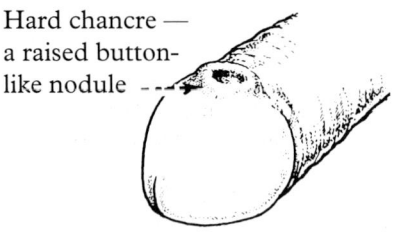

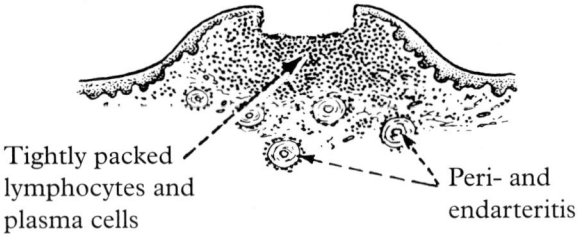

Diagnosis is by examination under dark ground illumination of serum taken from ulcer.

NB No neutrophilis: this is not an abscess. There is minimal tissue destruction and healing occurs without scarring.

The INGUINAL LYMPH NODES present clinically as painless, firm swellings due to proliferation of lymphocytes and plasma cells.

SECONDARY SYPHILIS

During the next 2 or 3 months, the spread of the organisms throughout the body causes secondary stage effects. These are a widespread rash (pox) of varying appearance, ulceration of mucous membranes, generalised lymphadenopathy, damage to various individual organs and tissues. There are constitutional effects - particularly fever and anaemia.

The essential pathology is the presence of very numerous spirochaetes accompanied by focal infiltration of lymphocytes, plasma cells and macrophages with mild arteritis. Infectivity is very high. Tissue destruction is minimal and healing occurs without scarring. A latent stage of long duration is followed in 35% of cases by tertiary syphilis.

TERTIARY (Late) SYPHILIS

The lesions which may occur at any time for many years after the healing of the secondary phase offer striking contrasts. This stage is characterised mainly by local destructive lesions, the result of cell-mediated immune reactions (T cells) causing necrosis of tissue. The main forms are:

1. **Gumma,** 2. **Syphilitic Aortitis** and 3. **Neurological Syphilis** (see page 77).

CHRONIC BACTERIAL INFECTION (GRANULOMAS)

TERTIARY SYPHILIS (continued)

1. **Gumma**
   This is a localised area of necrosis which may affect large parts of any organ or tissue but particularly bones, testis and liver.

2. **Syphilitic Aortitis**
   The arch and thoracic aorta is damaged with weakening of the media: this leads to ANEURYSM formation (see p. 235) which causes serious local pressure effects and may also rupture with severe haemorrhage.

3. **Neurological Syphilis**
   (a) **Meningovascular** — mainly affects the meningeal blood vessels and causes neurological impairment secondarily.

   (b) **Parenchymatous** —

(a) General paralysis of the insane — severe destruction of cerebral tissue

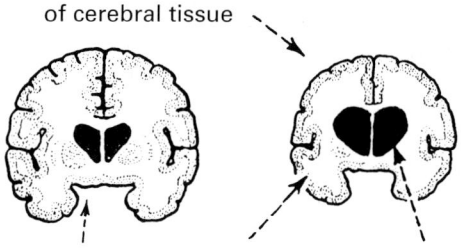

Normal Atrophy of convolutions Enlargement of ventricles

(b) Tabes dorsalis — the damage specifically affecting the posterior roots and columns of spinal cord — is associated with characteristic clinical symptoms due to loss of proprioceptive sensation in the legs

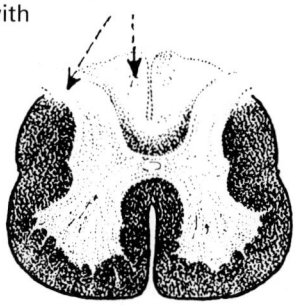

CONGENITAL SYPHILIS

Transplacental infection of the fetus occurs with the following possible consequences:
(a) abortion or stillbirth — many organs damaged
(b) birth of marasmic infant — organ and tissue damage at birth and in later childhood.

IMMUNITY IN SYPHILIS

Antibody production and diagnostic tests

1. *Screening tests*
   Antibodies of uncertain origin which bind to a phospholipid (cardiolipin): these are detected in Wasserman and VDRL (Venereal Diseases Reference Laboratory) tests.
2. *Specific diagnostic tests*
   Specific anti-treponemal antibodies: these are detected in Treponema immobilisation, haemagglutination and fluorescent antibody tests.

Cell-mediated delayed hypersensitivity also develops.
Sensitivity reactions are important in the mechanism of syphilitic damage to tissues.

VIRUS INFECTIONS

VIRUS INFECTIONS

Viruses, the smallest microorganisms in nature (measured in nm), are not visible by light microscopy but can be studied using the electron microscope (EM). The virus particle (*virion*: elementary body) consists of a central core of genetic material, either ribonucleic acid (RNA) or deoxyribonucleic acid (DNA) surrounded by a protein coat (capsid). The virus particle in itself does not contain the biochemical mechanism for replication; it is wholly dependent on the resources of the infected cell.

The diagram shows DNA virus using the host cell for replication: at the same time causing cell death.

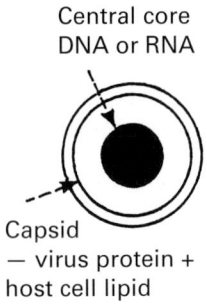

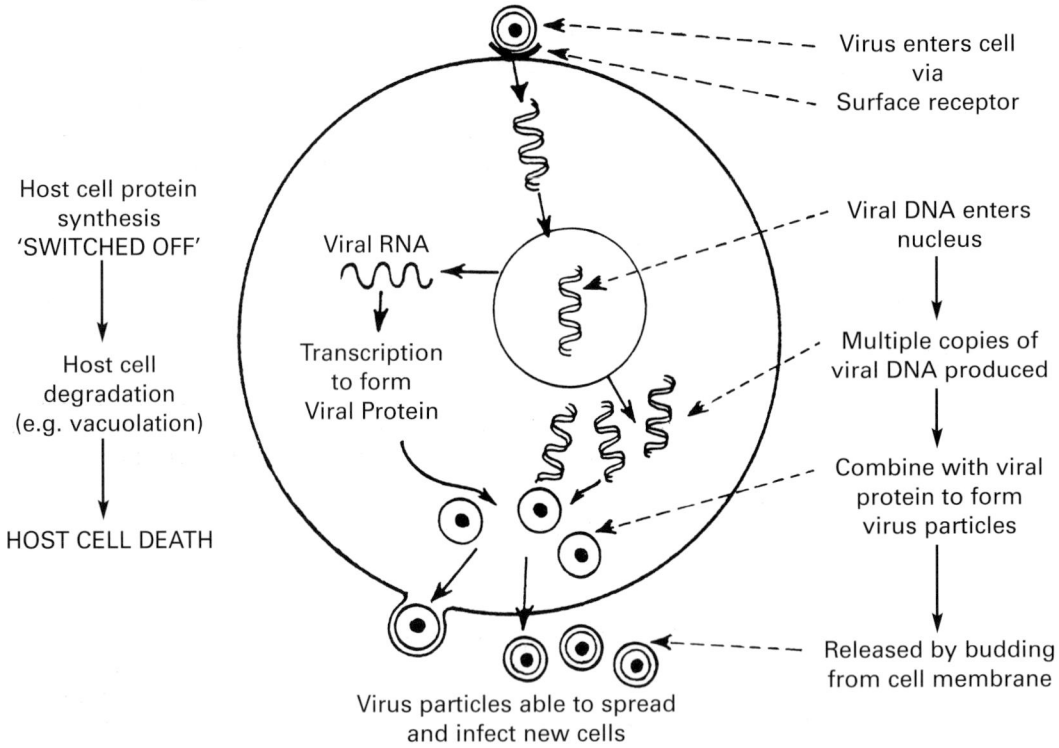

In addition to this direct cytopathic effect of the virus, damage to host may also be caused by:

(i) Side effects of the immune response,

(ii) Incorporation of virus into the cell genome severely affecting the intracellular metabolism.

RETROVIRUSES

An important variation occurs in a small group of RNA viruses. These contain an enzyme — **reverse transcriptase** — which, within the cell cytoplasm, is able (using the virus RNA as the template) to synthesise virus DNA which is then incorporated into the nuclear genetic material (note that messenger RNA is not required).

The virus DNA may remain there inactive for long periods. When activity is resumed, replication and cytopathic changes are effected as indicated in diagram.

Retroviruses are important agents in carcinogenesis and AIDS (see p. 106).

VIRUS INFECTIONS

ACUTE VIRUS INFECTION

The evolution of a typical acute virus infection can be understood in terms of virus replication, release and spread within the body, and of the host's reaction.

Typical evolution

Incubation period

Local lesion

Penetration of cells at site of infection
↓
Replication of VIRUS within CELLS LOCALLY
↓
CELL DEATH liberation of virus
↓
Virus spread to LOCAL LYMPH NODES
↓
Further replication of virus
Cell death

} Local symptoms. The common cold, Influenza, Enteritis (due to enterovirus) illustrate diseases of this type

---

Overt disease

Primary viraemia

Liberation of virus into blood stream
↓
VIRUS spread by blood to LYMPHOID TISSUES GENERALLY
↓
Further replication of virus

} General malaise and fever with lymph node enlargement

↓

Secondary viraemia

CELL DEATH
Liberation of virus into blood stream
↓
Virus spread, GENERALLY throughout the body with effects seen particularly in organs and tissues which possess specific receptors for particular viruses

} Specific symptoms referable to organ or tissue damage, e.g. poliomyelitis — nerve cells, infective hepatitis — liver cells, small pox — skin cells.

This typical evolution is produced by successive waves of virus. However, the great majority of virus infections are clinically latent or mild because virus replication and spread are prevented by the body's defence mechanisms. Severe overt disease occurs when there is a specially virulent virus or when the body's resistance is inadequate, especially in a primary infection.

Not all virus infections cause disease in this way, 3 important variations are:

(1) LATENT (2) ONCOGENIC (3) SLOW

VIRUS INFECTIONS

LATENT VIRUS INFECTION

A good example is the common 'cold sores' of the lips and face caused by the virus Herpes simplex (an enveloped DNA virus).

Initial infection

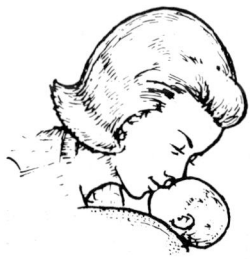

Mother (with herpes) kissing infant may result in trivial or unnoticed blister

VIRUS lies LATENT in cells locally

NOT INFECTIOUS TO OTHERS

Reactivation

At any time non-specific 'triggering' may occur e.g. associated with 'cold', 'flu', sunbathing

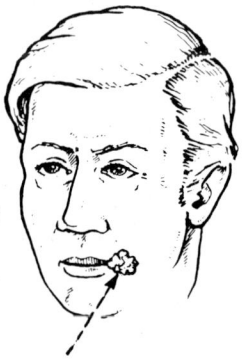

Recurrent cold sores INFECTIOUS TO OTHERS

Another example is **herpes zoster (shingles)**.

This is a painful affection of segmental sensory nerves and root ganglia due to infection by CHICKEN POX VIRUS **Varicella**.

Initial infection in childhood

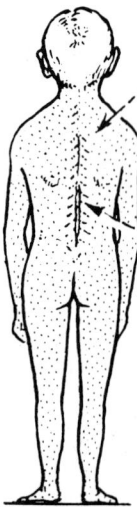

Generalised vesicular skin rash

↓

INFECTIOUS

RECOVERY but VIRUS DNA lies LATENT in DORSAL ROOT GANGLIA

↓

NOT INFECTIOUS

MANY YEARS LATER REACTIVATION OCCURS

↓

SHINGLES

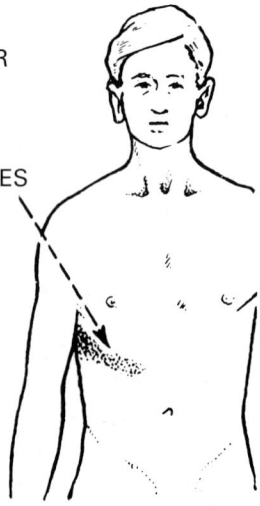

Virus moves down sensory nerve to skin. PAIN and vesicular rash usually confined to the distribution of a single sensory nerve e.g. intercostal

↓

INFECTIOUS

If the trigeminal nerve is affected serious damage to the eye may result.

VIRUS INFECTIONS

ONCOGENIC VIRUS INFECTION

In animals, viruses have been clearly proved to cause malignant tumours, and there is good evidence that some tumours in man are caused by viruses (see also p. 149).

Examples include the following:

(a) **The common wart** *verruca vulgaris* is due to infection by human papilloma viruses (HPV) and there is a close association of these viruses with **cervical carcinoma**.

(b) **The Epstein-Barr virus** (a member of the herpes group) causes glandular fever (infectious mononucleosis — a non-malignant condition) in young adults in Western societies. This virus is also closely associated with Burkitt's lymphoma (a malignant tumour) found in young Africans living in malarial areas and also possibly with Hodgkin's disease.

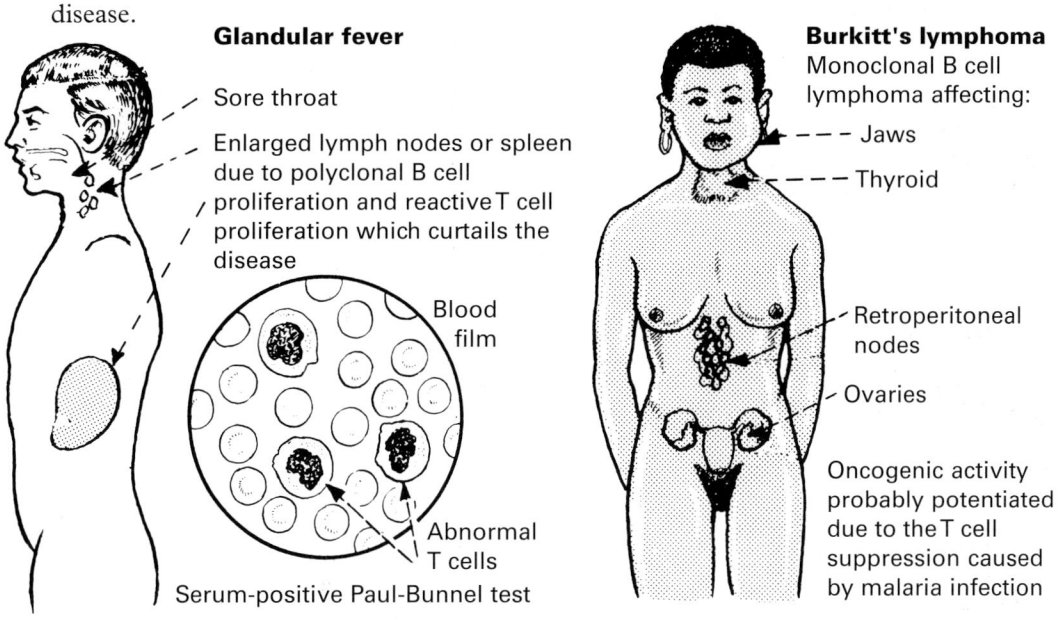

(c) T cell leukaemias are caused by specific retroviruses, i.e. human T cell Leukaemia-Lymphoma Virus (HTLV)

The mechanisms by which viruses cause tumours are illustrated on page 149.

SLOW VIRUS INFECTION

PRION DISEASE SCRAPIE in sheep and BOVINE SPONGIFORM ENCEPHALOPATHY (BSE) in cattle ('mad cow disease') after long incubation periods cause severe damage to the brain. KURU and CREUTZFELDT-JAKOB (CJ) disease are the human equivalents.

A new strain of CJ disease affecting young adults is related to BSE and may be transmitted by eating infected meat products containing offal.

The essential pathological changes consist of microscopic cerebral cystic degeneration.

The infective agents are very resistant to the usual sterilizing methods and, although they replicate, do not conform completely to the definition of a virus.

The name PRION has been given to agents of this type.

LENTIVIRUSES The progress of disease caused by LENTIVIRUSES (a type of retrovirus) is usually very slow. AIDS due to HIV infection is the prime example (see p. 106).

HOST/VIRUS INTERACTION

The reactions occurring in the host are important.

1. **Changes in the infected cells**

(a) Cell degeneration (with loss of function) leading to cell death.

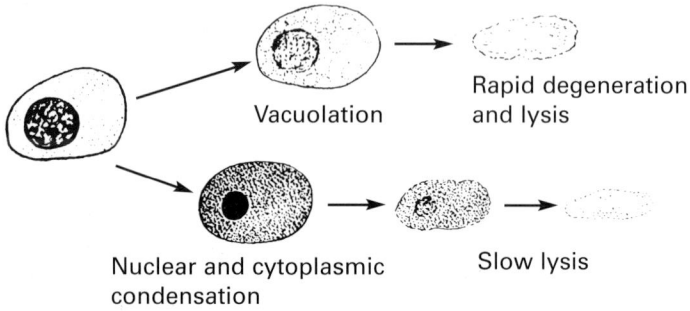

(b) Fusion of adjacent infected cells — giant cell formation, e.g. the Warthin-Finkeldy cell of measles

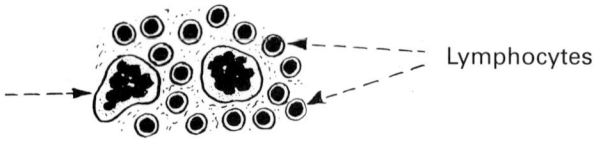

(c) Cell proliferation.

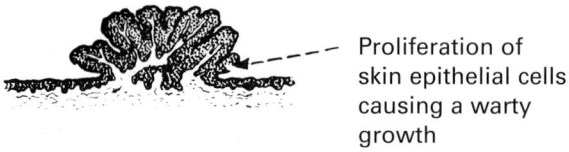

(d) Formation of 'inclusion' bodies within cytoplasm or nucleus: they consist of aggregates of virus and/or products of cell degeneration.

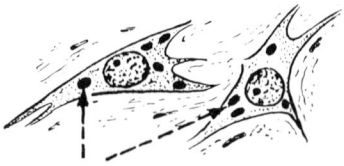

Diagnostic eosinophilic intracytoplasmic Negri bodies in nerve cells of the hippocampus in **RABIES**

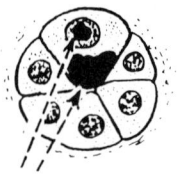

Nuclear and cytoplasmic inclusion in cytomegalic virus infection of salivary ducts

(e) No apparent change in cell but virus remains latent — reactivation later with continuous and slow release associated with gradually progressive disease.

(f) No apparent change but later malignant proliferation occurs, i.e. oncogenic infection.

HOST/VIRUS INTERACTION

REACTIONS IN HOST (continued)

2. **Interferon production** by the infected cells and specifically activated T lymphocytes. Interferons are a group of protein molecules - not antibodies. They represent the first and very important line of defence by interfering with the synthesis of viral protein and thus protect healthy cells.

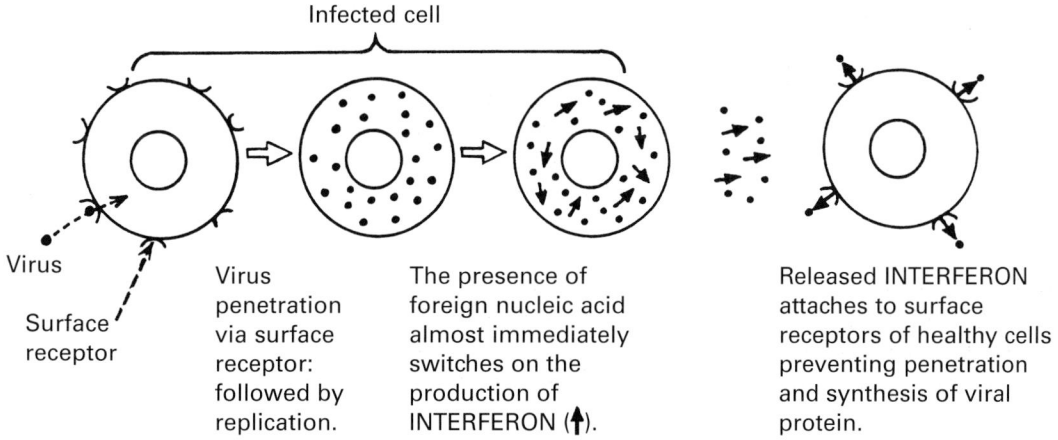

3. **The immune response** (see p. 89) begins 4–7 days after initial infection.

   (a) Antibodies to virus } limit initial infection but are very
   (b) Cell-mediated immunity } important in protecting against RE-INFECTION.
   (c) Occasionally virus antibody complexes cause special types of reaction in the host, e.g. inflammatory necrosis of arteries (arteritis), some forms of kidney damage, and the skin rashes of childhood viral infections.

4. **The inflammatory response**

   The vascular and exudative elements follow the usual pattern; **neutrophils** are **not** a feature unless there is considerable tissue necrosis or secondary bacterial infection. However, **macrophage** phagocytic activity is important in the defence against viral infection. There is often a relative **lymphocytosis**.

OPPORTUNISTIC INFECTIONS

This term is used for infections caused by organisms which are often nonpathogenic or of low grade virulence, occurring in individuals whose resistance to infection is impaired. They are occurring more frequently in modern medical practice because of the increasing use of powerful immunosuppressive drugs.

CAUSES OF LOWERED RESISTANCE

1. Congenital immunological deficiencies (rare).
2. Acquired

(a) *the result of disease:* HIV infection (AIDS); uraemia; liver disease; malignant tumours, particularly Hodgkin's disease and leukaemias;

(b) *the result of therapy:* e.g. immunosuppression in transplant surgery; immunosuppression — a side effect of tumour therapy; antibiotics — changing commensal populations; introduction of foreign material, e.g. heart valve prostheses; I.V. long lines in intensive care; tracheostomy.

Examples of infecting organisms

Bacteria → *Acinetobacter* wound infections: septicaemia

Staph. epidermidis on heart valves; low grade septicaemia

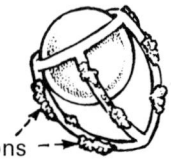

Vegetations on artificial heart valve

Protozoa

Pneumocystis carinii: a severe pneumonia (seen in AIDS cases particularly)

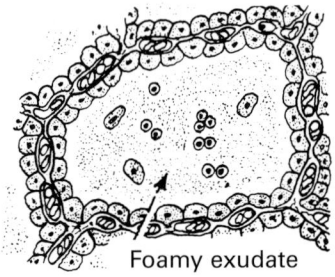

Foamy exudate

Viruses → Wart viruses: crop of warts around genitalia, e.g. Vulvar condylomata

Herpes virus group: generalised infections or severe organ damage e.g. Herpes encephalitis

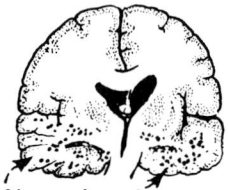

Necrosis

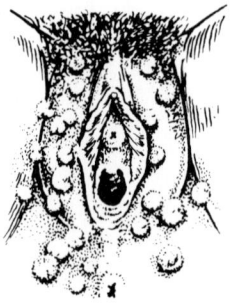

Fungi Apergillosis — lungs: septicaemia

Monilia (candidiasis) — mouth, oesophagus, bowel, anus: septicaemia; endocarditis.

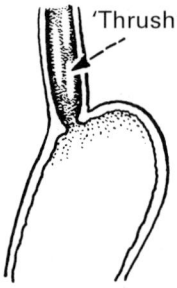

'Thrush'

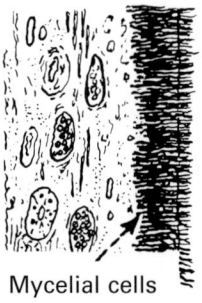

Mycelial cells

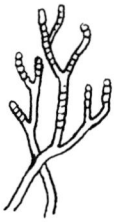

Monilia

INFECTION – GENERAL EFFECTS

The more general body reactions in infection are: FEVER and CHANGES IN METABOLISM.

FEVER (PYREXIA)

The body temperature rises above normal initially due partly to an imbalance between heat production and loss, but mainly due to a resetting at a higher level of the 'thermostat' mechanism in the hypothalamus. This results in:

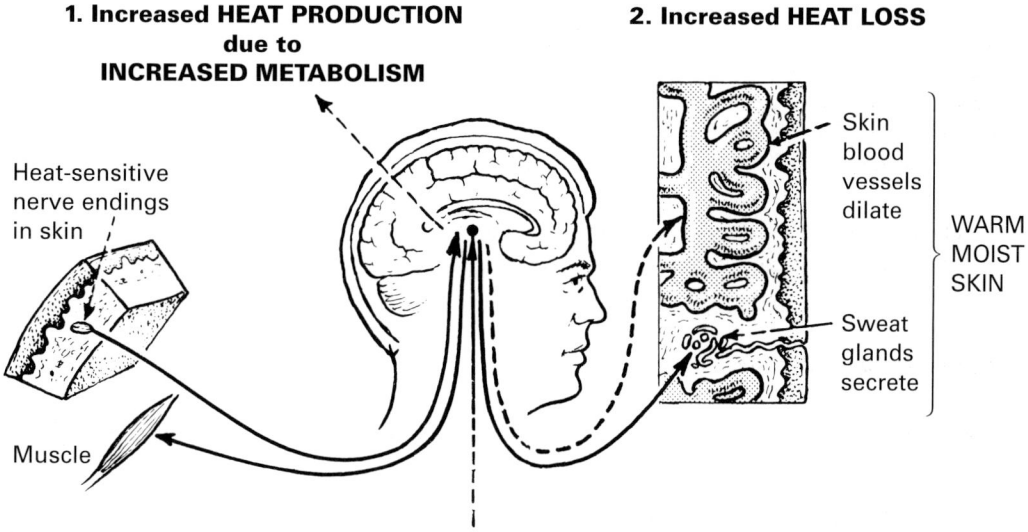

In early stages, when the temperature is rising internally, there may be a paradoxical feeling of cold with shivering (rigor).

Thermostat set at higher level due to pyrogens derived from (a) infecting organisms or (b) endogenous, derived from macrophages (e.g. interleukin-1) and polymorphs: the change is mediated by prostaglandin-E.

These changes are associated with an INCREASED PULSE RATE and a tendency to DEHYDRATION.

Pyrexia also occurs when there is:

(a) Considerable tissue necrosis, e.g. infarction and tumours

(b) Cerebral disease — especially in the region of the pons

(c) Heat-stroke — where the environmental temperature and humidity are high and there is excessive water and salt loss.

Hyperpyrexia [when the temperature exceeds 41°C (106°F)] is extremely dangerous because of damage to the nerve cells in the brain.

INFECTION – GENERAL EFFECTS

CHANGES in METABOLISM

Tissue breakdown is greatly increased, and in some infectious fevers there is a marked loss of body weight.

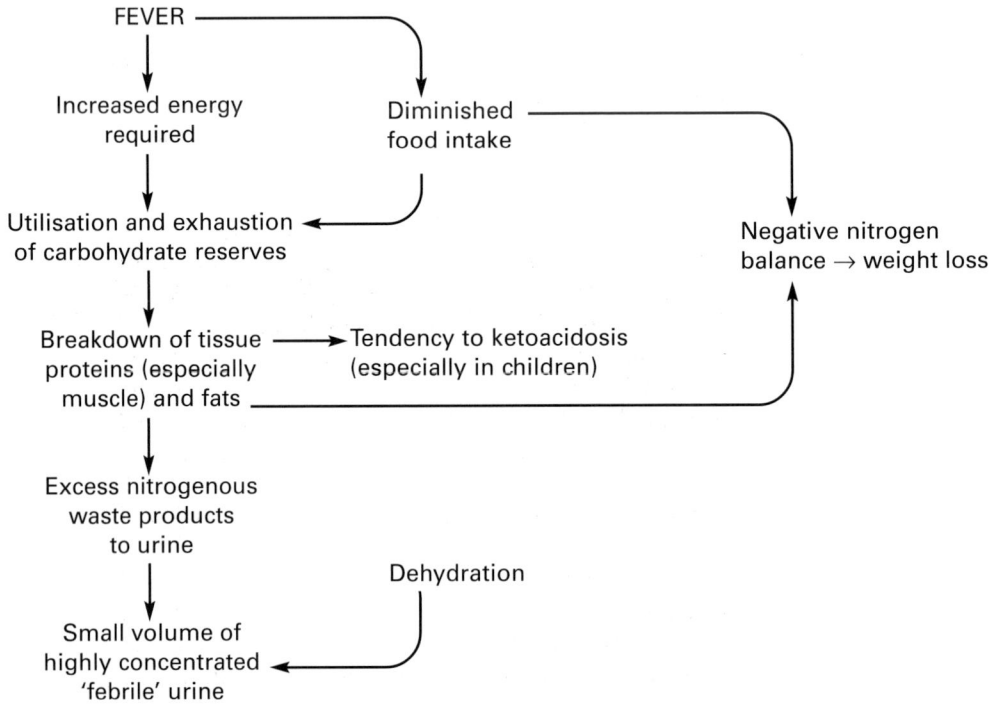

CHANGES in the BLOOD

(a) (i) **Neutrophil leukocytosis** - in acute bacterial infections.

(ii) **Lymphocytosis** — often in viral infections.

(iii) **Lymphopenia** — in typhoid fever and chronic debilitating infections.

(b) **Biochemical changes**

(i) **Non-specific** changes in plasma proteins → cause a rise in the **Erythrocyte Sedimentation Rate (ESR)**.

(ii) Specific antibodies are present in both bacterial and viral infections (See next chapter).

(iii) Acute Phase Reactants — a group of serum proteins which rise in response to inflammation: examples are C-reactive protein (used in diagnosis): complement components: and serum amyloid A protein: in long-standing chronic inflammation AMYLOIDOSIS may be a complication (see p. 24).

(iv) Other chemical changes are listed on page 36.

CHAPTER 5

IMMUNITY

Immunity 88
The Specific Immune Response 89
Antigen 90
Cellular Basis of the Immune Response 91
Genetic Influences on the Immune Response 92
Cell-Mediated Immunity 93
T Cell Activities 93, 94
Humoral Immunity — Immunoglobulins (Ig) 95
Immunoglobulins 96, 97
Immune Reactions 98, 99
Mononuclear Phagocyte System 100
Tolerance 101
Immunopathology 102
Hypersensitivity States 103, 104
Immune Deficiency States 105
Immune Deficiency States — AIDS 106, 107
Autoimmune Diseases 108–110
Applied Immunology 111
Applied Immunology — Tissue Transplantation 112

IMMUNITY

It has been known from historical times that a person who has recovered from an infectious disease, e.g. smallpox, is most unlikely to suffer from it again — even when exposed maximally — although he would remain susceptible to other infections.

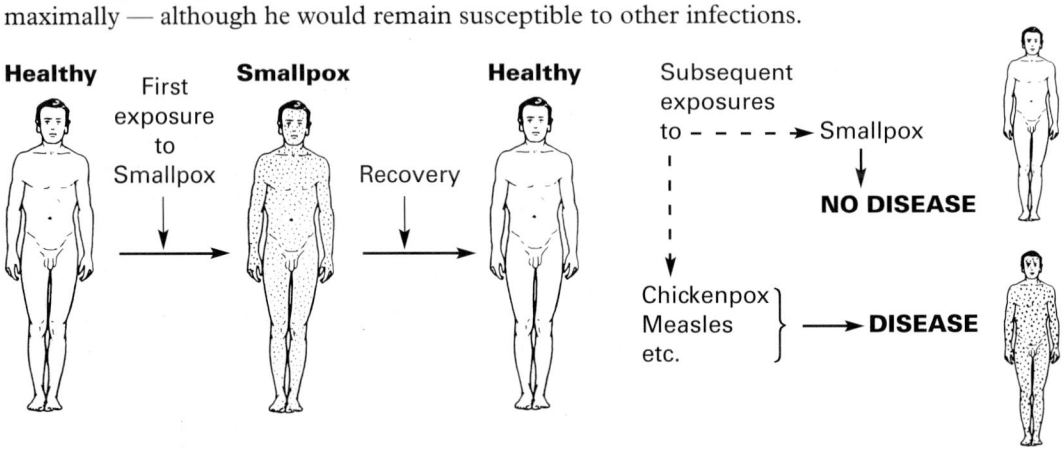

That is, during the recovery period he has ACQUIRED SPECIFIC IMMUNITY to smallpox but not to other unrelated infections.

Note: This immunity may extend to related infections: the use of the immunity against smallpox conferred by world-wide vaccination with cowpox (pioneered by Jenner in the 18th century) has completely eliminated smallpox throughout the world.

IMMUNITY — resistance to infection — also includes NON-SPECIFIC mechanisms, some of which have been mentioned previously.

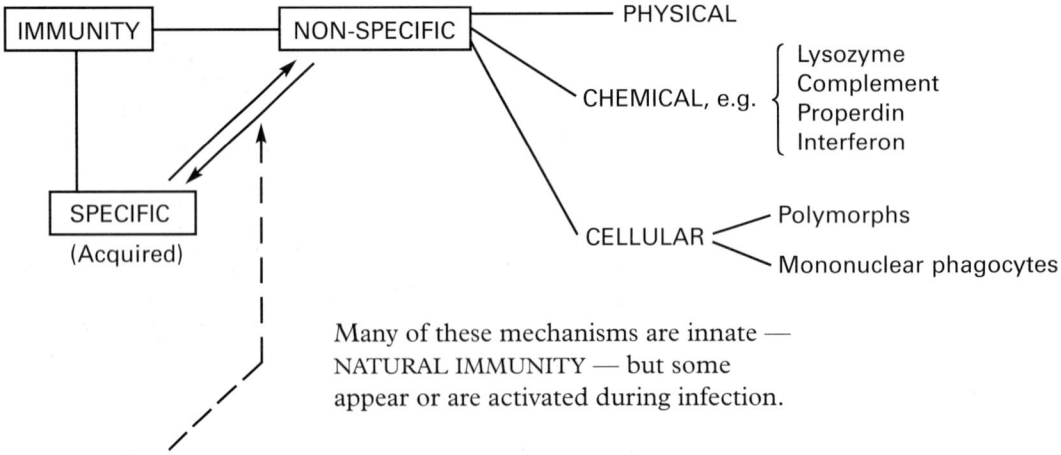

Note: CO-OPERATION. The specific and non-specific mechanisms are conveniently separated but they have important influences on each other.

The modern science of IMMUNOLOGY is engaged mainly in the study of the mechanisms involved in the establishment of specific immunity, i.e. the IMMUNE RESPONSE and its CONSEQUENCES.

THE SPECIFIC IMMUNE RESPONSE

The sequence of events in an infection is as follows:

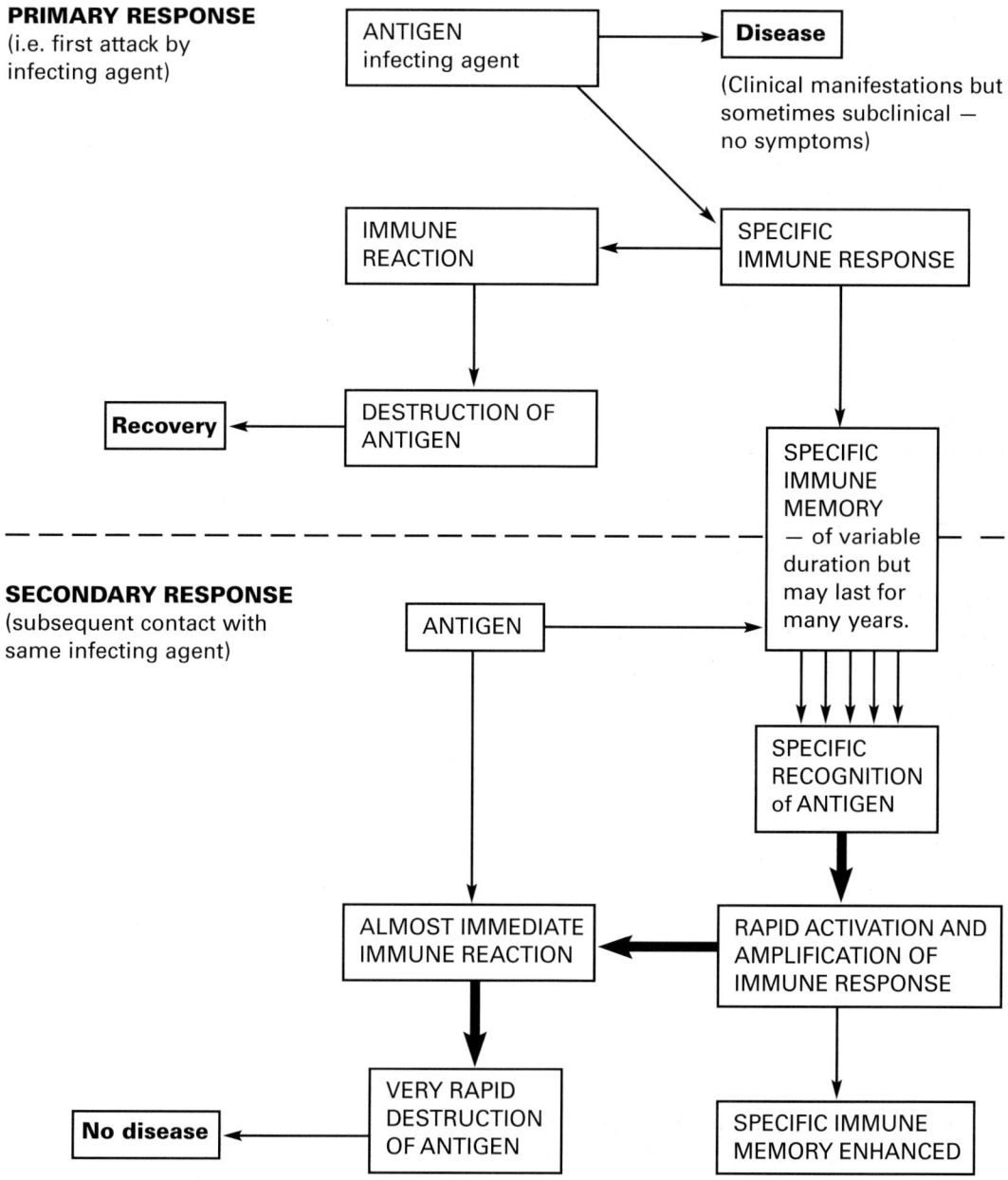

ANTIGEN

An antigen is any substance which provokes a specific immune response. The most familiar antigens are infectious agents such as bacteria and some viruses, but other substances foreign to the human body will stimulate the immune process. Most of them are of protein nature, but complex chemical substances such as some large carbohydrate molecules, lipoproteins and lipopolysaccharides will induce antibody formation. At the other end of the scale, immune reactions are provoked by fungi, protozoa such as malarial parasites, and helminths.

Many simple chemicals can act as HAPTENS. These are themselves unable to act as antigens inducing antibody formation but, if they become attached to a protein, antibody to the chemical may be induced.

Note: HAPTEN formation is the basis of many relatively simple chemicals causing ALLERGIC reaction (see page 102).

Antibodies are proteins, produced during an immune response, which bind to antigens. The union of antigen with antibody is a physicochemical reaction and takes place at specific sites on the antigen molecule — called DETERMINANTS. Their number influences the strength of the Ab/Ag binding.

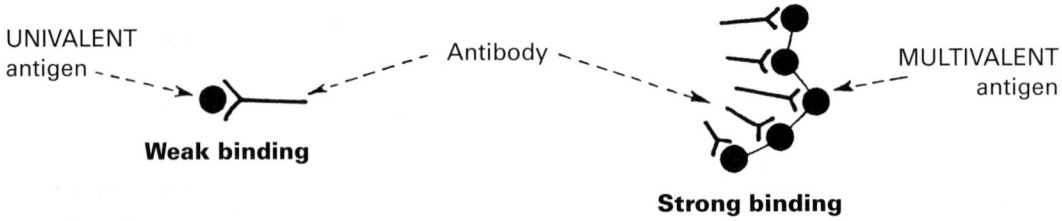

Cross-reactions

Complex antigens may have common determinant sites; this explains why the specific antibody to one may cross-react with other antigens. It may lead to confusion when immunological diagnostic tests are used in the laboratory.

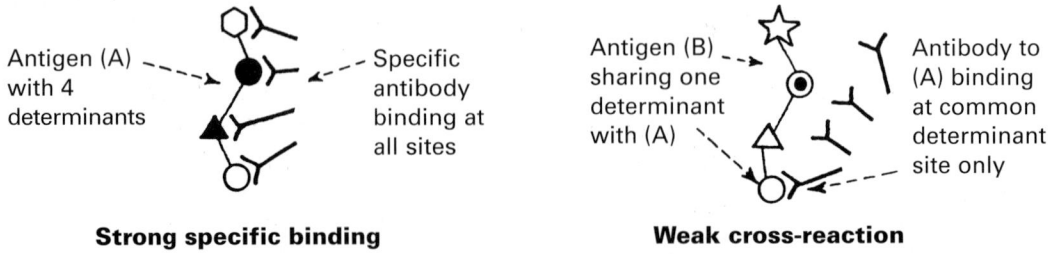

Antigens evoke the strongest response when they are introduced to the body parenterally, but some diseases are caused by surface absorption of antigen, e.g. gluten enteropathy (coeliac disease) and hay fever.

CELLULAR BASIS of the IMMUNE RESPONSE

The process is essentially an activity of the small lymphocytes of which there are two main types. They are indistinguishable by light microscopy using conventional stains but can be separated by the presence of different surface proteins on T and B cells.

Stem cells in MARROW

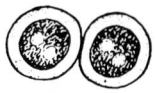

In man, to reach functional maturity, stem cells are processed mainly in the bone marrow. (First associated with the **B**ursa of Fabricius in the bowel of chicken)
∴ called **B lymphocytes**

In man and other mammals, to reach functional maturity, stem cells are processed in the **T**hymus
∴ called **T lymphocytes**

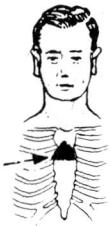

25%

70%

of
lymphocytes in the blood

The introduction of an antigen results in activation and proliferation of these two lymphocyte populations. This activity takes place in the lymphoid tissues.

'Resting' B cell **ANTIGENIC STIMULATION** 'Resting' T cell

Antigen

Activation

Transformation

Enlargement

Division
(Clonal proliferation)

Maturation

In germinal centre (not in blood)

Blast cells

Memory cells

In paracortical area and blood

Blast cells

Memory cell

PLASMA CELLS

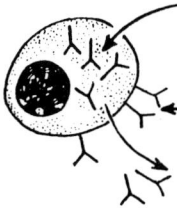

(i) Synthesis of specific antibody (Ig) within the cell

(ii) Cell surface Ig

(iii) Secretion of Ig into tissue fluids and blood.

The end result of the B cell response is the formation of humoral antibodies or
HUMORAL IMMUNITY
— protection against extracellular infection.

SPECIFICALLY SENSITISED LYMPHOCYTES

(i) Cytotoxic activity.
(ii) Production of messenger mediators (cytokines).

The end result of the T cell response is the formation of
CELL-MEDIATED IMMUNITY
— protection against intracellular organisms e.g. viruses and some bacteria (e.g. T.B.).

GENETIC INFLUENCES ON THE IMMUNE RESPONSE

The HUMAN LEUCOCYTE ANTIGEN (HLA) system, also known as the major histocompatibility complex (MHC), has an important role in the IMMUNE RESPONSE and DISEASE.

The genes controlling the system are in 2 major groups (Class I and Class II) on CHROMOSOME 6: each group has 3 genes which are highly polymorphic (i.e. show great variation within individual members of the same animal species). The multiple alleles of each gene encode for surface membrane glycoproteins.

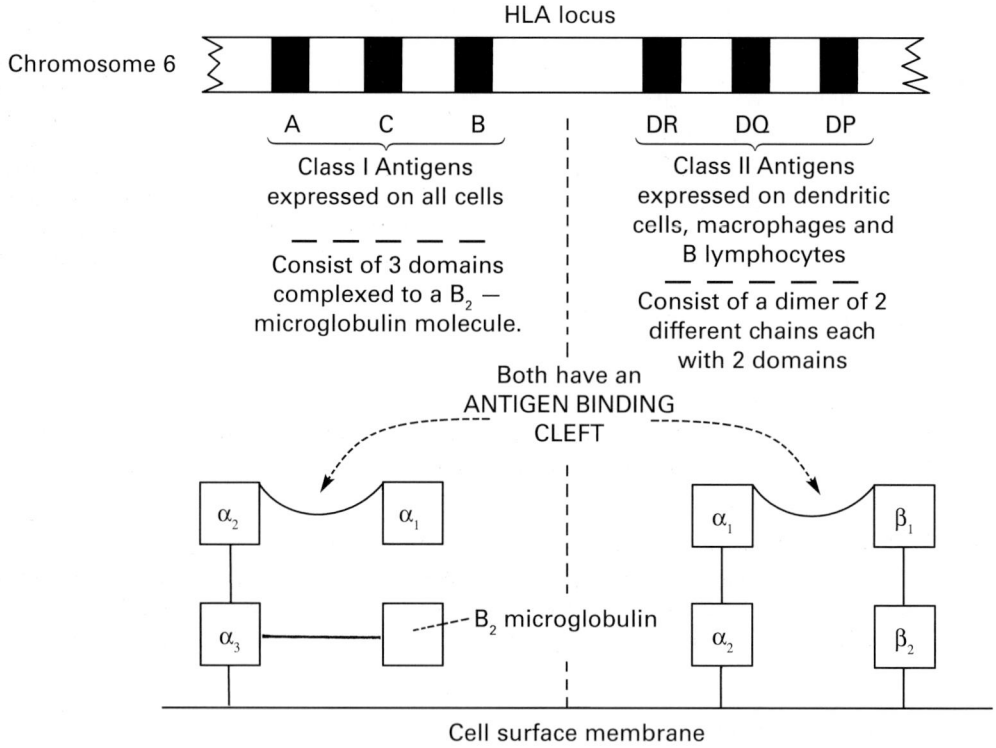

The important roles of HLA are:

(i) Presentation of peptides from foreign antigens to T lymphocytes
(Class I antigens to CD8 T cells,
Class II antigens to CD4 T cells).

(ii) They are the main stimulus to **graft rejection** in incompatible hosts. (The better the HLA match, the better the chance of graft survival.

(iii) There is a strong association with diseases — especially **auto-immune** disorders (page 108).
The most striking example is **ankylosing spondylitis** where >90% of patients carry the allele HLA B27.

CELL-MEDIATED IMMUNITY

Activation of T cells requires the involvement of ANTIGEN PRESENTING CELLS. Within these cells, foreign antigen is proteolytically digested to short peptides and then presented with HLA molecules to the T cell which possesses a specific receptor for that antigen.

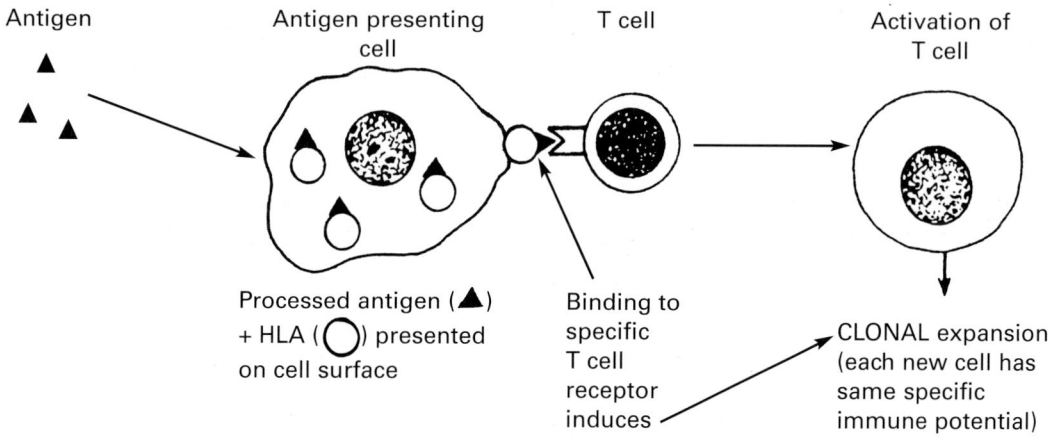

This cell mediated immunity (CMI) takes several days to develop.

TYPES of CELL

Two groups of T cells are recognised

(a) $CD4^+$ (helper) T cells react with antigens complexed to Class II MHC molecules.

(b) $CD8^+$ T cells react with antigens complexed to Class I MHC molecules.

T CELL ACTIVITIES

(a) **Regulation of immune response** — mainly by $CD4^+$ cells.

(b) **Delayed type hypersensitivity reactions** — mediated by cytokines (p. 94) released by $CD4^+$ T cells. Activation of other components of the immune system follows.

(c) **Specific lysis of cells** infected by virus, or of tumour cells — by $CD8^+$ T cells.

The following diagrams summarise these mechanisms.

(1) **Influence on B cells**

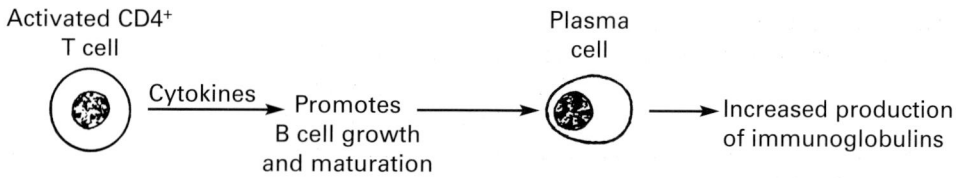

T-CELL ACTIVITIES

T CELL ACTIVITIES (continued)

(2) **Influence on other T cells**

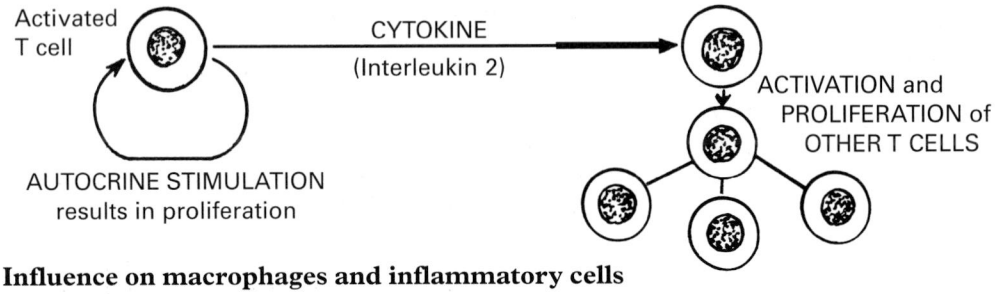

(3) **Influence on macrophages and inflammatory cells**

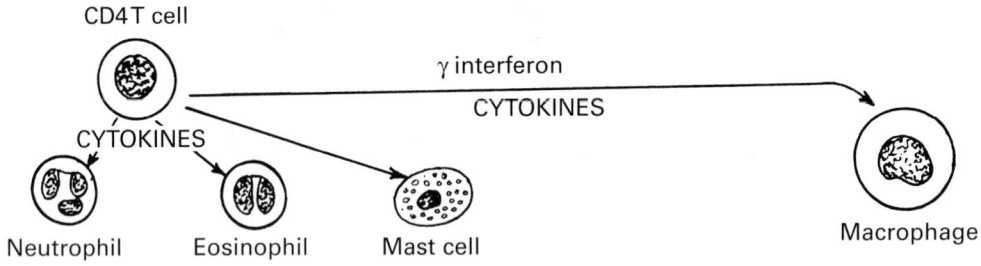

(4) **Cytotoxic activity against infected tissue cells**

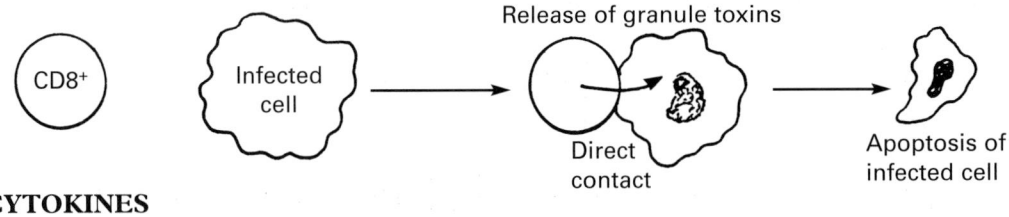

CYTOKINES

Immune reactions and inflammatory processes are interlinked. A list of the many chemical mediators is given on page 38.

CYTOKINES are a group of molecules released by T lymphocytes and other immune cells: they act as intercellular messengers with both stimulating and inhibiting effects. The group includes the INTERLEUKINS (IL), INTERFERONS and tumour necrosis factors. The diagram is a simplification of complex relationships.

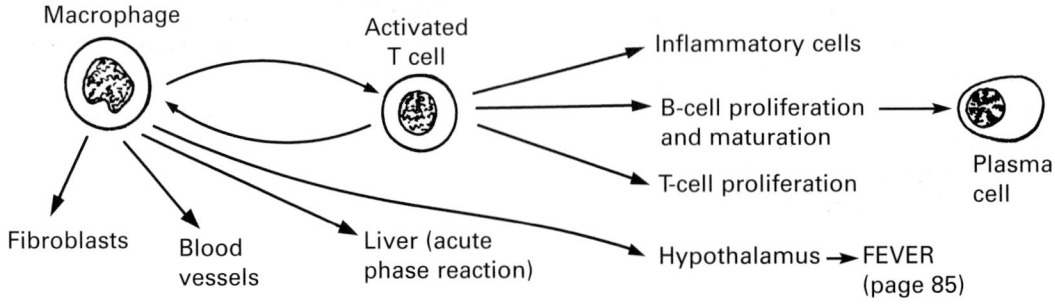

HUMORAL IMMUNITY – IMMUNOGLOBULINS (Ig)

The basic immunoglobulin is a protein molecule consisting of 2 pairs of polypeptide chains arranged in a particular way.

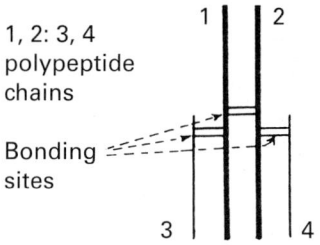

1 and 2 are **HEAVY** chains.
Differences in structure allow separation of five main Ig classes — IgG;A;M;D;E.

3 and 4 are **LIGHT** chains.
They exist in 2 forms — Kappa (κ) and Lambda (λ).
In any one molecule both chains are either κ or λ.

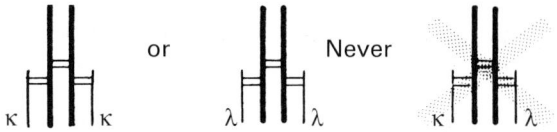

Note that the molecule has a hinge region which allows a better fit with the antigen surface and explains the symbols commonly used for Ig (,)

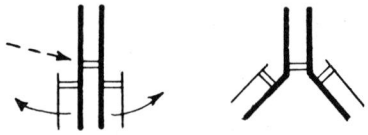

Enzymatic digestion (papain) splits the molecule into named fragments.

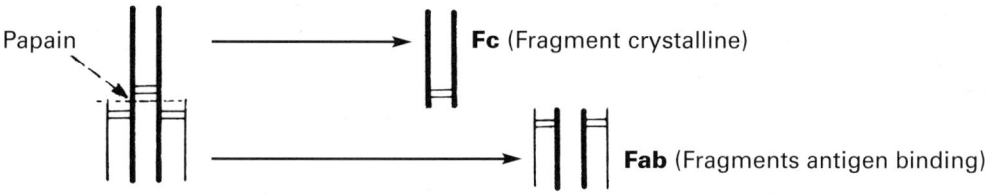

Fc is the *constant* part of the molecule and does not participate in antigen binding.

However, the Fc fragment is associated with secondary effects after binding has occurred, e.g. complement activation; attraction of inflammatory cells (chemotaxis) and particularly the facilitation of phagocytosis by macrophages which carry Fc receptors (opsonisation) (see p. 96).

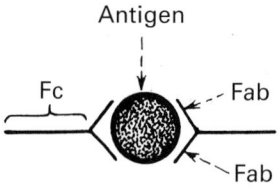

Fab are the *variable* parts of the molecule and are the site of antigen binding, the variation in amino acid content allowing a wide range of specific activity.

IMMUNOGLOBULINS

MAIN GROUPS

These groups are named according to the composition of the heavy chains.

IgM

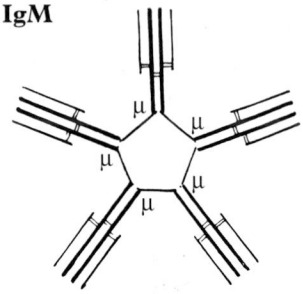

IgM (heavy chain = μ) is a polymer, joined by J chains, of five identical Ig molecules, therefore called macroglobulin. Although in low concentration in the blood, 0.5-2 mg/ml, it is the main Ig on the surface of B lymphocytes (before conversion to plasma cells) and is active in the early phase of the immune response. It neutralises viruses. In combination with complement, it is actively bactericidal and is especially effective in bacteraemia.
Note: The numerous (10) antigen-binding sites increase its efficiency.

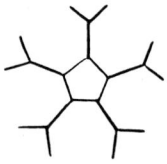

The natural blood group antibodies, anti-A and anti-B are M globulins.

IgG

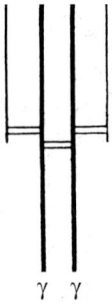

IgG (heavy chain = γ) is a single molecule with two antigen binding sites.

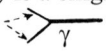

It is produced mainly in **secondary response**. IgG has the highest concentration of immunoglobulins in the blood — within a range of 8–16 mg/ml. Of its several activities, the important ones are:

(1) **Neutralisation of virus and toxins**

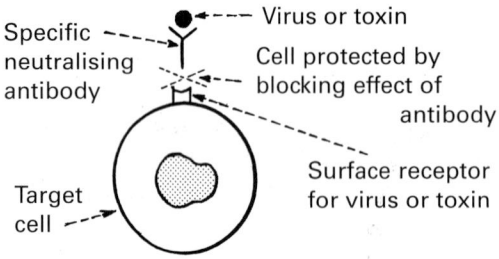

(2) **Opsonisation**

Specific antibodies attach bacteria to the cell surface by their Fc component and induce phagocytosis.

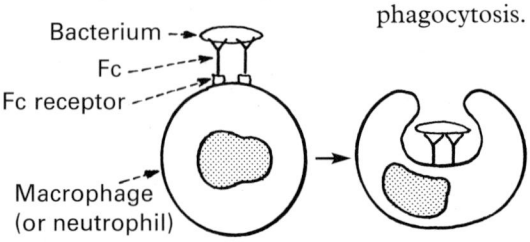

'Passive' transfer of IgG from mother to baby occurs via the placenta and colostrum. The immunity only lasts for a few months.

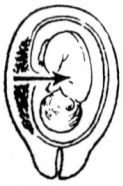

Transplacental passage of IgG

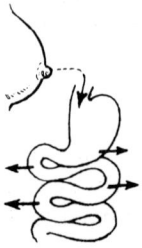

Colostrum, rich in IgG, absorbed from alimentary tract into the blood stream of the neonate.

IMMUNOGLOBULINS

IgA

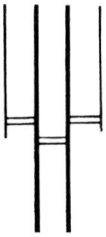

IgA (heavy chain = α) occurs in the blood (1.5–4 mg/ml) where its function is unknown.

It is the predominant immunoglobulin in secretions of eyes, nose, mouth, bronchi and gut. Its function is to protect mucous surfaces from antigenic attack and prevent access of foreign substances to the circulation and general immune system. It may neutralise toxins and prevent binding to mucous surfaces. IgA is a single molecule in the serum.

The diagram illustrates the local production of IgA in the gut.

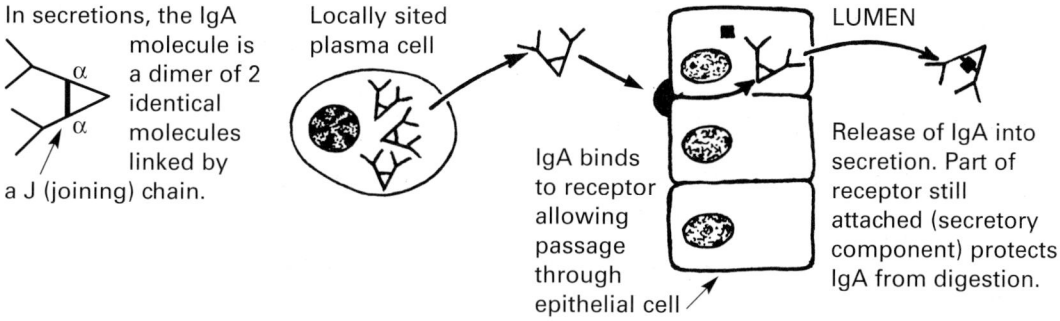

IgD (heavy chain Δ) of uncertain function: concentration in blood very low. Like IgM it is present on the surface of B lymphocytes prior to transformation.

IgE (heavy chain ε) — a single molecule similar to IgG and IgA.
It is sometimes called REAGIN: concentration in blood is low (20-500 ng/ml).
The serum level is raised in worm infestation and is probably protective.
Its main activity is mediated by MAST CELLS (or BASOPHILS); it is the principal mediator of atopic and anaphylactic disease.

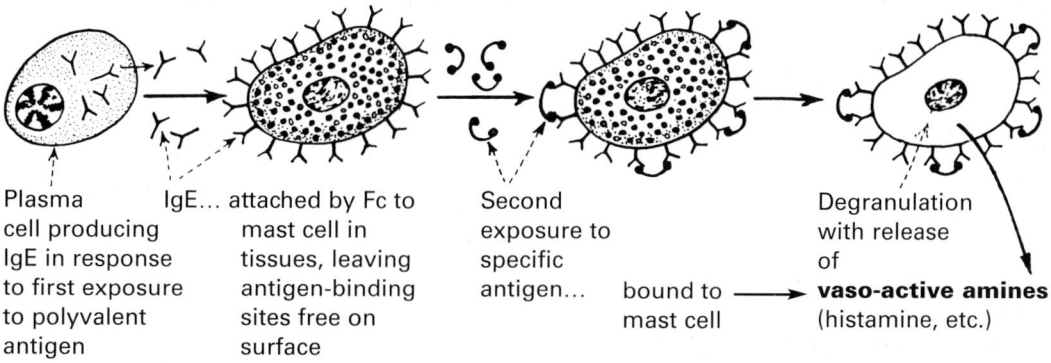

The range of antibodies is immense. B cells produce this vast number by rearranging the genes from the immunoglobulin light and heavy chains. The appropriate clone of plasma cells is stimulated by binding of antigen to the cell surface receptor (so-called clonal selection).

IMMUNE REACTIONS

ANTIBODY ANTIGEN COMPLEXES

When an antigen (Ag) binds with an antibody (Ab) an Ag/Ab complex is formed: this reaction is reversible in varying degree (Ag + Ab $\rightleftharpoons$ Ag/Ab)

The forces of attraction between Ag and Ab are increased by a 'good fit' between the determinants on the antigen surface and the antibody binding site.

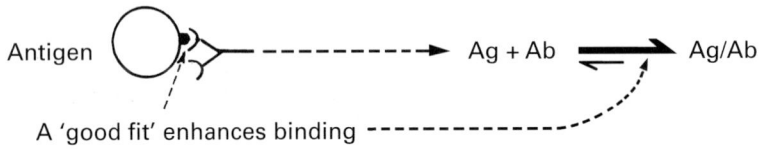

The consequences of Ag/Ab combination include:

1. PRECIPITATION

A soluble antigen is rendered insoluble by aggregation of the Ag/Ab complexes into a lattice.

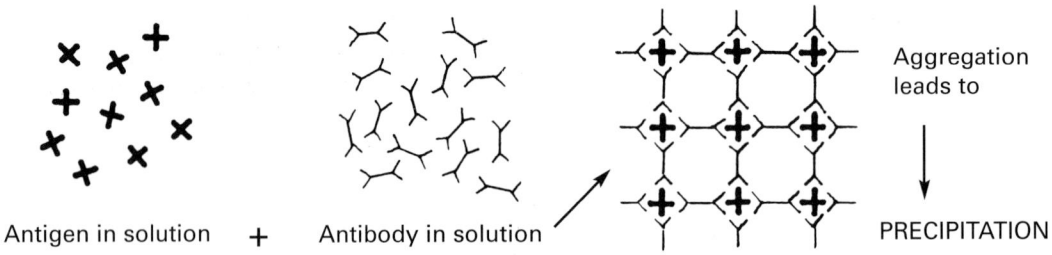

2. AGGLUTINATION

Particulate antigen, e.g. bacteria and red blood cells, are aggregated in the same way as in the precipitation reaction and the process is called AGGLUTINATION.

3. ANTI-TOXIC Effect

The Ag/Ab combination neutralises the toxic activity.

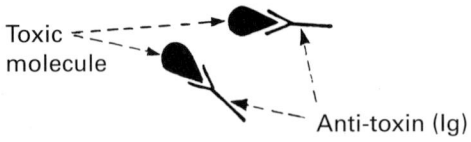

(see also page 96)

4. ENHANCEMENT of the non-specific defence mechanisms

(a) **Phagocytic activity** (Opsonisation) (See page 96 for details.)
Antibodies with this property are called **opsonins.**

(b) **Complement activation** (See next page for details of the mechanism.) The ultimate objective is to enhance the immune reaction by killing micro-organisms, by improving phagocytosis and mediating the inflammatory response.

IMMUNE REACTIONS

COMPLEMENT SYSTEM

Complement consists of nine main protein components present in inactive form in the blood.

The Fc part of the Ag/Ab complex binds to the first component, C1, and activates the cascade as follows:

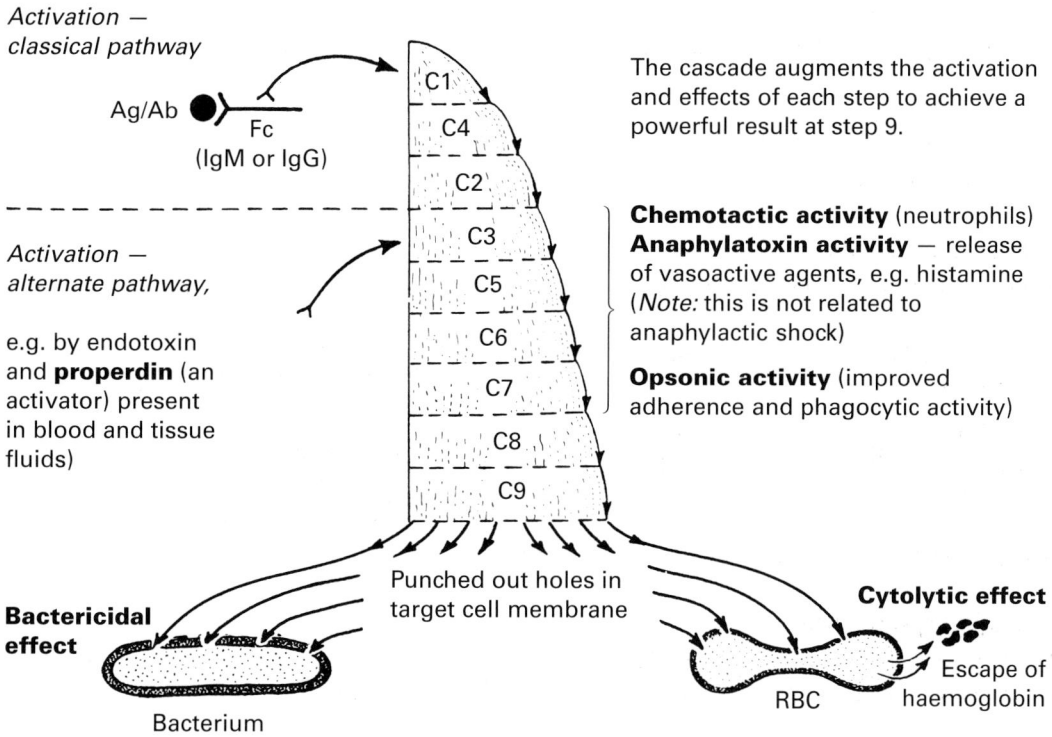

Activation of C by Ag/Ab complex is called **fixation of complement**. Using red cells as markers, this fixation can detect the presence of antigen or antibody in serum.

E.g. Test serum + antigen + C.
If serum contains antibody, C is fixed, otherwise it remains free.
Add sensitised RBC (coated with Ab).
Lysis of RBC ≡ complement still free ∴ no Ab in original serum.
No lysis = C was fixed by Ab in test serum.

MONONUCLEAR PHAGOCYTE SYSTEM

The cells of this system have important roles in many disease processes and appear throughout the book. Although their main functions are essentially *non-specific*, they have important roles in the immune response, particularly in cooperation with T lymphocytes. Found at many sites throughout the body, they are derived from

STEM CELLS in the bone marrow.

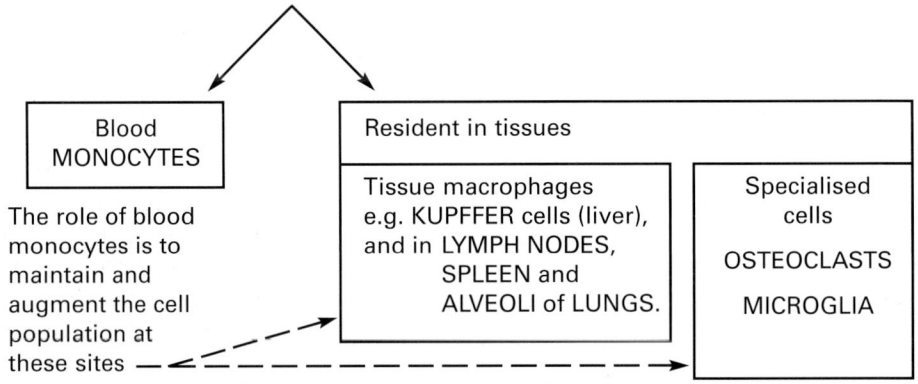

Historically, cells with varying degrees of phagocytic activity recognised at many of these sites were grouped into the **RETICULOENDOTHELIAL** system, but since reticulum cells are still ill-defined and endothelial cells have little phagocytic function the term is inappropriate and (although still used by some) has become obsolete.

Main functions

(1) PHAGOCYTOSIS — INFLAMMATION with indigestible antigen + immune response develop granulomatous reactions (page 43) ⇌ IMMUNE RESPONSE

Macrophage (non-specific effector cell) → Cytokines e.g. IL-1 → T lymphocyte → Cytokines e.g. IFN-γ → Macrophage

— STORAGE and METABOLIC PROCESSING e.g. iron and lipid metabolism

(2) SYNTHESIS of substances, e.g. complement components, interferon, proteolytic enzymes, pyrogens and growth factors.

(3) PRESENTATION of ANTIGEN by dendritic cells and activated macrophages.

The System in Disease

Primary disorders of the system are rare. Participation in many disease processes is well recognised and detailed mechanisms are being elucidated.

TOLERANCE

Humoral and cell-mediated immunity are specific active immune responses with a protective function.

In certain circumstances an antigen does not evoke these active responses. This is because the lymphocytes, although recognising the antigen, do not react — this is TOLERANCE.

Natural 'self' tolerance

The immune system recognises and tolerates its own tissues.

This tolerance is developed in the fetal and early neonatal periods, and prevents autoimmune diseases in normal individuals.

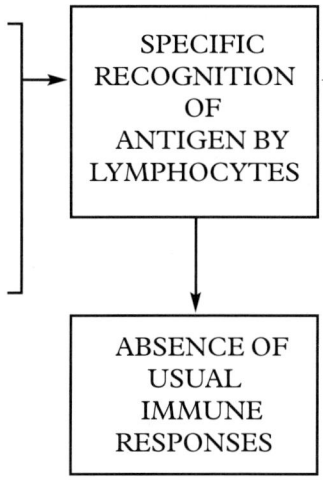

Acquired tolerance

After the neonatal period and throughout adult life, injections of soluble foreign antigens by selected routes (e.g. I.V.: mucosal) may induce tolerance in the adult.

This form of tolerance is the basis of desensitisation treatment in allergic disease and explains the absence of e.g. food hypersensitivity in normal individuals.

The mechanisms of inducing tolerance are not yet completely understood: main candidates are:

(1) **Clonal deletion** — in fetal life all lymphoid cells which recognise 'self' antigens are permanently eliminated by apoptosis. This mainly affects T cells and occurs in the **thymus**.

(2) **Clonal anergy** — T and B cells which recognise 'self' antigens in the periphery during development are 'switched off' but remain present in the body. This occurs during development and in adult life.

(3) **Active suppression** — under certain circumstances, contact with antigen stimulates lymphocytes which **suppress** other components of the immune system.

Tolerance is an important protective mechanism. When it breaks down, the serious effects give rise to **autoimmune disease** (see page 108).

IMMUNOPATHOLOGY

The complicated and delicately balanced immune mechanisms clearly have been developed to protect against antigens, particularly infections. When these immune reactions are upset, the protective mechanism can itself be a source of disease states.

There are three main categories: (1) hypersensitivity states, (2) immune deficiency states and (3) autoimmune diseases.

HYPERSENSITIVITY REACTIONS

Basically these consist of an exaggerated response by an individual to an antigen, following a previous exposure. Depending on the main type of immune response concerned, these are classified as follows:

(a) Those associated with *HUMORAL ANTIBODIES*
∴ immediate — types I, II, III

(b) Those associated with *CELL-MEDIATED IMMUNITY*
∴ delayed (24-72 hours) — type IV.

This classification is to some extent artificial. Hypersensitivity may start as an immediate humoral reaction but end in a mixed state with both humoral and cell-mediated activities.

Type 1 Anaphylaxis, atopy, allergy

This occurs within 20-60 minutes of exposure to antigen and is often referred to as 'immediate type hypersensitivity'.

All 3 terms have been used for this reaction. The basic mechanism is as follows.

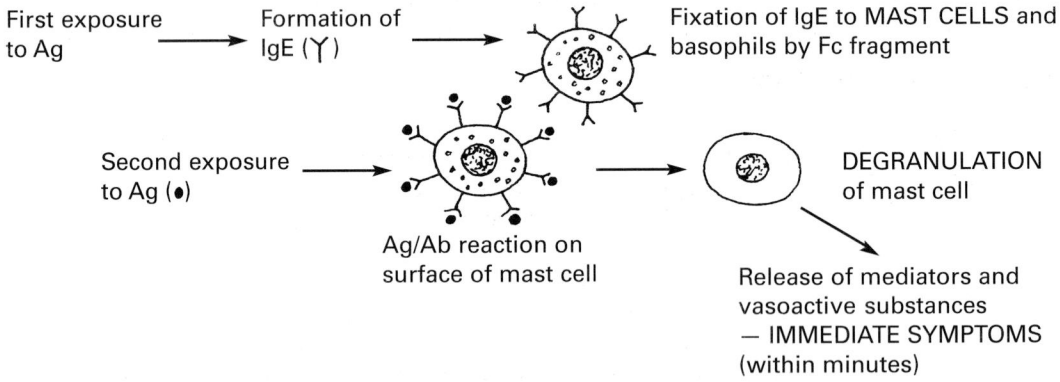

Antigens and 'allergens'

The most potent allergens are usually large molecules with molecular weights up to 40,000. Examples of common 'allergens' are pollen, house mite dust, cat fur and penicillin. Food allergy, e.g. to peanuts and milk, is uncommon.

Antibody

This is IgE. Plasma cells forming IgE are not normally found in the internal secretory surfaces of the body — tonsils, bronchi, gastrointestinal tract — but are present in large numbers in cases of allergy.

HYPERSENSITIVITY STATES

Mast cells

These have a wide distribution but are prominent in the same areas as the IgE-producing plasma cells, plus skin, bladder and synovial membranes. This explains the frequently used term 'target organs' when discussing hypersensitivity.

Clinical examples of Type I reaction

ANAPHYLACTIC SHOCK

1st injection of antigen e.g. penicillin or a bee sting → General sensitisation

— — — — — — — — — —

2nd injection of above → Acute collapse: bronchial constriction; vomiting; diarrhoea; perhaps a skin rash. May be fatal. Note that the antigens are injected — enter blood stream → basophils affected → widespread reaction

HAY FEVER

1st contact with grass pollen → Local sensitisation of conjunctiva and nasal passages

— — — — — — — — —

2nd contact with above → Irritation or swelling of conjunctiva with excessive watery secretion

ASTHMA

1st contact with house mite dust or animal dander → Local sensitisation of bronchi

— — — — — — — — —

2nd contact with above → Bronchial constriction and secretion of thick mucus cause dyspnoea (difficult breathing)

Chronic asthma may involve cell-mediated immunity with tissue destruction.

Eosinophils are a common finding in the tissues of patients with allergies. Allergic conditions are often familial with a genetic basis.

Type II — Cytotoxic type

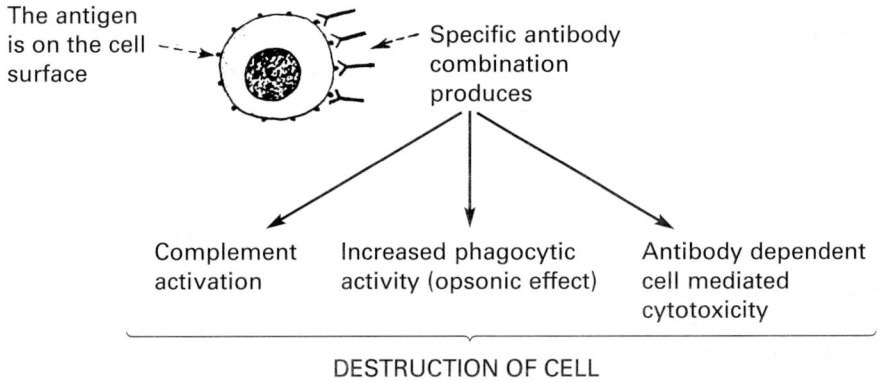

This cytotoxic reaction causes some forms of haemolytic anaemia [e.g. autoimmune HA (p. 406): Rhesus incompatibility (p. 407)] and some blood transfusion reactions.

In some auto-immune disorders antibodies of this type are directed against specialised cell surface receptors, e.g. Graves' disease or myasthenia gravis (see p. 110).

HYPERSENSITIVITY STATES

Type III — Immune complex (Arthus) type

The reaction is due to the consequences of specific direct antigen/antibody combination — particularly complement activation (p. 99) and platelet aggregation. The antibodies involved are IgG or IgM.

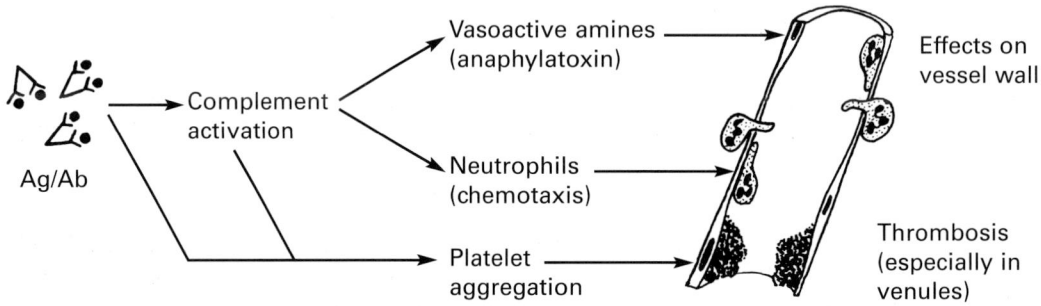

In most cases where there is Ag/Ab reaction, the immune complexes are removed from the circulation and hypersensitivity does not develop. In type III hypersensitivity, the Ag/Ab complexes aggregate in small vessels (e.g. renal glomeruli) and complement activation causes tissue damage. Serum sickness is a generalised form of this type of reaction. Type III hypersensitivity is also important as a cause of the tissue damage seen in systemic lupus erythematosis (SLE), see page 643.

Type IV — Cell mediated (delayed) type

This reaction is usually localised and is due to the activities of specifically sensitised T cells and activated macrophages. These reactions are often referred to as delayed type hypersensitivity (DTH) because they develop slowly over 24-72 hours. The classical example is the tubercle follicle; it is also concerned in other granulomatous diseases, the rejection of grafts and several autoimmune diseases (rheumatoid arthritis, diabetes mellitus and inflammatory bowel diseases).

The skin reaction to chemicals — **contact dermatitis** — is illustrative. This condition is now common due to the increasing use of chemicals in industry and for topical application. The chemical — often of a simple nature, e.g. nickel — acts as a hapten, evoking an immune response.

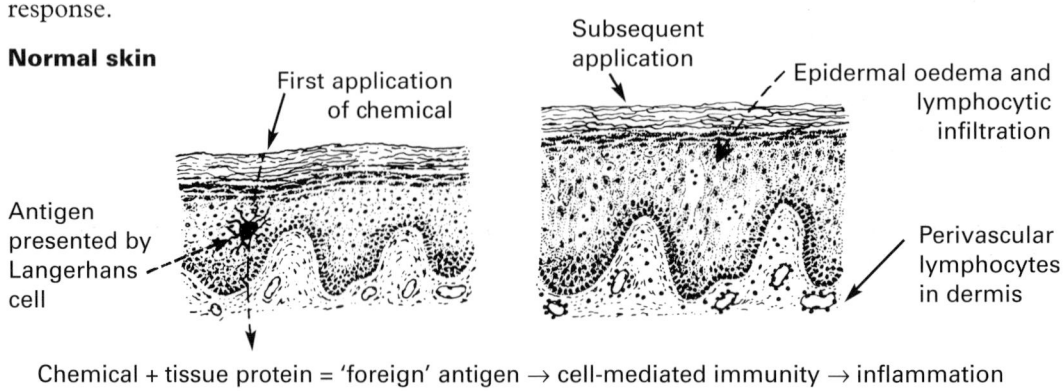

IMMUNE DEFICIENCY STATES

The systems involved are:

(1) **THE SPECIFIC SYSTEM** — humoral / cell-mediated

(2) **THE NON-SPECIFIC SYSTEM** — phagocytes / complement

Failure in any one alters the immune response. The deficiencies may be of a primary nature, commonly genetic in origin, or secondary to some other disease or circumstance. Equally, the alteration in any system may be quantitative or qualitative. In many of these deficiencies there is a failure in more than one system.

Primary (inherited) deficiencies of the specific system are rare. They include B cell, T cell and combined B and T cell deficits. B cell deficiency leads to infection by pyogenic bacteria. T cell deficits lead to infection by viruses, fungi and intracellular bacteria.

Secondary deficiencies of the specific system are common. Usually T cell activity is affected, resulting in deficient cell-mediated immunity and, later, B cell deficit occurs.

The acquired immunodeficiency syndrome (AIDS) is now a major world-wide public health problem. Other predisposing conditions and diseases include:

Malnutrition –
particularly with protein deficiency

Iatrogenic effects –
e.g. immunosuppressors: cytotoxics
corticosteroids

Infections –
acute viral
chronic bacterial
chronic protozoal, e.g. malaria

Chronic debilitating disease –
e.g. renal failure: diabetes mellitus

Malignant disease –
e.g. advanced cancer: lymphoma
Hodgkin's disease

→ IMPAIRED IMMUNITY → INFECTION often OPPORTUNISTIC (see p. 84)

Deficiencies of the non-specific system are rare. The disorders of neutrophil function are described on page 424.

IMMUNE DEFICIENCY STATES — AIDS

The acquired immune deficiency syndrome (AIDS) is a world-wide epidemic with large numbers of cases in sub-Saharan Africa and South East Asia. Globally, at least 20 million people are infected with the virus and at least 3 million have died.

The virus [human immunodeficiency virus (HIV)] is of the retrovirus group: it infects and destroys CD4 T-lymphocytes (macrophages are also infected).

The disease is slowly progressive and is usually ultimately fatal. Antiviral drugs, e.g. azidothymidine (AZT) and protease inhibitors may prolong survival. Progress is monitored by measuring the CD4 lymphocyte count and the viral count.

Infection	**Latent period**	**AIDS**
CD4 > 500 × 10^6. A symptomatic or a short febrile illness. Although the patient's cells contain HIV, tests for antibodies may be negative for up to several months.	CD4 — 200–500 × 10^6. Virus present in lymphocytes: may be persistent lymph node enlargement and fever.	CD4 < 200 × 10^6. Infections and tumours Infection — opportunistic, others Tumours — Kaposi sarcoma, lymphomas

The whole range of opportunistic infection (see p. 84), including disseminated virus infection (e.g. herpes simplex and cytomegalovirus), occurs.

The diagram shows the more common AIDS-associated diseases and sites:

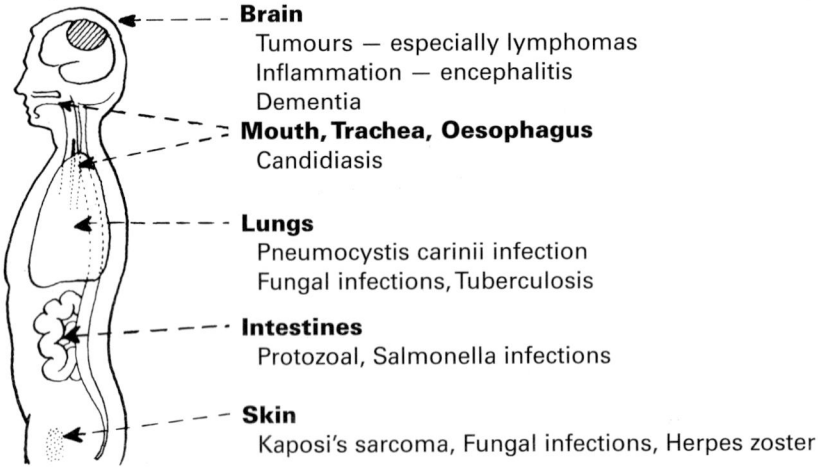

Blood Changes

Antibodies — Specific antibodies appear up to 6 months after infection and form the basis of the diagnostic test for HIV. The antibody titre may fall greatly late in the disease.

Immunoglobulins are usually elevated in the early stages.

CD4 lymphocytes are severely reduced, producing a lymphopenia.

IMMUNE DEFICIENCY STATES – AIDS

EPIDEMIOLOGY AND TRANSMISSION

Although the virus may be present in many body fluids and secretions, transmission is by the parenteral route, usually by (1) **sexual contact** or (2) **injection of blood** or **blood products**.

Transmission does not occur with normal social contact and there is a very low risk to medical or nursing personnel using normal procedures.

1. ***Sexual transmission***

(a) MALE HOMOSEXUAL PRACTICE: HIV in seminal fluid → via anorectal abrasion to passive partner.

(b) HETEROSEXUAL TRANSMISSION is less common except where there is a high prevalence in prostitutes and also in Africa.

Female to male — infectious genital secretions and blood → via penis to male (risk increased in uncircumcised).

Male to female — infectious seminal fluid and blood → to female cervix uteri and vagina.

In both sexes the risks are very considerably increased where there is genital ulceration or abrasion.

2. ***Transmission by blood***

The risk from blood transfusion and blood products has now been virtually eliminated by screening and sterilisation procedures (in the past many haemophiliacs were infected). The communal use of contaminated syringes and needles continues to be important among drug addicts.

Cellular mechanisms

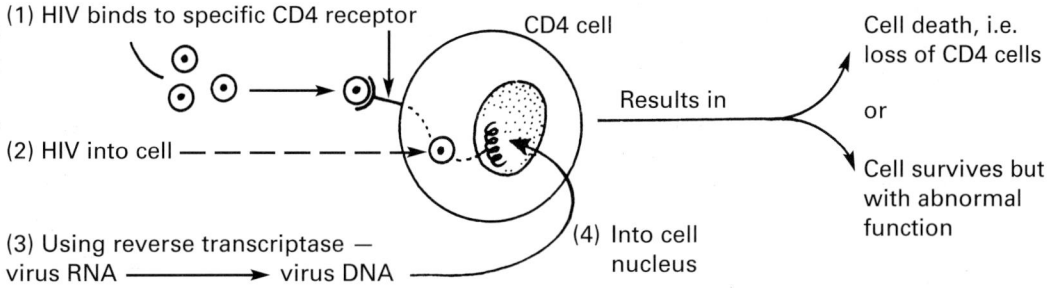

CD4 cell deficiency → During latent phase B cells may be stimulated, allowing antibody formation and lymph node enlargement.

CD4 cell deficiency → Gradual failure of immune effector mechanisms.

AUTOIMMUNE DISEASES

Autoimmune diseases result from, or are associated with, an immune response against the individual's own cells, or in some cases cell products. Although both humoral and cell mediated immunity are involved, it is thought that changes in the latter are of primary importance.

Aetiology

The aetiology of autoimmune diseases is not established, but clues to their genesis are available.

An increased FAMILIAL incidence of autoimmune diseases in general and of particular individual diseases

The overlapping of the incidence of antibodies and of the types of damage produced

suggest

an INBORN INSTABILITY OF IMMUNE TOLERANCE
particularly associated with inheritance of specific class II HLA antigens

The reasons for the breakdown of tolerance involve:

1. Antigenic abnormality and 2. Dysregulation of the immune response (particularly T cell activity).

(1) **Antigenic abnormality**

(a) Cell surface antigens modified by drugs or chemicals.
(b) Cell antigens modified by proteolysis associated with disease processes, particularly inflammation, when 'new' antigens are formed.
(c) Microbial cross-reacting antigens.

(2) **Immune dysregulation**

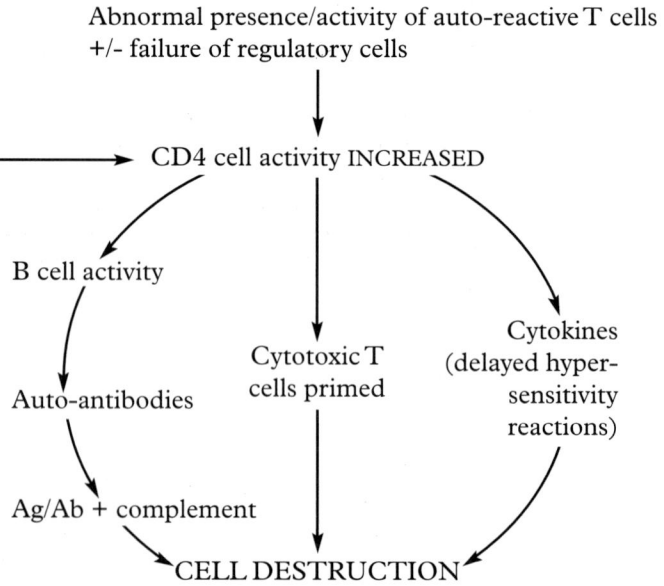

AUTOIMMUNE DISEASES

ORGAN-SPECIFIC

Antibody or cell mediated reaction to	Target Organ	Associated Diseases
(a) Thyroid cells and hormones, or (b) TSH receptor	Thyroid	Primary myxoedema Hashimoto's disease (auto-immune thyroiditis) Thyrotoxicosis (Graves' disease)
Parietal cells Intrinsic factor Intrinsic factor/ B12 complex	Stomach	Pernicious anaemia
Red blood cells	Red blood cells	Haemolytic anaemia
Pancreatic islet beta cells	Pancreas	Type 1 diabetes
Adrenal cortical cells ACTH receptor	Adrenal	Addison's disease
Parathyroid cells	Parathyroid	Primary hypoparathyroidism
Acetylcholine receptor	Voluntary muscle	Myasthenia gravis

NON-ORGAN-SPECIFIC

Antibody to	Target Organ	Associated Diseases
Mitochondria	Liver	Primary biliary cirrhosis
Smooth muscle	Liver	Autoimmune chronic hepatitis
Nuclear constituents — e.g. DNA IgG	Skin and muscles	The connective tissue diseases Dermatomyositis Rheumatoid arthritis Systemic lupus erythematosus (SLE) Progressive systemic sclerosis
Many other body proteins	Skin, kidney endocardium, blood vessels, joints	

AUTOIMMUNE DISEASES

Primary thyrotoxicosis (Graves' disease) and myasthenia gravis are of particular interest. In these diseases specific autoimmune antibodies combine with antigen on the cell surface and either stimulate or block the action of the physiological agent which would normally turn on the activity of the cell.

Stimulatory effect

In Graves' disease, excessive amounts of thyroid hormone are produced. LATS (long acting thyroid stimulator), an IgG auto-antibody, combines with antigen on the thyroid cell surface and produces changes mimicking those produced by TSH (thyroid stimulating hormone) — physiologically manufactured by the pituitary.

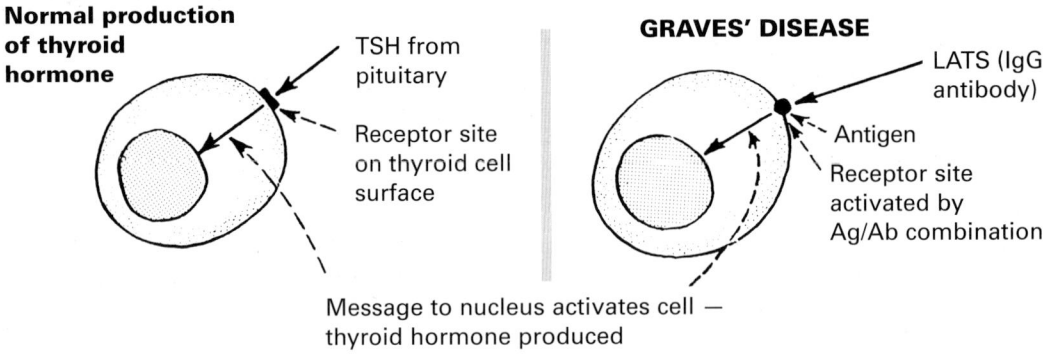

See also page 652

Blocking effect

In myasthenia gravis, the acetylcholine formed at the motor nerve endings is prevented from stimulating the muscle motor end plate due to the antibody blocking the specific acetylcholine receptors. The end plate is also damaged (Ag/Ab + complement).

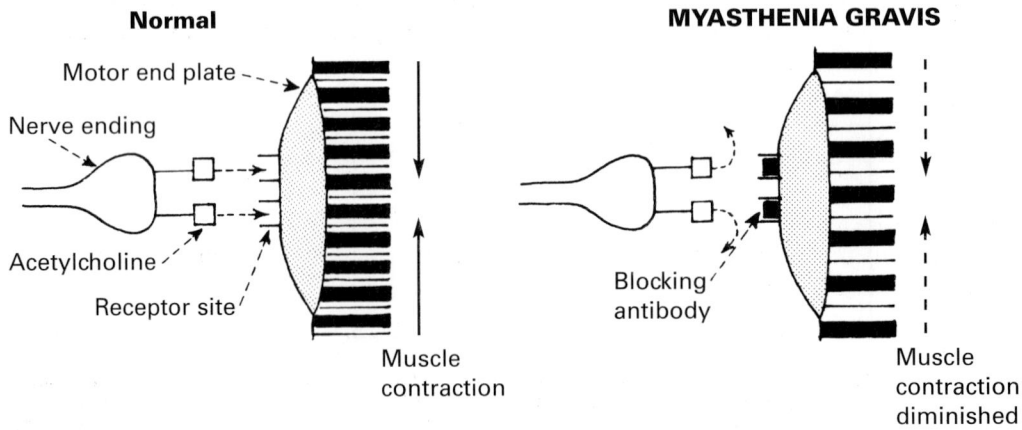

APPLIED IMMUNOLOGY

Immunohistochemical identification

Immunohistochemistry is now well established and allows identification of specific substances in histological sections.

Example:

(1) Monoclonal antibody to antigen (e.g. cytokeratin)

(2) Enzyme converts substrate to coloured reaction product

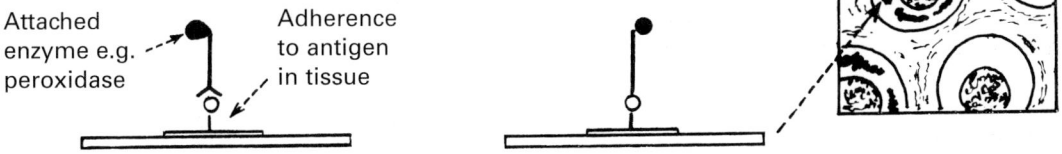

Slide containing cells with antigen.

Only cells containing cytokeratin contain coloured product e.g. Carcinoma cells.

This or similar techniques are used to identify a wide range of substances.

Flow cytometry

In this technique, cells in suspension are labelled by fluorescent markers, excited by a laser and counted electronically by passing them through a flow cytometer. This is the technique employed, among others, for monitoring $CD4^+$ counts in AIDS.

Prophylaxis and treatment of infections

1. **Passive immunisation** is the term used when antibody formed in one individual is given to another individual who is at risk of infection — the protection is temporary. Examples include:

   Pooled human γ-globulin → general protection → particularly useful in cases of immune deficiency.

2. **Active immunisation** is the term used when the infective agent is modified in some way to eliminate its harmful effects without loss of antigenicity. The subject's own immune response is activated. Examples include:

   TOXOID — e.g. tetanus toxin modified chemically.
   KILLED ORGANISMS — e.g. TAB (typhoid, paratyphoid A and B) vaccine.
   ATTENUATED ORGANISMS — e.g. viruses; cowpox, polio, measles.

Monoclonal antibodies

These are formed by immortalising a single clone of plasma cells, by fusion with myeloma cells, so that a large amount of identical antibody is produced.

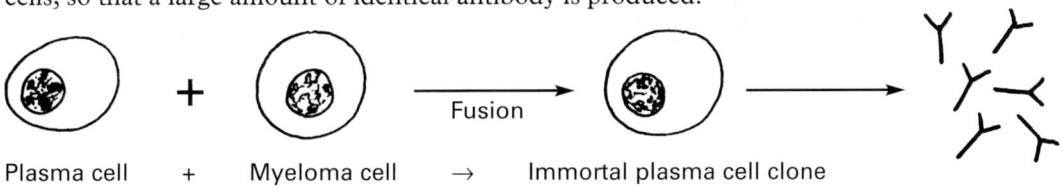

APPLIED IMMUNOLOGY – TISSUE TRANSPLANTATION

In the past, allografting (transplanting of tissues or organs from one individual to another of the same species) inevitably led to rejection of the graft by the host. Understanding of the mechanisms has allowed intervention so that nowadays successful survival of grafts is usual (e.g. 90% survival of renal transplants after 1 year).

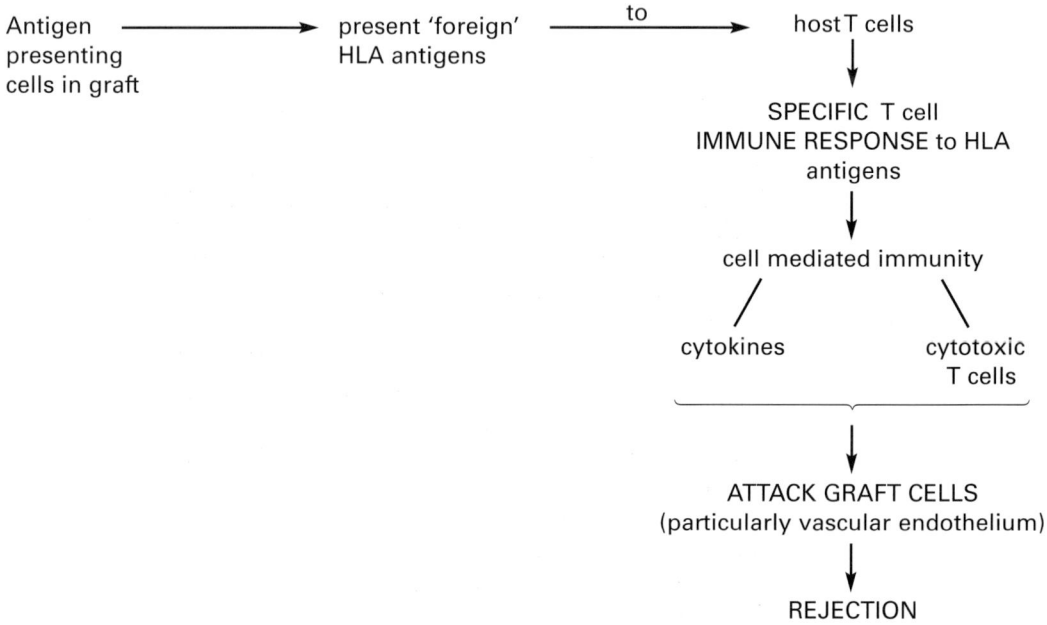

Rejection may also occur, very rapidly, if pre-existing antibodies are present (e.g. due to previous incompatible blood transfusion or pregnancy) — leading to activation of complement with haemolysis.

Usually rejection takes weeks while the cell mediated immune response is building up.

The remarkable improvement in transplant prognosis is due to:

(a) careful matching of HLA compatibility between donor and recipient,
(b) use of immuno-suppressive agents (particularly cyclosporin A),
(c) screening for the presence of pre-existing HLA and cytotoxic antibodies.

Paradoxically the pre-transplant transfusion of compatible blood improves the chances of graft survival.

GRAFT versus HOST DISEASE (GvHD)

When immunosuppressed individuals (e.g. leukaemia patients) undergo bone marrow transplantation, T cells from the graft proliferate in the recipient (host) and establish an immune response against the host tissues: the main target organs are the skin, the liver and the alimentary tract.

CHAPTER 6

NEOPLASIA

Neoplasia 114
Non-Neoplastic Proliferation 115
Neoplastic Proliferation 116
Neoplasms — Classification 117
Benign Tumours — Histology 118
Malignant Tumours — Histology 119
Benign Epithelial Tumours 120–122
Benign Connective Tissue Tumours 123, 124
Malignant Epithelial Tumours 125
Types of Carcinoma 126, 127
Malignant Connective Tissue Tumours 128
Sarcomas 129, 130
Other Tumour Types 131–134
Spread of Tumours 135
Lymphatic Spread 136, 137
Blood Spread 138, 139
Other Modes of Spread of Tumours 140
Effects of Tumours 141
Tumour Markers 142
Pre-Malignancy 143
Carcinoma in situ (Intraepithelial Neoplasia) 144
Carcinogenesis 145–148
Carcinogenesis — Viruses 149
Carcinogenesis — Heredity 150
Oncogenesis and Tumour Suppressor Genes 151
Oncogenes 152
Tumour Suppressor Genes 153
Carcinogenesis — Summary 154

NEOPLASIA

Cancer as a cause of death in the Western world (25%) is second only to heart disease. Knowledge of non-neoplastic proliferation is helpful in understanding neoplasia.

Physiological proliferation occurs

1. in somatic growth during fetal development → throughout CHILDHOOD → gradually diminishing → till ADULT MATURITY

   'explosive'

2. in tissues where constant proliferation is needed in RAPID CELL TURNOVER e.g. in
   (a) bone marrow (b) gut epithelium (c) skin

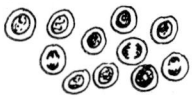

Constant supply of cells to blood

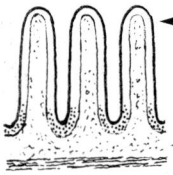

Cell loss on surface

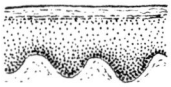

Proliferation at base

3. Proliferation at a much slower rate occurs in tissues where cell turnover is low e.g. LIVER, but will increase rapidly following injury.

Pathological proliferation is seen especially following tissue damage.

ENLARGEMENT of an organ due to increase in the parenchymal cell mass may be due to:
(1) an increase in the size and functional capacity of the individual cells — **hypertrophy**
or (2) an increase in the number of cells — **hyperplasia**
or (3) commonly a combination of (1) and (2).

The stimuli responsible are: (a) increase in functional demand
(b) increased trophic hormonal activity.

Physiological enlargement of organs is common and well illustrated by the increase in muscle bulk consequent upon training and the enlargement of uterus and breasts in pregnancy.

Pathological enlargement is the result of disease processes.

HYPERTROPHY (pathological)

Enlargement of the heart as a result of hypertension is a good example of hypertrophy: the result of the increased functional demands to maintain the high blood pressure is an increase in the size of the myocardial cells.

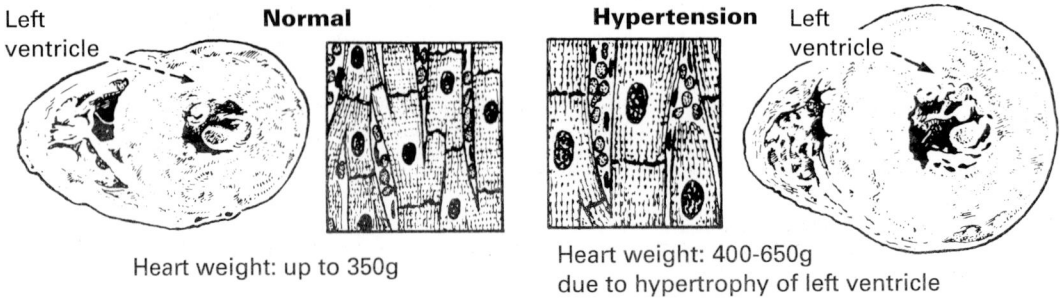

Heart weight: up to 350g

Heart weight: 400-650g due to hypertrophy of left ventricle

N.B. The process of hypertrophy *per se* does not involve proliferation, but there is often co-existent hyperplasia.

NON-NEOPLASTIC PROLIFERATION

HYPERPLASIA (pathological)

The two main causes are:

(a) *Chronic irritation* (and inflammation) e.g. in the skin, increased thickness results.

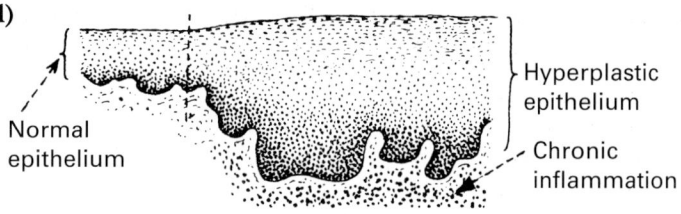

(b) *Imbalance of hormonal activity*, e.g. the irregular enlargement of the prostate in old age is due to hyperplasia of the component tissues.

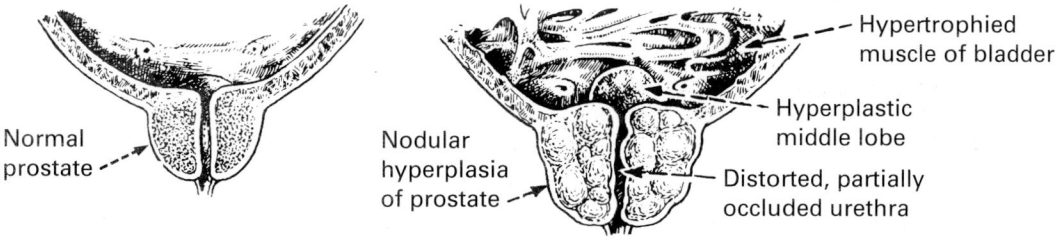

Note: If the abnormal stimulus is removed, the affected organ can return to normal.

METAPLASIA

This is a change from one type of differentiated tissue to another, usually of the same broad class but often less well specialised. The change is commonly seen in lining epithelia but occurs also in connective tissues and lining of serous cavities. There is frequently an associated hyperplasia.

e.g. (a) Change from mucus-secreting epithelium to stratified squamous epithelium as in the bronchial irritation associated with smoking.

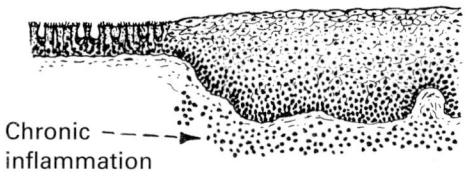

(b) Formation of bone in fibrous tissue — sometimes in healing process, e.g. prostatectomy scars.

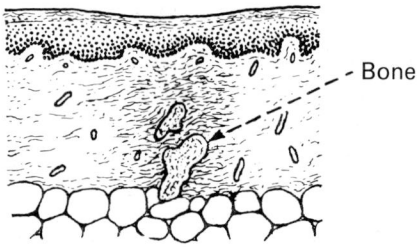

In some cases metaplasia is associated with chronic irritation, but the intimate causes are unknown in most instances. Lack of vitamin A however results in widespread squamous metaplasia of respiratory and salivary epithelium.

DYSPLASIA

This term refers to disordered growth which is frequently the precursor of malignancy. It is described on page 144.

NEOPLASTIC PROLIFERATION

A tumour is a proliferation of cells which persists after the stimulus which initiated it has been withdrawn. It is:

1. **Progressive**

e.g. Tumour of bone

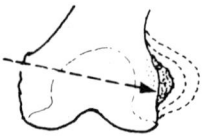

2. **Purposeless** e.g. Tumour of fibrous tissue

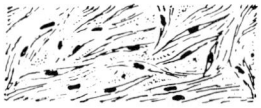

The fibres of a tumour of fibrous tissue have no regular arrangement and serve no useful purpose.

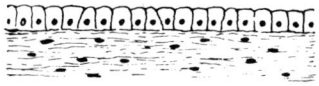

In normal fibrous tissue, the strands have a definite arrangement, supporting some structure such as an epithelial surface.

NB Individual cells of a tumour may exhibit function — the fibroblasts form collagen — but it has no purpose.

3. **Regardless of surrounding tissue,**

e.g. Smooth muscle tumour of uterus compresses normal tissues and distorts uterine cavity

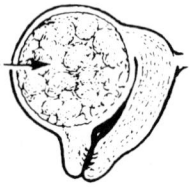

4. **Not related to needs of the body,**

e.g. Certain tumours of bone-marrow cells produce, needlessly, enormous numbers of leucocytes which enter the blood stream

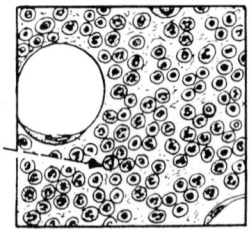

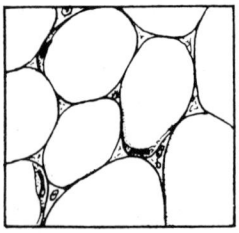

Normal

5. **Parasitic**

The tumour draws its nourishment from the body while contributing nothing to its function. It induces the body to provide a blood supply and, in the case of epithelial tumours, a supporting stroma.

Since the development of a neoplasm is independent of the normal processes in the body it is *autonomous* although its growth may to some extent be influenced by these prosesses.

NEOPLASMS – CLASSIFICATION

Tumours may be classified in two ways: (1) clinical and (2) histological origin.

1. **CLINICAL**

The tumour is classified according to its morbid anatomy and behaviour. Two main groups are recognised — *benign* (simple) and *malignant*. The contrast between these two groups is as follows:-

	BENIGN	**MALIGNANT**
Spread (the most important feature)	Remains localised	Cells transferred via lymphatics, blood vessels, tissue planes and serous cavities to set up satellite tumours (metastases)
Rate of Growth	Usually slow	Usually rapid
Boundaries	Circumscribed, often encapsulated	Irregular, ill-defined and non-encapsulated
Relationship to surrounding tissues	Merely compresses normal tissue	Invades and destroys normal tissues
Effects	Produced by pressure on vessels, tubes, nerves, organs, and by excess production of substances e.g. hormones. Removal will alleviate.	Destroys structures

In practice, there is a spectrum of malignancy. Some tumours may grow locally and destroy normal tissues but never produce metastases. Others will produce metastases only after a very considerable time while, at the other end of the spectrum, there are tumours which metastasise very early in their development.

2. **HISTOLOGICAL ORIGIN**

Although tumours may arise from any tissue in the body, they can be conveniently accommodated in five groups.

1. Epithelia.
2. Mesenchymal tissues including fibrous tissue, bone, cartilage and vessels.
3. Neuroectoderm.
4. Haemopoietic and lymphoid cells.
5. Germ cells.

The commonest tumours arise from tissues which have a rapid turnover of cells and which are exposed to environmental mutagens, e.g. epithelium of mucous membranes, skin, breast and reproductive organs and lymphoid and haemopoietic tissues.

BENIGN TUMOURS – HISTOLOGY

In general, the cells of benign tumours are well differentiated. They:

1. **Mimic the structure of their parent organ.**

e.g. In an adenoma (simple gland-forming tumour) of colon the cells arrange themselves in acini.

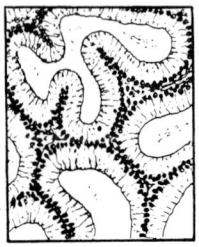

In a skin papilloma (wart) the squamous epithelium still forms a covering for underlying connective tissue

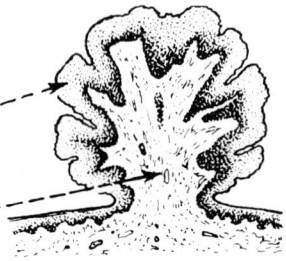

2. **Resemble the cells of their tissue of origin.**

e.g. The cells of a skin papilloma are squamous

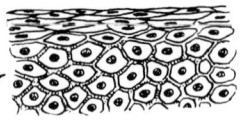

The cells of a myoma are muscle cells

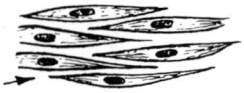

The cells of a chondroma are recognisable cartilage cells

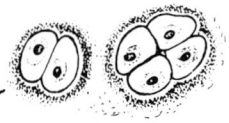

3. As in normal tissue, **show a remarkable uniformity in size, shape and nuclear configuration.**

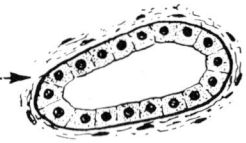

4. **Show evidence of normal function.**
This may be useless, e.g.

or

pathological, e.g. excess secretion of parathyroid hormone by a parathyroid adenoma.

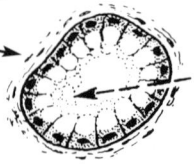

Mucous secretion in acinus of an adenoma

5. **Have relatively infrequent mitotic figures:** these are of normal type.

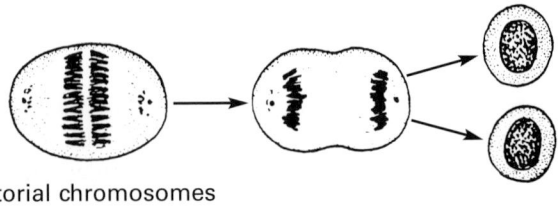

Division into two identical daughter cells.

Equatorial chromosomes

MALIGNANT TUMOURS – HISTOLOGY

The cells of malignant tumours tend to be less well-differentiated than those of benign tumours.

They:

1. **Generally show a haphazard arrangement.** → e.g. Carcinoma of breast

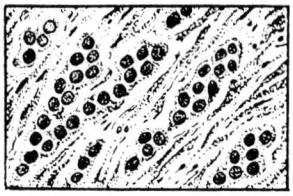

2. **Bear little resemblance to the cells of origin.**

3. **Tend to vary widely in size, shape and nuclear configuration, reflecting an increase in chromosomal number and DNA content (aneuploidy).** → e.g. Pleomorphic sarcoma

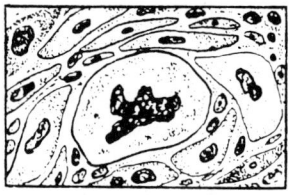

4. **Provide little evidence of normal function.** → e.g. Adeno carcinoma of bowel (Secretory activity very limited)

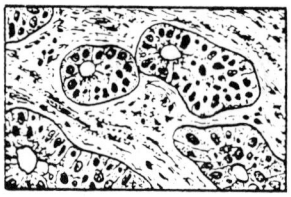

5. **Show frequent mitoses often of abnormal type.**

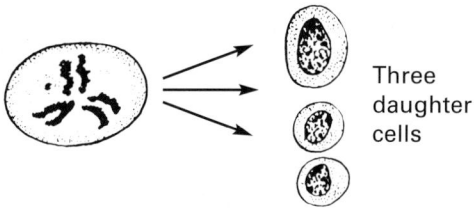

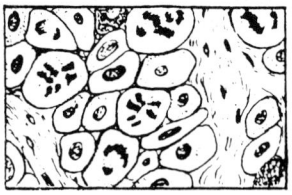

There is a spectrum within malignant neoplasms from slowly growing well differentiated examples to rapidly growing undifferentiated highly malignant tumours.

BENIGN EPITHELIAL TUMOURS

Benign epithelial tumours are essentially of two types: (1) papillomas and (2) adenomas.

PAPILLOMA

Papillomas take origin from an epithelial surface. As the epithelium proliferates it is thrown into folds which become increasingly complex.

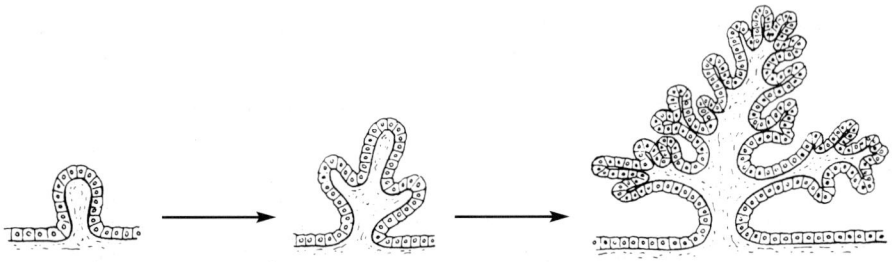

The epithelial proliferation is accompanied by a corresponding growth of supporting connective tissue and blood vessels.

Typical examples are found in the skin, e.g. the common wart.

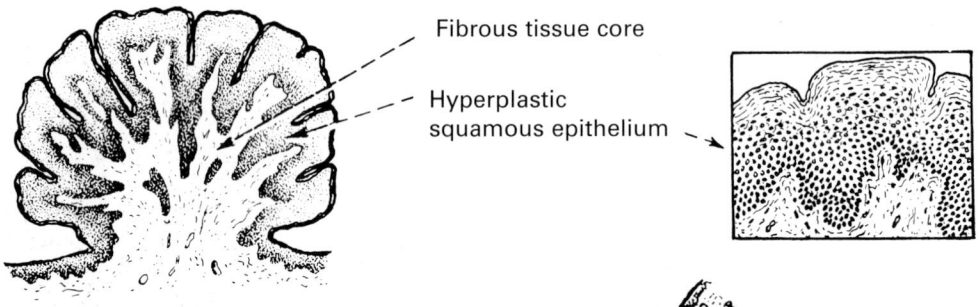

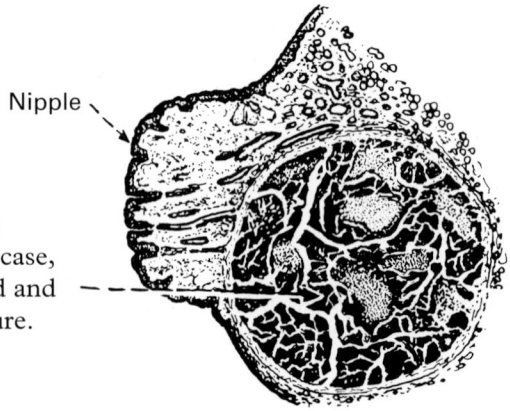

Papillomas may also form within ducts, e.g. in the breast. In such a case, the papilloma is much compressed and has an apparently complex structure.

In these benign tumours:

(a) The normal arrangement of epithelial cells is maintained, e.g. in skin papillomas the surface cells are squamous and proliferation is confined to the deepest layers.
(b) The relationship of epithelium to connective tissue is normal.
(c) Blood vessels are well formed.

BENIGN EPITHELIAL TUMOURS

ADENOMA

Adenomas are derived from the ducts and acini of glands, although the name is also used to cover simple tumours arising in solid epithelial organs.

Again the proliferation of epithelium of a gland causes the formation of tubules which ramify and become increasingly compound. The original communication with the parent gland duct or acinus tends to become lost.

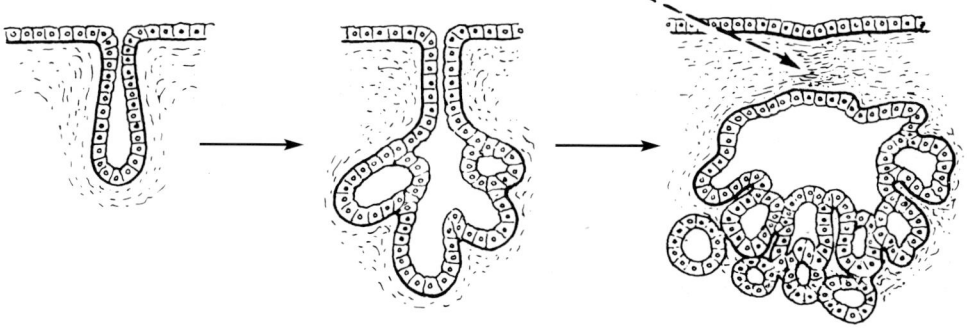

In the case of a hollow viscus, such as the intestine or gall bladder, the adenomatous proliferation, instead of growing down into the subjacent connective tissue, is usually pushed upwards into the lumen of the viscus.

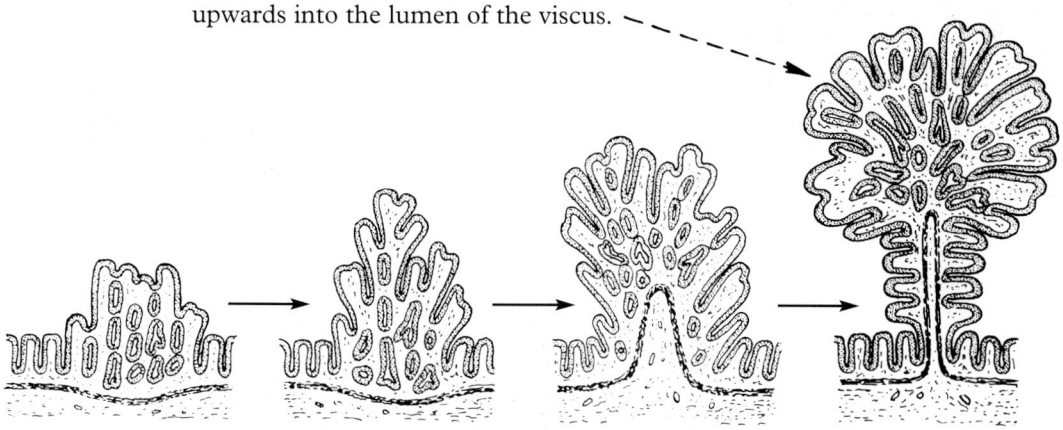

The growth therefore combines the features of a papilloma and an adenoma. The term adenomatous polyp is often applied in such a case.

BENIGN EPITHELIAL TUMOURS

ADENOMA (continued)
In the type which grows into the subjacent connective tissue, the progressive budding of the epithelium results in new acini which become nipped off from the parent acini.

In cases in which retention of secretion is marked, a cyst forms and the tumour is then called a **CYSTADENOMA** which may reach an enormous size, e.g. some cystadenomas of the ovary may be 30-40 cm in diameter, particularly those which secrete mucus.

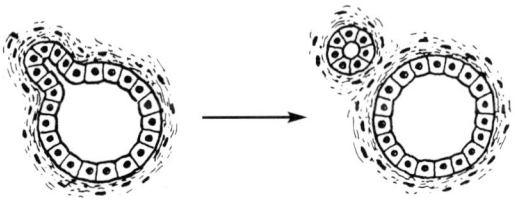

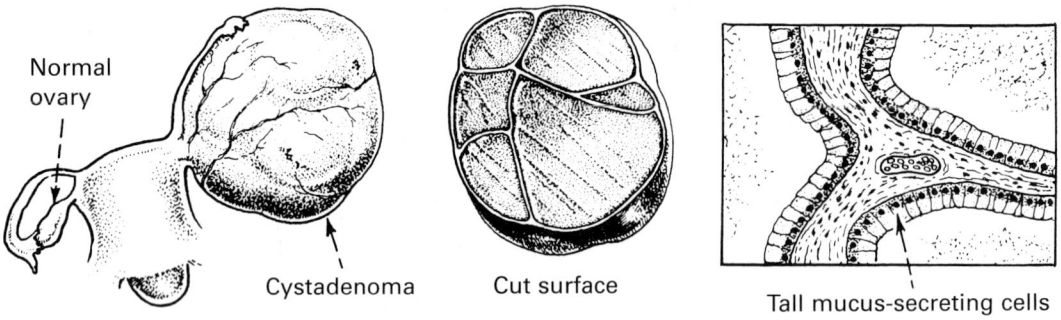

As in a hollow viscus, the proliferating epithelium may be heaped to form papillomas and the tumour then becomes a **PAPILLARY CYSTADENOMA**. These are also common in the ovary (see p.519).

FIBROADENOMA
In the breast the term is clinically useful for a small nodule consisting of a mixture of acinar elements and prominent supporting fibrous tissue. The histological appearances are variable depending on the distribution of the fibrous tissue (see also p.527).

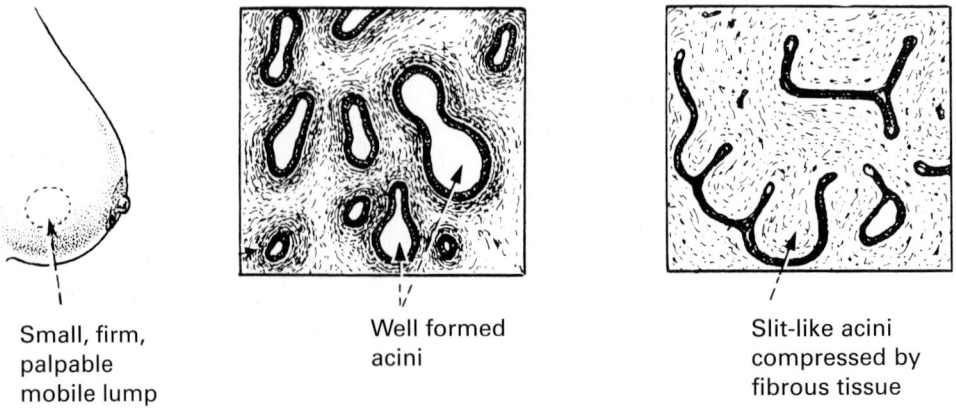

BENIGN CONNECTIVE TISSUE TUMOURS

Benign connective tissue tumours are composed of mature connective tissues - fat, cartilage, bone, nerves and blood vessels. They tend to form encapsulated rounded or lobulated masses which compress the surrounding tissues.

LIPOMA

Circumscribed masses of fat are commonly found in the subcutaneous tissue of the arms, shoulders and buttocks. Less commonly they occur in the deep soft tissues of the limbs or retroperitoneum, but at these sites they must be carefully distinguished from low grade liposarcomas. Lipomas very rarely arise from the viscera.

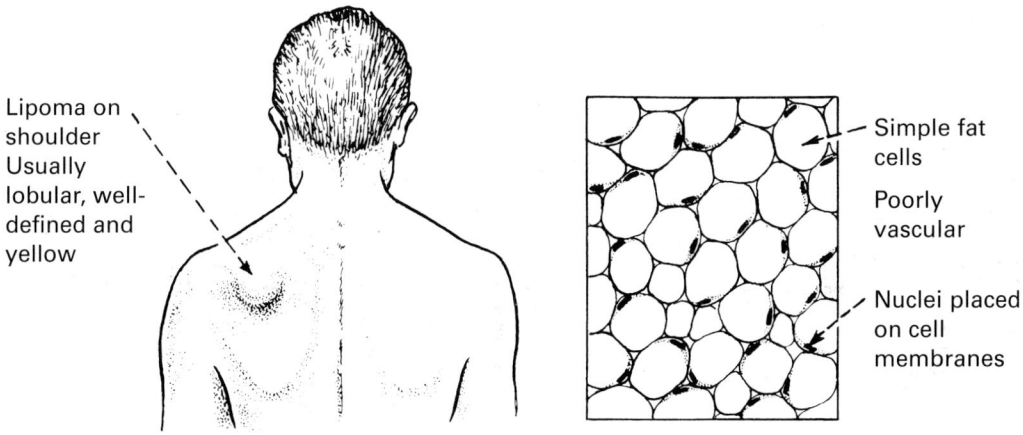

Sometimes lipomas may have projections into the surrounding tissues which make complete removal difficult.

CHONDROMA

A chondroma usually arises within the medullary cavity of the tubular bones of the hands and feet; it grows slowly, causing gradual expansion of the bone. Less commonly it occurs in long bones. Rarely multiple enchondromas appear in children and are associated with deformity: they occasionally become malignant.

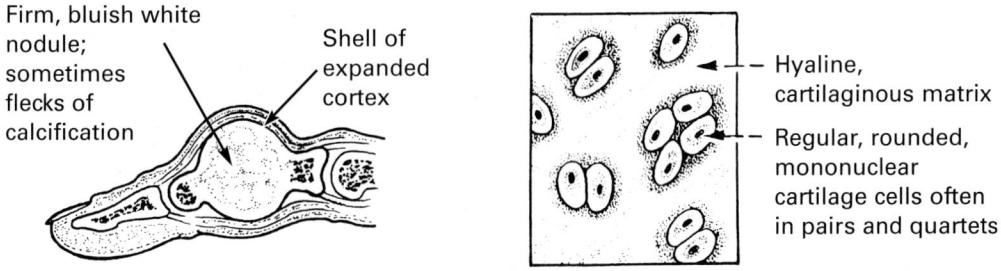

BENIGN CONNECTIVE TISSUE TUMOURS

OSTEOMA

This tumour is mainly found in the bones of the skull, although it may occur in long bones. Osteomas are relatively small but may produce severe symptoms because of their situation.

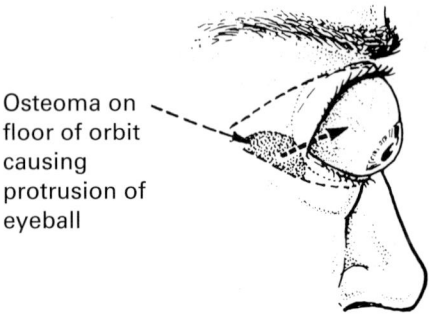

LEIOMYOMA

Simple tumours of muscle are derived from smooth muscle and the majority occur in the uterus where they are extremely common. They are firm, rounded masses which usually begin in the myometrium. Subsequently, they may move inward to the uterine cavity forming polypi, or towards the serous surface.

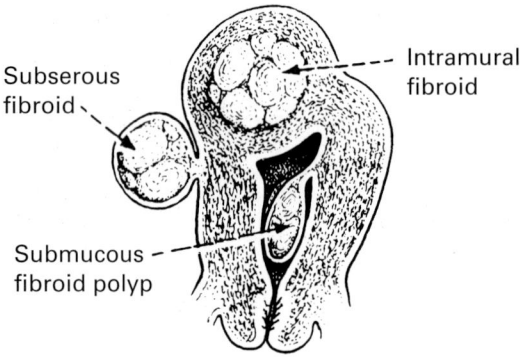

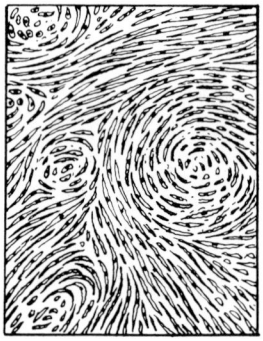

TUMOURS OF FIBROUS TISSUE

So-called fibromas are extremely rare but tumour like growths are fairly common. Examples are FIBROMATOSIS and KELOID (see p. 51).

Palmar fibromatosis, at first nodular, causes flexion deformities of fingers (Dupuytren's contracture) due to contraction of fibrous tissue within the palmar fascia. A similar condition may affect the plantar fascia.

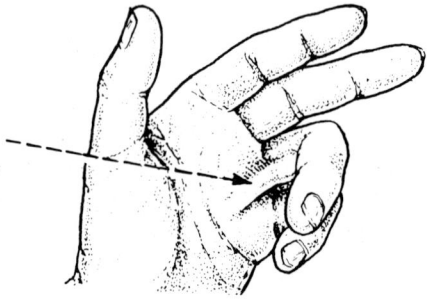

Benign tumours of PERIPHERAL NERVE and of VESSELS are described on pages 601 and 602.

MALIGNANT EPITHELIAL TUMOURS

Malignant epithelial tumours are known as **CARCINOMAS** (Greek *'karkinos'*: a crab), referring to the typical irregular jagged shape. This is due to invasion into adjacent normal tissues (p. 135).

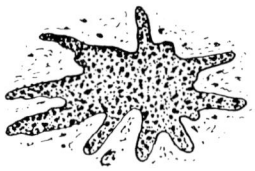

Types of CARCINOMA

Like benign epithelial tumours, carcinomas can arise from covering or glandular epithelium.

SQUAMOUS CELL CARCINOMA

This is commonly found on the skin, especially exposed surfaces, but also develops in other sites covered by stratified squamous epithelium, e.g. lips, tongue, pharynx, oesophagus and vagina. In addition, it may occur on surfaces covered by glandular type epithelium through metaplastic transformation as in the bronchus, gall bladder and uterine cervix. It frequently arises from areas of carcinoma-in-situ (p.144).

(1) It starts as a small papular mass

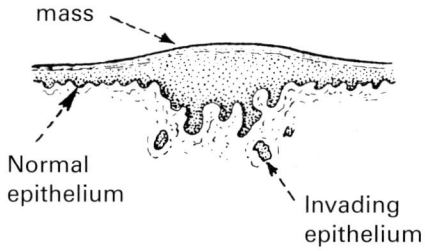

(2) The surface breaks down and a characteristic irregular ulcer is produced.

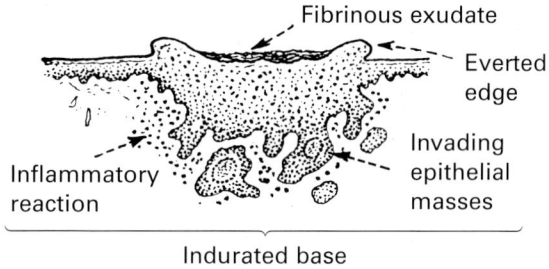

Histologically, it is composed of irregular strands and columns of invading epithelium which infiltrate the subjacent connective tissue. If well differentiated, the central cells of the invading masses show conversion into eosinophilic keratinised squames, while the outer layer consists of young basophilic cells. In cross-section, the appearance is typical.

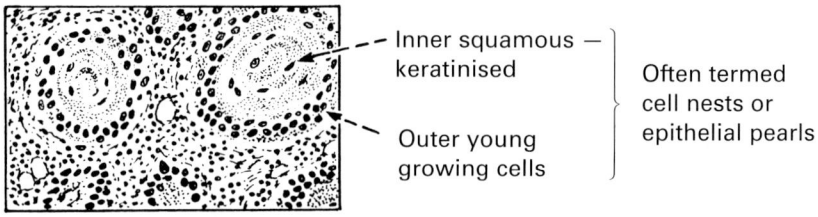

Squamous carcinoma of skin is typically well differentiated and slow growing. In contrast, uterine cervical carcinomas are poorly differentiated and spread early to draining lymph nodes.

MALIGNANT CONNECTIVE TISSUE TUMOURS

Malignant connective tissue tumours are referred to as Sarcomas (Greek *'sarkoma'*: flesh). They arise in soft tissue, in bone and rarely in viscera.

Sarcomas are far less common than carcinomas, but are second in frequency to leukaemias and lymphomas in childhood and early adult life.

Unlike the ill-defined infiltrative carcinomas, sarcomas are large well defined fleshy tumours. Naked eye assessment suggests that they are encapsulated, but histology shows that this is a false impression. Malignant cells do infiltrate between normal tissues at the margin, so that surgical 'shelling out' is almost inevitably followed by local recurrence from aggregates of cells remaining in the tumour bed.

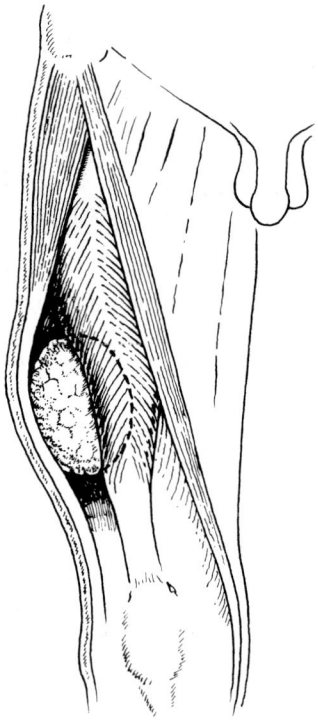

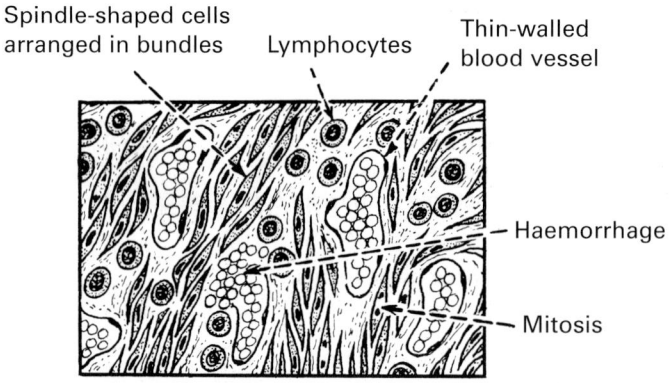

Most sarcomas consist of spindle shaped cells, although some are of round cell type. They are associated with the formation of many large thin walled blood vessels which are easily invaded by sarcoma cells. Blood borne metastases to lung are common.

SARCOMAS

Many different histological types of sarcoma have been described. The nomenclature is based on adding the suffix 'sarcoma' to the type of differentiation shown, e.g. chondrosarcoma, liposarcoma, leiomyosarcoma (cartilage, adipose tissue, smooth muscle).

In general, the grade of the tumour is of more prognostic importance than the precise histological type. Some of the commoner forms of sarcoma are described:

Malignant Fibrous Histiocytoma (MFH) is the commonest soft tissue sarcoma of adults. It occurs in the limbs and retroperitoneum and is rapidly growing with a poor prognosis. The histogenesis is uncertain; it is probably a tumour of primitive fibroblasts.

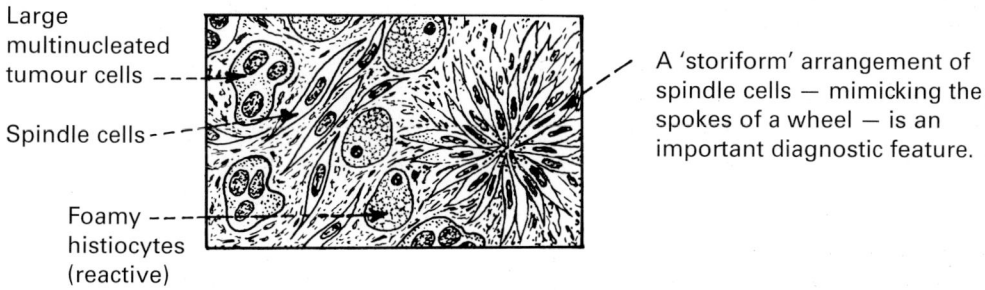

Liposarcoma

This tumour arises in soft tissues of the limbs and retroperitoneum. A number of sub types are described. Primitive fat containing cells (lipoblasts) are a feature.

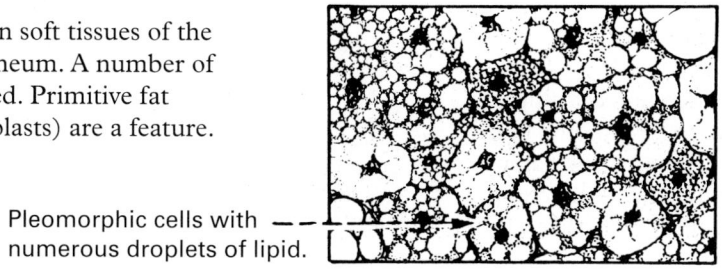

Well differentiated liposarcoma has an excellent prognosis and rarely metastasises. Pleomorphic and round cell liposarcomas are highly aggressive tumours which metastasise early.

SARCOMAS

MYOSARCOMA

There are two varieties:

1. Leiomyosarcoma

These rare tumours arise in the skin, deep soft tissues, the stomach and particularly in the uterus.

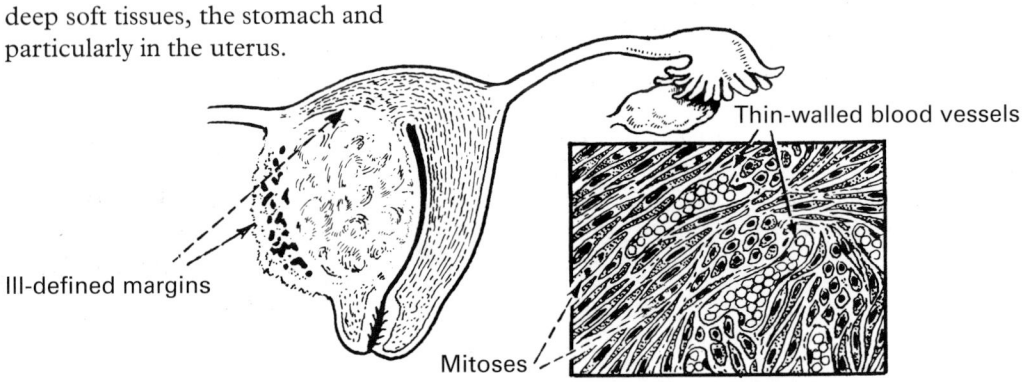

2. Rhabdomyosarcoma

This is a rare tumour occurring mainly in children. It occurs very rarely in skeletal muscles. More common but still rare are polypoid tumours in the bladder, uterus and vagina, sometimes called sarcoma botryoides (grape-like).

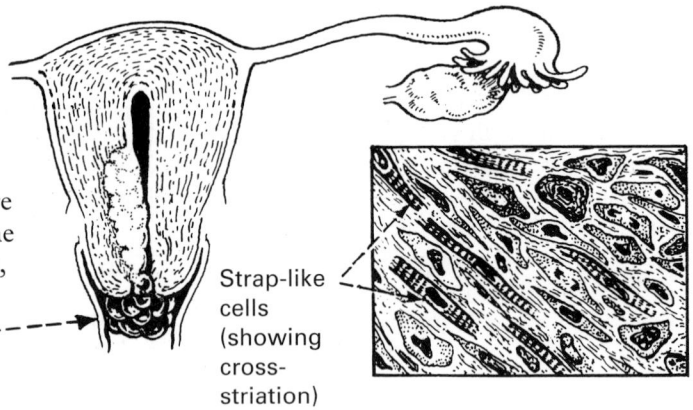

Pleomorphic or anaplastic sarcoma

Some sarcomas are so poorly differentiated that their histogenesis is not apparent. They are usually highly malignant.

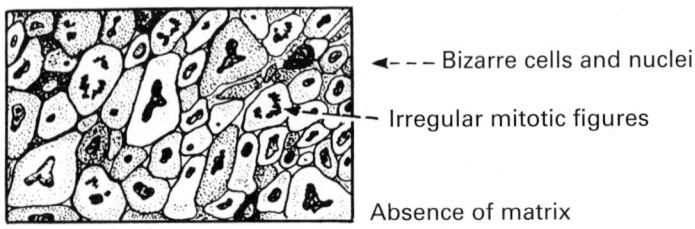

Immunocytochemistry, electron microscopy and cytogenetic analysis (demonstrating typical chromosome translocations) all help in reaching more specific diagnoses than can be reached by conventional histology alone.

Sarcomas of bone are described on page 631.

OTHER TUMOUR TYPES

TERATOMA

This is a tumour derived from totipotent germ cells. Most arise in the **ovary** (usually benign) and **testis** (**almost always malignant**): they may also occur at any site in the mid-line where germ cells have stopped in their migration to the gonads.

For example, **Benign cystic teratoma** is typically seen in the ovary.

It consists mainly of ectodermal structures such as skin and its appendages and neural tissue. Frequently respiratory epithelium, intestinal epithelium, bone and cartilage are present.

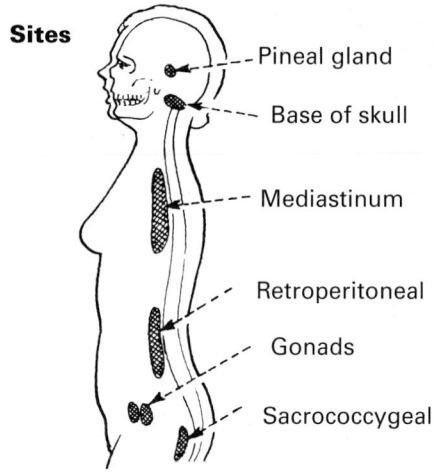

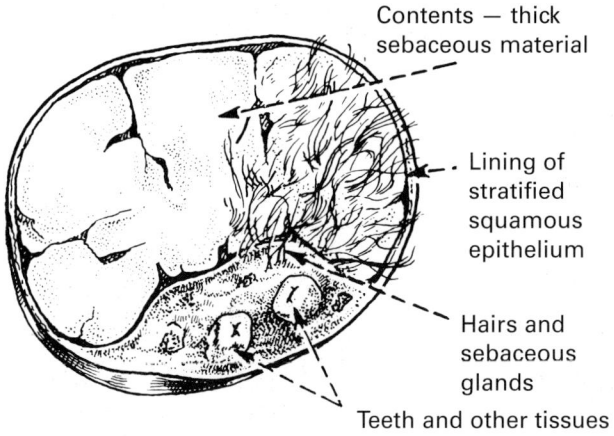

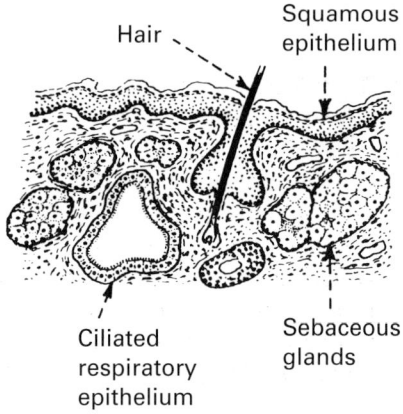

Testicular Teratomas are described on page 539.

MIXED TUMOURS

A number of tumours show differing histological patterns of epithelial and connective tissue components. The commonest is the MIXED PAROTID TUMOUR (PLEOMORPHIC ADENOMA)
— presenting as a lobulated, firm, slow growing lump.

The stromal elements arise from metaplasia of myo-epithelial cells.

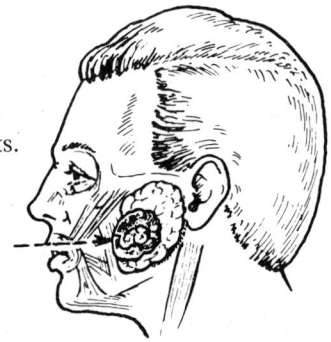

Malignant mesothelioma (page 288), synovial sarcoma (page 641) and the very rare carcino-sarcoma show similar variable patterns.

OTHER TUMOUR TYPES

HAMARTOMA

A hamartoma is a tumour-like but non-neoplastic malformation consisting of a mixture of tissues normally found at the particular site.

The commonest forms of hamartoma are those composed of blood vessels and those involving pigment cells of the skin.

Hamartomas are also found involving the peripheral nerves - neurofibromatosis and its variants — the intestinal tract, congenital polypi, and in many other organs. Tuberous sclerosis is a condition in which hamartomas are present in many of the organs.

Although hamartomas are not neoplastic, true tumour growth may develop from a hamartoma.

Hamartoma	**True neoplasm**
Developmental abnormality.	New growth.
Present and often visible at birth.	Most occur in adults.
Enlargement continues until physiological growth ceases (i.e. on reaching adulthood).	Growth is progressive, autonomous and not related to stages of body development.
Condition is essentially benign.	May be malignant.

It will be appreciated that the borderline between hamartoma and some types of benign neoplasm is ill-defined and the distinction is often not of practical importance.

HAEMANGIOMA

Two main varieties exist:

1. **Capillary angioma**

These are common in the skin as 'birth-marks' which vary in size. Occasionally they may be found in internal organs. They are well defined, deep red or purple. A single artery provides a supply separate from the surrounding tissue.

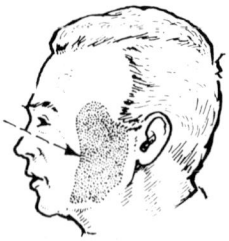

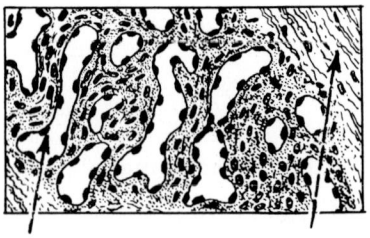

2. **Cavernous angioma**

This type is usually confined to internal organs and quite often found in the liver. Like the capillary variety they are well defined and deep purple. Similar tumours are found involving the lymphatic system but less commonly.

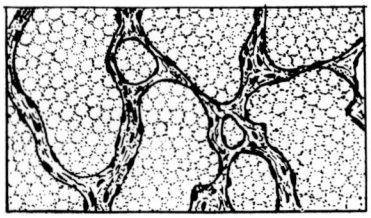

OTHER TUMOUR TYPES

BENIGN PIGMENTED NAEVUS or LENTIGO (Melanocytic naevus or mole)
Benign pigmented naevus is one of the commonest forms of hamartoma. The term 'naevus' means a birthmark, but most naevi are acquired in childhood and adolescence.

During fetal life melanin-pigment-forming neuroectodermal cells migrate to the skin and are found in small numbers in the basal layer of the skin.

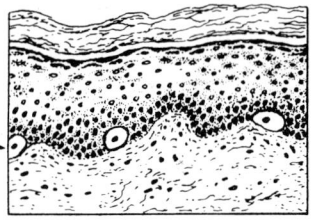

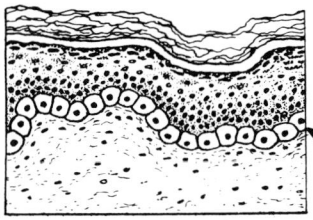

The common congenital pigmented mole is the result of an abnormality in migration, proliferation and maturation of these neuroectodermal cells. A continuous layer of pigmented cells is found adjacent to the basal epidermal cells.

The resulting naevi vary in size and appearance, varying from small flat macular brown areas or smooth papular lesions to warty hairy excrescences. Pigmentation is variable.

Sometimes proliferation of the 'naevus' cells is a striking feature and this varies in degree and extent:

Junctional naevus
In this case proliferation is local and confined to the dermoepidermal junction

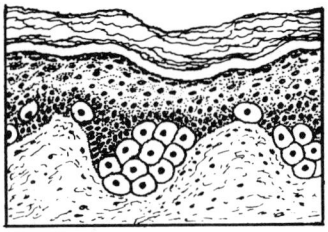

Compound naevus
Proliferation is found in the dermis as well as the junctional area.

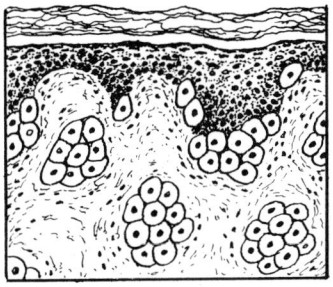

Intradermal naevus
Proliferation is wholly in the dermis.

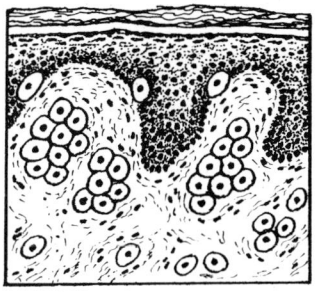

Blue naevus is another variation in which melanocytes are arrested in migration in the dermis.

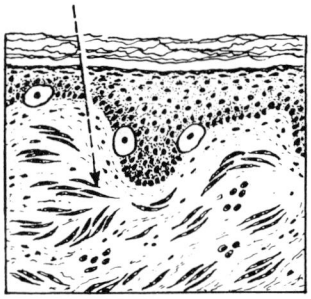

Active proliferative activity may extend into adult life, but the great majority of these lesions undergo a degree of involution. One feature which differentiates them from the malignant change is that the deeper the cells penetrate the dermis the smaller they become and the less active.

OTHER TUMOUR TYPES

MALIGNANT MELANOMA

Malignant proliferation of melanocytes usually arises de novo but some melanomas arise from pre-existing naevi. Exposure to SUNLIGHT (the U.V. component) is the most important aetiological factor.

1. *Chronic* — over many years — especially relevant in the elderly.
2. *Acute* — causing burning. This is particularly important.

Sites

1. Skin of (a) face, soles of feet, palms of hands, nail beds,
   (b) legs (women) and (c) trunk (in men).
2. Mucous membranes of mouth, arms and genitalia — rare.
3. Eye and meninges — rare.

Some growths are amelanotic (non-pigmented). The rate of growth is variable.

Four types of growth may occur:

1. *Lentigo maligna* — an 'in situ' lesion occurring on the face of the elderly. It may spread at one edge and regress at another.

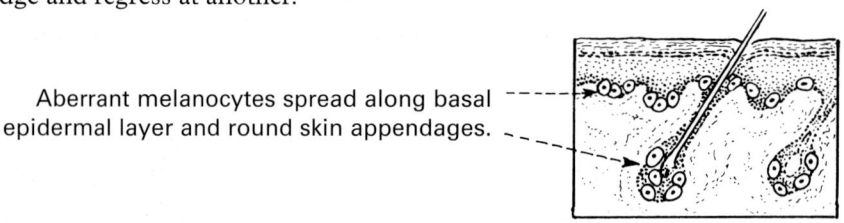

It may not reach the invasive stage before the patient dies of 'natural causes'.

2. *Superficial spreading melanoma* — occurs on female leg, male trunk. It accounts for 50% of all skin melanomas in northern countries.
3. *Acral lentiginous melanoma* — found on palms of hands, soles of feet and mucous membranes.
4. *Nodular malignant melanoma* — usually on trunk. It invades early and ulceration is common.

Types 2, 3 and 4 occur in younger adults, and all can have an in situ stage.

The essential features of malignant melanoma are:

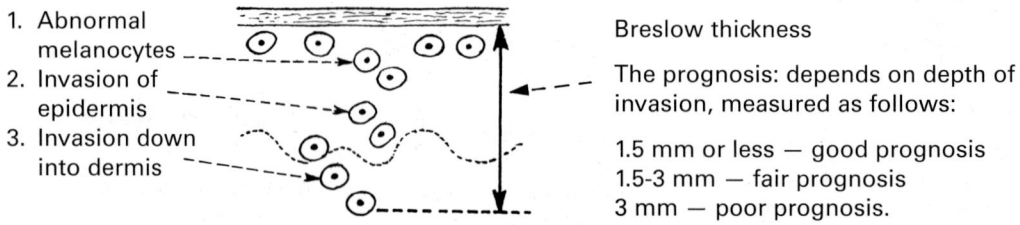

SPREAD OF TUMOURS

Tumours spread by several routes.

1. Local invasion.
2. Lymphatic spread.
3. Blood (Haematogenous) spread
4. Transcoelomic spread.
5. Perineural spread.
6. Intraepithelial spread.

LOCAL SPREAD

The proliferating cells break through normal barriers.

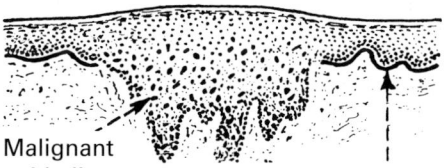

Malignant epithelium breaks through basement membrane and subjacent connective tissue

Further spread is by penetration between normal tissues.

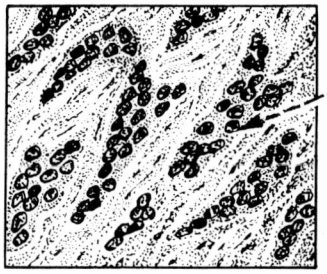

Malignant cells permeating spaces

An important principle is that these permeating tumour cells take the line of least physical resistance.

Growth of malignant cells may stimulate the production of new collagen fibres which are sometimes converted into dense fibrous tissue → contracts and fixes the growth to surrounding structures

e.g. Carcinoma of breast →

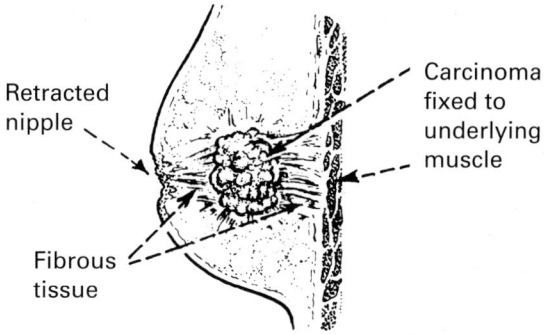

The following diagram illustrates the basic mechanisms of cancer cell invasion.

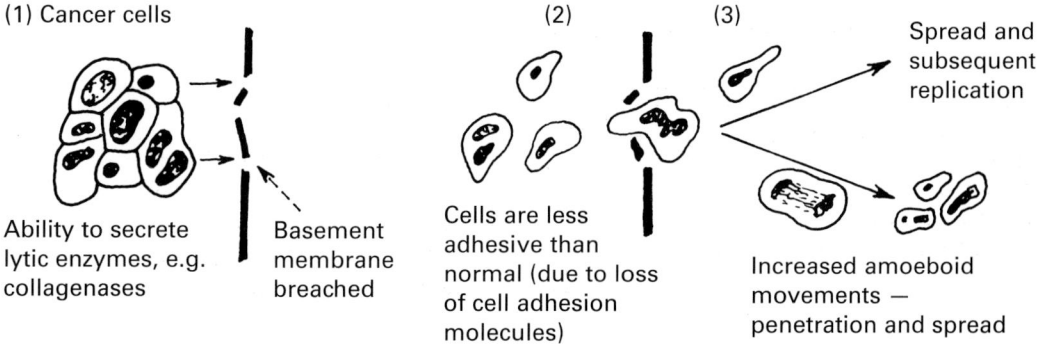

LYMPHATIC SPREAD

LYMPHATIC SPREAD

This is the commonest mode of spread of carcinomas, but rarely of sarcomas. Malignant epithelial cells easily invade lymphatic channels from the tissue spaces.

Groups of cells form emboli in the lymph stream and are carried to the nearest node.

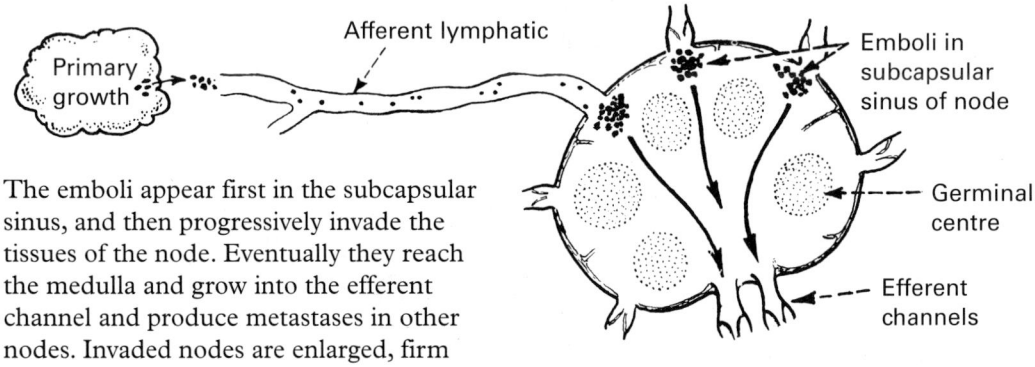

The emboli appear first in the subcapsular sinus, and then progressively invade the tissues of the node. Eventually they reach the medulla and grow into the efferent channel and produce metastases in other nodes. Invaded nodes are enlarged, firm and white.

Microscopic emboli can escape notice at operation. They account for recurrence of growth in many cases.

Growth of carcinoma cells in a node may result in occlusion of afferent and efferent channels. Lymph flow is thus diverted and this has two effects:

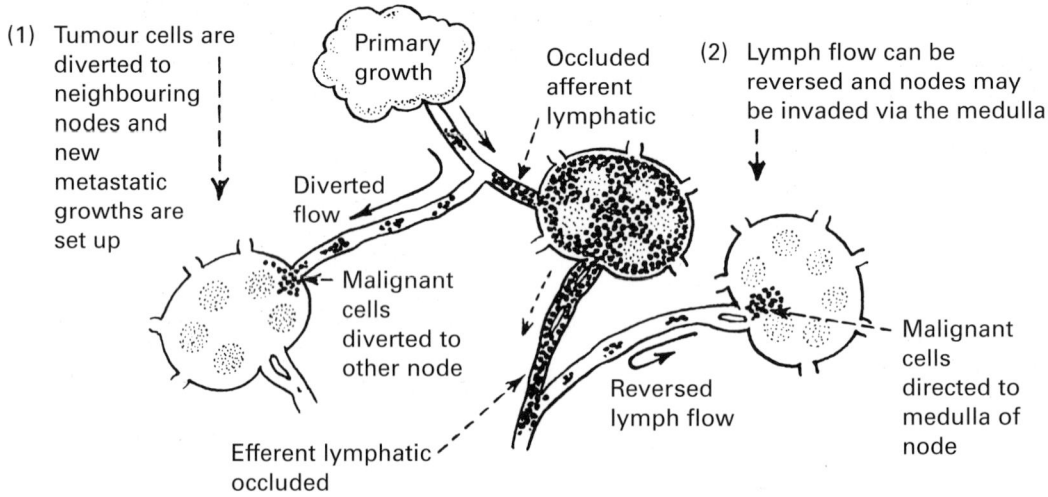

This accounts for the spread of carcinoma in a diverse and often irregular manner.

LYMPHATIC SPREAD

LYMPHATIC SPREAD (continued)

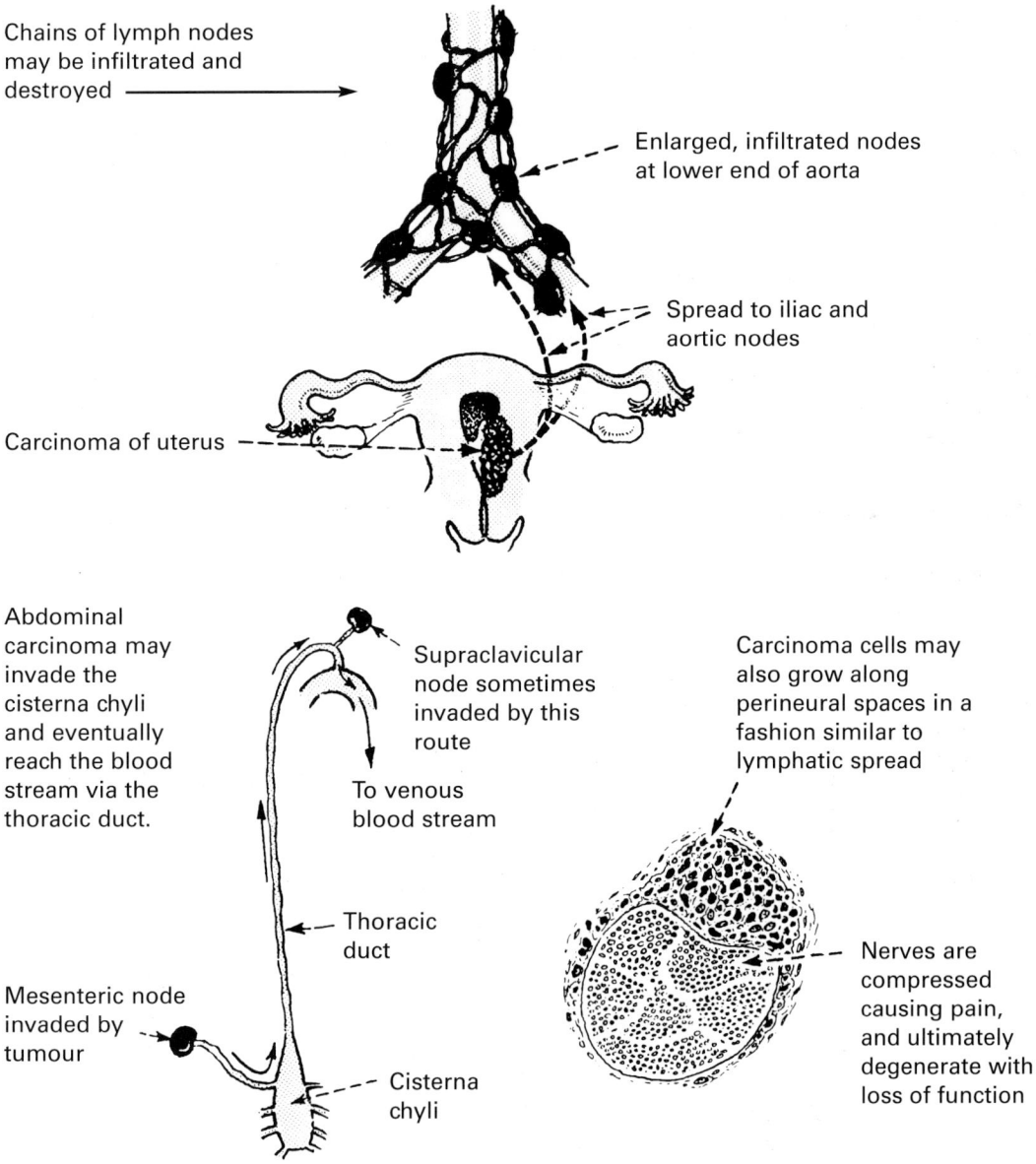

Although lymphatic embolism is of major practical importance, tumour cells may also grow along lymphatic channels in continuous solid columns — **lymphatic permeation**.

BLOOD SPREAD

Both carcinomas and sarcomas spread by the blood stream. The entry of malignant cells into the blood is via invasion of VENULES and by lymphatic embolism through the thoracic duct into the subclavian vein.

Carcinoma cells invading the thin wall of the vessel and entering the lumen.

The following are possible sequels:

1. Tumour embolism to lungs (systemic circulation).
2. Embolism to liver (portal circulation).
3. Embolism via pulmonary veins to systemic ARTERIAL circulation. (Primary and secondary lung tumours.)

4. Thrombosis within the lumen: consisting of a mixture of cancer cells and coagulum.

Cancer cells

Fibrin

Subsequent embolism as in 1, 2, 3 above.

VIA LARGER VEINS

Occasionally tumour thrombus is propagated from venules into larger veins. This is classically seen in RENAL CARCINOMA.

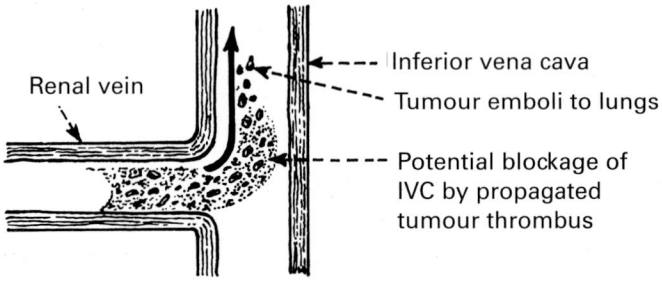

Larger veins e.g. superior vena cava may suffer compression effects in 2 ways:

(1) Compression by tumour: vein may ultimately be obliterated.

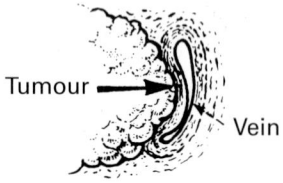

(2) Lumen reduced by growth of fibrous tissue stimulated by the neoplasm.

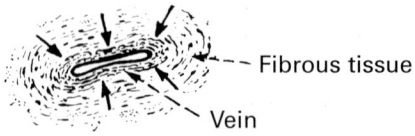

Rarely, a malignant process may be complicated by thrombosis of distant veins (thrombophlebitis migrans). This is not due to malignant invasion of the veins but is caused by the action of circulating thromboplastins formed by the tumour.

ARTERIAL SYSTEM

Direct invasion of arteries and arteriolar lumens is very rare because of the physical barrier provided by the thick muscular and elastic walls.

BLOOD SPREAD

DESTINATION of EMBOLI

This depends on the anatomical damage of the vessel invaded.

(1) **Portal venous system** – emboli pass to liver

(2) **Systemic venous system** – emboli pass to lungs. There are exceptions (see 'Retrograde Spread' below).

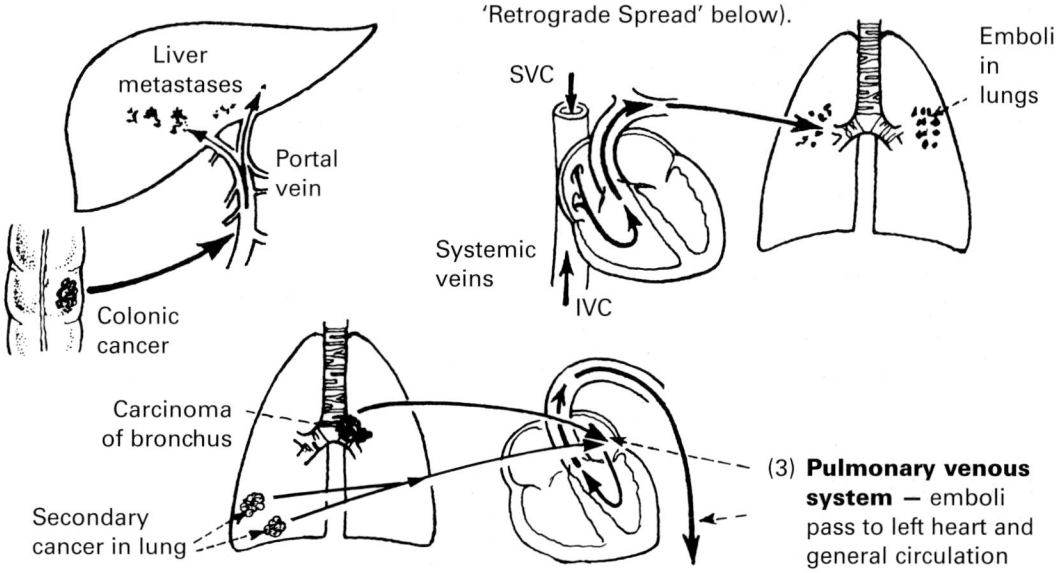

(3) **Pulmonary venous system** – emboli pass to left heart and general circulation

RETROGRADE VENOUS SPREAD

As in lymphatics, growth of tumour within a vein may cause reversal of blood flow. In addition, reversal of flow is apt to happen in certain areas of the body where veins form a rich plexus and are deficient in valves, e.g. in the pelvis and around vertebrae. Changes in intra-abdominal and intrathoracic pressures easily induce changes in blood flow in these channels. It is for this reason that secondary tumours are relatively common in vertebral bodies.

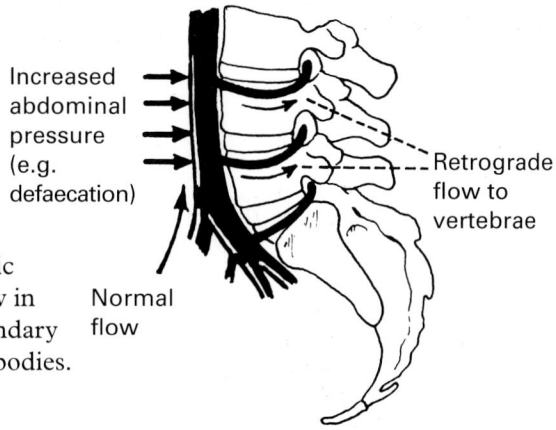

FATE of CARCINOMATOUS EMBOLI

SEED and SOIL ANALOGY

The distribution of carcinomatous emboli is determined in part by anatomy, but many complex factors both in the 'seed' (the cancer cell) and the 'soil' (the potential metastatic site) are at play in the establishment of metastases at particular sites. They include surface properties of the cancer cells e.g. increased expression of **integrins** and their **receptors** present in the endothelial cells at the metastatic site. Variation in the host IMMUNE RESPONSE is also important.

OTHER MODES OF SPREAD OF TUMOURS

TRANSCOELOMIC SPREAD (via SEROUS SACS)

This is an important and frequent route of spread in the peritoneal and pleural cavities. It also takes place in the pericardial sac.

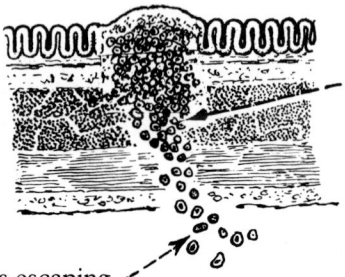

Carcinoma cells penetrate the wall of the stomach and extend to the serous surface.

Carcinoma cells escaping into peritoneal cavity where 'seeding' occurs.

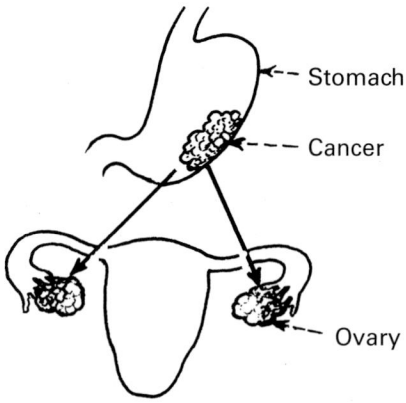

As malignant cells sink in the peritoneal cavity, they will settle in various sites. They may cause an inflammatory reaction with fibrin formation. This can cause adhesions between organs, e.g. loops of bowel.

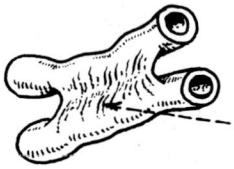

Fibrous adhesions

Gastric cancer can spread to both ovaries (so-called KRUKENBERG TUMOUR).

INTRA-EPITHELIAL SPREAD

This form of spread may occur where carcinoma develops in a gland or its duct, e.g. in the breast. Carcinoma cells spread in the areolar skin. (Paget's disease of the nipple.)

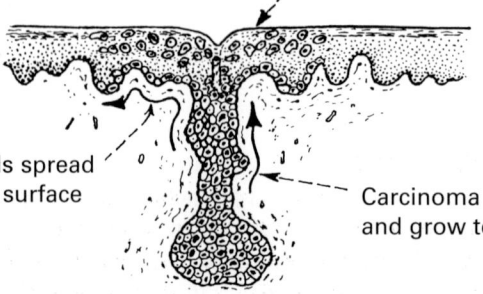

Carcinoma cells spread laterally in the surface epithelium.

Carcinoma cells fill the duct and grow towards the surface

EFFECTS OF TUMOURS

BENIGN TUMOURS

(a) The localised tumour mass may compress neighbouring structures causing loss of function and (b) benign endocrine tumours may produce excess hormones.

A Pituitary Adenoma is illustrative:

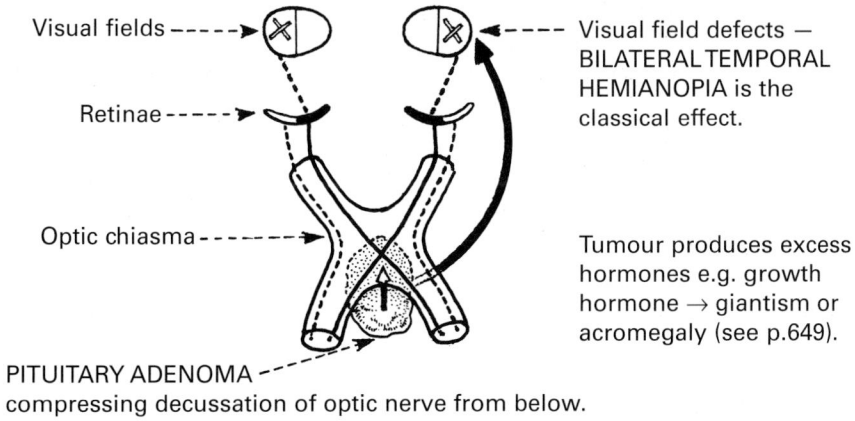

MALIGNANT TUMOURS

(a) **Local effects**
A tumour may narrow a hollow viscus e.g causing intestinal obstruction, ulceration and bleeding leading to anaemia.
E.g. 'ring' cancer of colon

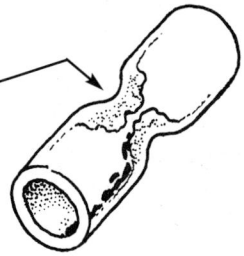

(b) **Involvement of neighbouring structures**
Direct spread compresses adjacent viscera, blood vessels and nerves — LUNG CARCINOMA is illustrative (see p.348).

(c) **Effects of distant metastases**
These are very numerous and variable. Two illustrative examples are given.

1. Metastases to bone cause pain (e.g. vertebral) and pathological fracture.

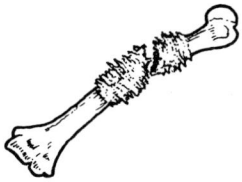

2. Metastases to the brain causing epilepsy, stroke, etc. (see p.597).

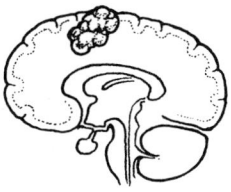

NON-METASTATIC COMPLICATIONS

Patients with cancer often have severe weight loss (cachexia), loss of appetite and fever. These are probably due to release of cytokines (e.g. TUMOUR NECROSIS FACTOR) from tumour cells. Other complications include myopathy and neuropathy. Relapsing thrombosis of distant veins (thrombo-phlebitis migrans) is due to release of thromboplastins.

TUMOUR MARKERS

Tumour cells produce substances, many of which are proteins which are helpful in diagnosis and monitoring of treatment.

(a) Product enters blood stream (and/ or urine) where it can be measured.

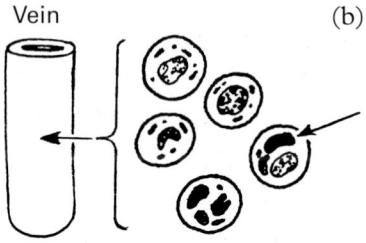

(b) Histological diagnosis is improved by identifying the specific product using immuno-staining in the cytoplasm of the tumour cells.

Some examples are:

Tumour Marker	Tumour
Human chorionic gonadotrophin (HCG)	Choriocarcinoma, Teratoma of testis
αFeto-protein (αFP)	Hepatocellular carcinoma, Teratoma of testis
Prostate specific antigen, Prostatic acid phosphatase	Prostatic carcinoma
Carcino-embryonic antigen	Gastro-intestinal and other cancers
Calcitonin	Medullary thyroid carcinoma
5-hydroxyindole-acetic acid (5HIAA) in URINE [metabolite of 5-hydroxy-tryptamine (5HT-SEROTONIN)]	Intestinal carcinoid

Monitoring Treatment

Blood levels of tumour markers reflect the effects of treatment.
Example:- **Testicular teratoma**

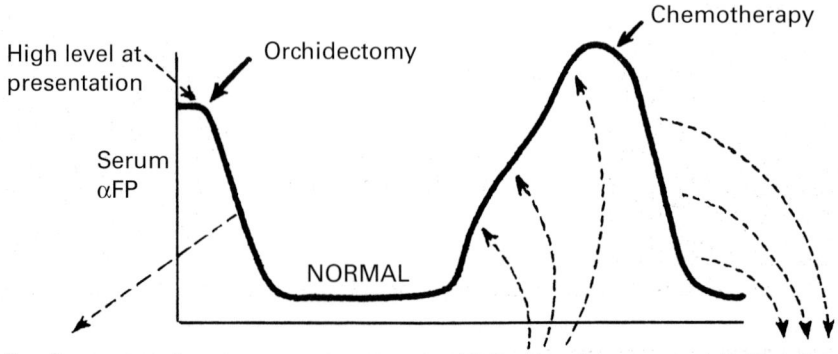

PRE-MALIGNANCY

The pathological conditions which are associated with the development of malignancy fall into 3 groups, (1) Benign tumours, (2) Chronic Inflammatory conditions and (3) Intraepithelial neoplasia.

1. **MALIGNANT TRANSFORMATION OF BENIGN TUMOURS**

(a) **Colonic cancer** is a good example in that many arise from a benign adenoma.

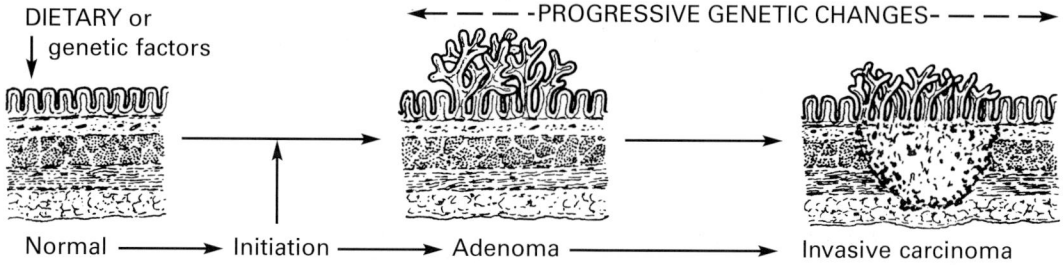

(b) In Familial adenomatous polyposis (Polyposis coli) the transformation to cancer in one or more of the very numerous adenomas is inevitable (p.333).

2. **CHRONIC INFLAMMATORY CONDITIONS**

The inflammation has to be very long standing and transformation to cancer is RARE. Examples are:

(a) In **Ulcerative colitis**, repeated epithelial damage and repair increase the risk of cancer.

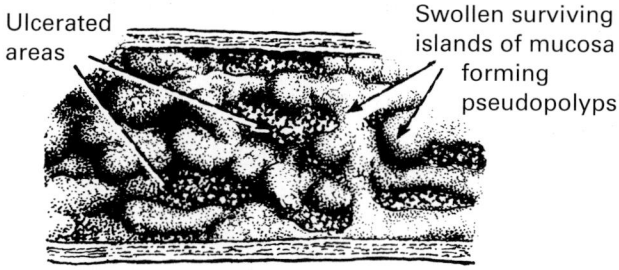

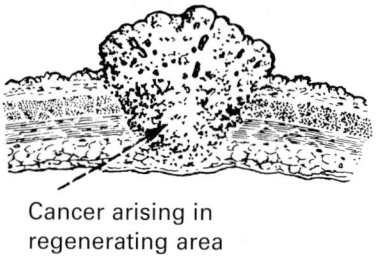

(b) In **Hashimoto's disease** — an auto-immune thyroiditis — the uniformly enlarged thyroid contains many proliferating lymphoid follicles and lymphocytes.

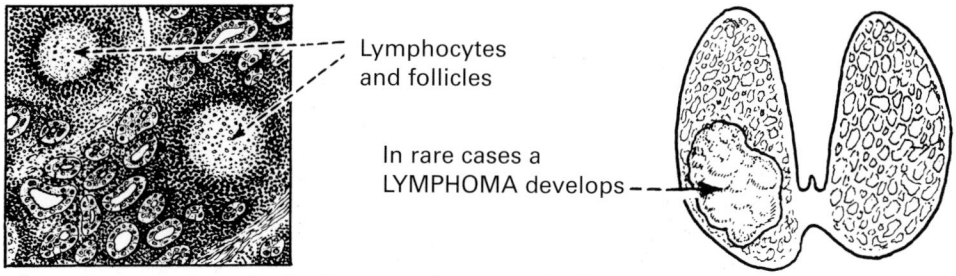

Apart from the evolution of colonic cancer from an adenoma, most malignancies arise de novo.

3. **INTRA-EPITHELIAL NEOPLASIA** is common and a very important pre-cancerous condition at several sites.

CARCINOMA IN SITU (INTRAEPITHELIAL NEOPLASIA)

This represents an intermediate stage in the production of a cancer. All the cytological features of malignancy are present, but the cells have not invaded the surrounding tissues. It is frequently found in the cervix uteri at the junction of ecto and endocervix.

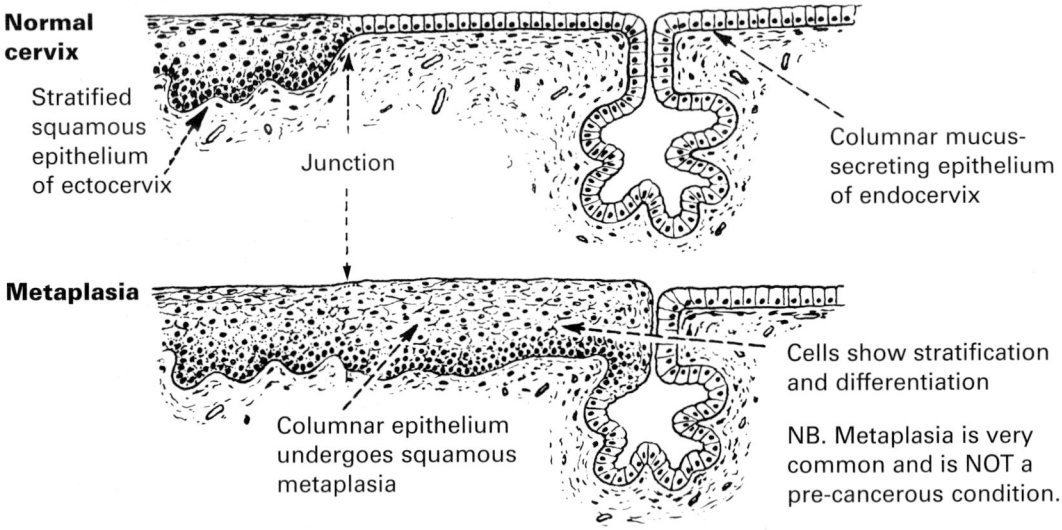

In the cervix, the abbreviation CIN (cervical intraepithelial neoplasia) is universally used. There are 3 grades of severity.

(1) CIN 1
(mild dysplasia)

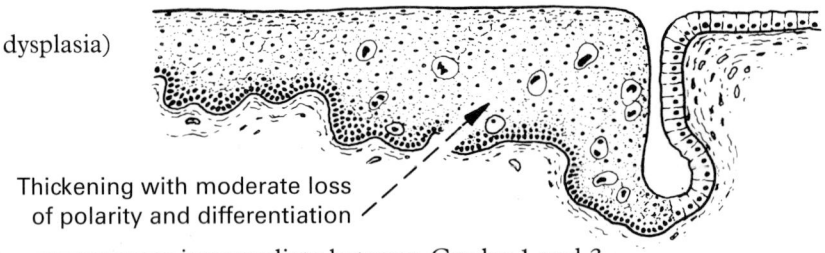

(2) CIN 2 — appearances intermediate between Grades 1 and 3,
(3) CIN 3 (Carcinoma-in-situ)

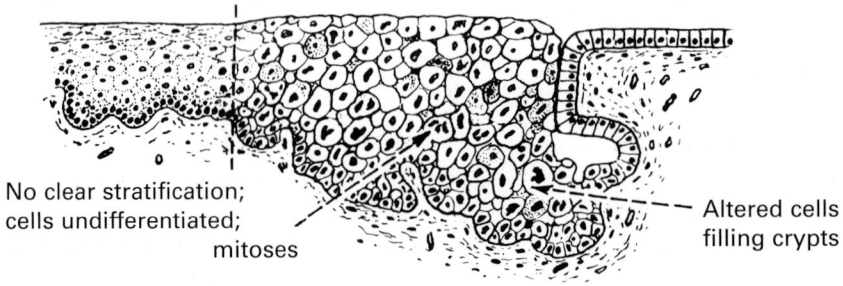

These premalignant conditions may revert to normal, but most commonly they become truly malignant and invade the surrounding tissues. The determining factors are unknown.

The concept of progressive premalignant proliferation applies equally in other organs (e.g. breast, stomach, bronchus, prostate, mouth, vulva)

CARCINOGENESIS

Malignant tumours are due to UNCONTROLLED PROLIFERATION of cells.

Most tumours are MONOCLONAL i.e. are derived from a single transformed cell.

This concept is well illustrated in MULTIPLE MYELOMA — a malignant tumour of plasma cells.

All the tumour cells produce the same immunoglobulin — including the same light chain.

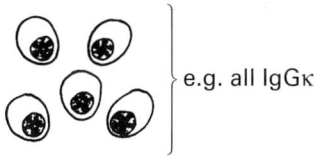

See also page 96.

In contrast, an inflammatory infiltrate of plasma cells is POLYCLONAL...

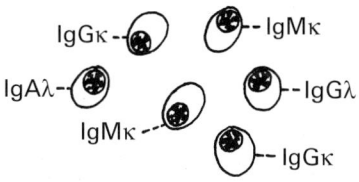

...producing various immunoglobulins and light chains.

CLONAL EVOLUTION

In time, some cells undergo further mutations which are passed on to their progeny. This is called clonal evolution or progression and explains the morphological variations seen in tumours. Some of the subclones grow more rapidly and metastasise more readily while others are so abnormal that proliferation is not possible and the clone dies out.

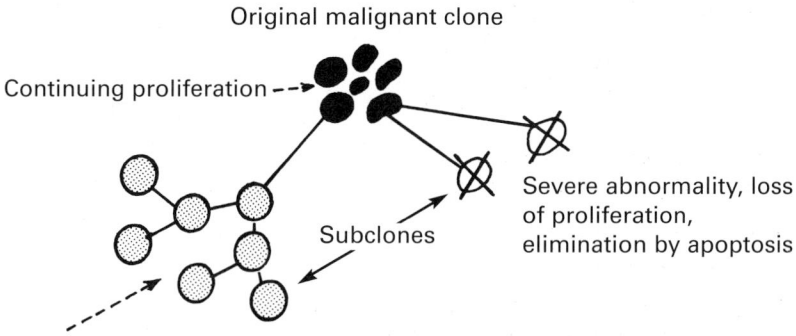

Nuclear morphology and DNA content

In histological sections these abnormalities are indicated by variations in nuclear density (usually increased), size and shape (i.e. PLEOMORPHISM).

The term 'POLYPLOIDY' is used when the nuclear DNA is increased by exact multiples of the normal.

'ANEUPLOIDY' indicates irregular increases in DNA content.→ 

CARCINOGENESIS

A number of factors, both environmental and genetic, contribute to a cell undergoing malignant change. This should be regarded as a multistep sequence (see p. 154).

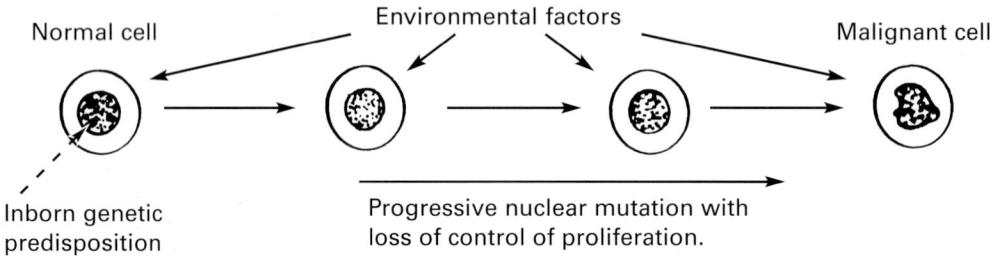

ENVIRONMENTAL FACTORS

The 3 major environmental factors which induce tumours are 1. Chemical carcinogens, 2. Radiation and 3. Viruses.

CHEMICAL CARCINOGENESIS

Historically, chemical agents were the first to be associated with cancer. Now, many are recognised in (a) industrial processes, (b) social habits and (c) diet.

Industry	Tumour	Chemical Responsible
Aniline dyes	Bladder cancer	Naphthylamine
Insulation e.g. shipbuilding, building	Mesothelioma, lung, laryngeal cancer	Asbestos
Mineral oil and tar	Skin cancers	Benzpyrene and other hydrocarbons
Plastics	Angiosarcomas of liver	Vinyl chloride monomer
Wood dust	Cancer of nose and sinuses	?

Social Habits

Cigarette smoking is strongly associated with the development of many cancers, including lung, mouth, larynx and bladder. Chewing tobacco greatly increases the risk of oral cancer. It is likely that air pollution, e.g. combustion products of petrol and diesel, also contributes to carcinogenesis.

Diet

Chemicals in food may be carcinogenic. Nitrosamines may be formed by the action of bacteria on ingested nitrites. AFLATOXINS are produced by fungi (Aspergillus flavus) and by contaminating foodstuffs may cause liver cancer.

Note: Chemical carcinogens may act in 2 ways:

1. Directly at the site of application or portal of entry e.g. skin and lung cancers.
2. After modification, either at the sites of metabolism or excretion e.g. liver and urinary tract tumours.

CARCINOGENESIS

CHEMICAL CARCINOGENESIS (continued)

This is a multistep process of long duration.

The stages of **initiation** and **promotion** are important and are exemplified in experimental skin carcinogenesis.

(1) **Normal skin**

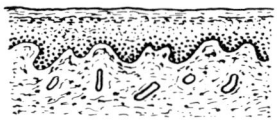

Application of carcinogen e.g. Benzpyrene (a mutagen) → (2) **INITIATION** Skin appears normal but important changes have occurred in the cell's DNA.

(3) **PROMOTION** — initiated by co-carcinogens e.g. croton oil, turpentine. (These agents are not mutagenic but act by stimulating cell proliferation.) Visible surface and histological changes are seen.

(a) Keratosis and papilloma formation

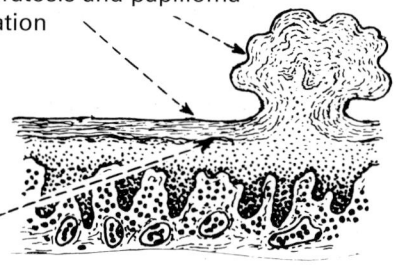

Proliferation of epithelium

(b) Dysplasia i.e. cytological features of malignancy, but no invasion (see p. 144).

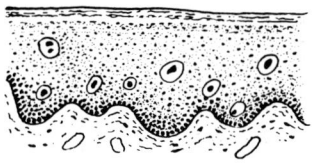

These stages are reversible

(4) **Appearance of MALIGNANT TUMOUR** — [An irreversible change]

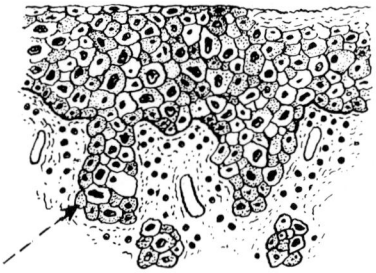

Breech of basement membrane: **INVASION**

The order of application of these agents is important. No tumour follows application of promotor alone, or promotor *followed* by initiator.

In rodents, these changes take months; in humans the time scale is years and is exemplified in the skin, cervix uteri, bronchus, urinary bladder, colon and breast.

CARCINOGENESIS

RADIANT ENERGY

The potential dangers from irradiation give much cause for concern.

Source of Radiation	Tumours	Type of Radiation
Sunlight	Melanoma, Carcinoma of skin	Ultraviolet (non-ionising)
Nuclear explosions (e.g. atom bombs, Chernobyl)	Leukaemia, carcinomas of lung, breast, thyroid	
Therapeutic irradiation	Various carcinomas, sarcomas, leukaemia	Ionising
Mining radioactive substances e.g. Uranium	Lung carcinomas	Ionising
X-ray workers (historical)	Skin cancer, leukaemia	X-rays Ionising

Effects of Irradiation on Cells

The ionising effect of radiation damages the cell's DNA, especially during cell proliferation, ranging from single gene mutation to major chromosome damage, including breaks, deletions and translocations.

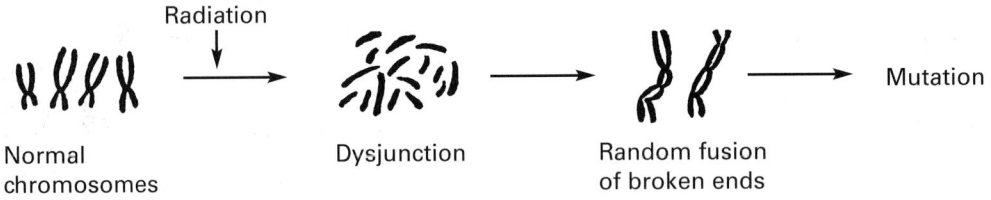

Proliferating cells are particularly vulnerable. Marrow, gastro-intestinal mucosa are highly sensitive.

Ultraviolet light is of low energy and mainly affects the skin. The 'PYRIMIDINE DIMERS' formed by UV light are normally excised by DNA repair mechanisms. In **xeroderma pigmentosum**, these are deficient leading to numerous skin tumours.

CARCINOGENESIS – VIRUSES

Viruses have long been known to cause cancer in animals (e.g. the mouse mammary tumour virus — the Bittner milk factor).

In recent years viruses have been shown to contribute to the development of some human cancers.

Virus	Type	Tumour type
Epstein-Barr (E.B.V.)	DNA	Burkett's lymphoma, nasopharyngeal cancer, Hodgkin's disease, post-transplantation lymphomas
Hepatitis 'B'	DNA	Hepatocellular carcinomas
Human papilloma virus (HPV)	DNA	Cervical, penile, anal carcinoma
Human 'T' cell leukaemia virus (HTLV-1)	RNA (Retrovirus)	T-lymphoblastic leukaemia

Mode of action on oncogenic viruses

The essential feature is addition of new DNA to the nucleus of host cells resulting in mutants, but the way in which this is achieved differs in the two types of virus.

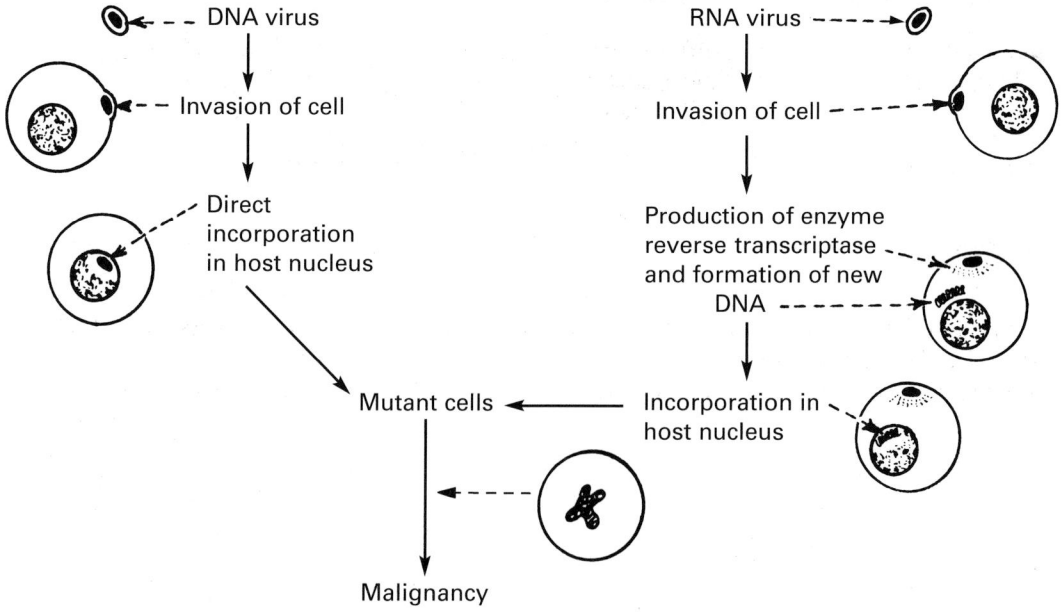

CARCINOGENESIS – HEREDITY

The inherited genetic influences in cancer are now well recognised.

1. There is a high risk of cancer in some uncommon syndromes inherited as Mendelian traits.

Illustrative examples are:

(a) **Familial adenomatous polyposis coli** (APC). An autosomal dominant condition. Numerous polyps occur in the colon in late childhood (10–14 years) and inevitably lead to adenocarcinoma in early middle age (30–45 years). The APC gene responsible lies on chromosome 5.

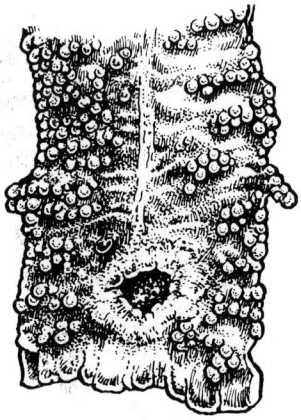

(b) **Xeroderma pigmentosum.** An autosomal recessive trait where failure of DNA repair mechanism leads to skin cancer.

(c) **Neurofibromatosis** — multiple neurofibromas (NF) — with a 1% risk of sarcoma, is due to a defect of NF-1 gene on chromosome 17.

(d) **Retinoblastoma** — an autosomal dominant (Rb gene on chromosome 13), (p. 153).

2. A less well defined, but strong familial tendency, is seen with some common tumours. For some the gene is identified e.g. BRCA-1 gene, chromosome 17-60% risk of breast or ovarian cancer by 50 years.

3. In some families, there is a high risk of several types of cancer. In the rare Li-Fraumeni syndrome, childhood sarcomas, breast cancer in young women, and many other cancers are seen. This is due to a germ-line mutation of the p53 gene (p. 153).

Illustrative Family Tree:

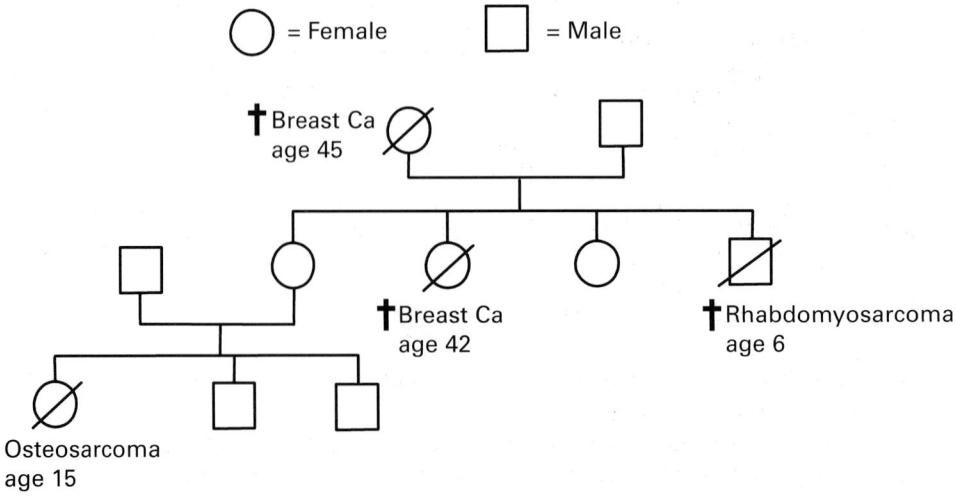

ONCOGENES AND TUMOUR SUPPRESSOR GENES

Cellular proto-oncogenes are NORMAL genes which STIMULATE cell division. Tumour suppressor genes are NORMAL genes which INHIBIT cell division. Their normal activity during somatic growth and in regeneration and repair takes place during the G_1–G_0 phase of the cell cycle and is strictly controlled.

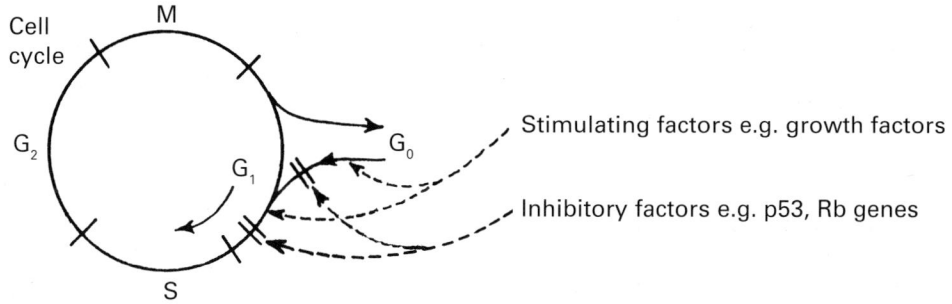

In cancer cells the normal controls are defective so that the balance between factors stimulating and inhibiting cell growth is permanently lost, resulting in increased proliferation.

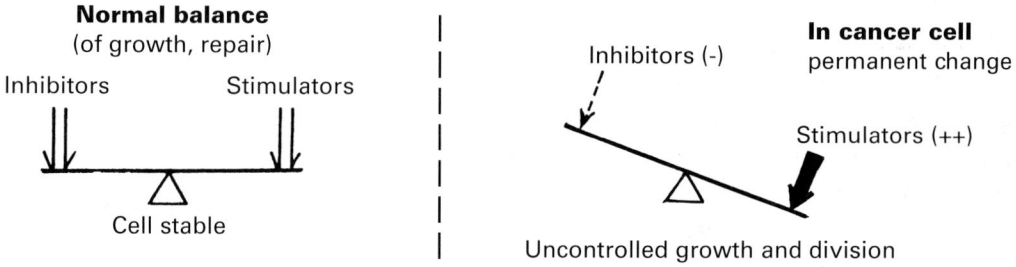

Cellular proto-oncogenes code for a number of proteins involved in cell proliferation:

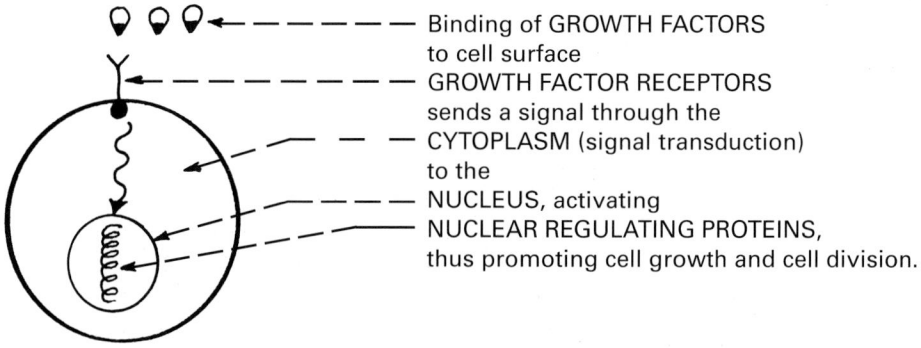

In the cancer cell, these normal genes are permanently changed to ONCOGENES and proliferation is uncontrolled.

Mutation or overexpression of genes which normally control APOPTOSIS (page 4) are increasingly recognised in many tumours e.g. overexpression of *bcl-2* inhibits apoptosis in Follicle Centre Lymphoma (page 448).

ONCOGENES

The production and activity of ONCOGENESIS is complex and there are many ways in which they are activated.

The following are a few illustrative examples.

1. **Production of excess NORMAL protein**

(a) Gene amplification e.g. neuroblastoma (*myc* type gene)

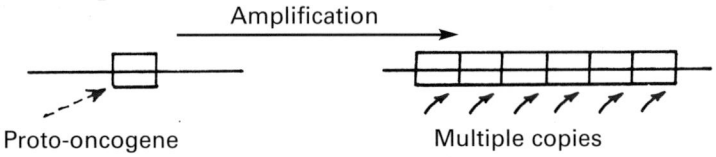

(b) Increased mRNA transcription due to chromosomal translocation e.g. in Burkett's LYMPHOMA chromosomes 8 and 14 are involved.

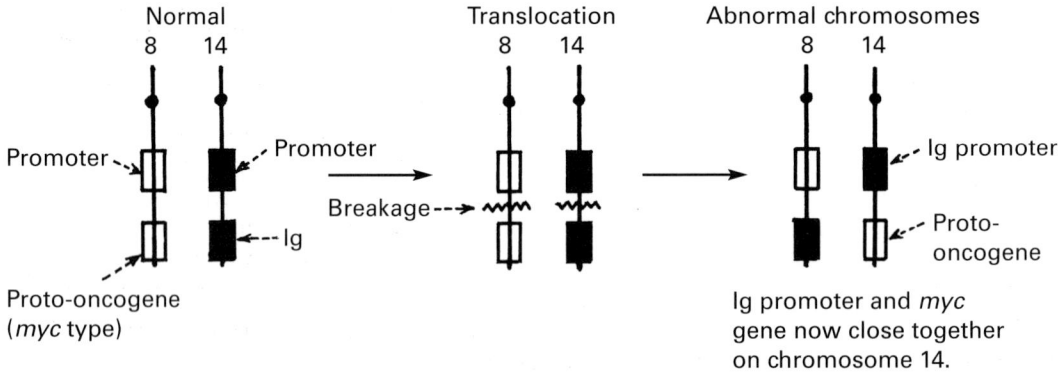

The myc oncogene is now under the influence of the Ig gene control and is permanently switched on.

2. **Production of FUNCTIONALLY ABNORMAL PROTEIN**

A point mutation of the proto-oncogene produces a protein with an altered function so that over-stimulation occurs.

Altered growth **factor receptor function** is an example.

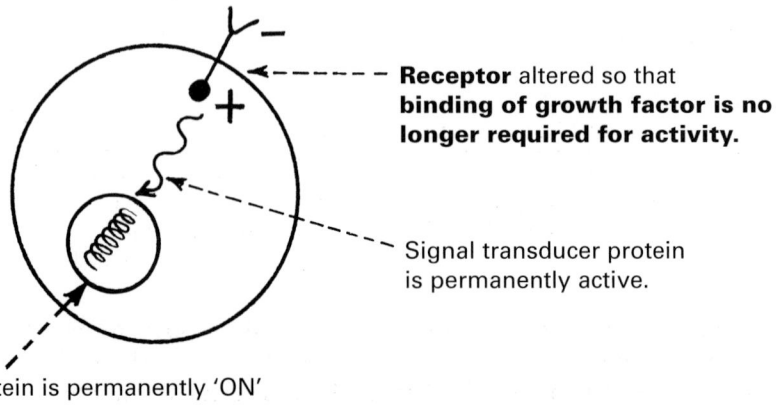

TUMOUR SUPPRESSOR GENES

Tumour suppressor genes are normal genes which switch off cell proliferation by acting on the cell cycle in G_1. Their biological role is much broader than simply suppressing tumour function, but the name reflects how they have been discovered.

Loss of *both* copies of a tumour suppressor gene is required for cancer to develop. In contrast, only one copy of a given oncogene needs to be activated to cause excess proliferation.

Examples are:

Tumour suppressor gene	Chromosome	Tumours
P53	17	Carcinoma of Lung and breast: Sarcomas
Retinoblastoma (Rb)	13	Retinoblastoma, Sarcoma: some carcinomas
NF1	17	Neurofibromas, malignant peripheral nerve tumours
APC	5	Colonic carcinoma
WT1	11	Wilm's tumour, bladder cancer, breast cancer: rhabdomyosarcoma

p53 gene: This gene codes for a nuclear phosphoprotein, which is expressed in increased amounts following cellular damage e.g. **irradiation.**

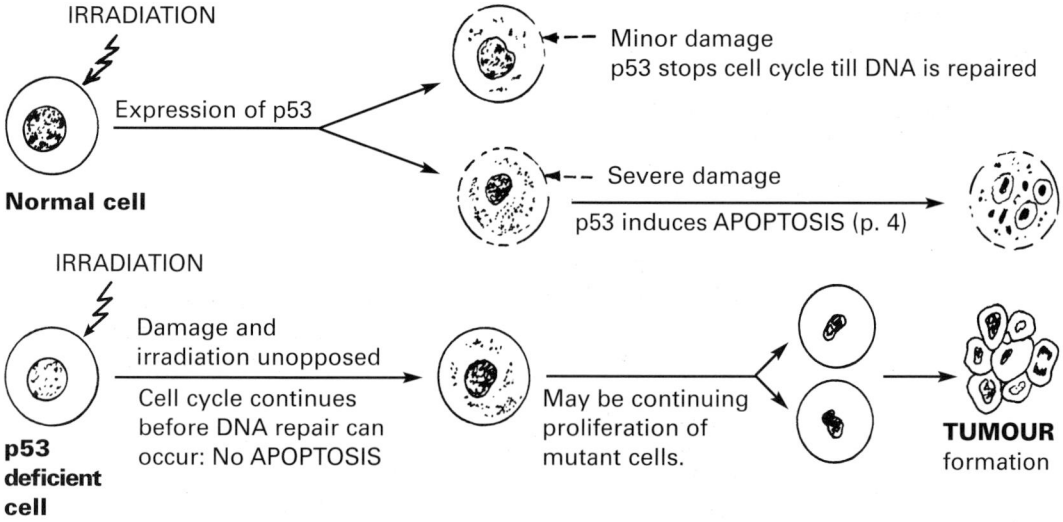

p53 has been called the 'Guardian of the genome'. Abnormalities of p53 are found in at least 30% of all cancers.

Germ line p53 mutation is a feature of the Li-Fraumeni syndrome.

CARCINOGENESIS – SUMMARY

The MULTISTEP STAIRWAY to MALIGNANCY

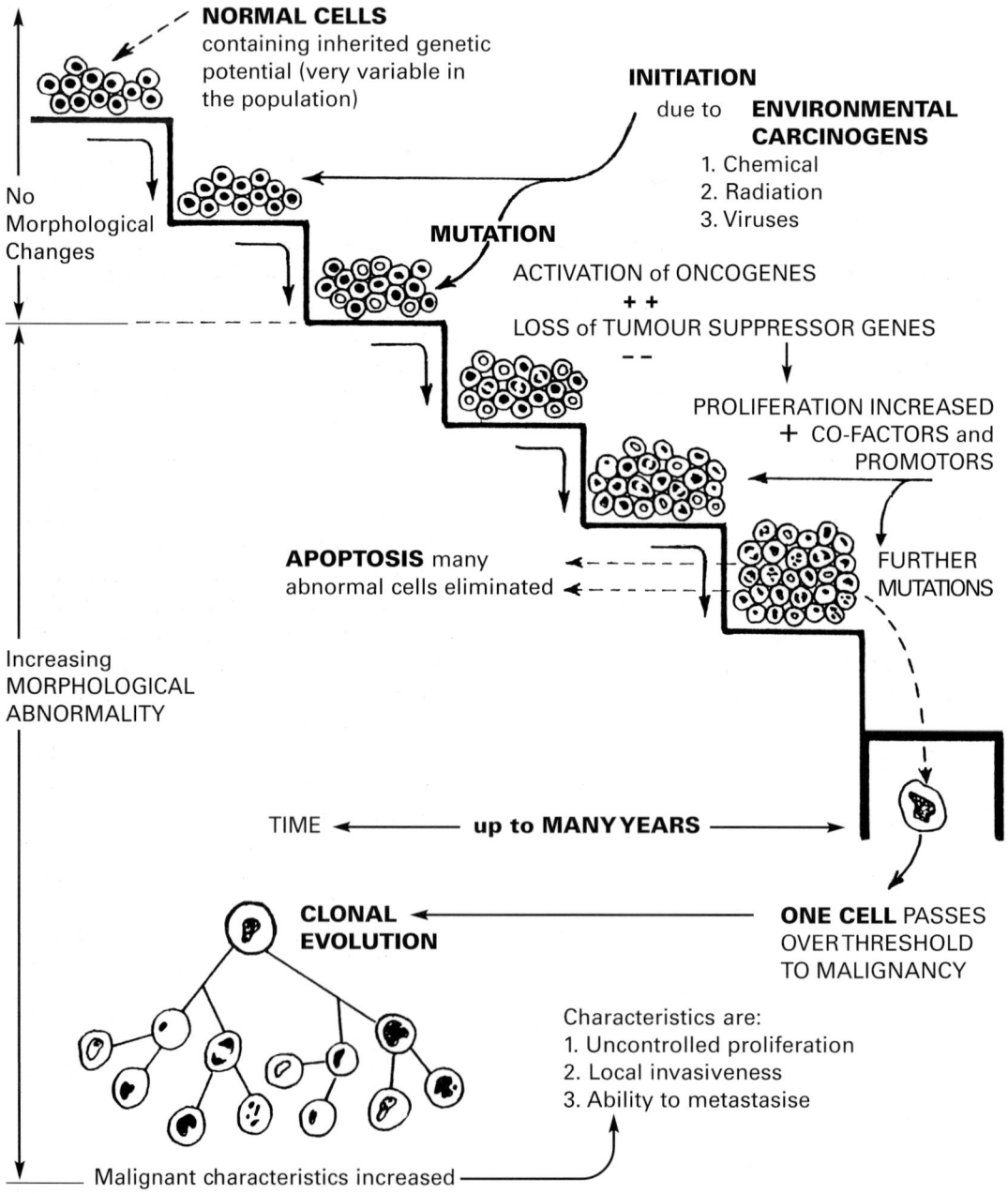

CHAPTER 7

CARDIOVASCULAR DISEASES

General Considerations 156
Factors Leading to Thrombosis 157, 158
Common Sites and Types of Thrombus 159, 160
Sequels of Thrombosis 161
Embolism 162, 163
Arterial Obstruction 164
Important Sites of Infarction 165
Normal Tissue Fluid Circulation 166
Oedema 167
Shock 168–172
Shock — Individual Organs 173–176
Shock — Individual Organs: Outcome 177
Cardiac Function 178
Heart Failure 179–184
Effects of Heart Failure 185
Acute Pulmonary Oedema 186
Heart Failure 187, 188
High Output Cardiac Failure 189
Diseases of Arteries — Arteriosclerosis 190
Atheroma (Atherosclerosis) 191
Atheroma — Complications 192
Atheroma — Aetiology 193–195
Atheroma — Aetiology: Current Interventions 196
Hypertension 197,198
Hypertension — Essential and Secondary 199
Hypertension 200, 201
Ischaemic Heart Disease 202
Myocardial Infarction 203–209
Chronic Ischaemic Heart Disease 210
Ischaemic Heart Disease 211, 212
Miscellaneous Affections of the Myocardium 213–215
Rheumatic Fever 216–218
Valvular Heart Disease 219
Mitral Valve Disease 220, 221
Aortic Valve Disease 222, 223
Infective Endocarditis 224, 225
Cardiac Arrhythmias 226, 227
Congenital Heart Disease 228
Diseases of the Pericardium 229, 230
Cardiac Tumours 230
Diseases of Arteries 231–233
Aneurysms 234–237
Arterial Diseases — Miscellaneous 238
Diseases of Veins 239
Thrombophlebitis 240
Varicose Veins 241–243
Diseases of Lymphatics 244
Lymphatic Obstruction 245
Vascular Tumours 246, 247
Kaposi's Sarcoma 248

GENERAL CONSIDERATIONS

Cardiovascular diseases are the commonest cause of death in Westernised communities. The main forms are:

1. **Ischaemic heart disease.** 2. **Cerebrovascular diseases.**

Some general abnormalities of the circulation require to be discussed first.

THROMBOSIS

A thrombus is a mass formed from blood constituents within a vessel or the heart during life. Blood clotting is a physiological protective mechanism but thrombosis is a pathological process with serious consequences.

MECHANISM OF FORMATION

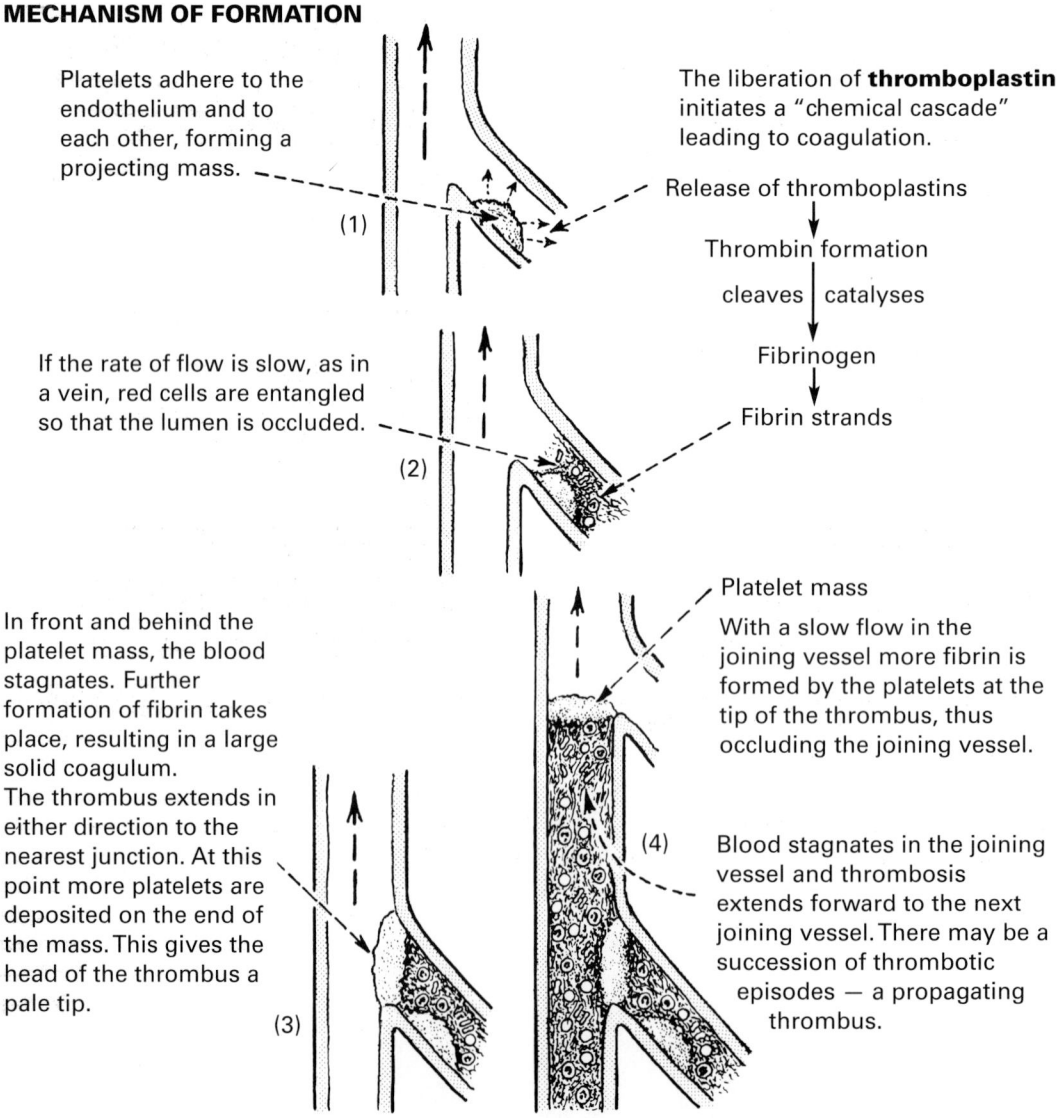

FACTORS LEADING TO THROMBOSIS

The 3 MAIN factors leading to thrombosis are known as Virchow's triad: they are closely concerned with local changes in the coagulability of the blood (see pages 425 et seq.).

1. ALTERATIONS OF BLOOD FLOW

The main effect is to bring platelets into contact with the vessel wall. This results from:
Slowing of blood flow, e.g. in cardiac failure or during bed rest. With slowing, the normal axial stream of blood cells is lost and white cells and platelets fall out of the main stream and accumulate in the peripheral plasma zone.

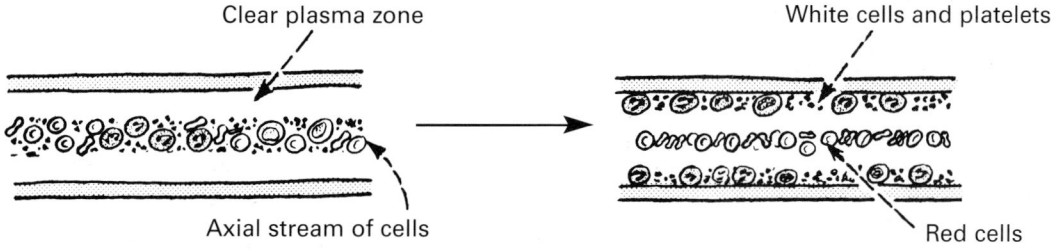

Turbulence, e.g. by deformation of vessel wall or around venous valves.

Local increase in lumen, as in varicose veins or aneurysm, causes eddies and platelets and white cells fall out of main stream.

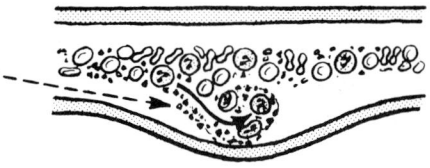

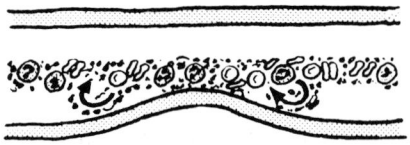

Swelling or compression of vessel wall by disease. Eddies form in front and behind obstruction.

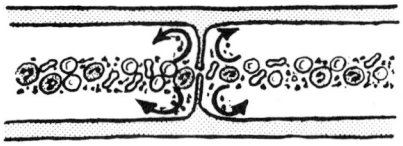

Eddies form around valves if flow slows.

These changes in flow and shear stress cause altered endothelial function with increased production of agents which promote thrombosis (page 158).

FACTORS LEADING TO THROMBOSIS

2. DAMAGE TO ENDOTHELIUM OF VESSEL

This leads to platelet adhesion and aggregation. Common causes are:

(a) Disease in vessel wall e.g. atheroma.

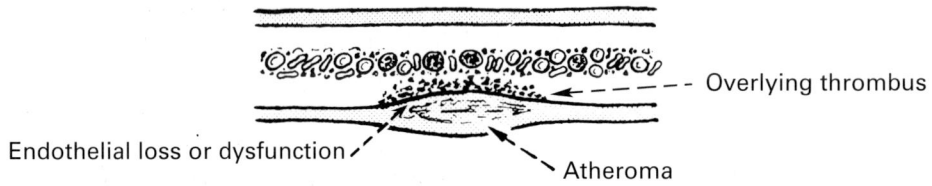

(b) Toxins from nearby inflammatory processes.
(c) Local compression of vessels (e.g. during operations).

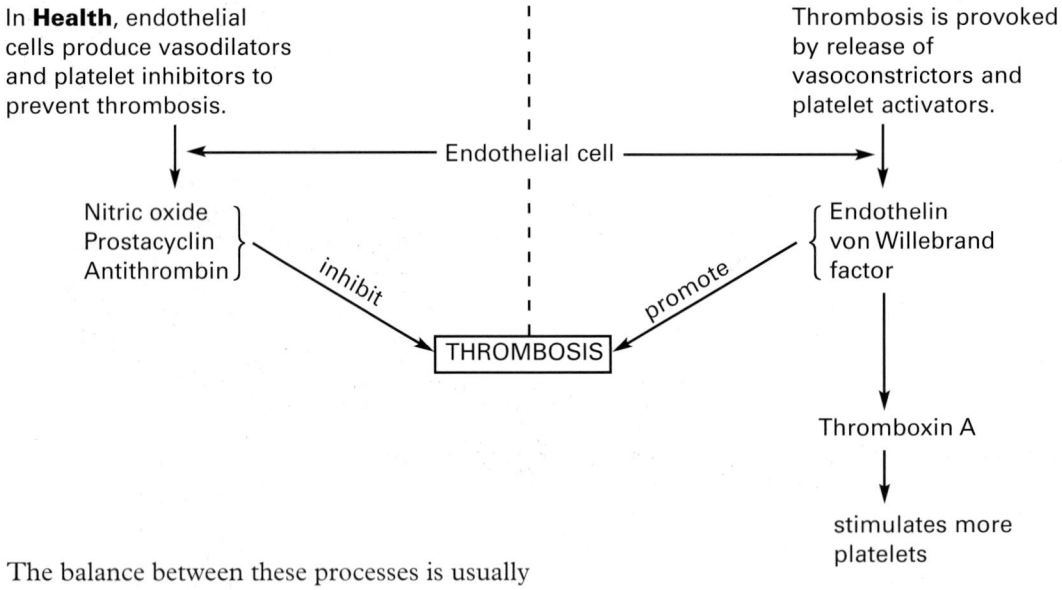

The balance between these processes is usually AGAINST THROMBOSIS.

3. CHANGES IN COMPOSITION of the BLOOD

(a) INCREASE in platelets, fibrinogen and prothrombin after operations and childbirth: usually after 5–10 days.
(b) INCREASE in platelet adhesiveness – again after surgery.
(c) Rare inherited abnormalities of thrombosis inhibitors – e.g. antithrombin C deficiency: protein C deficiency.
(d) Miscellaneous factors e.g. oral contraceptives, smoking, some cancers.

COMMON SITES AND TYPES OF THROMBUS

ARTERIAL

Thrombi are common in arteries as a complication of **atheroma**. Forming in a rapid circulation, the thrombus consists mainly of PLATELETS (WHITE thrombus).

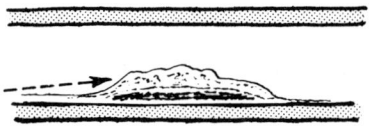

Common sites include:

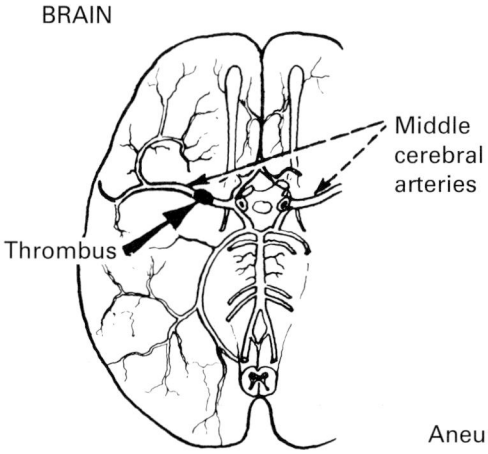

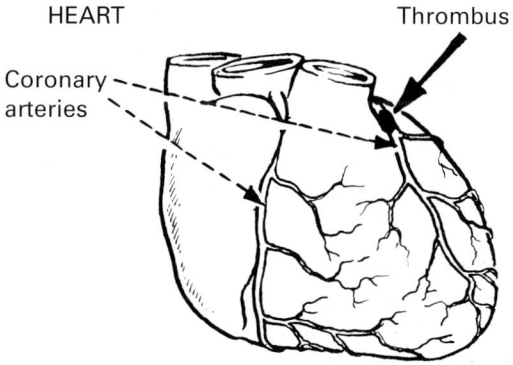

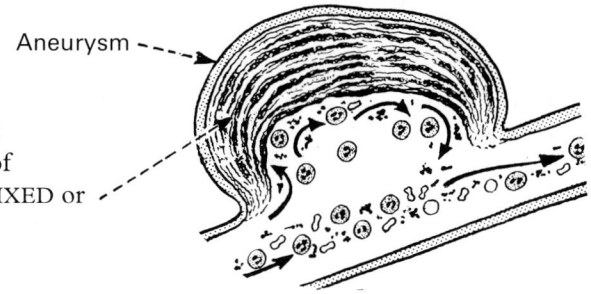

Thrombus formation is common in the walls of **aneurysms**, consisting of layers of red and white thrombus (MIXED or LAMINATED thrombus).

VENOUS

Systemic venous thrombosis is common because of the slow blood flow and lower pressure. It consists of red cells, platelets and fibrin (RED thrombus).

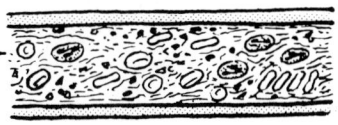

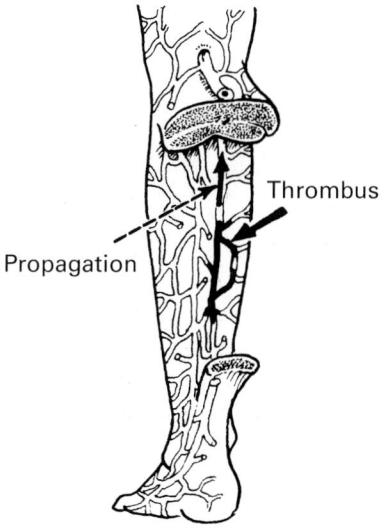

It is most common in the deep veins of the calf and frequently propagates in the femoral and iliac veins — from where it may embolise to the lungs (p.162).

Bed rest, operations and cardiac disease are predisposing conditions.

Portal thrombosis is a rare complication of abdominal disease e.g. hepatic cirrhosis.

COMMON SITES OF THROMBOSIS

CAPILLARY

Thrombi, composed mainly of fused red cells, form when capillaries are damaged, usually in acute inflammatory processes.

Capillaries are occluded by fibrin thrombi in cases of disseminated intravascular coagulation (DIC – see page 430).

CARDIAC

Thrombi may be seen in the ATRIA (especially in the auricles in ATRIAL FIBRILLATION); in the VENTRICLES and on the heart VALVES.

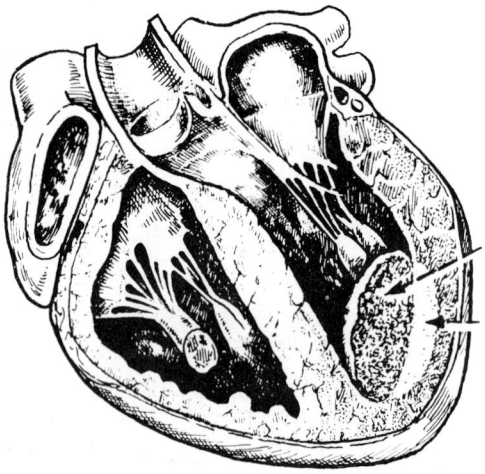

Red and pale thrombi occur in ventricles, especially the left: such thrombi are usually secondary to INFARCTION of the ventricular wall.

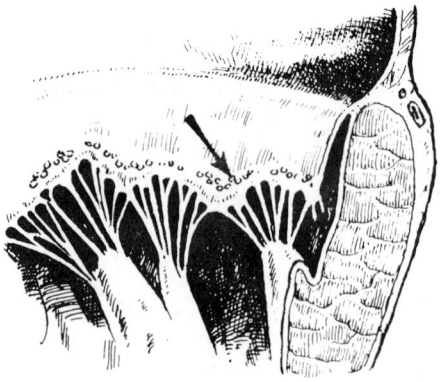

Thrombi of pale variety occur on the heart valves in rheumatic endocarditis.

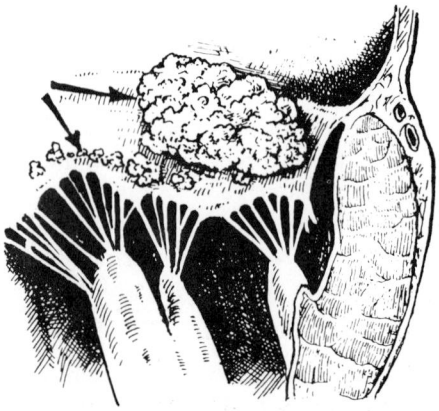

Sometimes infective endocarditis occurs and the thrombi are larger, mixed, friable and contain masses of micro-organisms.

SEQUELS OF THROMBOSIS

1. **FIBRINOLYSIS**
   Many small thrombi are completely removed by the **Fibrinolytic System** which exists to limit thrombosis.

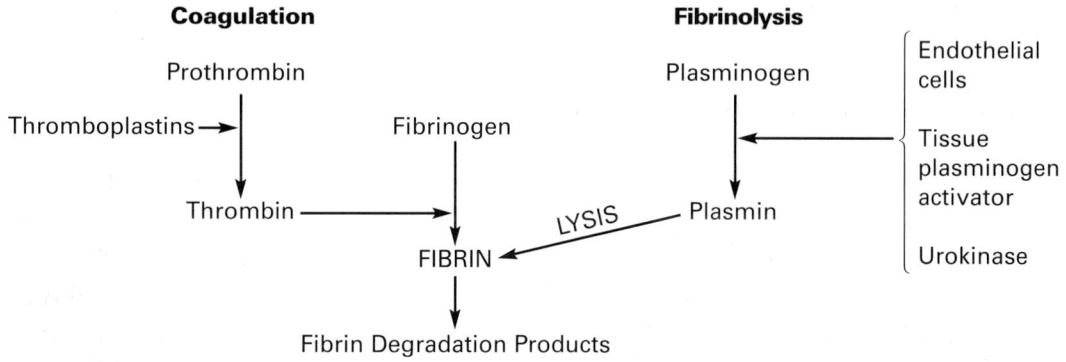

2. **ORGANISATION**
   Capillaries grow into the point of thrombus attachment within a day or two. Fibroblasts and phagocytic cells accompany the capillaries, and gradually the thrombus material is dissolved and replaced by a fibrovascular tissue. At the same time endothelium covers the ends of the thrombus, thus limiting the thrombotic process.

Ultimately, the branching capillaries may be converted into one or two stouter vessels which may partially restore the circulation through the vessel— RECANALISATION.

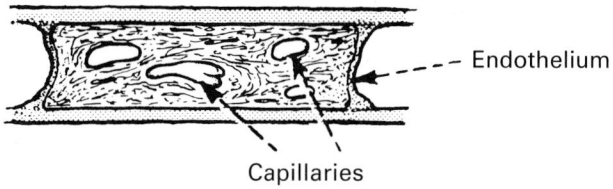

3. **CALCIFICATION**
   In diseased vessels, organisation may not take place. The thrombus shrinks, calcium salts are deposited and convert it into a phlebolith — seen in X-rays.

4. **INCORPORATION**
   A mural thrombus, e.g. in a large artery, may be covered by endothelium and incorporated in the vessel wall. This process may be important in the formation of atheroma.

5. **EMBOLISM**
   Part of the thrombus may be detached and carried along in the blood stream to impact in a distant vessel. This is extremely important clinically.

PROPHYLAXIS and THERAPY of thrombosis aims at:

1. Reducing coagulability utilising (a) anticoagulants aimed at specific sites in the coagulation cascade e.g. warfarin derivatives, heparin (see p. 431) and (b) inhibiting specific prostaglandin synthesis e.g. aspirin.
2. Encouraging fibrinolysis, using fibrinolysins.

EMBOLISM

An embolus is any abnormal mass of matter carried in the blood stream and large enough to **occlude some vessel**.

The commonest emboli are derived from material generated within the vascular system e.g. fragments of thrombus or material from atheromatous plaques. (Less common emboli are described on next page.)

1. **Pulmonary thrombo-embolism**

   Emboli from the systemic veins (especially deep venous thrombosis) pass through the right side of the heart to the pulmonary circulation. The consequences depend on the size of the embolus and the patient's previous health.

   (i) **Massive** embolus → blocks main pulmonary artery trunk → acute total circulatory block → SUDDEN DEATH.

   (ii) **Moderate** embolus

   With a double blood supply — pulmonary and bronchial arteries — and a vast anastomosis, obstruction of a pulmonary artery branch does not necessarily cause infarction. When there is pre-existing circulatory stagnation within the lung, the arrival of an embolus in the pulmonary arterial tree will cause infarction.

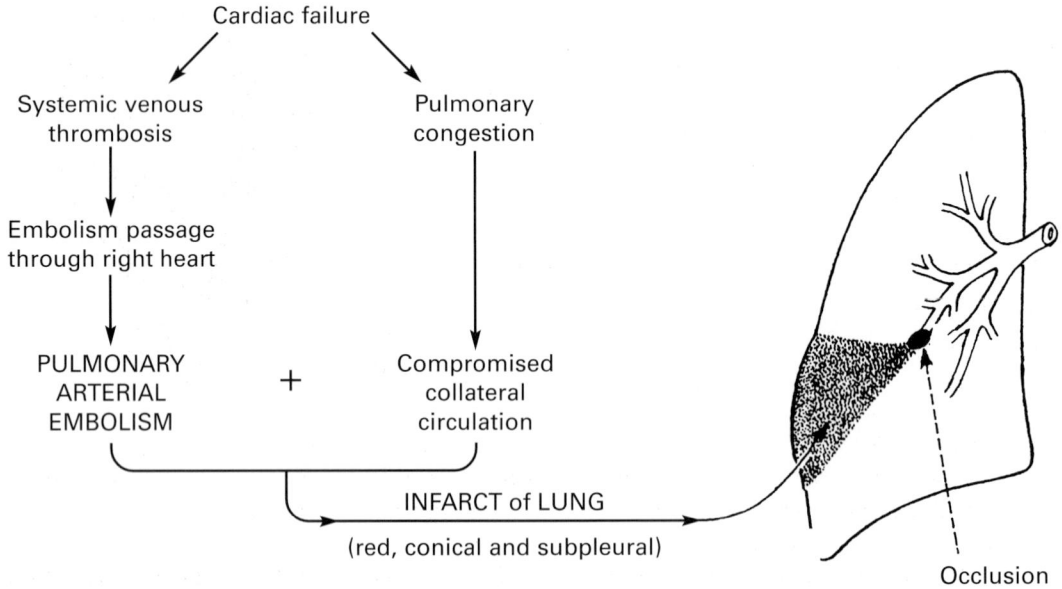

   (iii) **Small** emboli

   Many are removed by the fibrinolytic system and are asymptomatic. However, repeated minor emboli may result in pulmonary hypertension.

   Repeated small emboli → blockage of peripheral pulmonary arterial branches → **pulmonary hypertension**.

2. **Emboli of the arterial system** are derived from the heart or the larger arteries which have become atheromatous. The results of arterial obstruction are very important.

EMBOLISM

EMBOLISM — Other forms

Matter entering the vascular system may be
(a) *Solid* e.g. tumour cells, bacterial clumps, fat, parasites.
(b) *Gaseous* — air
(c) *Liquid* e.g. amniotic fluid with fetal derived matter.

Fat embolism

This may occur when a long bone is fractured, usually 24–72 hours later. Fat globules enter torn veins and pass to lungs; obstruction of pulmonary blood flow may be sufficient to cause *anoxia*. Cerebral symptoms are common due to anoxia but also the arrival in the brain of fat particles which have passed through the lung capillaries.

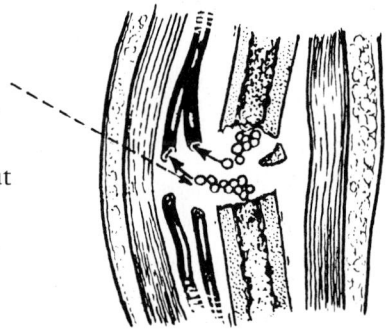

Amniotic fluid embolism

During parturition, amniotic fluid may enter a uterine vein, especially after manipulations or with certain obstetric treatments. Vernix, hairs and squames enter the circulation. In addition to embolic phenomena, there are also coagulation disorders (page 430).

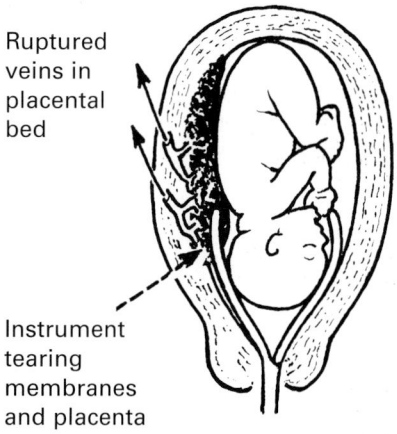

Embolism in drug addicts

Lung lesions occur in addicts using intravenous injection due to particulate matter (e.g. talc).

Gas embolism

This occurs mainly in 2 forms:

(a) *Single embolism*
Atmospheric air may enter the blood when a neck or intracranial vein is incised. Inspiration induces a suction effect by causing a negative pressure in the veins. As a result of frothing in the right ventricle, cardiac action is seriously impaired.

(b) *Multiple embolism,* in 'Caisson disease'
This occurs in persons working in barometric pressures of several atmospheres, e.g. diving to great depths. The atmospheric gases go into solution in high concentration in the blood and tissues. If decompression occurs too quickly, these gases 'boil' off and appear as bubbles in the circulation. The oxygen is taken up by the tissues but insoluble gases cause widespread 'embolism', especially in the nervous system and bone.

ARTERIAL OBSTRUCTION

Arterial obstruction is usually due to thrombosis or embolism and may be (i) partial or complete, (ii) acute or slowly progressive.

The effects depend on the local anatomy, particularly on the presence of an anastomotic collateral circulation.

Occlusion of end arteries

These may have (a) no collaterals (e.g. splenic artery),
(b) capillary anastomoses (e.g. renal and coronary arteries),
(c) arterial anastomoses which are too small to maintain circulation (e.g. superior mesenteric artery).

Result:

Obstruction → anoxia of tissues → necrosis (INFARCT — a 'stuffing' of tissue — Latin).

INFARCTS

An infarct is an area of necrosis due to ischaemia. It is often found at the periphery of an organ e.g. the kidney.

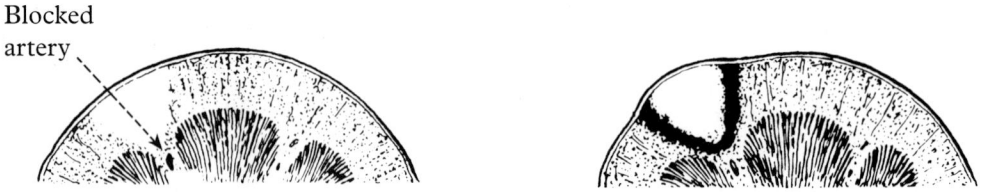

After 12 hours: Area is pale. Degenerative changes already seen with electron microscope or histochemical tests.

After 36 hours: Area shows pallor and swelling due to coagulative necrosis. The surrounding tissues are congested.

Healing

This takes place slowly. Capillaries and fibroblasts replace the necrotic tissue. Collagen is formed, contracts and results in a depressed scar.

IMPORTANT SITES OF INFARCTION

The HEART, the LUNGS and the BRAIN are the most common sites. Less common are the SMALL INTESTINES (with serious effects) and the kidney and spleen (less serious).

IMPORTANT SITES OF INFARCTION

HEART

Infarction is almost always due to coronary arterial thrombosis complicating atheroma.

Cardiac action is immediately upset, eddies form, the endocardium may be damaged and a thrombus form on the inner surface of the infarcted area. The damage may extend to the external surface causing pericarditis.

If the patient survives, the infarct heals by fibrosis.

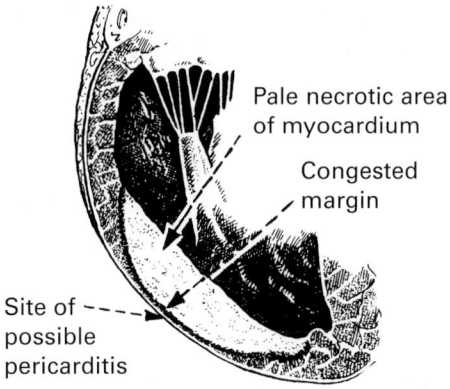

BRAIN

Infarcts are commonly due to thrombosis of diseased vessels or to embolism from the left heart or carotid arteries, e.g. MIDDLE CEREBRAL, posterior cerebral and basilar arteries.

The usual changes of infarction take place, but the necrosis is colliquative – **cerebral softening.**

Infarction may occur without arterial occlusion in severe, prolonged hypotension (shock).

Parts of the brain at the junction of arterial territories are affected (boundary zone or watershed infarcts) (see page 176).

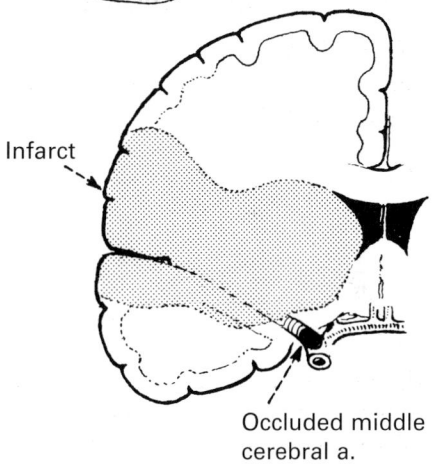

INTESTINE

Infarction may follow thrombosis of or embolisation to the mesenteric arteries. The sequence of changes usually seen in solid organs is altered by the effects of anastomoses and, in the later stages, by **bacterial invasion.**

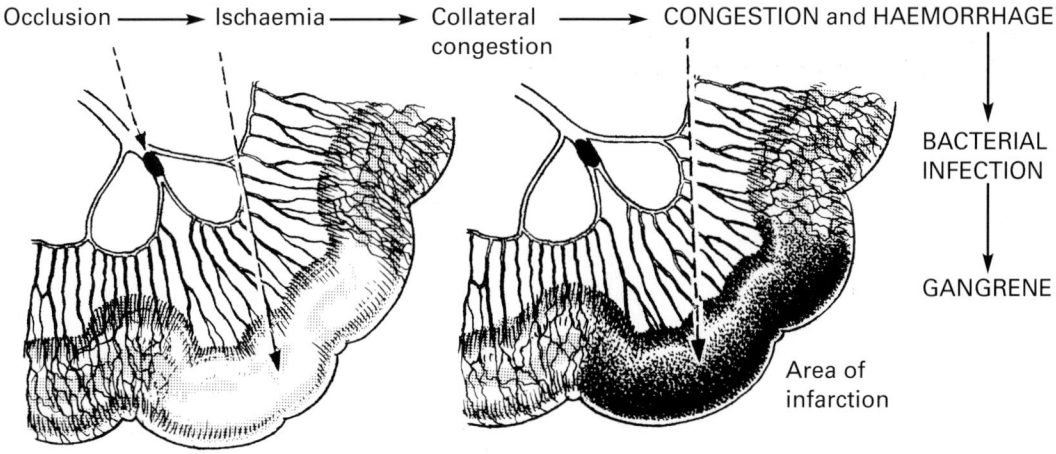

NORMAL TISSUE FLUID CIRCULATION

There is a continuous interchange of fluid between blood and tissues. Some fluid enters the lymphatics before eventually returning to the blood stream. Two main forces operate pressure gradients controlling the fluid movement.

1. ***Hydrostatic pressure,*** i.e. capillary blood pressure (BP) encouraging the passage of fluid through the capillary wall, = 35 mm mercury.
2. ***Protein osmotic pressure,*** (OP), i.e. the plasma proteins encourage the retention of fluid in the capillaries to maintain osmotic equilibrium. This pressure is equivalent to 25 mm mercury.

At the arterial end the blood pressure is greater than the osmotic pressure and fluid is forced out of the capillary. The reverse is true at the venous end and fluid is attracted into the vessel.

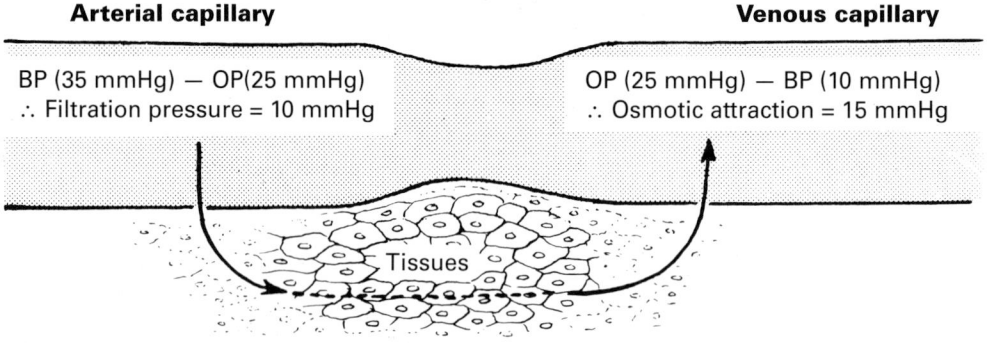

A small amount of fluid enters lymphatics. This is partly the result of tissue pressure and partly due to osmotic attraction of proteins in the lymphatic system.

In addition to those forces operating at capillary level, there are other mechanisms which influence the movement of fluid within the body in a general manner.

1. **Fluid intake**
   Intake via the gut or parenterally may exceed the ability of the kidneys to eliminate water.
2. **Integrity of the kidneys**
   Damage to the renal parenchyma may diminish the elimination of fluid.
3. **Hormone activity**

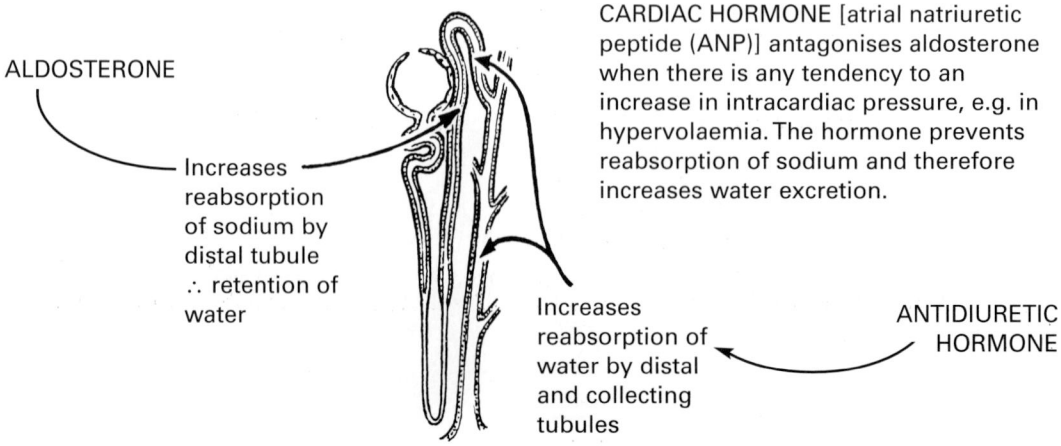

OEDEMA

Oedema is an accumulation of excess fluid in the extravascular tissues. It can be local or generalised. A wide variety of causes of oedema can be explained by their effects on the pressure gradients described on the previous page.

DECREASE in blood osmotic pressure
(usually due to HYPOALBUMINAEMIA)

Common causes:
Liver disease — deficient synthesis.
Renal disease — protein loss.
Starvation.

INCREASE in venous pressure
(hydrostatic pressure ↑)

Common causes:
Cardiac failure.
Venous obstruction in lower limbs.

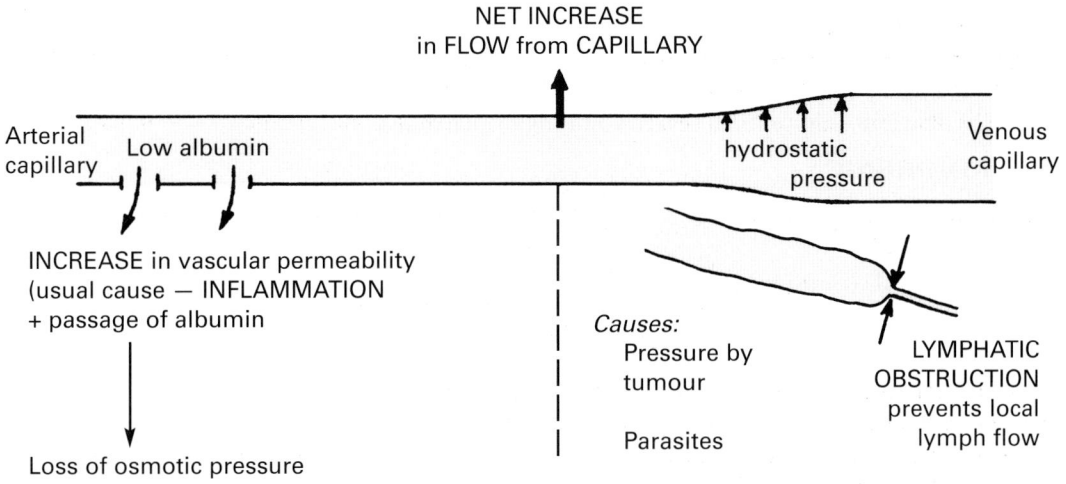

More than one factor may apply:

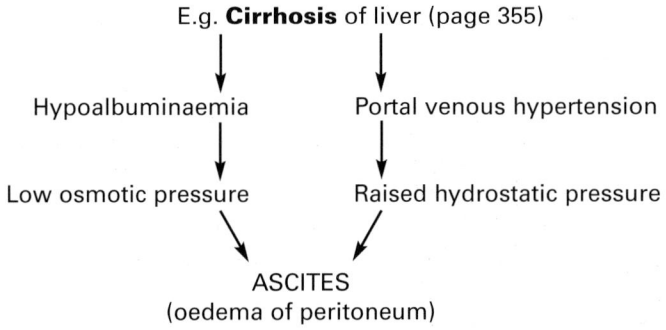

Cerebral (p. 551) and pulmonary oedema (p. 186) are life threatening and are dealt with separately.

SHOCK

Shock is a condition in which the vital functions of the body are depressed due to a severe and acute reduction in cardiac output and effective circulating blood volume. There is progressive cardiovascular collapse characterised by hypotension, hyperventilation and clouding of consciousness. Subsequently there is oliguria.

CAUSES

There are many causes, conveniently grouped under 4 main headings:

1. HYPOVOLAEMIC (i.e. diminished blood volume)
Associated with:

(a) **Trauma**
- (i) Severe haemorrhage — external or internal
- (ii) Severe injury — especially fractures of bones and crushing of tissues
- (iii) Burning — especially where extensive surface damage allows loss of a large amount of exudate.

(b) **Dehydration** — in cases of severe vomiting or diarrhoea.

2. **CARDIOGENIC**
Acute diseases of the heart — especially myocardial infarction — in which there is a sudden fall in cardiac output.

3. **BACTERIAL (Septic, bacteraemic, endotoxic)**
In serious bacterial infections (especially Gram-negative organisms, e.g. *E. coli* and *bacteroides*).

4. **ANAPHYLAXIS** — a severe immune hypersensitivity reaction (p. 102).

EFFECTS

The loss of effective circulating blood causes tissue and cell damage and, at the same time, initiates reactive changes in the circulation.

These two mechanisms combine to cause the shock syndrome.

The main consequences of shock are:

1. Low cardiac output.
2. Hypotension.
3. Impaired tissue perfusion.
4. Cellular hypoxia.

SHOCK

REACTIVE CHANGES — EARLY STAGE

These changes are concerned with the maintenance of an adequate cerebral and coronary circulation and are effected by a redistribution of the blood in the body as a whole.

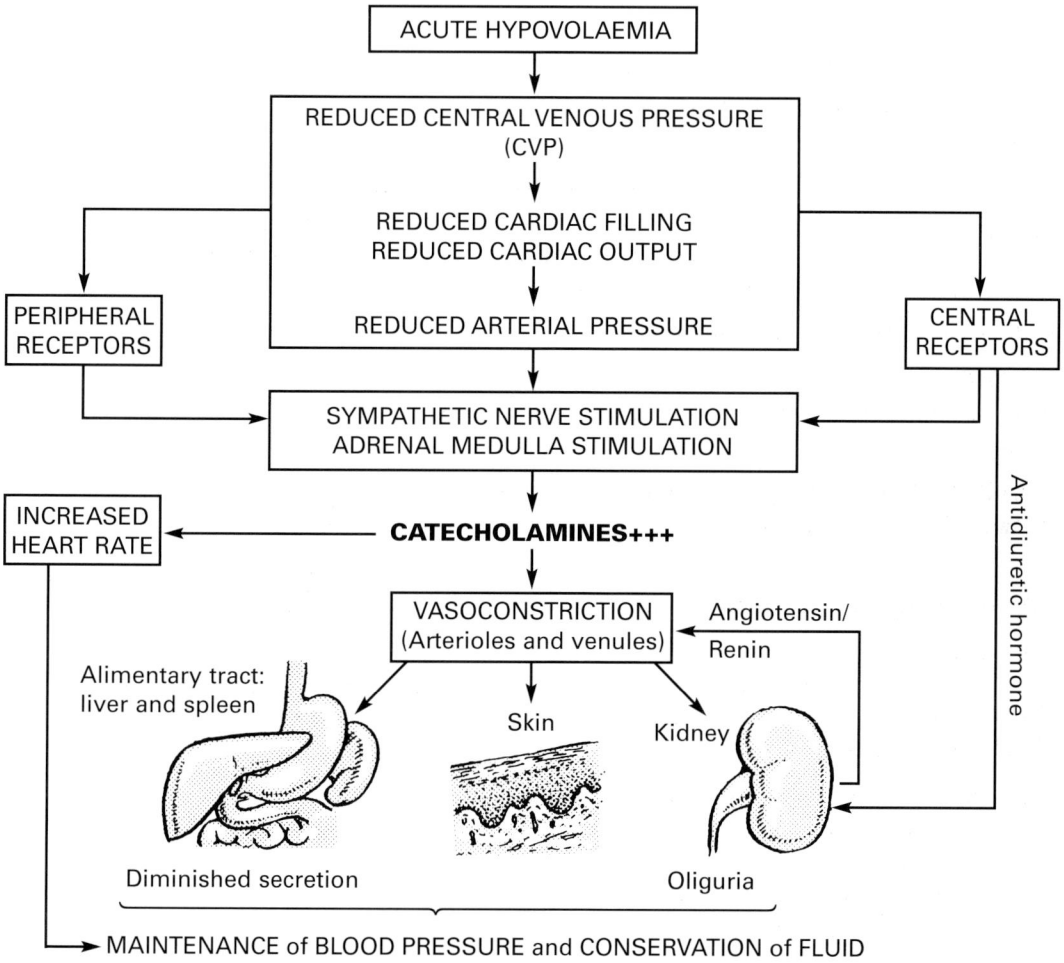

Note: Salt and water are retained due to aldosterone from the adrenal cortex.

At the same time, the circulations in the brain and heart are protected by autoregulatory mechanisms. They are not subject to the generalised vasoconstriction.

Instead:

DILATATION of → CEREBRAL and CORONARY → ARTERIES — maintains satisfactory flow down to blood pressures of 50–60 mmHg

If the loss of circulating fluid volume is great, the limits of the compensatory mechanism are exceeded and the patient goes into a state of severe shock.

SHOCK

ADVANCED STAGE (Decompensation)

The patient is now listless, pale and cold, the face is pinched and the lips blue. The pulse is rapid and weak and the blood pressure is low.

Conditions in Vascular bed

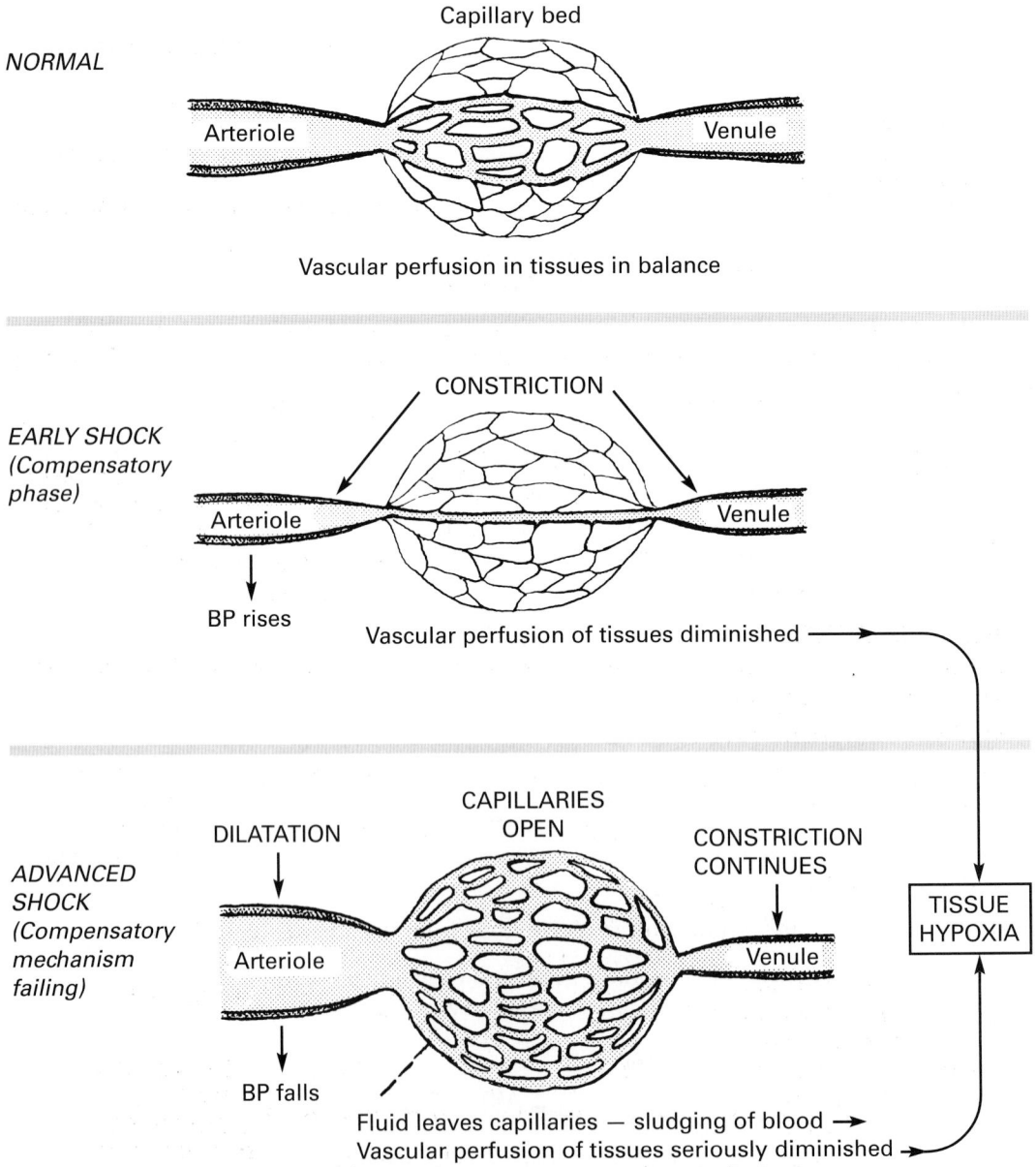

SHOCK

ADVANCED STAGE (continued)

Thus, from the beginning of the shock process, all the body tissues, with the exception of the brain and the heart, suffer from hypoxia. This sets up vicious circles which aggravate the condition:

1.

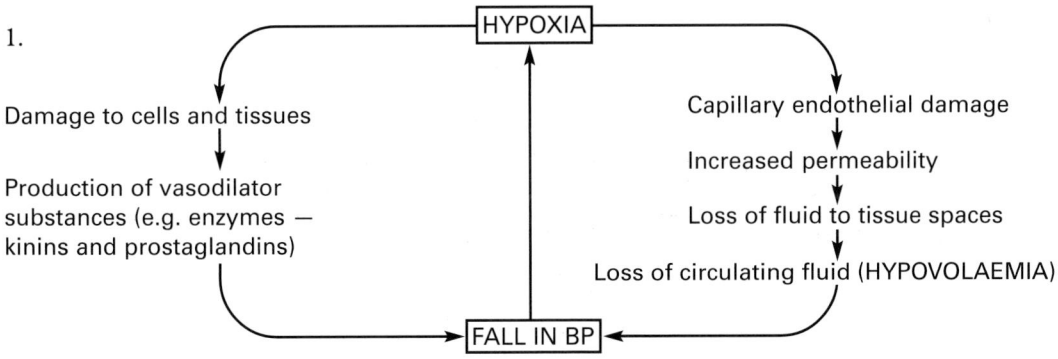

2. When the blood pressure falls below 50–60 mmHg, the autoregulatory control of the cerebral and coronary circulation fails. Serious damage to the brain (p. 169) and heart may occur.

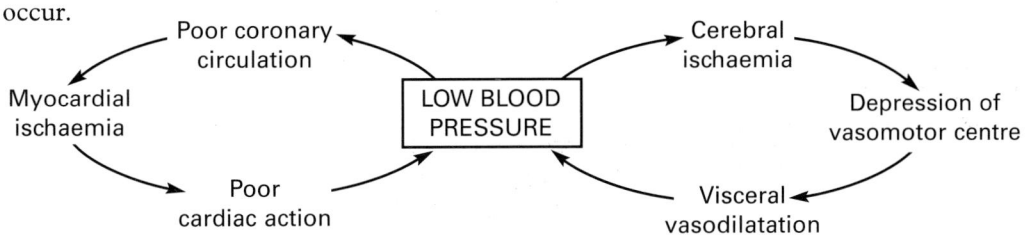

CHANGES IN THE BLOOD AND CELL METABOLISM

As well as these basic circulatory disturbances, important changes in the blood and cellular metabolism occur in shock.

Blood coagulation system

Acute hypoxia → Damaged endothelium → Coagulation cascade triggered → May proceed to formation of FIBRIN → Disseminated intravascular coagulation (DIC) syndrome

Cellular metabolism

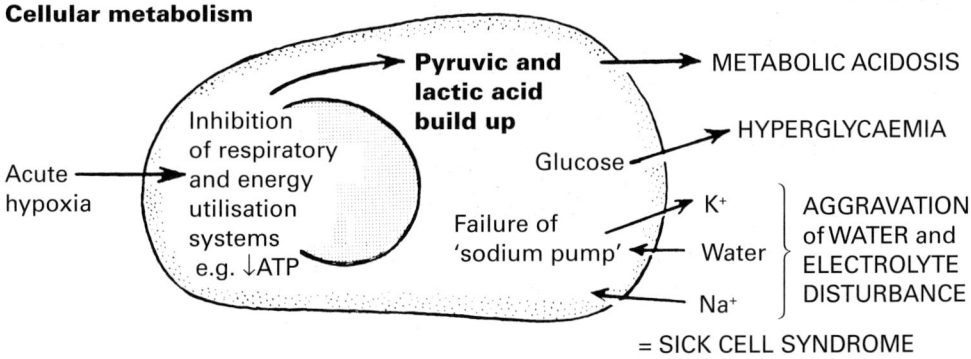

SHOCK

BACTERIAL SHOCK (ENDOTOXIC)

Causes

1. *Bacteria* — The GRAM-NEGATIVE BACTERIA, especially the coliform group, are the commonest causes, and the shock is caused by ENDOTOXIN (lipopolysaccharide). Other organisms can also produce shock e.g. staphylococci, streptococci and meningococci.
2. *Associated conditions*
   (a) Serious primary bacterial infection e.g. septicaemia, peritonitis – potentiated by deficiency in immune status (p. 64) and liver disease where detoxification is impaired.
   (b) Bacterial shock may complicate pre-existing shock due to other causes, e.g. burns.
   (c) Bacterial shock may complicate relatively trivial surgical procedures, especially in the gastrointestinal and urinary tracts in the presence of infection.

Mechanism

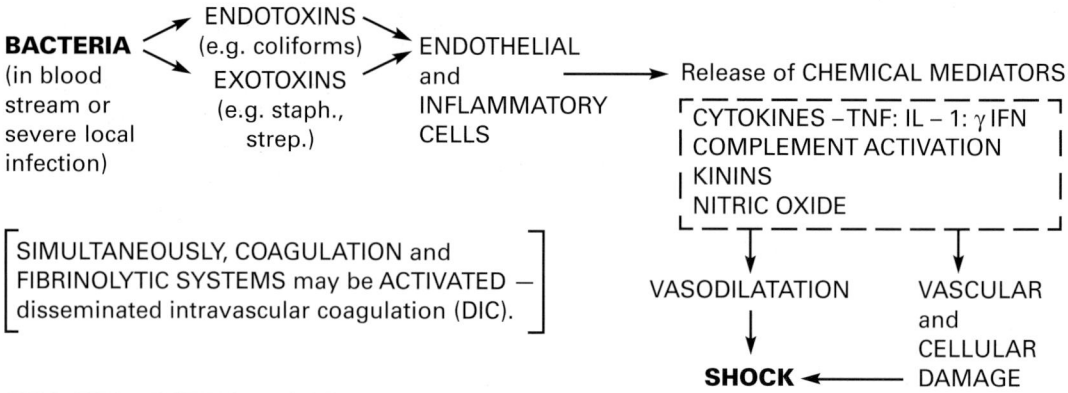

SHOCK in BURNS and SCALDS

Mechanism

1. The immediate reaction is NERVOUS — PAIN, and stimulation of afferent nerves, followed by
2. An INFLAMMATORY RESPONSE evoked by the burnt tissues.

   Massive exudation and loss of PROTEIN-RICH fluid (sludging of blood in capillaries) ⟶ HYPOVOLAEMIA ⟶ SHOCK

The mechanism explains why the SEVERITY of the shock is roughly proportional to the exuding SURFACE AREA and not to the depth of the burn, and why PLASMA transfusion is indicated.

Other factors are chemical mediators derived from the burnt tissues.

3. Complications which aggravate the shock
   (a) Infection: Burnt tissues ⟶ Susceptible to infection esp. Staph.aureus, Strep.pyogenes, Gram-neg. bacilli (e.g. Pseudomonas) ⟶ BACTERIAL SHOCK may be superimposed
   (b) Anaemia: Haemolysis of red cells at burnt site and later if sludging is severe ⟶ ANAEMIA

SHOCK – INDIVIDUAL ORGANS

HEART

There are two main ways in which heart failure may be associated with shock.

1. In hypovolaemic and bacteraemic shock, heart failure is a *COMPLICATION*.
2. In cardiogenic shock, acute heart failure is the *CAUSE* of shock.

Mechanisms

Impaired respiratory function → HYPOXIA

Poor coronary circulation when BP falls to critical level → HYPOXIA

Chemicals released from damaged tissue (esp. pancreas) → Depresses activity of myocardium

Peripheral vasoconstriction → Increases strain on myocardium → may be focal necrosis

Mechanism

Acute fall in cardiac output → Tissue HYPOXIA → SHOCK reaction → Further cardiac damage → Acute fall in cardiac output

Note: Venous return to heart (CVP) not reduced
Fluid replacement *not* required

The commonest condition is myocardial infarction

LUNGS

Respiratory function is seriously disturbed in 2 main ways:

Circulatory changes in the lung (especially in septic/traumatic shock). These occur when compensatory mechanisms are failing. There is congestion and oedema, patchy to begin with but becoming confluent. At autopsy the lungs are heavy and wet. This condition is called 'shock lung' or adult respiratory distress syndrome (ARDS).

Early patchy changes throughout the lungs:

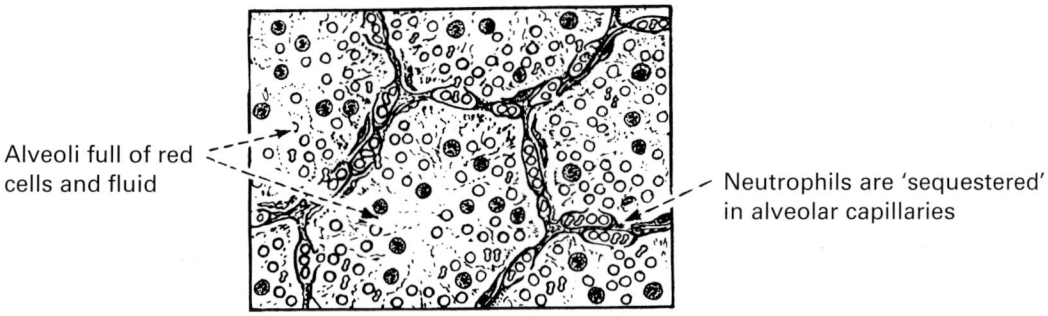

SHOCK – INDIVIDUAL ORGANS

Circulatory changes in the lung (continued)

The mechanisms initiating and progressively augmenting the damage are complex and interacting:

1.

ENZYMES and VASO-ACTIVE SUBSTANCES
from damaged tissues

+

ENDOTOXINS from Gram-ve sepsis

+

Damaging agents (e.g. superoxides) from sequestered neutrophils

AUGMENTING FACTORS

(a) Oxygen therapy

(b) Some forms of drug therapy

(c) Cardiac failure with pulmonary oedema

(d) Disseminated intravascular coagulation

↘ ↙

DAMAGE alveolar epithelium and capillary endothelium

↓

ALVEOLAR OEDEMA and HAEMORRHAGE

2. There may also be:

(a) Patchy ALVEOLAR COLLAPSE and
(b) Formation of HYALINE MEMBRANES

Epithelial damage

↓

Cessation of surfactant action

↙ ↘

Alveolar collapse Hyaline membranes

3. If the patient survives, the organisation is followed by fibrosis: the end result in severe cases may be a combination of fibrosis, emphysema and bronchiolectasis.

SHOCK – INDIVIDUAL ORGANS

KIDNEYS

The secretory function of the kidneys is always disturbed in shock. This is due to the general circulatory collapse and hypotension, but it may be aggravated by the secretion of renin and angiotensin by the kidney, aldosterone by the adrenal and antidiuretic hormone by the posterior pituitary. These hormones are secreted in an attempt to retain fluid and restore the blood volume, but by inducing vasoconstriction they will tend to increase renal damage.

Mechanism

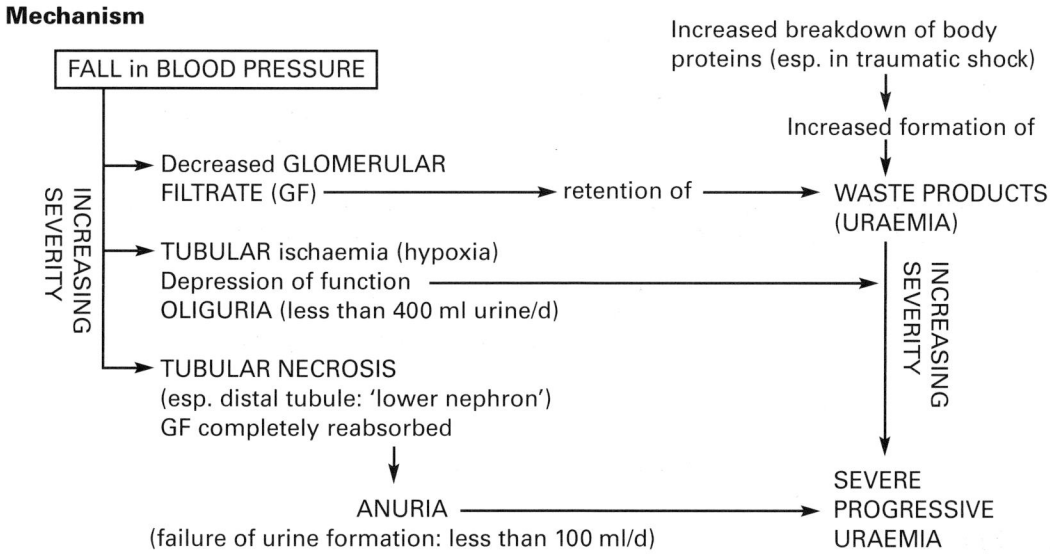

In such cases, at post mortem the kidneys are pale and swollen and the architectural markings are blurred

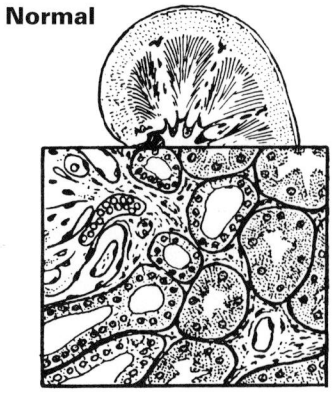

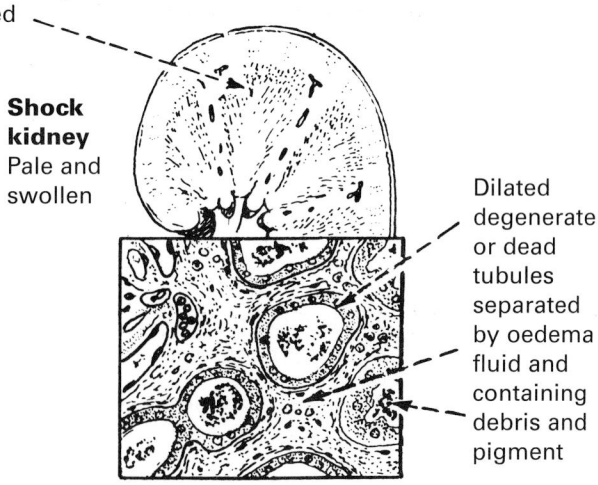

In even more severe shock the entire cortex may become necrotic (acute cortical necrosis).

SHOCK – INDIVIDUAL ORGANS

BRAIN

During the compensated phase of shock, relatively mild cerebral ischaemia is associated with changes in the state of consciousness. When the blood pressure falls to below 50–60 mmHg, the brain suffers serious ischaemic damage which can amount to actual infarction in the 'boundary zones' of the cerebral cortex (and cerebellum).

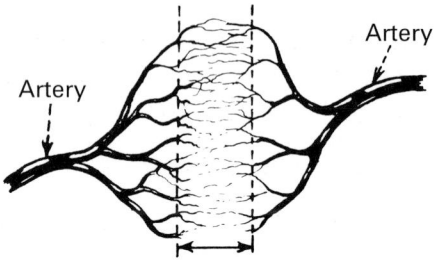

Boundary zone
(Sluggish circulation)

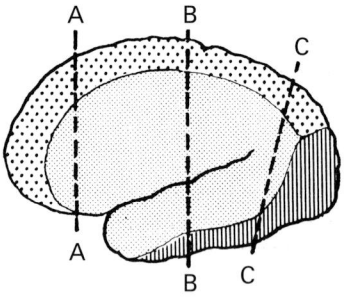

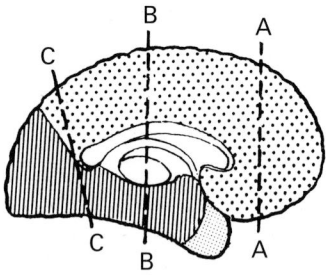

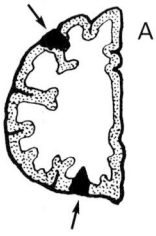

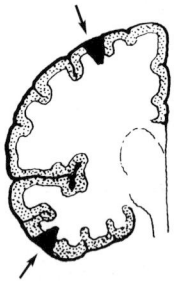

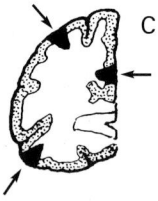

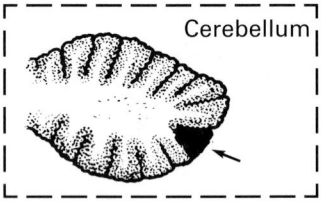

There may also be more diffuse cerebral damage.

ALIMENTARY TRACT

The stomach and duodenum are particularly vulnerable — acute ulceration (Curling's or 'stress' ulcers) which may perforate is a serious complication of shock.

Ischaemia → necrosis → ulceration → perforation.

SHOCK – INDIVIDUAL ORGANS: OUTCOME

LIVER

The liver acinus is supplied by portal venous blood and hepatic arterial blood: in shock, Zone 3 of the hepatic acinus is vulnerable to anoxia (see page 342).

Shock → reduced arterial blood supply → ANOXIA.

May proceed to Zone 3 necrosis (i.e. microcirculatory periphery).

Note: In endotoxic shock, damage to cholangioles (cholangiolitis) may lead to cholestatic (obstructive) jaundice.

The OUTCOME of SHOCK

There are 3 possibilities, depending on several factors:

1. RECOVERY after convalescence, which may be long.
2. SURVIVAL with permanent damage to various organs.
3. DEATH

Factors favouring recovery	Factors favouring progression of shock
1. AVAILABILITY of EARLY TREATMENT of (a) the INITIATING CAUSE (b) the HYPOVOLAEMIA	1. DELAY in TREATMENT 2. FAILURE to REMOVE the INITIATING CAUSE
2. Youth	3. Old age
3. Good general health	4. Poor general health
	5. Pre-existing Cardiovascular and Lung disease
	6. Onset of Complications, esp. Infection and Organ damage

IRREVERSIBLE SHOCK

Theoretically, at some stage in its evolution, shock becomes irreversible due to the severity of vascular impairment and tissue damage. In medical practice, no certain indications are available as to when this point is reached. Measurements of blood pressure and central venous pressure indicate the severity of the vascular disturbance, but many severe cases respond to modern sophisticated treatment. However, the basic essentials remain the early transfusion of fluid and the removal of the original cause of the shock.

CARDIAC FUNCTION

The essential function of the heart is to provide the pumping action in a closed circulation.

Comparison with a simple mechanical system is useful and valid provided that it is appreciated that the animal system is infinitely more sophisticated with delicate built-in controls and balances which influence the inotropic (intrinsic contractility) activity of the heart.

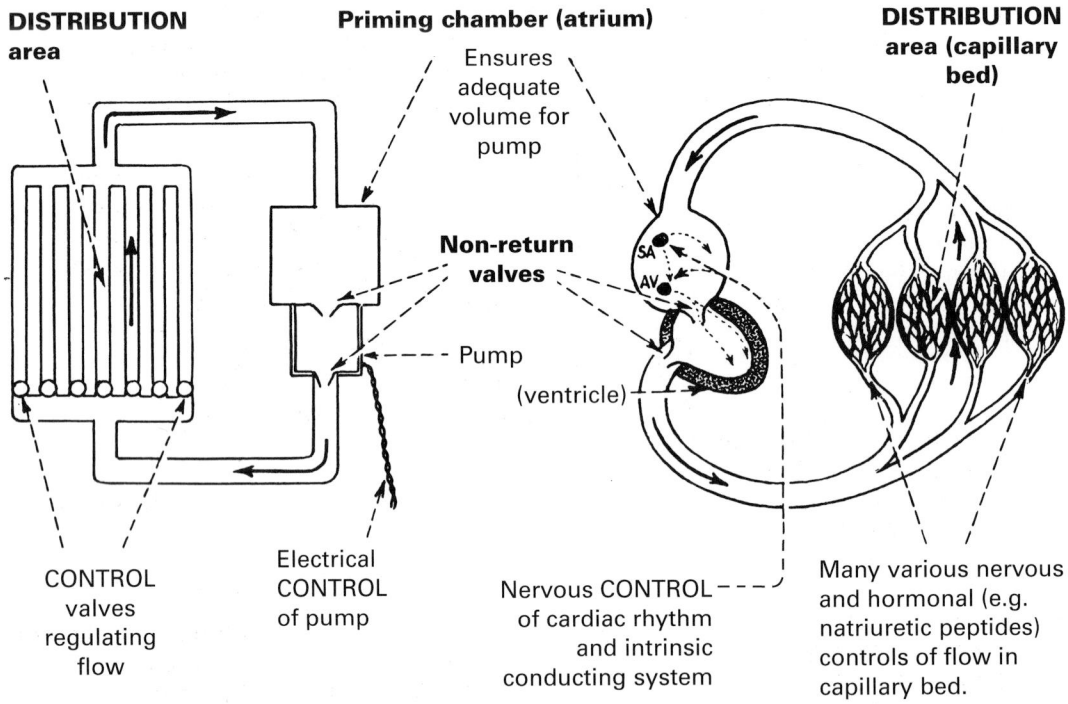

The pump is the essential part of the system: it has to be flexible to accommodate any changes required in the distribution side of the system.

In the animal circulation, very great reserves of ventricular muscle power are available to meet the wide range of metabolic activity required in the distribution area.

HEART FAILURE

Heart failure is very common and occurs when the ***ventricular muscle*** is incapable of maintaining a circulation adequate for the needs of the body (usually assessed in terms of O_2 requirement) — producing symptoms on exercise and at rest.

Although, in the last analysis, heart failure is the result of myocardial failure, it is useful to separate the situations in which heart failure occurs into two main groups:

1. Diseases PRIMARILY affecting the MYOCARDIUM (PUMP)

(a) ISCHAEMIC HEART DISEASE
This is the most common and a very serious disease of the heart. The primary disease — atheroma and thrombosis — in the coronary arteries leads to

MYOCARDIAL DAMAGE...
...FIBROSIS or INFARCTION

(b) INFLAMMATION and TOXIC DEGENERATION of the MYOCARDIUM (MYOCARDITIS)

(c) INFILTRATIONS of the MYOCARDIUM and CARDIOMYOPATHIES

2. Diseases of other cardiac and circulatory components leading secondarily to muscle failure.

(a) CONTROL MECHANISM DEFECTS

Valvular disease increases work load

Nodes

Cardiac arrhythmias (inefficient pumping action)

Bundle of His

(b) DISTRIBUTION DEFECTS

SYSTEMIC HYPERTENSION

Chronic lung disease causing pulmonary hypertension

Increased work load

LOSS OF MYOCARDIAL EFFICIENCY
INITIATION OF COMPENSATORY MECHANISMS

↓

FAILURE OF COMPENSATORY MECHANISMS

↓

Further LOSS OF MYOCARDIAL EFFICIENCY

↓

HEART FAILURE

HEART FAILURE

ACUTE and CHRONIC

Assignment to a particular category depends on the **suddenness of onset** and **rate of development**.

The causative diseases and the effects are different.

	Acute	**Chronic**
Time factors	Instantaneous Sudden (Hours — a few days)	Weeks Months
Causal diseases	(a) ACUTE CORONARY ARTERIAL OCCLUSION with infarction or arrhythmia (b) Pulmonary embolism (c) Severe malignant hypertension (d) Acute toxic myocarditis (e) Acute valve rupture	(a) Ischaemic heart disease (b) Hypertension (c) Chronic valvular diseases (d) Chronic lung diseases (e) Chronic severe anaemia
Effects	SUDDEN DEATH May be no time for compensatory mechanisms to be initiated. Acute pulmonary oedema is common. May be acute ischaemic effects in brain and kidneys.	Compensatory mechanisms fully developed — hypertrophy and dilatation. Chronic oedema and chronic venous congestion.

Acute and chronic failure are at opposite ends of a spectrum but may merge into each other in two ways.

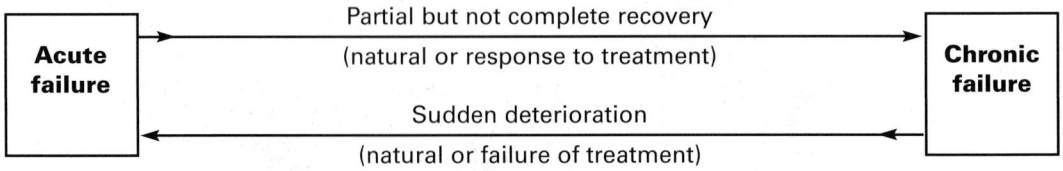

HEART FAILURE

LEFT, RIGHT and COMBINED VENTRICULAR FAILURE

Since the initiating causes and symptoms are referable to either the left or right ventricle, from a clinical point of view it is convenient to consider heart failure as affecting one or other side of the heart.

The pulmonary circulation
A low pressure system
Systolic arterial pressure = 24 mm Hg
Pressure gradient, artery/vein = 8 mm Hg

The systemic circulation
A high pressure system
Systolic arterial pressure = 120 mm Hg
Pressure gradient, artery/vein = 90 mm Hg

Right ventricular mass and coronary blood supply < Left ventricular mass and coronary blood supply
1:4 (approx.)

MAIN CAUSES OF:

Right ventricular failure

Usually secondary to disease elsewhere, causing obstruction to pulmonary blood flow.

(a) LUNG DISEASE e.g. emphysema, fibrosis, malignancy

(b) Some forms of cardiac valve disease, esp. MITRAL STENOSIS

(c) Congenital heart disease
(d) As a CONSEQUENCE of LV FAILURE

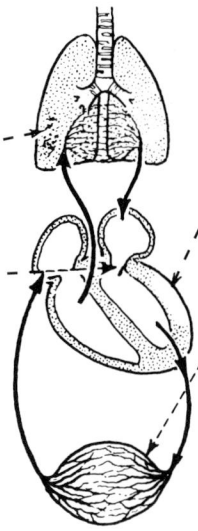

Left ventricular failure

1. Muscle weakness — ISCHAEMIC HEART DISEASE (due to coronary artery disease)

2. Excessive work load — SYSTEMIC HYPERTENSION
Since these causes are so prevalent, LV failure is much more common than RV failure.

Less common causes are:

Aortic valve disease

Mitral incompetence

Congenital heart disease.

However, it should be remembered that in health the function of both ventricles is closely integrated in that they have the same capacity, pump virtually synchronously and are constructed in such a way that layers of muscle fibres pass from one ventricle to the other.

This simplification of a very complex arrangement of muscle fibres shows layers passing between the two ventricles.

Superficial layer RV } ——
Deep layer LV }

Superficial layer LV } - - - -
Deep layer RV }

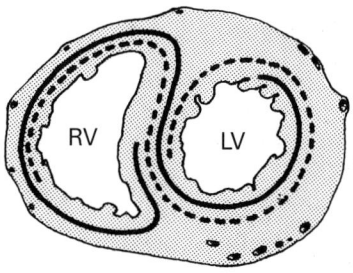

Thus the action of each ventricle is not isolated; it both influences and is influenced by the action of the other. Therefore, in addition to the combined failure which arises as a consequence of left ventricular failure, cases which begin and progress as combined failure are not uncommon.

HEART FAILURE

COMPENSATORY MECHANISMS

The myocardial reserve is provided by three main mechanisms:

1. **Increased rate of pumping**
2. **Dilatation** of the ventricular chambers (due to increased muscle stretching) } are designed to meet the normal physiological reserves
3. **Hypertrophy** is added to these when the pumping load exceeds physiological levels.

In the heart under pathological strain, all three mechanisms are operative and can compensate for considerable derangement.

DILATATION

In physiological conditions, the volume of the ventricular chamber at the end of diastole directly influences the pumping force of the ventricular muscle thus:

The larger the chamber size
(i.e. the longer the initial fibre length
(i.e. the greater the fibre stretch) } the greater the contracting force.

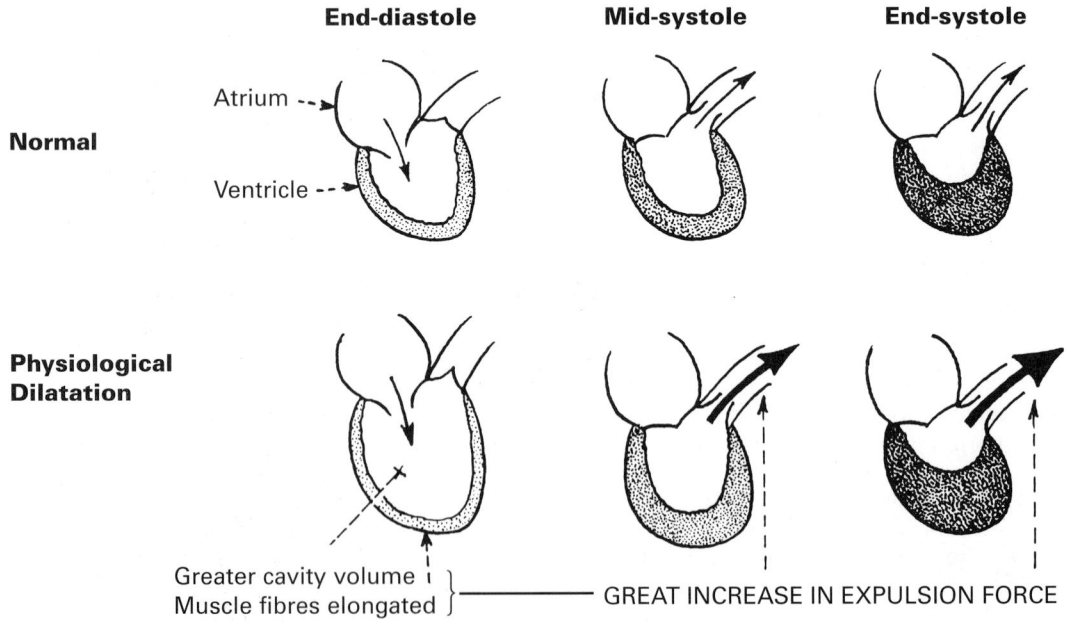

This physiological dilatation also compensates in cardiac disease.

HEART FAILURE

Compensatory mechanisms — Dilatation (continued)

In cardiac disease, particularly in cases of valvular incompetence, dilatation which occurs passively to accommodate the regurgitated blood is an important factor.

Aortic valve incompetence is a good example:

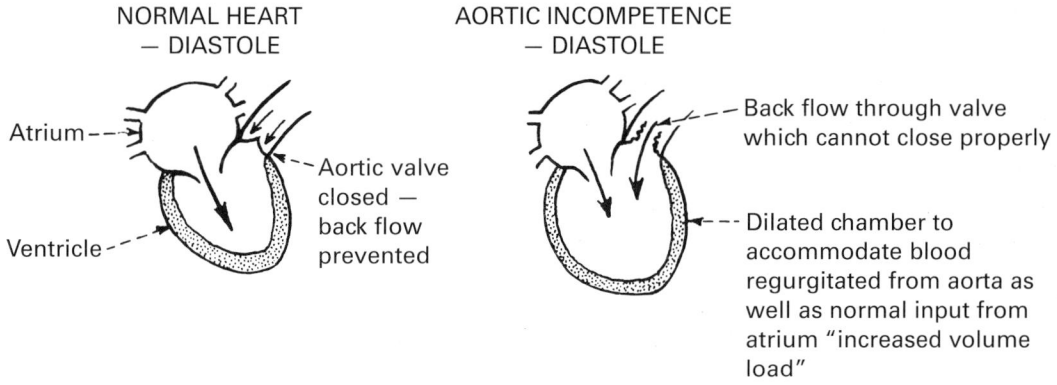

HYPERTROPHY involves an increase in muscle fibre bulk; the increased muscle mass is able to deal with a greater work load. In its pure form, hypertrophy is seen best in cases of increased pressure load.

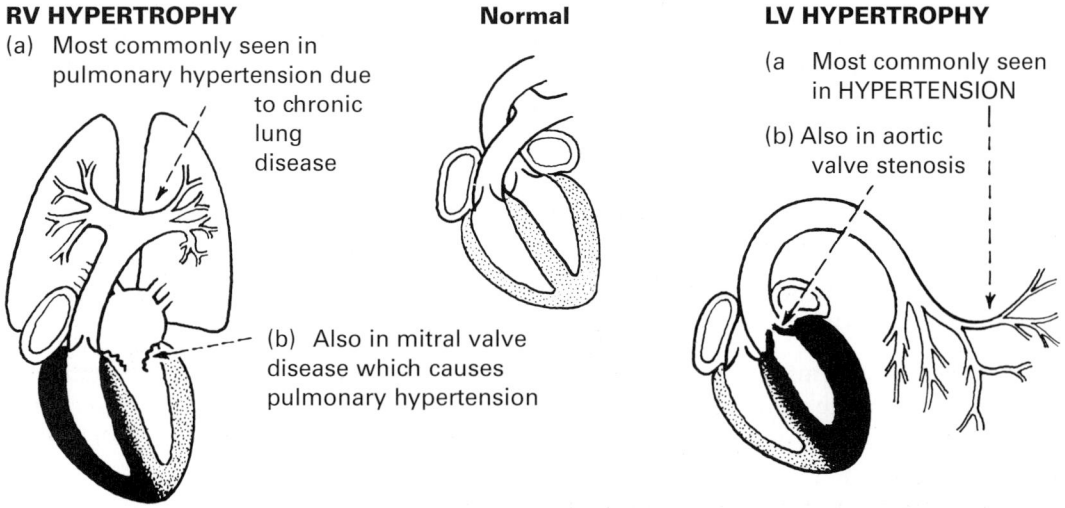

At first the blood supply to the hypertrophied muscle increases to meet the increased metabolic requirements. Later, severe hypertrophy leads to hypoxia and reduced function.

HEART FAILURE

FAILURE of COMPENSATORY MECHANISMS

The increased efficiency derived from all three mechanisms is limited, and beyond this limit serious deficiency ensues — HEART FAILURE.

Beyond the critical limit:

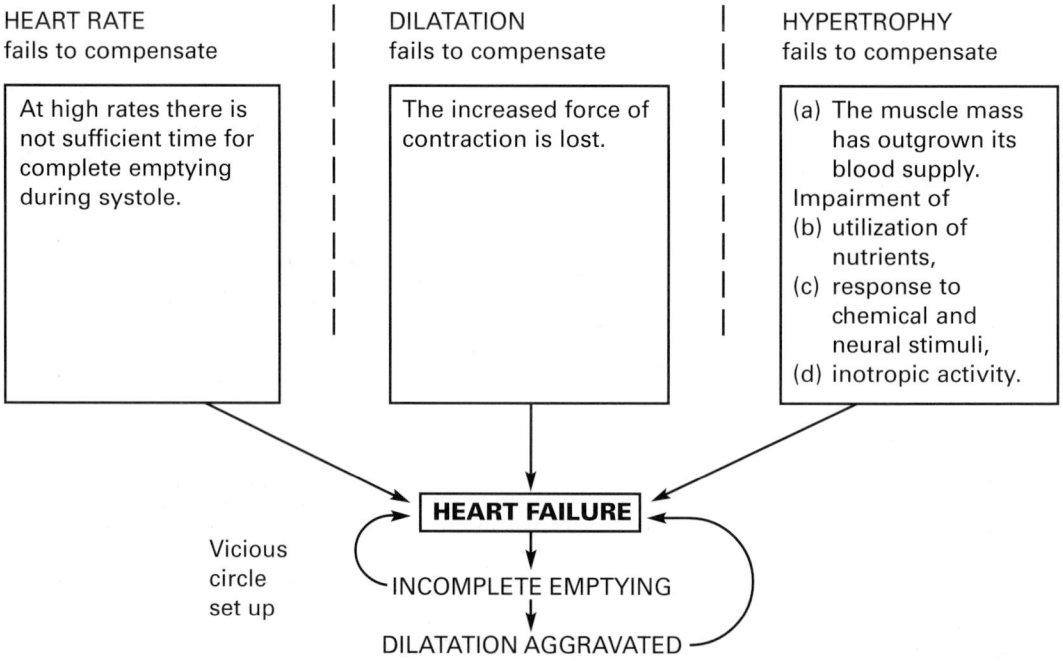

Thus in most cases of heart failure there is CARDIAC ENLARGEMENT due usually to a combination of hypertrophy and dilatation.

The **effects** and **symptoms** of heart failure are seen in the peripheral organs and are due to HYPOXIA and VENOUS CONGESTION.

(a) In the chronic forms of heart failure, the **weakness and fatigue** which are such common symptoms are probably effects mainly of **hypoxia**, but damage to organs is more difficult to define since the effects of venous congestion and water retention are added.

(b) Venous congestion and oedema are important.

Breathlessness (dyspnoea) is almost a constant concommitant of cardiac failure and is essentially due to venous congestion and fluid retention within the lungs.

In severe failure, particularly when bed rest is obligatory, *hypostatic pneumonia* and *pulmonary embolism* (from leg vein thrombosis) may be serious and terminal complications.

EFFECTS of HEART FAILURE

Left ventricular failure is the initiating event in most cases of combined failure.

The main effects are the results of:

(a) low output
(b) 'backward' pressure

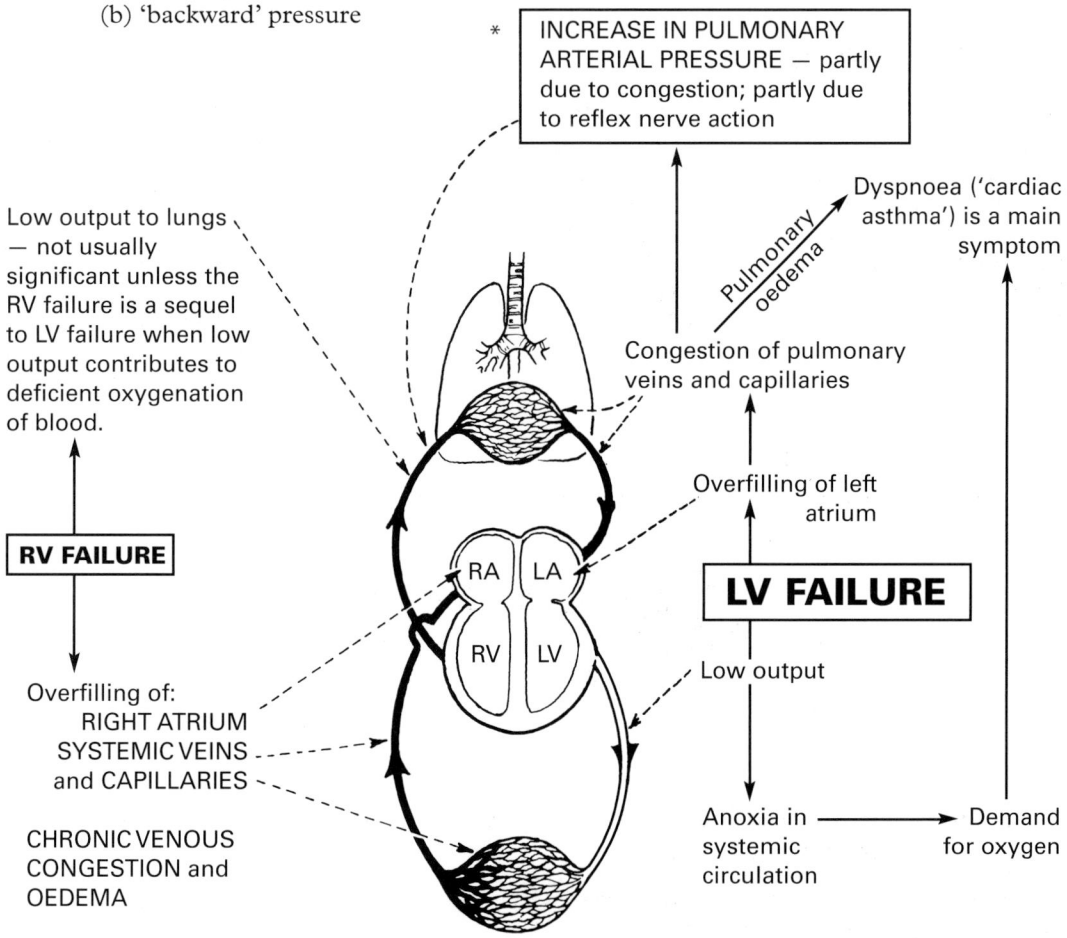

Cyanosis is the result of excess reduced haemoglobin in capillaries and venules.

*The increase in pulmonary arterial pressure is important because in most cases of chronic LV failure it eventually leads to RV failure (combined failure).

ACUTE PULMONARY OEDEMA

In **acute left ventricular failure**, accumulation of fluid results in dyspnoea and hypoxaemia.

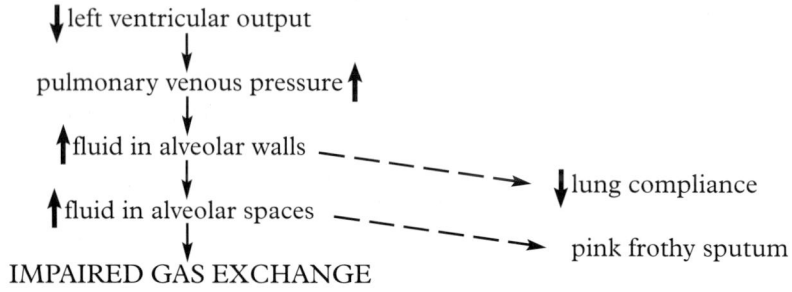

CHRONIC VENOUS CONGESTION of the LUNGS

The results from chronic combined (congestive) failure and/or chronic left ventricular failure:

The lungs are bulky, congested and brownish in colour.

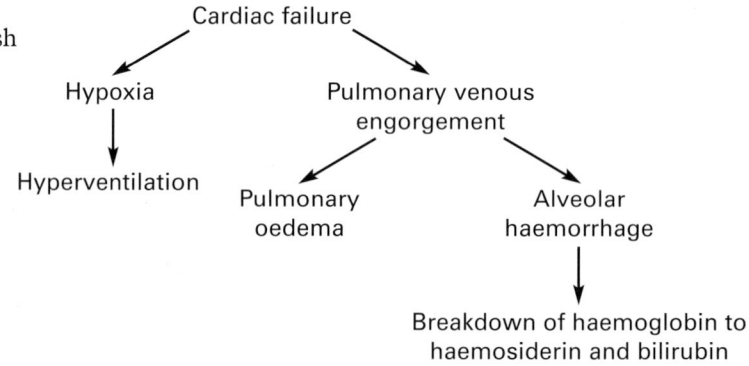

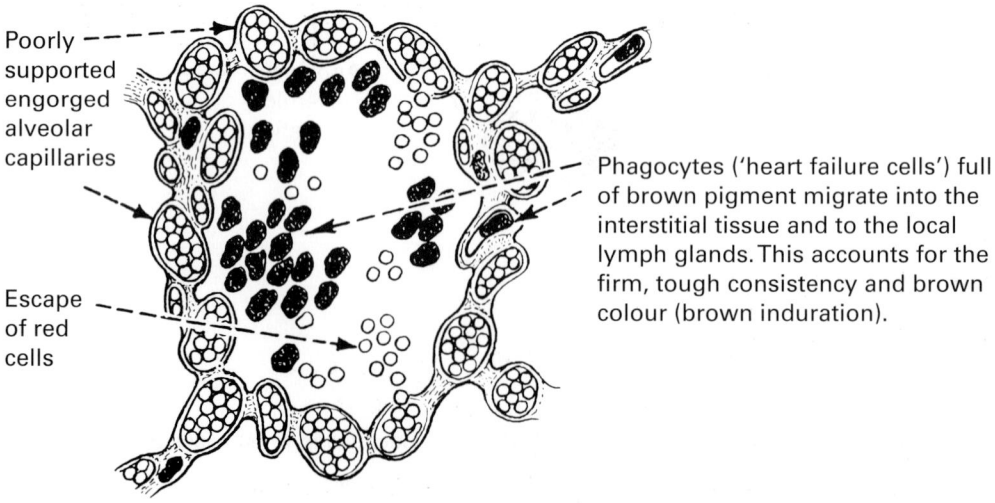

At post mortem, application of potassium ferrocyanide and hydrochloric acid to the lung results in a blue colour (Prussian blue reaction) indicating the presence of haemosiderin.

HEART FAILURE

CHRONIC VENOUS CONGESTION

Congestion of the systemic venous circulation is a result of right heart failure whether secondary to left heart failure or lung disease (*cor pulmonale*).

The basic mechanism is:

CHRONIC CARDIAC FAILURE

↓

REDUCED left ventricular output
+ MITRAL valve incompetence

↓

chronic **PULMONARY VENOUS CONGESTION**

+ increased pulmonary arterial pressure

↓

LUNG DISEASE

↓

increased pulmonary vascular resistance

↓

RIGHT VENTRICULAR FAILURE

↓

TRICUSPID valve incompetence

↓

SYSTEMIC VENOUS CONGESTION

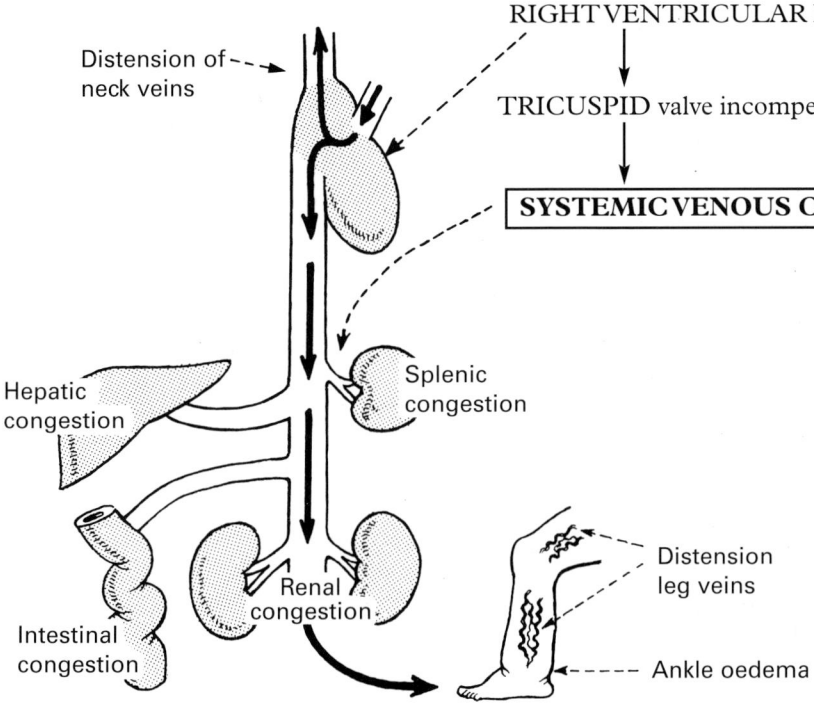

Pleural effusion is also a common effect (see page 287).

HEART FAILURE

CHRONIC VENOUS CONGESTION (continued)

Because of the increase in venous blood, the organs become swollen and purplish. With long continued over-distension, the walls of the venules show reactive thickening and there is mild interstitial fibrosis of the organs, giving them a very firm consistency. These changes are seen typically in the kidney and spleen.

The **liver** shows striking changes: Mechanical distension of the veins causes enlargement of the liver so that it can be felt below the costal margin.

The parenchymal cells furthest from the arterial blood supply, i.e. around the hepatic venules (centrilobular), undergo degeneration with atrophy and ultimately disappear. Cells nearer the arteries show an accumulation of fat.

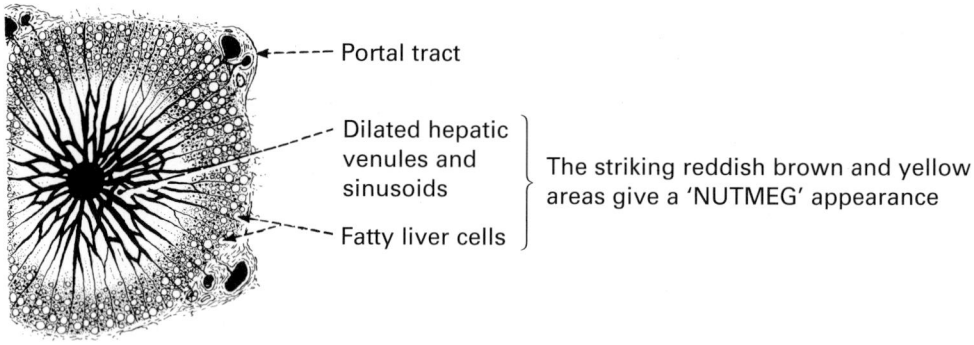

Much of the liver parenchyma may be destroyed. If the patient has periods of remission, the remaining liver cells may undergo compensatory hyperplasia. This results in small, irregular, pale nodules alternating with areas of fibrosis — so-called cardiac cirrhosis. It is not a true cirrhosis and does not cause hepatic failure.

FLUID RETENTION

This is related to the REDUCED OUTPUT from the LEFT VENTRICLE: the mechanism involves retention of sodium and water.

Reduced LV output → renin released → angiotensin is activated

↓ Reduced KIDNEY perfusion → Fall in glomerular filtration

↓ adrenal cortex stimulated → aldosterone secreted

→ RETENTION of SODIUM and WATER

↓

contributes to OEDEMA — for which there are 2 main mechanisms in heart failure:

(1) **Overfilling of venules** → Increased hydrostatic pressure

(2) **Retention of water and electrolytes** → Increased total body fluid

→ Oedema of dependent parts where pressure is greatest

Pleural effusion (p.287) and ascites (p.167) are also common effects of fluid retention in congestive cardiac failure.

HIGH OUTPUT CARDIAC FAILURE

LOW and HIGH OUTPUT FAILURE

By definition, in cardiac failure, output is low in respect of body requirements, and in most cases this output is lower than the usual normal output. Such cases are called **Low Output type.**

In a few conditions, the cardiac failure complicates a pre-existing state in which the output before failure was greater than normal. In these cases, the output is not sufficient to meet the body requirements but may still be higher than the normal. Such cases are called **High Output type.**

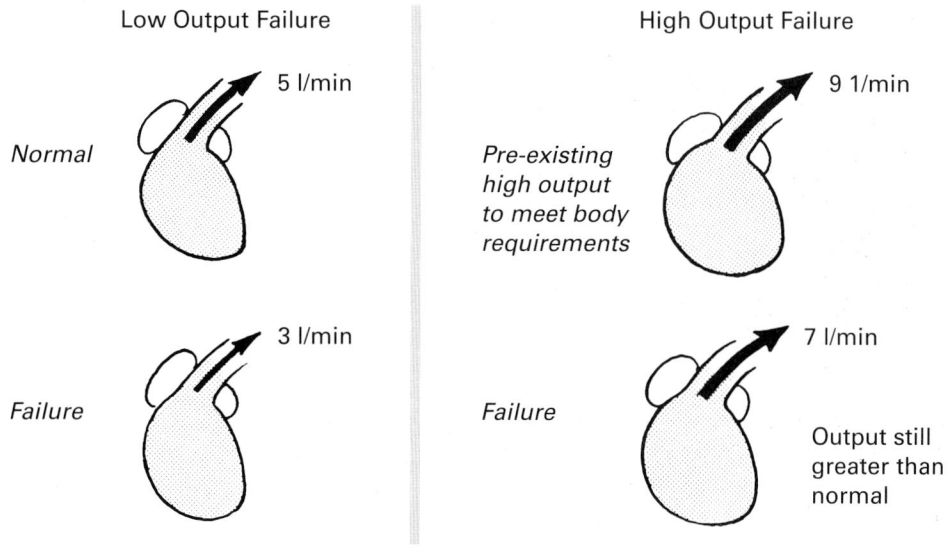

Causes

The common types of failure:

HYPERTENSIVE
ISCHAEMIC HEART DISEASE
VALVULAR HEART DISEASE
MYOCARDITIS

Diseases associated with increased blood volume:

CHRONIC ANAEMIA
ARTERIOVENOUS SHUNTING
or increased vascularity of tissues
e.g. PAGET'S DISEASE OF BONE
(rare and only if very severe);
HYPERTHYROIDISM;
following TRANSFUSION OVERLOAD.

In both types of failure, venous overfilling is an important sign, but in high output failure venous overfilling is usually present before failure ensues, reflecting the increased blood volume.

DISEASES OF ARTERIES – ARTERIOSCLEROSIS

Arterial diseases are very common and are important because of their serious effects, especially on the heart and brain.

Normal age related vascular changes:

ARTERIOSCLEROSIS (hardening of the arteries)

This is a generalised degeneration of the specialised muscle and elastic tissue of the media, and replacement by fibrous tissue, proteoglycan and calcium salts. There is also intimal proliferation.

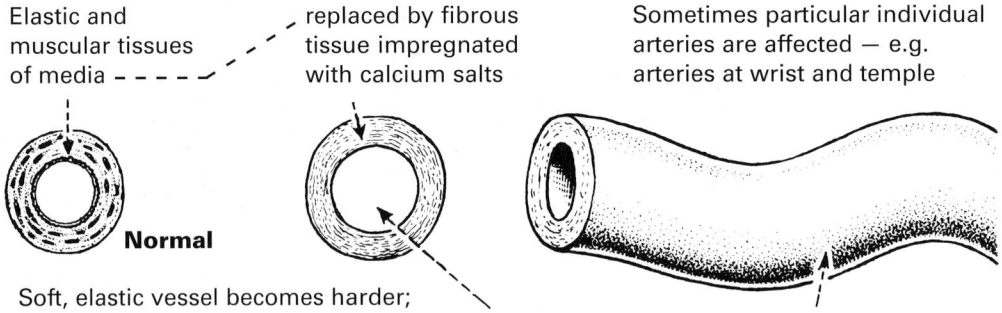

HYALINE ARTERIOLOSCLEROSIS affects the small branches of the arterial system (arterioles) — especially in the kidney.

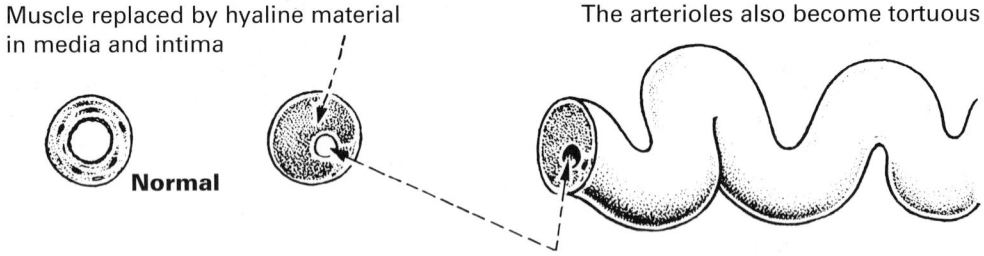

This is due to entry of blood plasma under the endothelium with protein deposition; gradual replacement by collagen occurs. The process is called **plasmatic vasculosis.**

Note that the lumen is usually narrowed so that ischaemia may be an important complication.

Note: Arteriosclerosis is aggravated by HYPERTENSION and DIABETES MELLITUS.

In a variant of arteriosclerosis (Monckeberg), seen in the very elderly, calcium salts are very heavily deposited in the media particularly of the leg arteries. The X-ray appearances are striking but there is no significant loss of lumen unless atheroma co-exists or is superimposed.

ATHEROMA (ATHEROSCLEROSIS)

Atheroma is a common disease in Westernised countries, of gradual onset but progressive. It is commonly seen in the middle aged and elderly but the earliest changes are present in adolescents. It is often asymptomatic but it may cause serious disease or death from complicating thrombosis. The lesions represent patchy deposition of lipid within plaques deep in the intima. The evolution of the disease is described in 3 phases.

(Vessel opened longitudinally)

EARLY PROLIFERATIVE PHASE

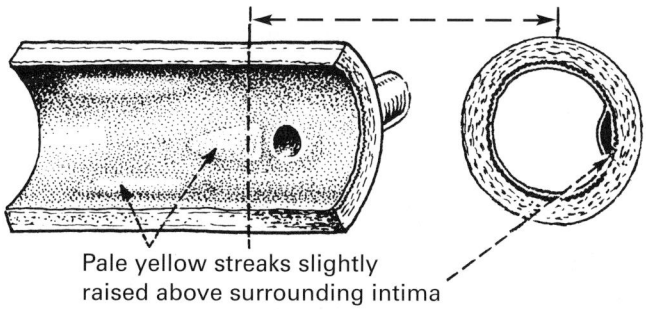

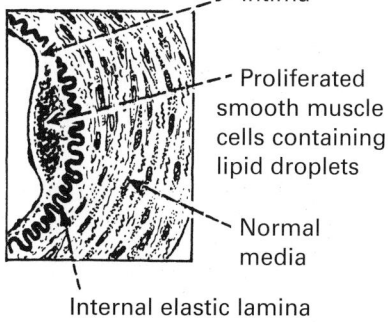

PROGRESSING PHASE

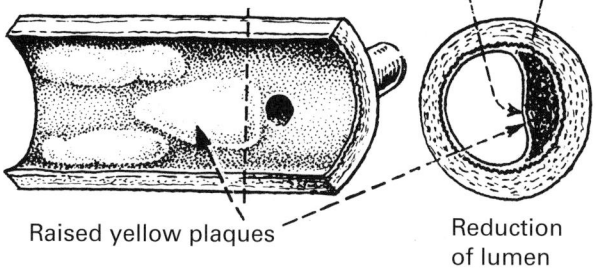

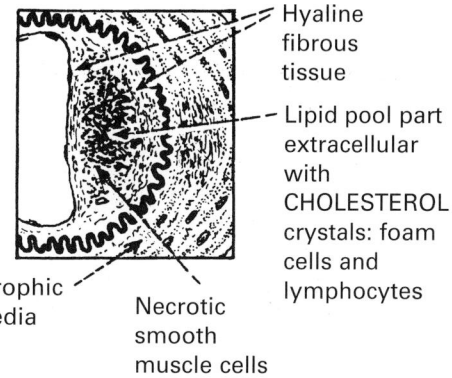

LATE ULCERATIVE PHASE

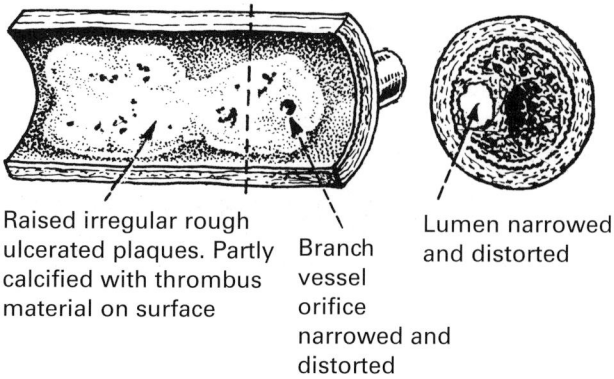

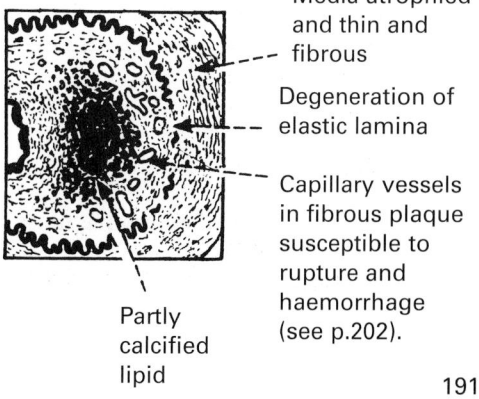

ATHEROMA – COMPLICATIONS

Fibrosis in the intima and media weaken the wall and may lead to aneurysm formation (see p.234), but the most important complication of atheroma is THROMBOSIS.

Local factors at the site of the atheromatous plaque are important:

1. Intimal roughening or distortion with eddying of flow
2. Thin, easily damaged intimal surface
3. Rupture of new capillaries in plaque with haemorrhage into the plaque

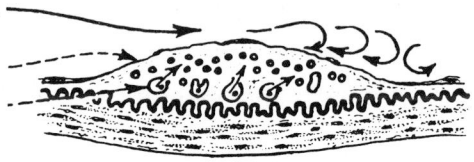

In addition, general factors influencing blood coagulability are important, e.g. smoking affecting vessel contractility and platelet function.

Results

(1) Medium and small arteries – coronaries, cerebrals

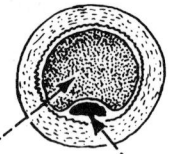

Usually occlusion by red thrombus

Atheromatous plaque

(2) Larger arteries – aorta, carotids. Lumen usually too large to be completely occluded

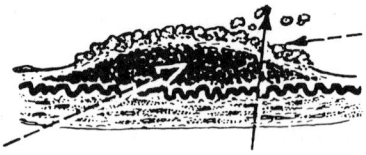

Paler platelet thrombus on intimal surface

Small emboli may be detached – esp. to kidney, legs and brain.

The important sites of atheroma and the effects due to complications are:

CEREBRALS (Circle of Willis or branches) CAROTIDS	**Acute local ischaemia** — cerebral infarction (stroke). Chronic ischaemia of brain — multi-infarct dementia.
CORONARIES	**Acute infarction.** **Chronic ischaemia of myocardium with fibrosis.**
ABDOMINAL AORTA	**Aneurysm** — embolism to legs.
RENAL ARTERIES	**Chronic ischaemia of kidneys.**
Visceral arteries	Acute or chronic ischaemia of bowel.
Lower limb arteries (Upper limb arteries are rarely affected)	With severe atheroma, chronic ischaemia with claudication occurs and gangrene may develop.

In severe cases of atheroma, most of these sites may be affected, but not uncommonly, one particular artery may be much more severely damaged than the others, e.g. coronaries, cerebrals.

ATHEROMA – AETIOLOGY

The cause of atheroma is complex and multifactorial. There are many risk factors, the most of which are illustrated in the classical victim — the HEAVY SMOKING, HYPERTENSIVE, OBESE, SEDENTARY MALE.

The various risk factors exponentially increase with AGE. They are considered in 3 groups:

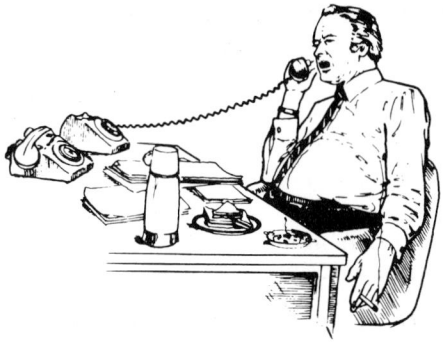

1. **ENDOGENOUS**
   - (a) *SEX* — male > female.
   - (b) *HEREDITY*
     - (i) Family history of premature heart disease.
     - (ii) Familial hyperlipidaemias.
   - (c) *PERSONALITY* — Type A.
2. **ENVIRONMENTAL**
   - (a) *SMOKING.*
   - (b) *DIET* — rich in saturated fats and cholesterol.
   - (c) Lack of exercise.
   - (d) Low socio-economic group status.
3. **DISEASES**
   - (a) *HYPERTENSION.*
   - (b) Hyperlipidaemia.
   - (c) Diabetes Mellitus.
   - (d) Severe obesity.
   - (e) Increased fibrinogen levels.

Modification of some of these risk factors has led to a fall in mortality especially in higher socio-economic groups. Avoiding smoking, dietary improvement and exercise seem most important.

These background factors may act as follows:

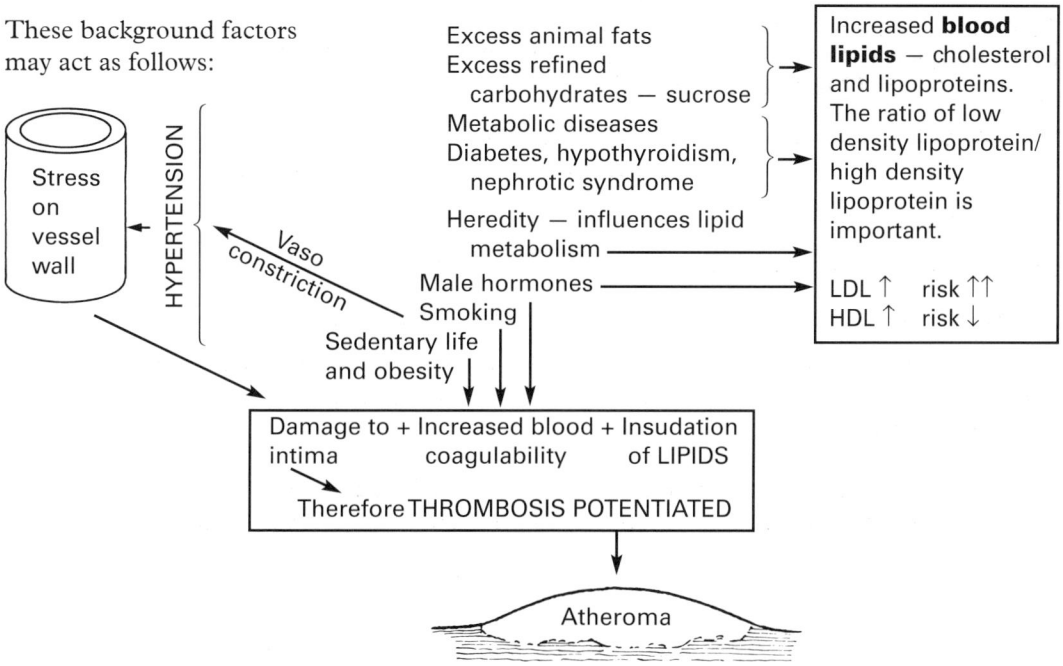

ATHEROMA – AETIOLOGY

1. **Endothelial Damage**

There is a preferential distribution of lesions, e.g. arch of aorta, coronary arteries, cerebral arteries, carotids, abdominal aorta.

This is determined by local mechanical stresses which potentiate local endothelial damage.

e.g. **Areas of lateral and shearing stresses and turbulence** at acute bends or branching – in aorta, carotids, abdominal aortic branches.

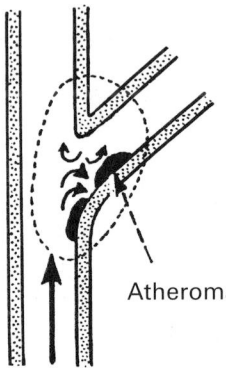

e.g. **Poor support**

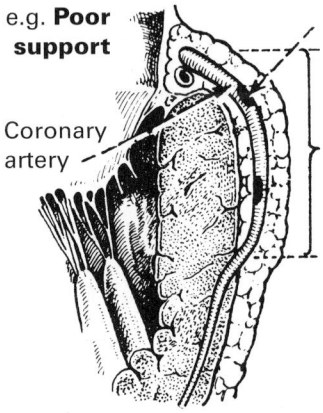

Other factors may contribute to endothelial damage as follows:

HYPERTENSION → ENDOTHELIAL CELL DAMAGE

INCREASED PLASMA LDL (particularly oxidised forms) → FREE RADICALS → ENDOTHELIAL CELL DAMAGE

SMOKING → Increased plasma FIBRINOGEN + → PLATELET AGGREGATION

INFLAMMATION → CYTOKINES (macrophage-T-lymphocyte interaction) → GROWTH FACTORS

ENDOTHELIAL CELL DAMAGE → PLATELET AGGREGATION → GROWTH FACTORS → INTIMAL SMOOTH MUSCLE proliferation → DEFICIENT METABOLISM OF LIPIDS — esp. LDL (see next page) ? overloading of clearance mechanisms → **ATHEROMA**

2. **Lipid Deposition**

This is related to (a) the ability of the intima to metabolise lipids and (b) the types of lipid.

The ability of the intima to metabolise lipids:

Normal

Intima is metabolically active: nourished by diffusion of gases and soluble chemicals including soluble lipids from lumen under filtration pressure.

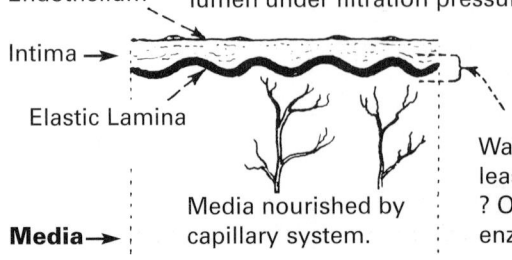

Atheroma

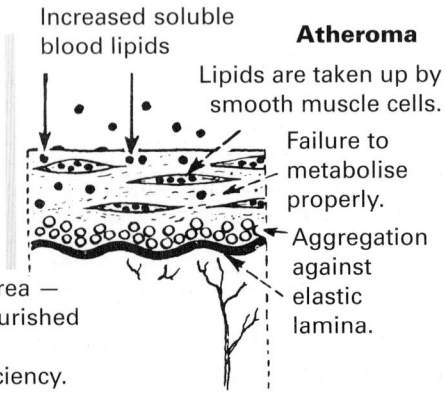

ATHEROMA – AETIOLOGY

LIPID METABOLISM in ATHEROGENESIS

As has been indicated previously, CHOLESTEROL and CHOLESTEROL-containing LIPOPROTEINS play an important role in atherogenesis.

The main cholesterol-containing lipoproteins are graded according to their density: the density divisions are arbitrary and represent overlapping averages.

Density → ↓ related to molecular size	Very low density lipoprotein **VLDL**	Low density lipoprotein **LDL**	High density lipoprotein **HDL**
	Large molecule	Medium	Small molecule
CHOLESTEROL CONTENT	Moderate	**HIGH** **LDL** accounts for 70% of plasma cholesterol	Low

Atheroma is specifically associated with high blood LDL levels (as well as total CHOLESTEROL levels).

LIPID METABOLISM is complex, involving many enzyme systems, receptors and binding molecules (ligands): all with feed-back controls.

The following is a much simplified summary indicating the 3 main sites of activity:

1. **MUSCLES and ADIPOSE TISSUES**

   There are 2 main sources for the supply of TRIGLYCERIDES required for local metabolism:

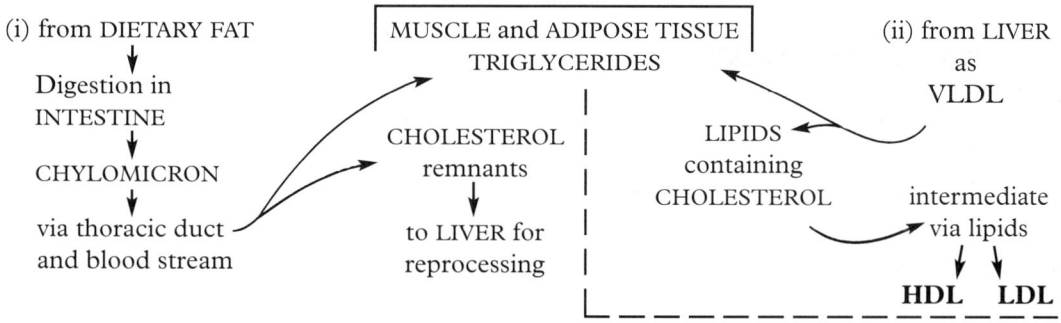

2. The **LIVER** is the main site of synthesis and reprocessing of lipids.

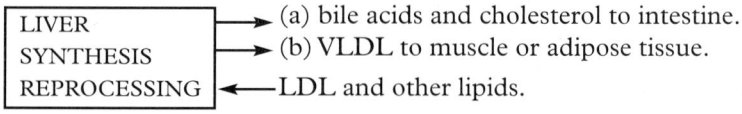

3. The **SOMATIC CELLS** generally require CHOLESTEROL for the synthesis of cell membranes and steroids. LDL is the main source.

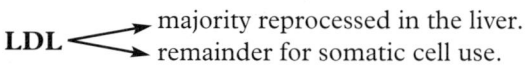

The plasma levels of LDL are conditioned by the delicate balance of these various activities. An understanding of them gives some indication of potential intervention sites.

ATHEROMA – AETIOLOGY: CURRENT INTERVENTIONS

The 2 classical theories of atherogenesis were proposed in the 19th century.

1. The association of high blood cholesterol (and LDL) levels with atheroma gives support to the INSUDATION theory (Virchow). It stated that at sites of intimal damage insudation of lipid occurred and resulted in fat accumulation and fibrosis.
2. The THROMBOTIC theory (Rokitansky) proposed that thrombotic encrustation at the site of intimal injury initiated the atheromatous plaque and that the lipid was derived from the thrombus material (particularly platelets).

Formation of a plaque from platelet thrombus:

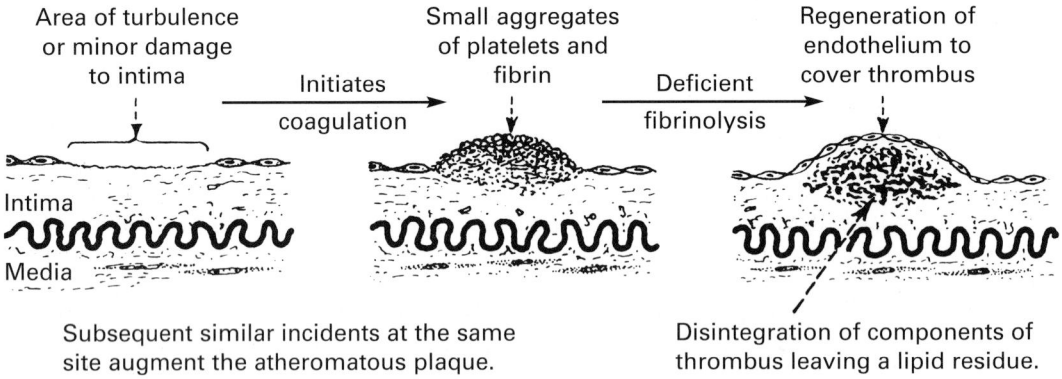

ATHEROMA — SUMMARY

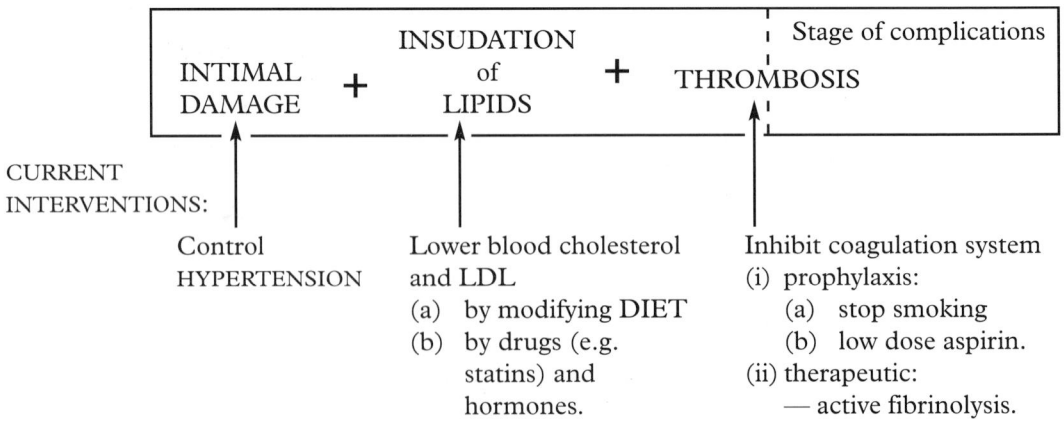

HYPERTENSION

High blood pressure (BP) is important because it increases the risk of cardiovascular disease, especially:—

1. **Left Ventricular Hypertrophy** } → Cardiac failure.
2. **Ischaemic Heart Disease** } → Sudden death.
3. **Stroke** — Cerebral haemorrhage or Infarction.

Blood pressure is a continuous variable within the population. It is determined essentially by 2 variables:

BLOOD PRESSURE = CARDIAC OUTPUT × TOTAL PERIPHERAL RESISTANCE.

Mechanisms of normal maintenance of BP and the effect of age

The systolic pressure is governed by (a) cardiac action (b) the ELASTICITY and DISTENSIBILITY of the CONDUCTING ARTERIES.	Increasing AGE is normally associated with ARTERIOSCLEROSIS – loss of distensibility →	∴ Increased SYSTOLIC pressure
The diastolic pressure is maintained by the **RESISTANCE (TONE)** of arterioles (a subsidiary factor is blood viscosity)	ARTERIOLOSCLEROSIS — increased resistance →	∴ Increased DIASTOLIC pressure

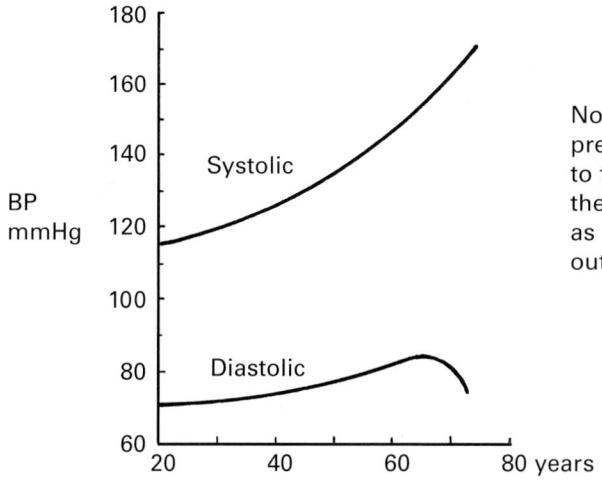

Note: Diastolic pressure tends to fall after the 7th decade as cardiac output falls.

Because of the wide range in the normal population, the definition of high BP is arbitrary. The risk of complications progressively increases with BP, including within the normal range. The levels of **systolic** and **diastolic** pressure are both risk factors.

Systolic BP > 160 mmHg and Diastolic BP > 95 are generally accepted as **Hypertension.**

Modern therapy is effective in lowering BP. The decision whether or not to treat depends on the level of BP and the presence of other risk factors for cardiovascular disease.

HYPERTENSION

Aetiology

The following diagram illustrates the physiological mechanisms controlling Blood Pressure. They are presented in 2 groups but are complex and interconnected with feed-back controls.

1. **Autonomic Nervous System**
   (a) External environment
   (b) Internal environment
   e.g. baroreceptors

2. **Hormones**
   (a) Pituitary/Adrenal
   (b) Renal

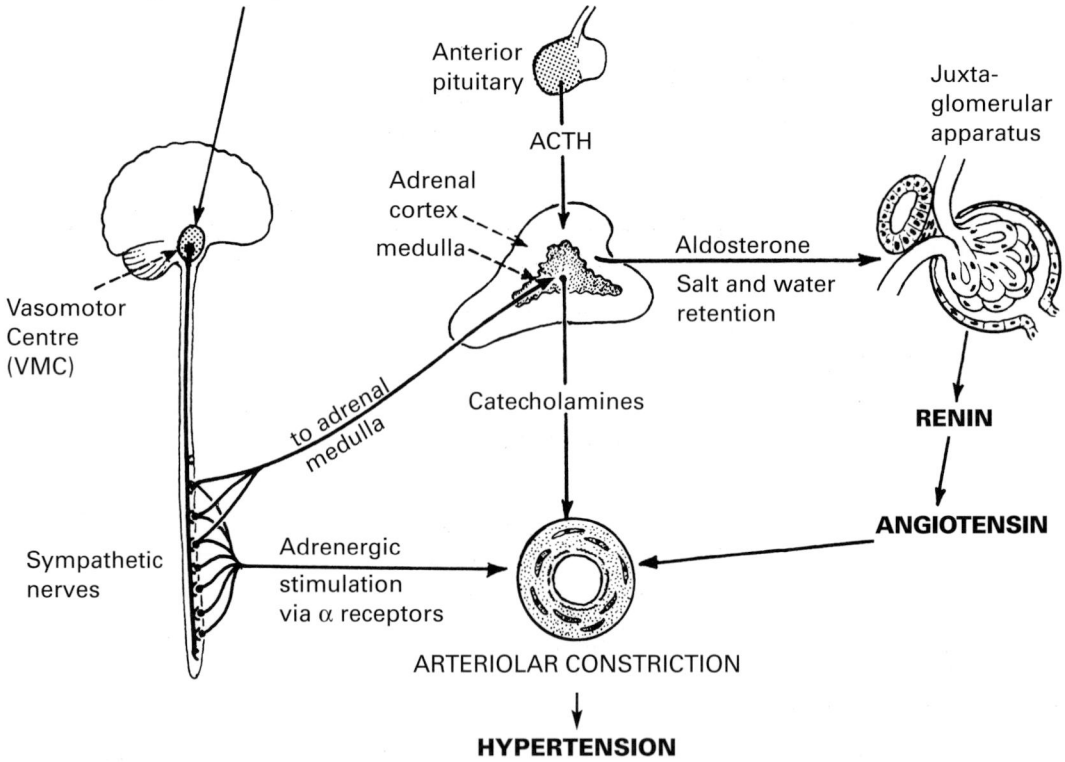

Note: **Nitric oxide** (NO) and **Endothelin** are both produced physiologically by endothelial cells. They have powerful opposite effects.

Nitric oxide ———— vasodilatation (short-acting).
Endothelin ———— vasoconstriction (long-acting).

Their role in hypertension is not yet clear.

HYPERTENSION – ESSENTIAL AND SECONDARY

ESSENTIAL HYPERTENSION

In 90–95% of cases of hypertension no obvious cause is found — this is ESSENTIAL hypertension — (a diagnosis of exclusion).

A number of aetiological factors may be implicated:

1. Genetic predisposition — polygenic inheritance.
2. Racial e.g. black > white.
3. Sodium homeostasis: increased **salt intake**.
4. Stress — sympathetic nervous overactivity.
5. Lack of exercise.

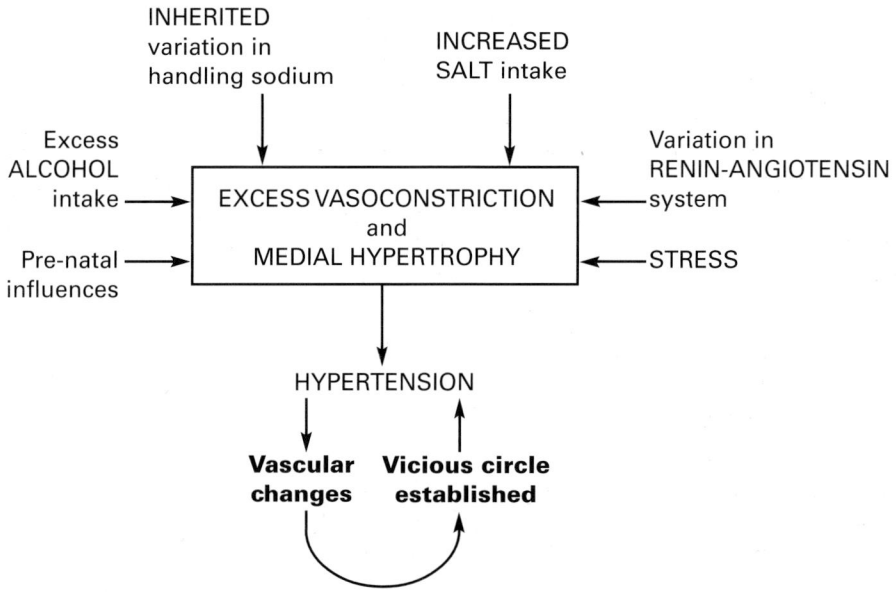

SECONDARY HYPERTENSION

5–10% of hypertension is a complication of other diseases. They are broadly classified as:

(a) *Kidney diseases* e.g. chronic renal failure, renal artery stenosis, polycystic kidneys, diabetic nephropathy. The mechanism is usually renal ischaemia with activation of the renin–angiotensin system.

(b) *Endocrine disorders* — Cushing's syndrome — corticosteroid excess;
Conn's syndrome — aldosterone excess;
Phaeochromocytoma — catecholamine excess.

(c) *Coarctation of aorta* — aortic narrowing → renal perfusion impaired → renin–angiotension activation.

(d) *Eclampsia* and pre-eclampsia in pregnancy.

(e) *Drugs* e.g. steroids: oral contraceptives.

HYPERTENSION – ESSENTIAL AND SECONDARY

CLASSIFICATION — BENIGN and MALIGNANT

In the classification of hypertension, in addition to the aetiology, two other main factors are considered.

(1) **Rate of Progress**		(2) **Height and rapidity of rise of the BP**	
Chronic — over many years	+	Usually only mild or moderate very slow rise. (*NB* the very old may have considerably higher BP without ill-effects)	**Benign** — during long course but eventually may have serious effects
Rapid (acute) — months or 1–2 years	+	Usually very high and rapidly rising BP, e.g. 120 + diastolic	**Malignant** — serious damaging effects

Summary

Essential (90–95%) — Benign or Malignant

Secondary (5–10%) — Benign, Malignant

COMPARISON of BENIGN and MALIGNANT HYPERTENSION

	Benign	**Malignant**
Aetiology	Usually ESSENTIAL If secondary, commonly of endocrine type	A few cases arise out of benign essential. Majority are SECONDARY TO RENAL DISEASE
Age	Begins younger than 45 years but is prolonged into 6 and 7 decades	Young adults 25–35 years
Sex	Female > Male	Female = Male
Prevalence	VERY COMMON — at least 15% of population in Western societies	Rare
Course	VERY SLOW — many years	RAPID — months to 1–2 years
Blood pressure	Diastolic 90–120 mm Hg Very slow rise	120+ Rapid rise

HYPERTENSION

COMPARISON of BENIGN and MALIGNANT HYPERTENSION (continued)

VASCULAR CHANGES

	Benign	Malignant
Arteries	Accelerates ARTERIOSCLEROSIS; POTENTIATES ATHEROMA	Accelerates arteriosclerosis; causes INTIMAL FIBROUS THICKENING
Arterioles	Hyaline thickening	FIBRINOID necrosis of vessel wall and thrombosis, especially affecting kidney and abdominal viscera

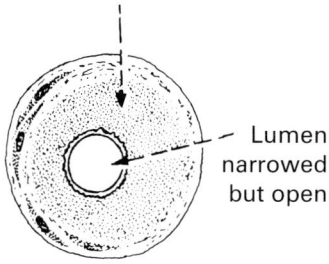

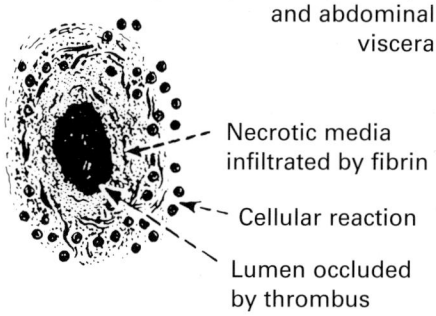

EFFECTS and MAIN COMPLICATIONS in VARIOUS ORGANS

Heart	Hypertrophy of left ventricle	Hypertrophy of left ventricle ± focal myocardial necrosis
Heart failure	Common	Acute heart failure
Cerebral haemorrhage	Due to rupture of damaged artery — 30% of cases	Encephalopathy (fits and loss of consciousness) due to cerebral oedema and haemorrhage.
Kidney	Varying degrees of NEPHROSCLEROSIS but usually *not* serious.	Severe renal damage — death in uraemia
Eyes	Arterial narrowing — retinal exudation.	Papilloedema; arterial narrowing; haemorrhage and exudates.

The effects and complications are proportional to the height of the blood pressure. Therefore drug treatment which lowers the BP lowers the incidence of complications, but the diseased vessels do not return to normal and organ perfusion may be inadequate at levels of BP which would usually be considered physiological.

NB Modern drug therapy has greatly reduced the morbidity and mortality from malignant hypertension.

ISCHAEMIC HEART DISEASE

Cardiac ischaemia is the major cause of death in affluent Western societies. It is almost always due to **atheroma** of the **coronary arteries** causing narrowing or occlusion. The effects may be of sudden or gradual onset.

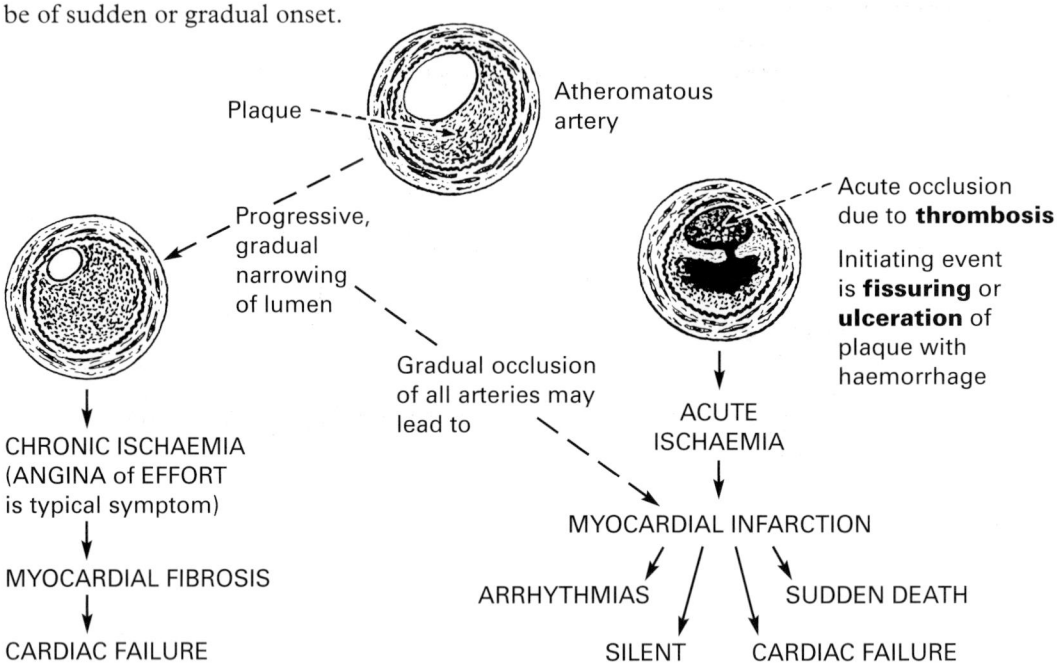

Distribution of atheromatous plaques

(1) There may be only a few plaques, but because the sites of predilection are in the proximal parts of the arteries (usually within 3 cm of the origin from the aorta), the effects of occlusion are serious.

or (2) Very numerous plaques throughout the arborisation on the surface of the heart. *Note:* The small terminal arteries penetrating the myocardium are usually not affected

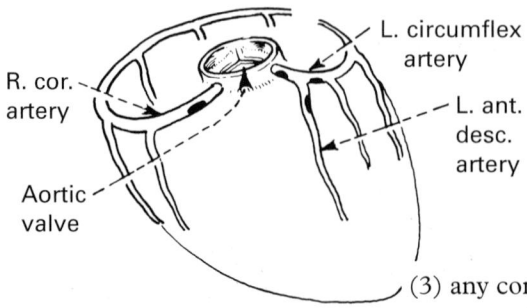

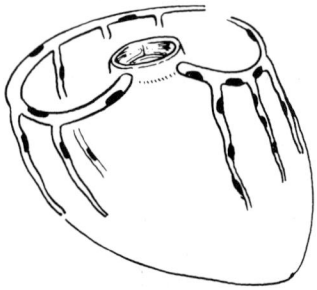

(3) any combination of (1) and (2).

The site of ischaemic damage usually represents the distribution area of the diseased arterial branch.

MYOCARDIAL INFARCTION

REGIONAL INFARCTION

90% of cardiac infarcts are regional in distribution. The 3 common ones are illustrated in order of frequency.

(1) LEFT CORONARY ARTERY – ANTERIOR DESCENDING BRANCH

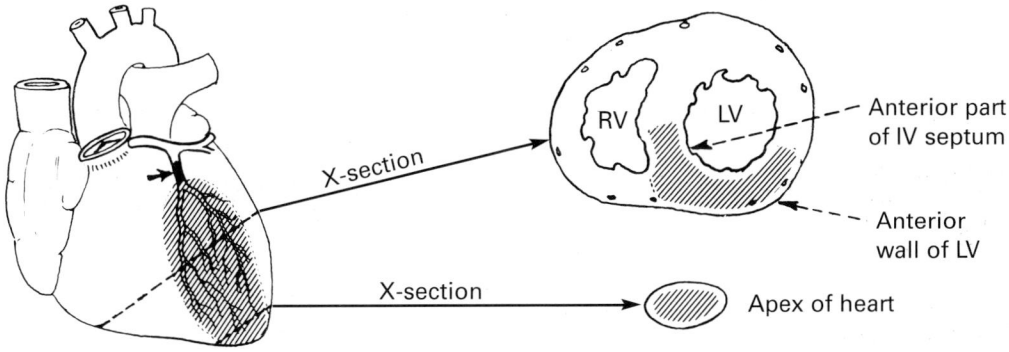

(2) RIGHT CORONARY ARTERY

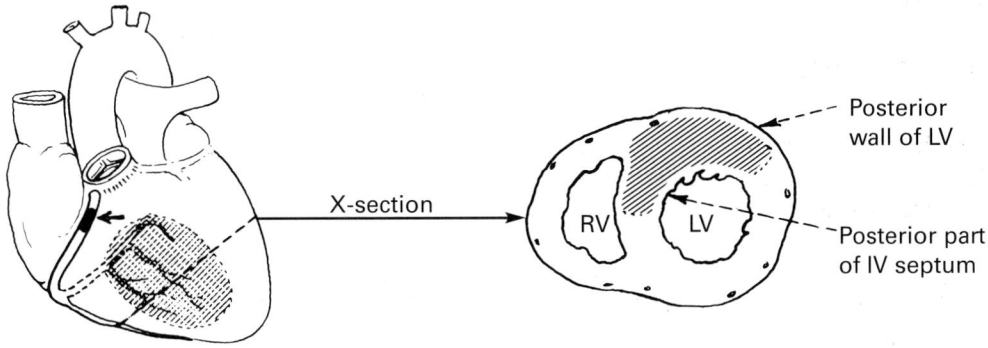

(3) LEFT CORONARY ARTERY – CIRCUMFLEX BRANCH

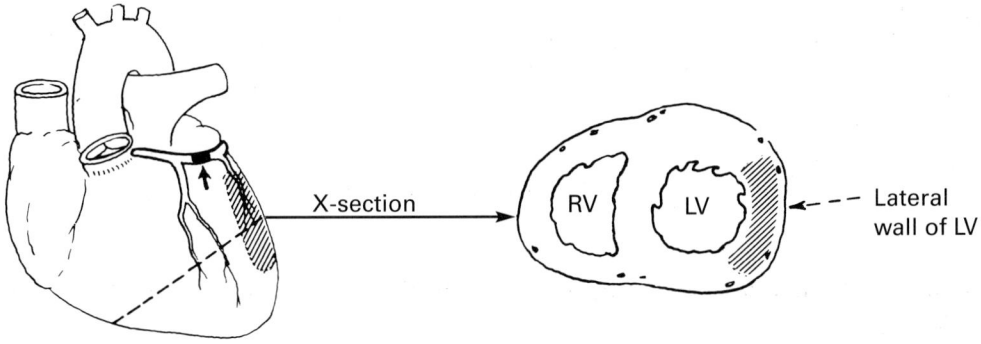

MYOCARDIAL INFARCTION

EXTENT OF DAMAGE

This depends on:

1. The inherited individual anatomical variation in distribution area, e.g. the calibres of the right coronary artery and the circumflex branch of the left coronary artery show considerable variation and are usually inversely related.

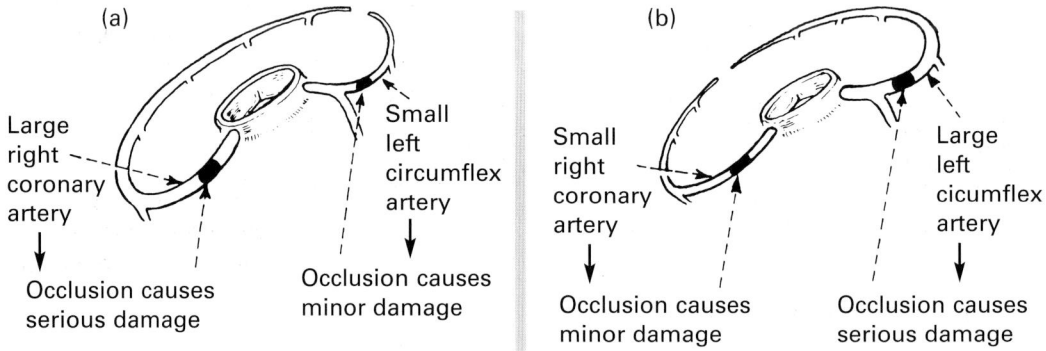

2. The efficiency of any anastomosis in the deprived distribution area. Gradual narrowing of an artery allows time for increased anastomosis to the deprived distribution area to develop, and so old age tends to be associated with improved anastomoses.

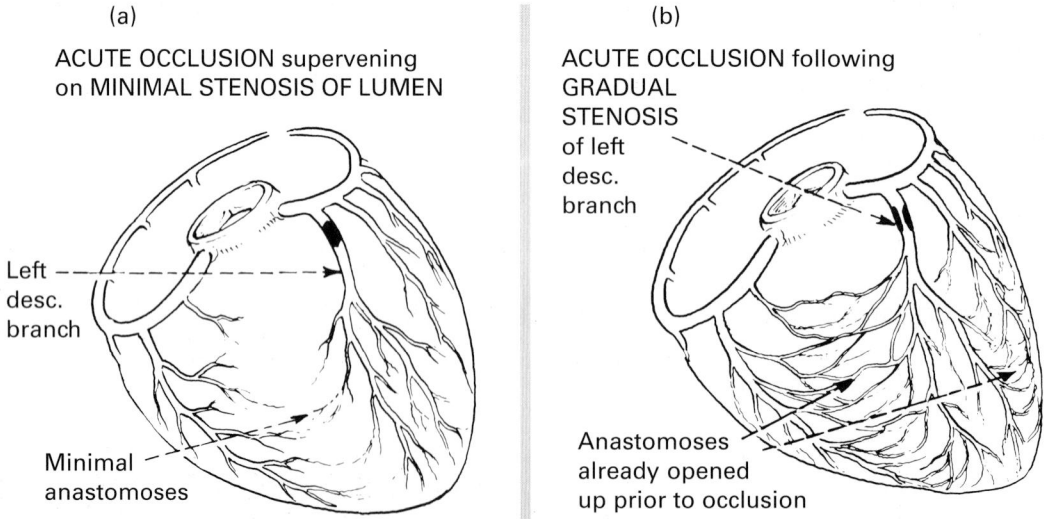

COMPLETE OCCLUSION is usually accompanied by myocardial infarction.

COMPLETE OCCLUSION may be accompanied by only minor damage.

MYOCARDIAL INFARCTION

GLOBAL OR CIRCUMFERENTIAL SUBENDOCARDIAL INFARCTION

This type is not uncommon. It occurs round the circumference of the left ventricle under the endocardium in cases of severe stenosis of all the coronary arteries and is often due to hypotension. The coronaries are usually not thrombosed.

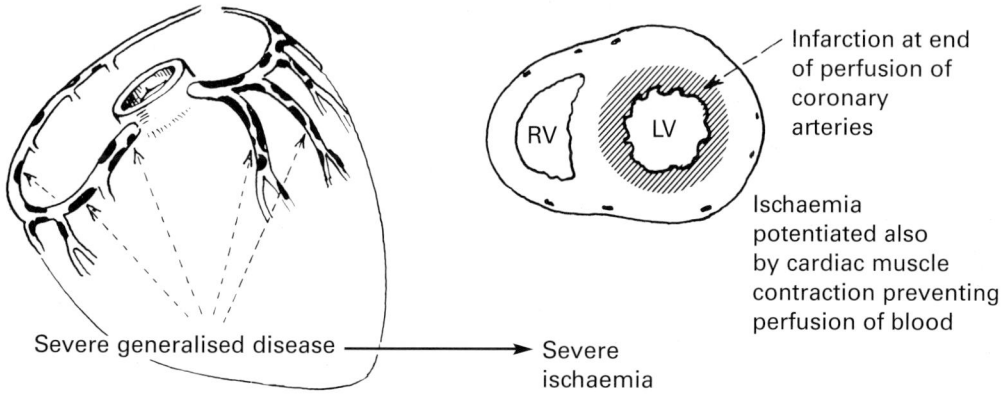

Global infarction is a serious condition which is not always detected by ECG.

MICROSCOPIC FOCAL INFARCTION

This is necrosis of single or small groups of muscle fibres at the margins of areas of myocardium previously damaged by ischaemia and is a component of progressive chronic ischaemia.

The **time scale** of the pathological changes following acute infarction are illustrated.

1. During the first 24 hours changes are minimal.

Time			
0–24 hrs	Minimal change	Slight blotchiness (congestion and pallor) of infarcted area	Slight separation of fibres; slight increase of leucocytes between fibres; slight disturbance of cell cytoplasm

MYOCARDIAL INFARCTION

Time			
24 hrs –3 days	Definite changes in dead muscle	Dead muscle, paler yellow Note: Usually a thin layer of healthy muscle under the endocardium 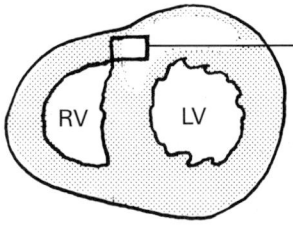	Dead muscle fibres have lost striations and nuclei; cytoplasm glassy pink (H & E staining); capillary congestion at margin; neutrophils and macrophages increasing in number 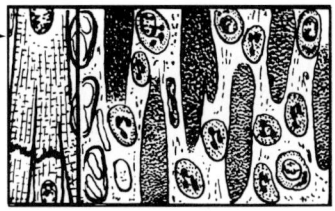
3–10 days	Healing (organisation) commencing	Margin of congestion (redness) appearing round dead muscle and resorption of muscle becoming visible at the edges 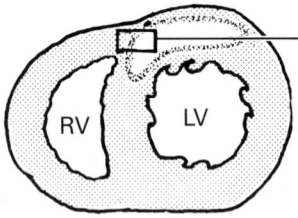	Muscle fibres splitting up and being resorbed; granulation tissue at edges; neutrophils still present 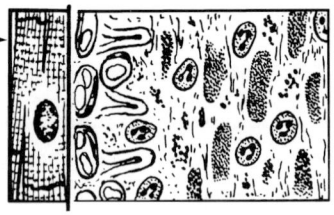
Weeks – months	Scar tissue – healing complete	White fibrous tissue 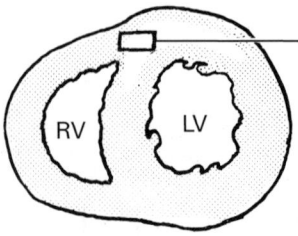	Scar tissue – may be occasional surviving muscle fibres embedded 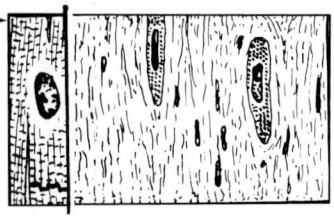

These changes represent the uncomplicated continuous process of healing. However, complications are frequent, producing serious, often fatal, effects.

MYOCARDIAL INFARCTION

Time	COMPLICATIONS
Minutes, hours	1. **ARRHYTHMIAS** (a) *Ventricular fibrillation*, i.e. cardiac arrest (especially liable at onset of infarction and during first few days). (b) *Block of impulse conduction in Bundle of His and/or its branches* — usually causes slowing of ventricular rhythm or upsets the balance of ventricular contraction. 2. **CARDIAC FAILURE** 3. **CARDIOGENIC SHOCK** Associated with large infarcts.
Days	4. **THROMBOTIC COMPLICATIONS** (a) ***MURAL THROMBOSIS*** 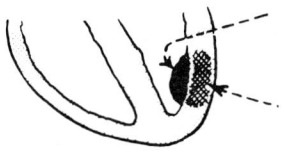 Thrombus may form on endocardium over site of infarction: potential EMBOLISM to Brain Intestine Kidney Lower limbs (b) ***ATRIAL THROMBOSIS*** 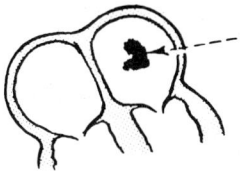 Thrombus may form in atrial appendages — especially if atrial rhythm is disturbed (c) ***LEG VEIN THROMBOSIS*** 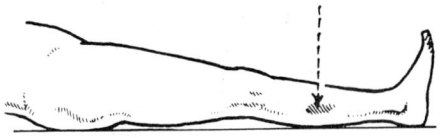 Due to recumbancy and venous stasis → **Pulmonary embolism** may be FATAL

MYOCARDIAL INFARCTION

Time	**COMPLICATIONS (continued)**
3–14 days	5. **RUPTURE OF HEART** Potentiated by: (a) infarction of whole wall thickness (b) unusual increased neutrophil activity before organisation is established → softening of dead muscle (myomalacia cordis) **Sites affected and results** (i) *MURAL MYOCARDIUM* 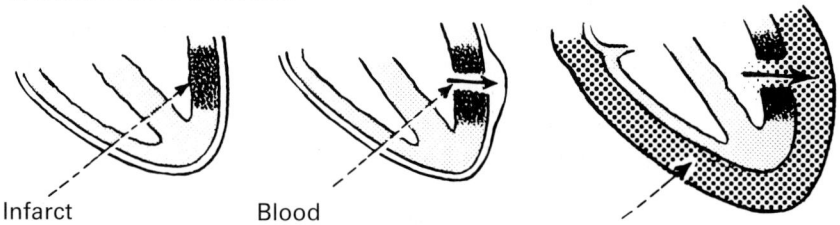 Infarct Blood passing through ventricular wall into pericardial sac Pericardial sac is distended with blood (tamponade); heart action impeded — DEATH (ii) *PAPILLARY MUSCLE* 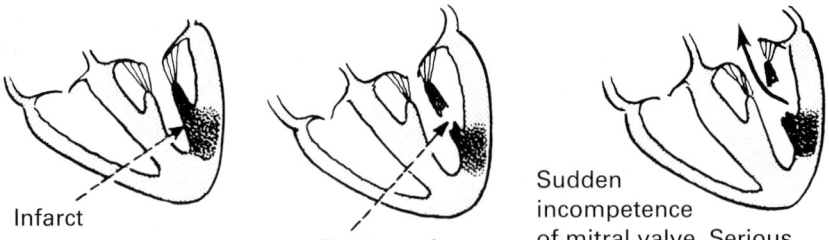 Infarct Rupture of muscle Sudden incompetence of mitral valve. Serious aggravation of cardiac pumping load; acute failure → often DEATH. (iii) *INTERVENTRICULAR SEPTUM* 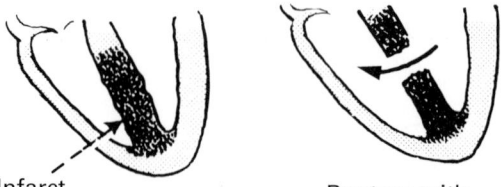 Infarct Rupture with interventricular communication → Rapid combined ventricular failure → DEATH

MYOCARDIAL INFARCTION

Time	**COMPLICATIONS (continued)**
3–14 days	6. **ACUTE PERICARDITIS** This may complicate the infarct.
Weeks	7. **CHRONIC HEART FAILURE** At the stage of fibrosis, chronic heart failure may supervene (+ ANGINA PECTORIS). 8. **DRESSLER'S SYNDROME** An auto-immune disorder with **pericarditis** and **pleurisy**, related to the release of antigens from damaged heart muscle.
Months	9. **CARDIAC ANEURYSM** 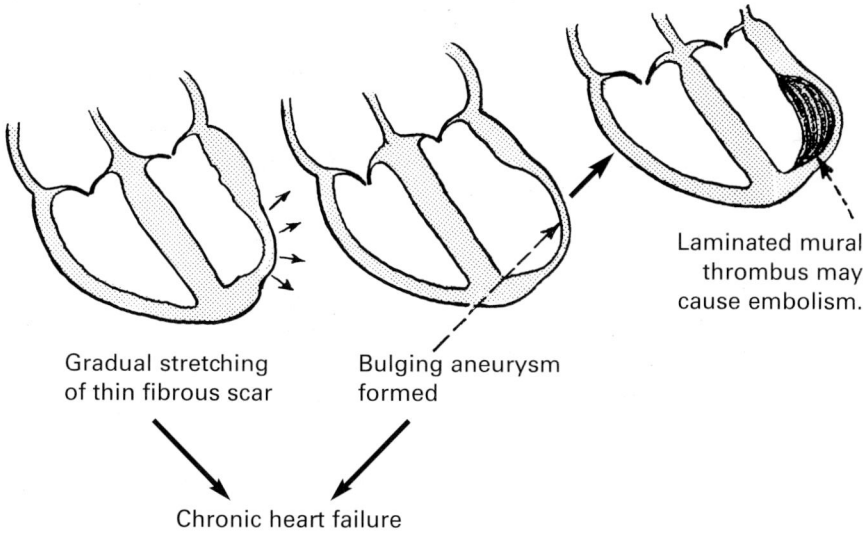
At any time	10. **RECURRENCE OF INFARCTION** Due to further thrombotic occlusion of a coronary arterial branch.

CHRONIC ISCHAEMIC HEART DISEASE

The basic pathological process is replacement of the myocardial fibres by fibrous tissue which is laid down in two main ways depending on whether the coronary insufficiency is due to severe generalised stenosis or is the result of local infarction following thrombosis.

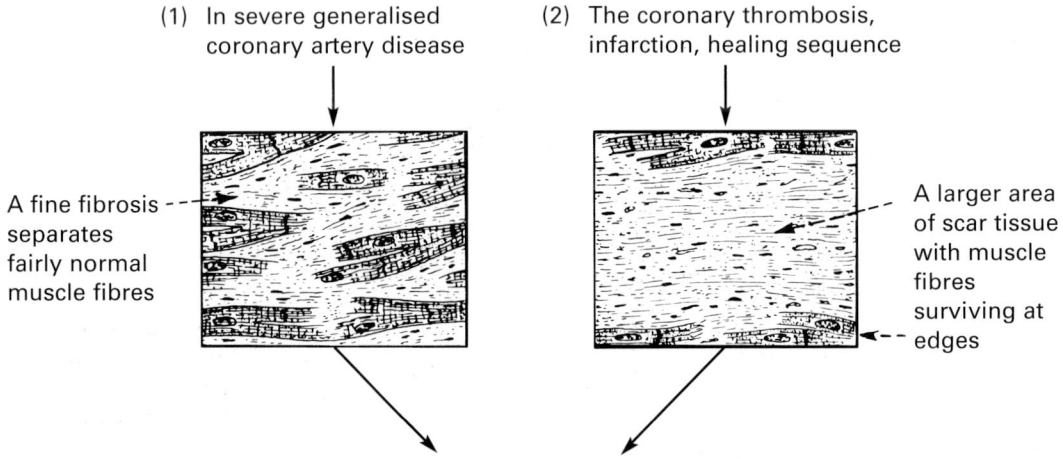

However, in many cases both mechanisms are present and lesions merge indistinguishably into each other.

Myocardial fibrosis tends to be progressive, reflecting the progression of the atheromatous narrowing of the arteries.

Myocardial hypertrophy from any cause is an important contributory factor in many cases.

Greater muscle mass → Greater blood supply required → Greater susceptibility to ischaemic damage

Thus hypertension, which causes left ventricular hypertrophy, is an important background factor.

ISCHAEMIC HEART DISEASE

CLINICAL, LABORATORY and ELECTROCARDIOGRAPH (ECG) EFFECTS

Cardiac Pain is caused by muscle ischaemia as follows:

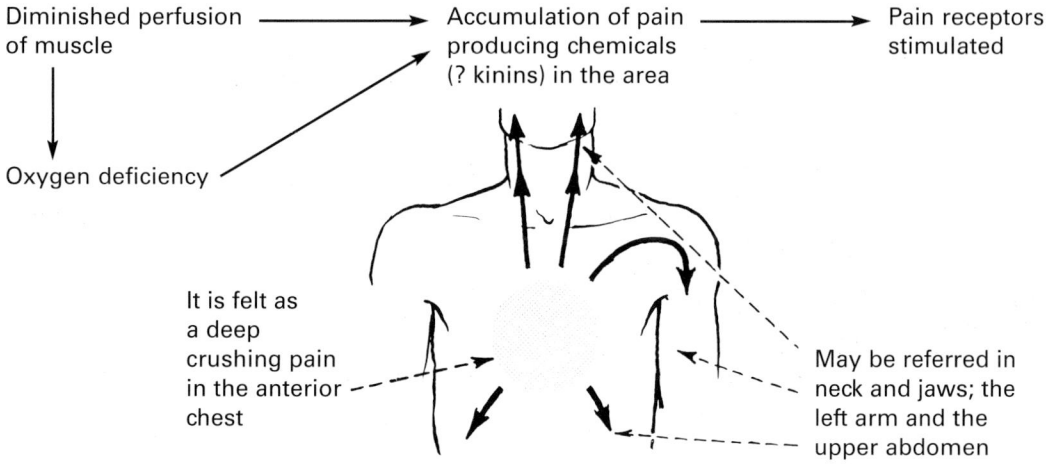

It occurs in 3 main circumstances:

1 **In acute infarction** — especially in the early phases before necrosis is complete. It is usually a continuous pain — not relieved by rest.

2. **In chronic myocardial ischaemia without infarction,** e.g. ANGINA PECTORIS — episodes of cardiac pain brought on by temporary ischaemia.

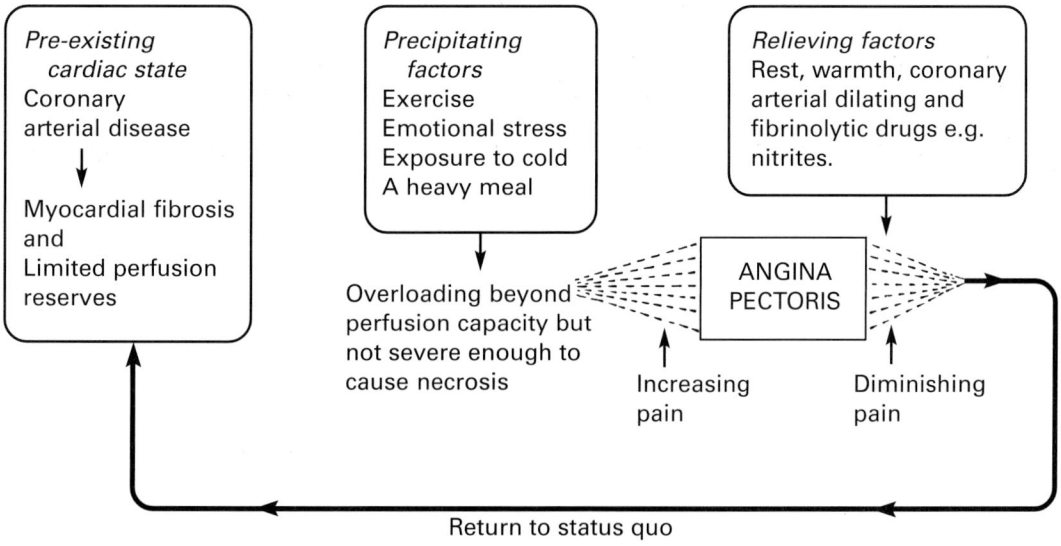

3. *Note:* The term **Crescendo Angina** refers to rapidly increasing anginal pain over a period of a few days without treatment, usually leading to myocardial infarction. It is due to developing thrombus or plaque rupture.

ISCHAEMIC HEART DISEASE

CLINICAL, LABORATORY and ECG EFFECTS (continued)

The blood in myocardial infarction

Leucocytosis
12–15,000/mm^3
lasting not more
than one week

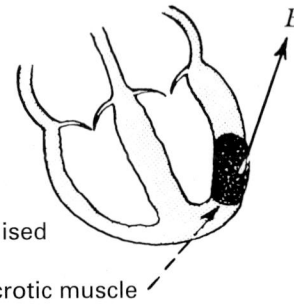

Neutrophils mobilised
from marrow by
chemotaxis of necrotic muscle

Enzyme changes
Enzymes liberated from necrotic muscle.
Two commonly used in diagnosis:

1. Myocardial creatine kinase (CKMB) is specific for cardiac muscle.
   Peak in 24 hours; falls in 72 hours.
2. Serum glutamic oxaloacetic transaminase (SGOT). Non-specific for cardiac muscle.
   Peak in 48–72 hrs; falls over 5 days.

These changes do not occur in angina pectoris since by definition necrosis has not occurred.

The Electrocardiogram (ECG)

The ventricular changes in ischaemia are reflected in the portion of ECG representing ventricular activity, i.e. the QRST complex. During excitation, contraction and restitution, the electrical potentials across the membranes of necrotic muscle fibres are strikingly different from healthy muscle. The ECG changes may be subtle but three common patterns are illustrated.

Normal

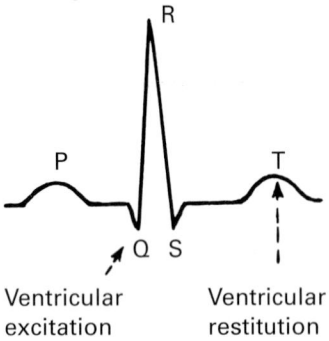

Infarction

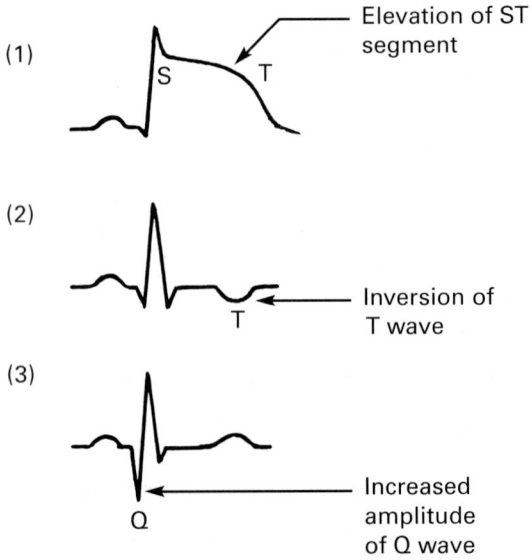

MISCELLANEOUS AFFECTIONS OF THE MYOCARDIUM

MYOCARDITIS

Inflammation of the myocardium is rare but may be caused by a variety of agents. The process is usually acute and may be generalised, regional or focal; most patients have chest pain but recover well: less commonly heart failure develops. Some patients die suddenly.

Agents	Special features	Basic pathology
Viruses E.g. coxsackie B group	Usually generalised: interstitial inflammation the main feature	Muscle fibre damage — necrosis and lysis of individual or small groups
Bacteria — pyogenic Direct invasion either from infected valves or by blood-stream.	Focal suppuration Neutrophils ++	
Toxins (incl. chemicals) Classical example — diphtheria toxin circulating in blood. Also in other severe infections e.g. typhoid, pneumonia	Usually generalised: muscle damage the main feature	Interstitial oedema and inflammatory cellular infiltrate

Immunological

E.g. rheumatic fever — myocarditis is an important component of the disease (see p.216 for details of special pathology).

CARDIOMYOPATHY

This term refers to diseases of cardiac muscle when ischaemia, hypertension, valvular disease and inflammation have been excluded. Genetic influences are important.

3 main forms are recognised:

1. **Dilated (congestive) Cardiomyopathy**

All the chambers of the heart are dilated and hypertrophied

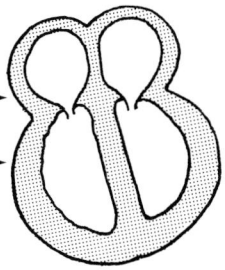

This is an uncommon condition which is familial in a minority of cases. Patients present clinically with unexplained heart failure usually between the ages of 30 and 60 years.

MISCELLANEOUS AFFECTIONS OF THE MYOCARDIUM

CARDIOMYOPATHY (continued)

2a. **Hypertrophic Cardiomyopathy**

This can occur at any age, but young adults are often affected. There is often a family history presenting usually as an autosomal dominant pattern. At least 6 genes may be involved, e.g. β-myosin heavy chain.

The effects include:

SUDDEN DEATH: CARDIAC FAILURE: EMBOLI from mural thrombus.

Muscle hypertrophy is often of a particular anatomical component of the heart: histologically the enlarged muscle fibres show a striking irregularity of orientation.

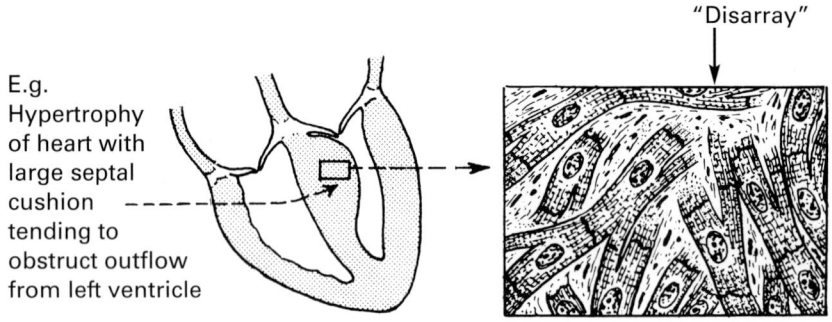

2b. **Restrictive Cardiomyopathy**

In this form the myocardium does not relax properly in diastole; this restricts ventricular filling and **cardiac output is reduced.**

A similar problem is seen in **Endomyocardial Fibrosis** — a disease of childhood seen mainly in Africa.

Other myocardial disorders include:

(i) Amyloidosis (page 24).
(ii) Haemochromatosis (page 355).
(iii) Drugs e.g. alcohol, adriamycin, cocaine.

MISCELLANEOUS AFFECTIONS OF THE MYOCARDIUM

FATTY INFILTRATION (ADIPOSITY)

The right ventricle is most commonly affected — fatty tissue penetrates between the muscle fibres but only in very severe cases contributes materially to cardiac insufficiency.

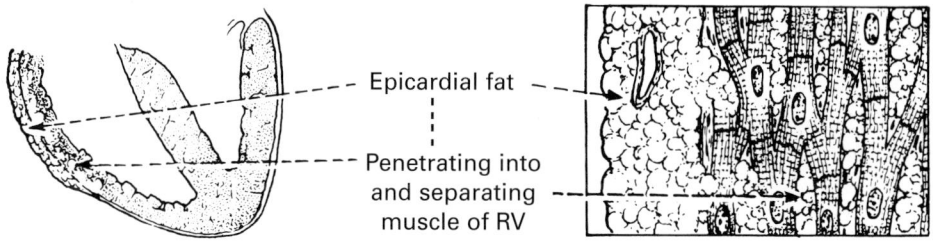

FATTY CHANGE

This reflects serious metabolic disturbance of the muscle cell and is usually caused by the action of toxins or hypoxia, particularly secondary to severe anaemia.

The muscle cells contain microscopic deposits of lipid; the change may be diffuse or in cases of severe anaemia may present as a dappled mottling under the endocardium (thrush breast).

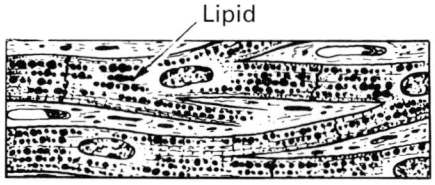

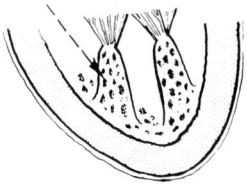

ATROPHY OF HEART

This occurs in cases of chronic starvation and generalised inanition associated with the terminal stages of cancer. The presence of lipofuscin in the muscle cells may give the heart a striking brown appearance.

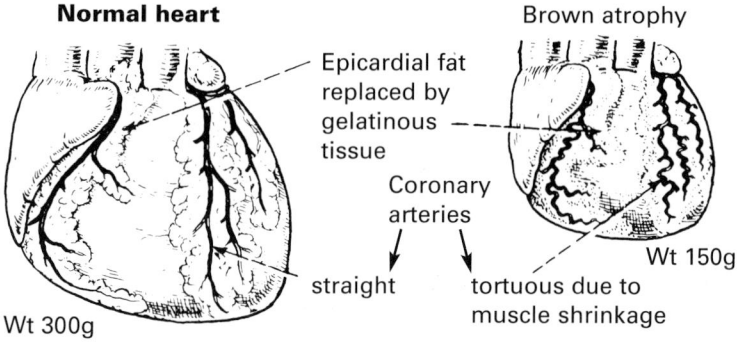

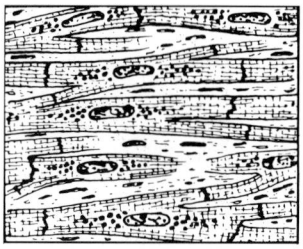

Thin muscle fibres with pigment (lipofuscin) deposition

RHEUMATIC FEVER

In rheumatic fever (acute rheumatism), a disease of children and young adults, inflammation affects the connective tissues at many sites, of which the **heart** is the most important.

Aetiology

There is a strong association with streptococcal sore throat. The streptococcus is important because it may share antigens with human tissues, particularly heart muscle and cardiac valves.

In the current most plausible theory, the inflammation is regarded as being due to immunological cross-reactions in genetically predisposed individuals since streptococci are not found at the various local sites and the disease follows some 2–4 weeks after the throat infection.

Mechanism

Throat infection due to β-haemolytic streptococcus (Group A) → IMMUNE RESPONSE → Cell mediated and ANTIBODIES to STREPTOCOCCAL ANTIGENS → CROSS-REACTION with CARDIAC and connective tissues of SUSCEPTIBLE individuals

In addition to the cardiac damage, the disease is manifest in the following ways:

1. **General manifestations** include:
   Fever with sweating and malaise: raised ESR and C-reactive protein: neutrophil leucocytosis.
2. **Indications of inflammation at local sites**
   (a) *Joints and adjacent musculofascial tissues* – causing ARTHRITIS with effusion, muscle pains and weakness.
   (b) *Serous membranes* – pericardial and sometimes pleural effusion.
   (c) *Skin* (i) a rash (erythema marginatum).
   (ii) small subcutaneous palpable nodules over bony prominences subject to pressure.
   (d) *Central nervous system* – chorea (involuntary spasmodic muscular movements).

The basic process is a non-specific inflammation in which exudation of a fibrin-rich fluid is a major component.

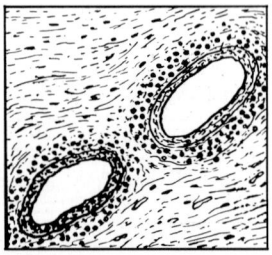

Joints and connective tissues

Oedema – fibrin-rich fluid: perivascular inflammatory **cellular infiltrate**

Subcutaneous skin nodules

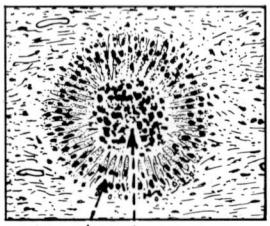

Central core of necrotic cell debris: mononuclear cells tending to a spindle shape and arranged in a pallisade. The surrounding tissues show the usual nonspecific inflammation.

RHEUMATIC FEVER

CARDIAC MANIFESTATIONS

The inflammation is widespread throughout the heart, i.e. there is PANCARDITIS. It is convenient to consider the effects on the three anatomical cardiac layers separately — pericardial, myocardial and endocardial.

1. **Pericarditis** occurs during the acute phase of the illness and is an important cause of pericardial effusion.
2. **Myocarditis** is common during the acute phase and is usually mild: it is rarely severe enough to cause cardiac failure. The histological picture is striking and the presence of the Aschoff body is characteristic.

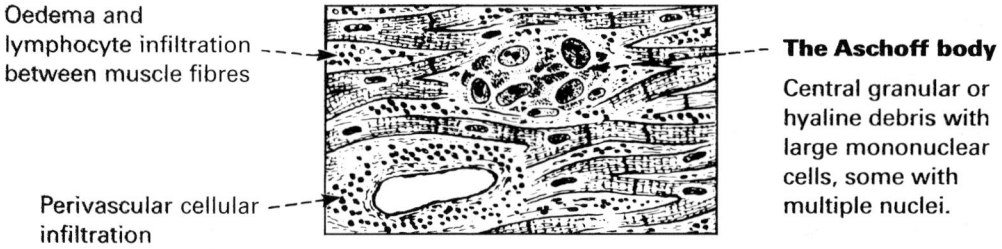

3. **Endocarditis.** Although there is a widespread histological inflammation, gross changes are seen usually on the endocardial sites subject to the greatest pressures and traumas, i.e. in the left side of the heart at the points of valve closure and at any sites of jet effect in the blood flow. The basic inflammation is complicated by ulceration of the valve surface followed by platelet and fibrin thrombosis in the form of small 'vegetations'.

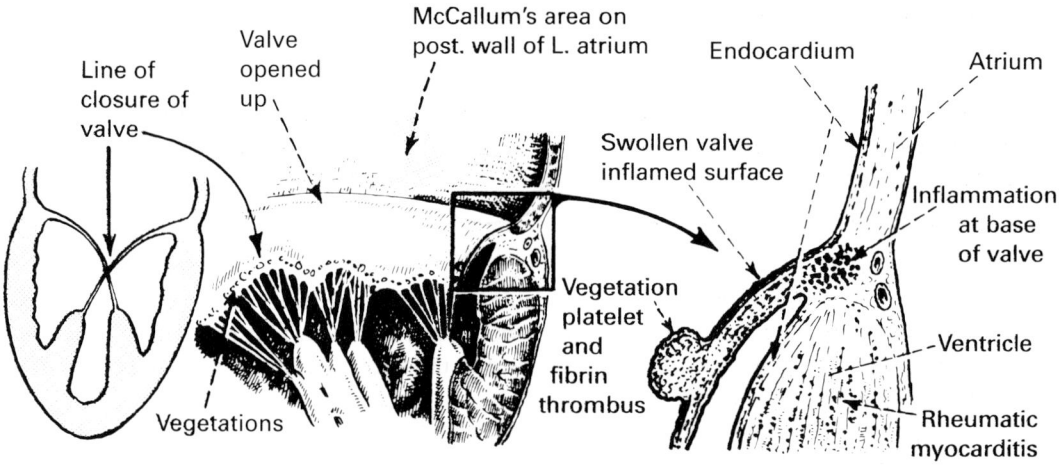

MITRAL VALVE DISEASE

Mitral disease (continued)

Incompetence may follow from the rheumatic process by a similar slow mechanism.

In addition it may develop acutely due to other quite different causes:

1. In cases of left ventricular failure when severe dilatation occurs.

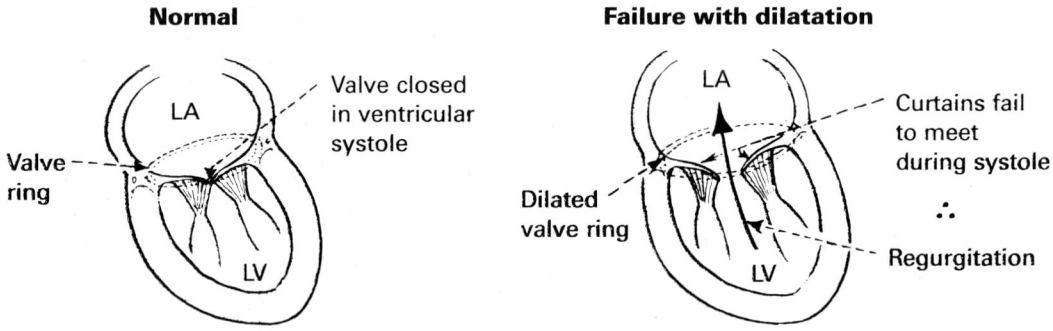

2. Necrosis with rupture of papillary muscle in acute myocardial infarction.
3. It may result from myxoid degeneration of the valve – the 'floppy valve syndrome'. More cases of this condition are now being recognised using modern non-invasive techniques to study cardiac valve function in life.
4. Infective endocarditis (see page 224).

The mechanical effects of mitral disease

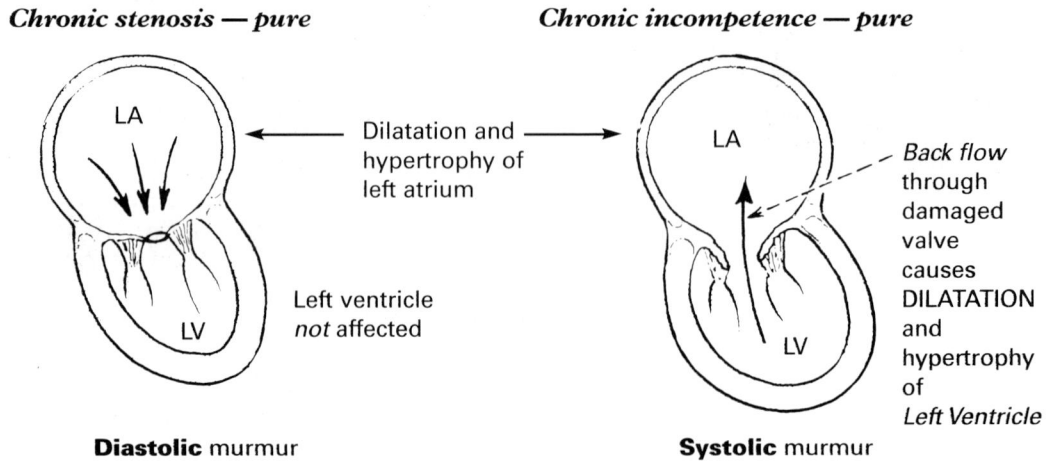

In rheumatic heart disease, pure stenosis is not uncommon; combined stenosis and incompetence is often seen.

MITRAL VALVE DISEASE

Mitral disease (continued)

In mitral disease, the back pressure in the left atrium is transmitted to the pulmonary veins and by raising pulmonary arterial pressure causes effects on the right side of the heart.

(a) **Compensated phase**

(1) Left atrial dilatation

↓

(2) Pulmonary congestion

↓

(3) Right ventricular hypertrophy

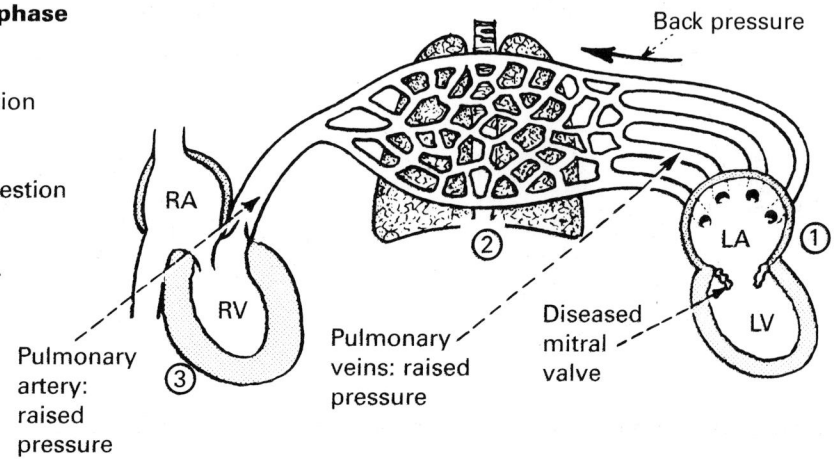

(b) **Congestive cardiac failure**

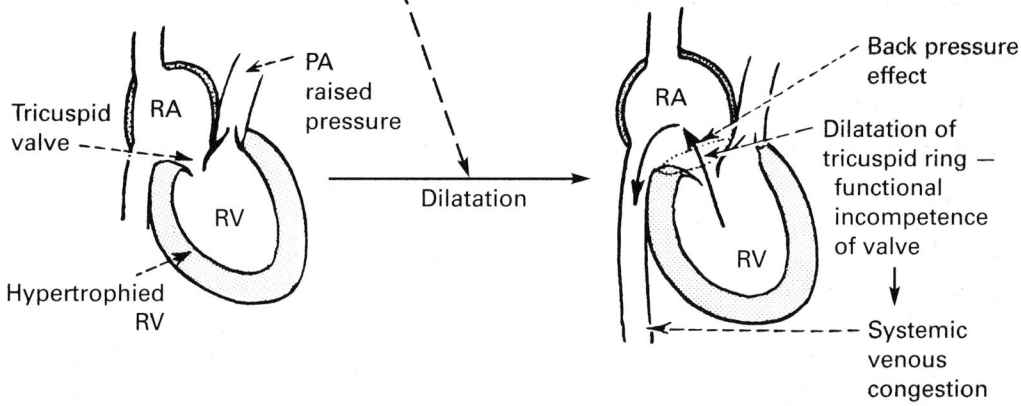

(3) Right Ventricular Hypertrophy → (4) Dilated RV → (5) Dilated RA

In the acute types of mitral incompetence, the sudden change in the intracardiac haemodynamics very seriously aggravates the heart failure already present due to the primary disease.

Complications of chronic mitral disease

1. Atrial fibrillation is common.
   Fibrillation → Thrombosis in atrial appendage → Systemic embolism
2. Infective endocarditis.

AORTIC VALVE DISEASE

STENOSIS

The main causes are RHEUMATIC SCARRING and CALCIFICATION occurring in a CONGENITALLY ABNORMAL VALVE (usually bicuspid) or one previously damaged by rheumatism or endocarditis (bacterial), but in elderly people there may be no obvious pre-existing disease.

Changes in the valve

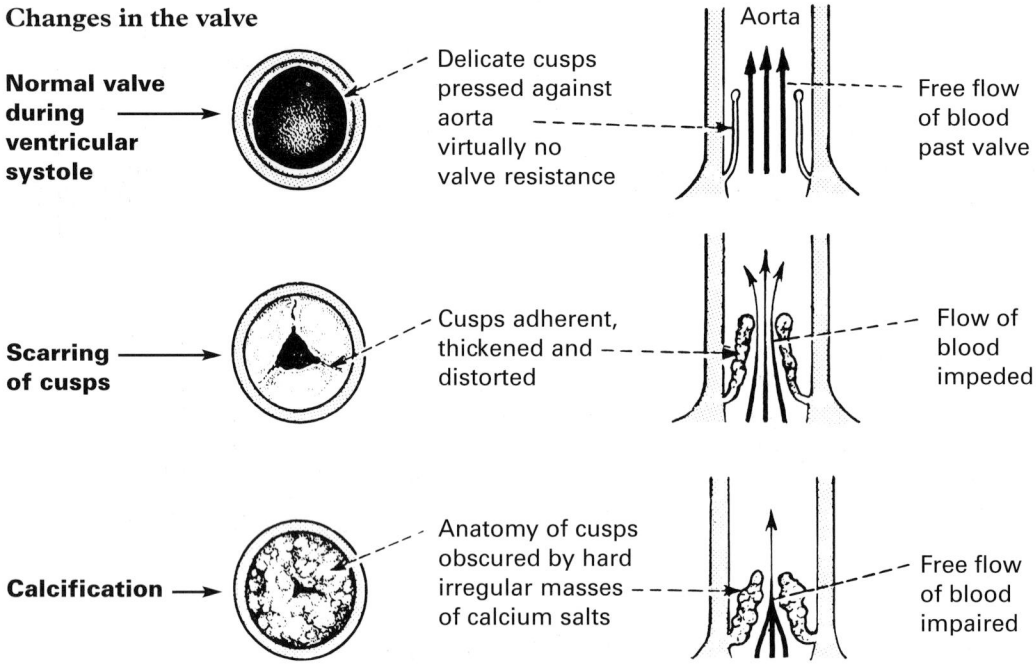

Effects

The main effect is pure HYPERTROPHY of the left ventricle to overcome the valve resistance,
e.g. 600 g
(normal — 300 g)

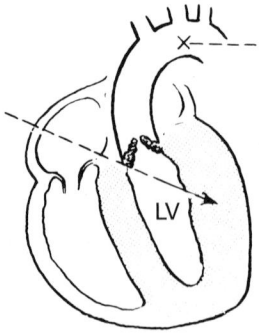

Low pulse pressure may reduce coronary supply, rendering the hypertrophied muscle susceptible to ischaemic damage.
The heart often remains in this 'compensated' state for years but eventually failure develops with dilatation.

Ejection Systolic murmur

However SUDDEN DEATH (without pre-existing signs of failure) is a definite risk at any time, but particularly during exercise in cases of aortic stenosis.

In adults, severe aortic stenosis usually requires valve replacement.

AORTIC VALVE DISEASE

INCOMPETENCE

The main causes are scarring of the cusps due to rheumatic or infective endocarditis: less commonly dilatation of the valve ring due to disease (e.g. in ankylosing spondylitis: Marfan's syndrome) or degeneration in very old age.

Changes in the valve

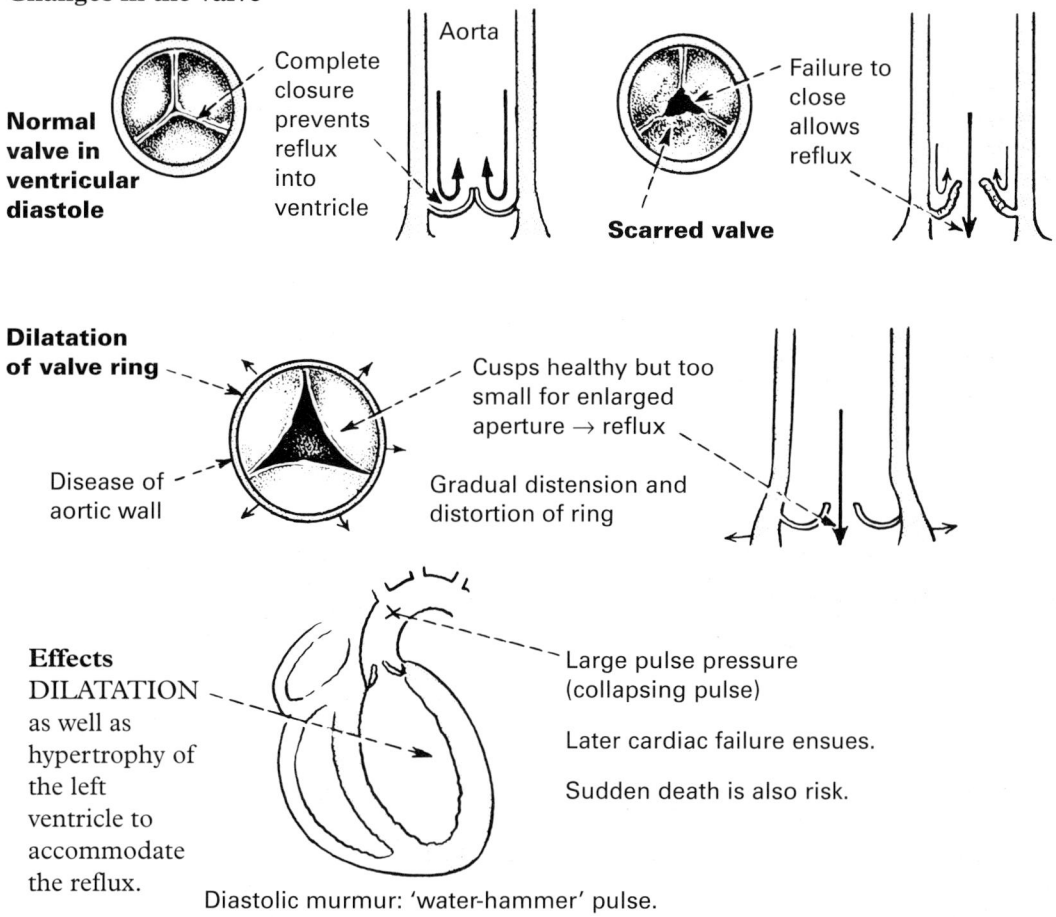

Aortic stenosis and incompetence often exist together and the effects are compounded.

TRICUSPID AND PULMONARY VALVES

Diseases of these valves on the right side of the heart are not common. However functional tricuspid incompetence due to severe cardiac dilatation is an important end stage in progressive cardiac failure.

Progressive failure → Dilatation → TRICUSPID INCOMPETENCE → Right atrial failure → Severe systemic venous congestion (congestive cardiac failure)

INFECTIVE ENDOCARDITIS

This is a disease of the heart valves particularly: the mural endocardium is only occasionally affected by late spread from the valves.

In the classical situation, bacteria settle on previously diseased valves. In drug abusers using the intravenous route, normal valves may be affected.

There is a spectrum between 2 extremes classically called acute and subacute and the disease evolves in one of 2 main patterns depending on the type of bacteria.

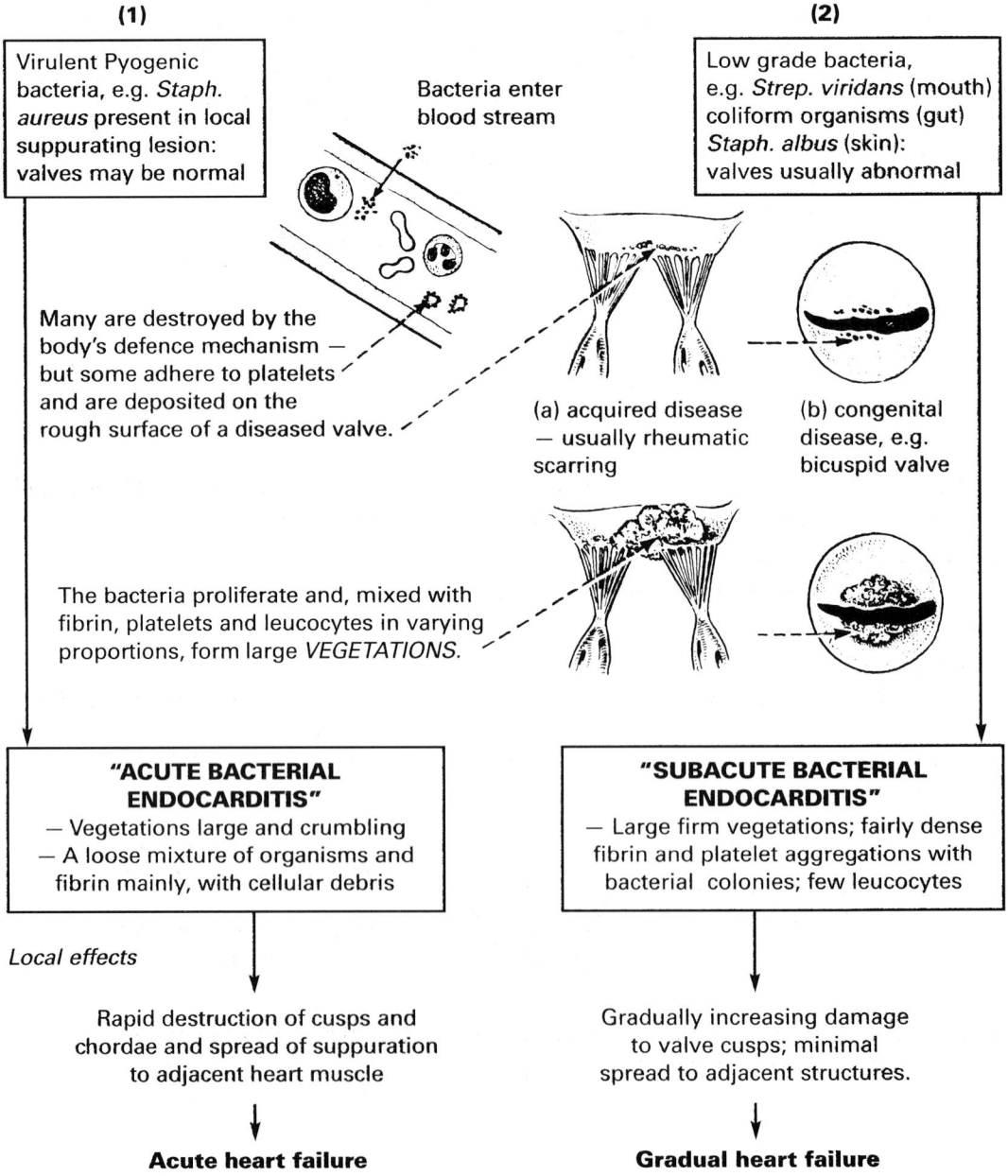

INFECTIVE ENDOCARDITIS

In addition to the local effects, the course of the disease is influenced by other important complications.

So-called

	"Acute bacterial endocarditis"	**"Subacute bacterial endocarditis"**
1. *Embolic effects*	Suppurative lesions (pyaemic abscess) in important organs, e.g. brain and kidneys	Usually bland microinfarction, e.g. in skin — splinter haemorrhage in nail beds; 'embolic' nephritis — causing haematuria; glomerular damage due to antigen–antibody complexes causing focal glomerulitis
2. *Toxic — systemic effects*	Severe Pyrexia Leucocytosis	Moderate Continuous low grade pyrexia Leucocytosis ± Splenomegaly Anaemia (partly haemolytic)
	Rapid course	Slow course
	Leading to DEATH	

This classical situation is nowadays modified by immunosuppressive drugs, antibiotics and intracardiac prostheses including catheter lines from peripheral veins.

Immunosuppression
This allows opportunistic infection by a much wider range of organisms, e.g. bacteria not usually pathogenic, and fungi.

Antibiotics
1. Their effects blur the distinction between the two types and allow healing but often with serious scarring of the valve.
2. The structure of the vegetation is important; in some cases the bacterial colonies are protected from the antibiotic.

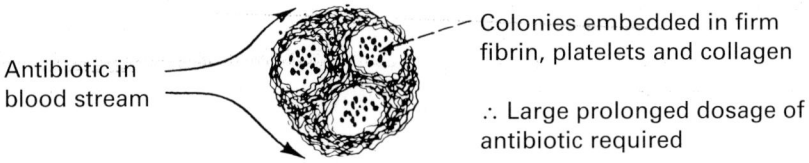

Cardiac prostheses and catheter lines act as a focus for bacterial growth and infective endocarditis is a serious complication.

CARDIAC ARRHYTHMIAS

CARDIAC ARRHYTHMIAS and DISEASES of the CONDUCTING SYSTEM

Of the wide variety of cardiac arrhythmias which have now been studied in detail using the electrocardiograph, the majority are due to (A) functional disturbances of the intrinsic excitability of the cardiac muscle at various sites or of the cardiac neurohumoral controls; only a minority are due to (B) organic disease of the conducting system itself. Organic heart disease particularly of ischaemic type is a common concomitant.

(A) **Important disorders of cardiac muscle excitability**

1. **Atrial fibrillation**
   In this common disorder, continuous incoordinate movement of the atrial muscle completely negates its role as a priming pump and the atria become functionally inert. There is no specific pathological change in the atrial wall, but atrial dilatation associated with cardiac disease is usually a precondition.

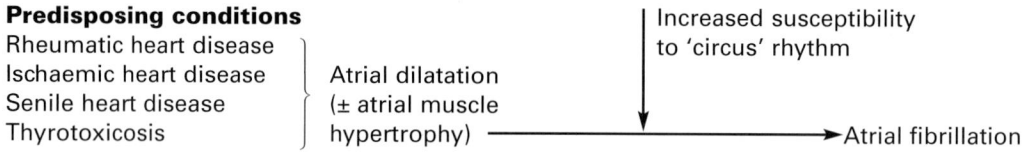

There are two main effects:

(i) *Contribution to cardiac failure*

(a) loss of atrial contraction to priming of ventricles

(b) *NB* causes increased *irregular* ventricular rate

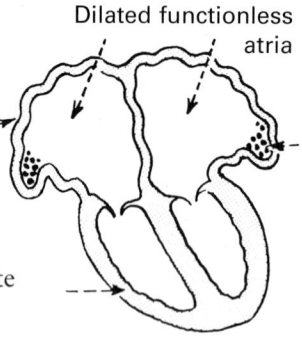

(ii) *Intra-atrial thrombosis and embolism*

Small thrombi forming in atrial appendages

Embolism to vital organs — brain, kidney, intestines (also legs) from left atrium. Pulmonary embolism from right atrium.

2. **Ventricular paroxysmal tachycardia and fibrillation**
   These very serious conditions are usually superimposed upon and aggravate pre-existing severe myocardial disease — usually ischaemic in type. In fibrillation, a form of cardiac 'arrest', cardiac function ceases; it is the terminal event in many fatal diseases.

CARDIAC ARRHYTHMIAS

Cardiac arrhythmia (continued)

(B) **Diseases of the conducting system**
The usual disorder is slowing of the impulse and it is most often associated with organic disease in the adjacent cardiac tissue.

Associated conditions

Cardiac ischaemia — Acute infarction / Fibrosis } are the most common and important

Others are — myocarditis, calcification around the valve rings and drugs, e.g. digitalis, propranolol.

Sites of disorder **Effects**

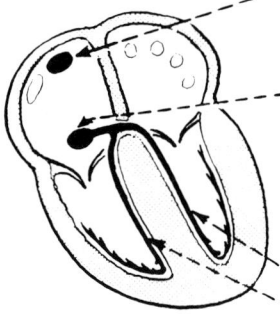

SA node — Very rarely affected

AV node and Bundle of His — *Heart block*
1st degree: only mild delay in conduction
∴ no effect on ventricular rate
2nd degree: moderate delay, missed ventricular beats
3rd degree: complete block idioventricular rhythm established, 35 or less per min

Left and right bundles — *Bundle branch block*
Causes loss of efficiency of ventricular contraction

The 3 important components of arrhythmias are:
Tachycardia, bradycardia and irregularity.
The effect of any arrhythmia on cardiac function depends essentially on its effect on ventricular output.

Tachycardia
pulse rate over 160/min → Diastolic time too short to allow adequate ventricular filling; also impairment of coronary flow → Low cardiac output → Failure

↓ Seriously aggravated by **Irregularity**

↑

Bradycardia
— pulse rate less than 35/min → Low cardiac output

CONGENITAL HEART DISEASE

Developmental abnormalities of the heart are relatively common; clinically significant defects occur in 7–11 per 1000 live births and the rate is significantly higher in stillbirths. The severity varies from minor aberrations to complex distortions incompatible with life. Many patients now live normal lives after cardiac surgery.

Aetiology

This is often obscure. Hereditary factors are of limited importance; possible environmental factors are complex and numerous.

Examples include: virus infection, e.g. rubella; teratogen, e.g. thalidomide (historically); altitude at birth (patent ductus arteriosus is commoner at high altitudes).

The initial damage which is sustained during the early formative stages in the 2nd and 3rd months of pregnancy is modified by later fetal and postnatal growth and development.

Single anatomical abnormalities occur, but often there are multiple defects which are associated in groups of which the more common are given specific names.

Abnormal development occurs:

(1) At the emergence of the great vessels

↓

Stenoses cause impedence to blood flow

(2) During formation of the septa between right and left sides and following failure of closure, e.g. ductus and foramen ovale.

↓

Abnormal apertures allow shunting of blood

This is a huge subject:

Fallot's tetralogy illustrates these main points:

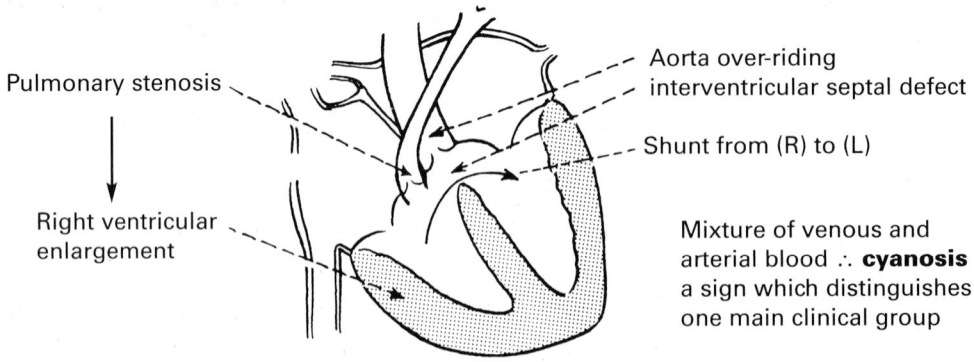

Often complications — pulmonary hypertension, increased blood volume polycythaemia, and infective endocarditis – increase the disability.

Surgical repair is the ideal treatment.

DISEASES OF THE PERICARDIUM

PERICARDITIS

Pericarditis is commonly a complication of diseases of the heart or adjacent structures or of generalised disorders; primary (or idiopathic) inflammation where no cause is found also occurs.

In **acute pericarditis**, fibrin exudation is common: sometimes exudation of serous fluid is the main feature. Haemorrhage may be superadded in cases of uraemia and tumour infiltration. Purulent pericarditis complicating bacterial infections is rare.

Fibrinous pericarditis

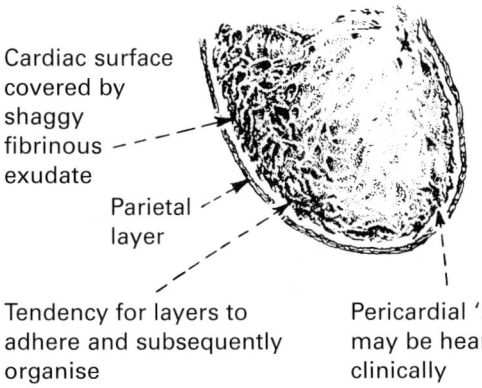

Pericarditis with effusion

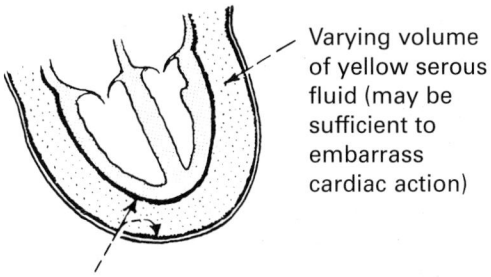

Diseases which may lead to pericarditis

(a) *Intrinsic heart disease*

(i) myocardial infarction

(ii) acute rheumatism (pancarditis)

(iii) trauma — esp. surgical

(iv) myocarditis — — pericarditis frequently occurs in Coxsackie B virus infection

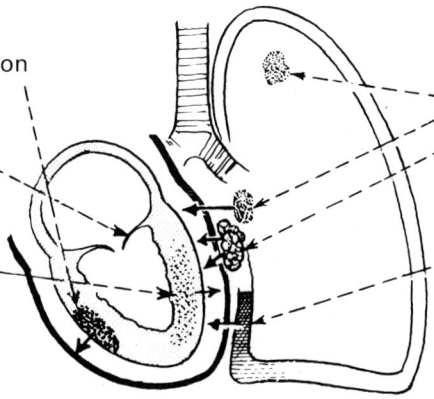

(b) *Diseases in lungs, pleura and mediastinum*

(i) tuberculosis

(ii) carcinoma

(iii) pneumonia complicated by empyema — bacterial infection is now rare due to antibiotic treatment.

(c) *Generalised disorders* (mechanism not known)

(i) uraemia
(ii) connective tissue diseases
(iii) hypothyroidism

DISEASES OF THE PERICARDIUM

CHRONIC PERICARDITIS is usually the result of recurrent attacks of rheumatism or allied diseases; occasionally it is insidiously chronic throughout. The basic changes are organisation and calcification. In extreme cases, cardiac function is impaired.

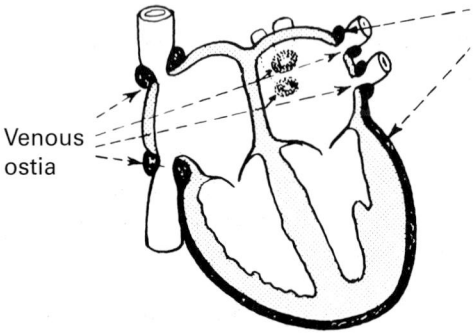

Dense fibrous calcified tissues — causing close adherence of the pericardial layers; preventing proper cardiac filling;
— this extreme condition is called **constrictive pericarditis.**

PERICARDIAL HAEMORRHAGE occurs most commonly as a result of **cardiac rupture** complicating **acute infarction**. The other main cause is rupture of **aortic aneurysm** back into the pericardium. The pericardial sac becomes distended with blood (tamponade) and death follows rapidly due to compression of the heart. Tamponade may also occur with very large pericardial effusions.

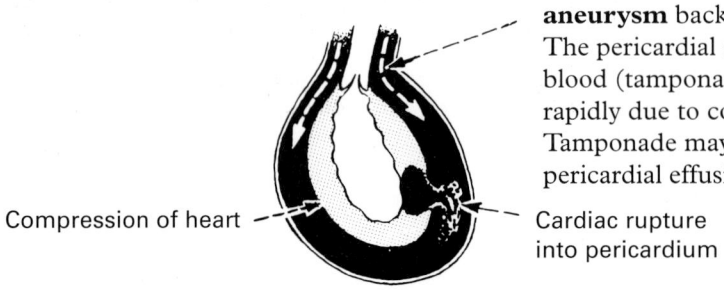

CARDIAC TUMOURS

Primary tumours in the heart are very rare. Secondary tumours, especially from the lungs, affecting the pericardium by direct spread and the heart by blood spread are fairly common and represent terminal stages in malignant disease.

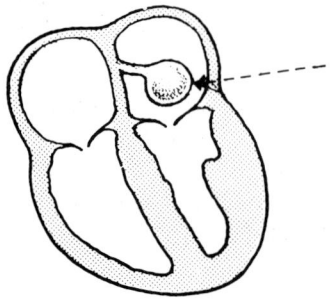

The so-called cardiac 'myxoma' is a rare condition affecting usually the left atrium in which a smooth, pale, soft, rounded mass is attached by a pedicle to the endocardium. It can cause serious effects by occluding the mitral valve opening or by embolisation.
Mesothelioma may present primarily in the pericardium.
Rhabdomyomas are occasionally seen in childhood associated with tuberous sclerosis

DISEASES OF ARTERIES

ARTERITIS

(a) Associated with specific infectious diseases, e.g. tuberculosis and syphilis. The endarteritis and periarteritis, sometimes complicated by thrombosis, augment the damage caused by the infecting organisms.

(b) Arterial necrosis and inflammation of less certain or unknown aetiology – generally known as arteritis or vasculitis. This group may affect large, medium or small arteries.

Polyarteritis nodosa

This is a disease affecting the medium and small arteries and arterioles. In the acute phase, there are signs of generalised illness with fever, etc., but the disease often becomes chronic and relapsing so that all stages of the arterial lesion may be present at the same time.

The typical lesion is a focal necrosis of the arterial wall.

In microscopic polyarteritis, a form of glomerulonephritis is associated with affection of afferent arterioles.

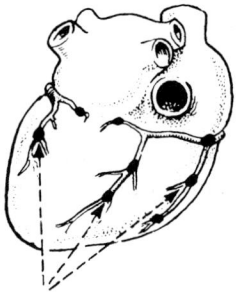

Heart showing focal 'nodose' distribution

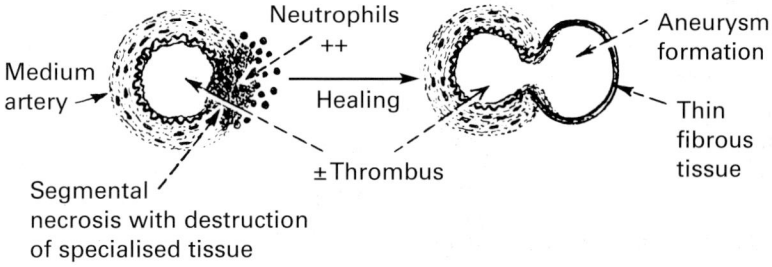

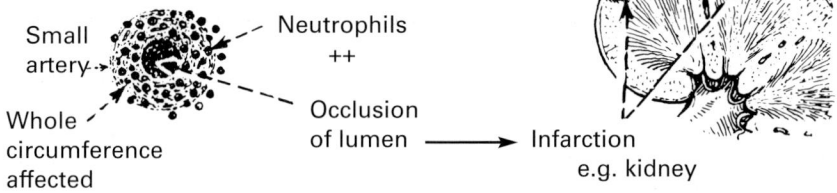

Any artery may be affected, but damage to the HEART, KIDNEYS, BRAIN and GUT is particularly important. When the arteries supplying peripheral nerves are affected symptoms of 'neuritis' may be striking.

Other forms of arteritis with some characteristics related to polyarteritis nodosa may occur as *primary disease processes*, e.g. *Wegener's granulomatosis* in which destructive lesions of the nasal mucosa, the lungs and the kidneys result from arteritis.

Arteritis may also complicate other conditions (usually the *connective tissue diseases*, see p. 642), e.g. rheumatoid arthritis, systemic lupus erythematosus (SLE).

DISEASES OF ARTERIES

Aetiology

The aetiology of most cases of arteritis remains unknown: in some of these conditions there is a strong presumptive evidence that hypersensitivity reactions, due to antigen/antibody complexes (Arthus, i.e. Type III), damage the vessel wall. The antigens, a wide variety of agents, include drugs and microbial (esp. viral) components.

In some cases there is a further association with hypersensitivity reactions of the anaphylactic (Atopic, i.e. Type I), and eosinophilia may be a feature (e.g. in some cases of allergic **asthma**).

Anti-neutrophil cytoplasmic antibodies (ANCA) occur frequently in various types of vasculitis. They are auto-antibodies to enzyme constituents e.g. myeloperoxidase and elastase.

Capillaries and venules may also be damaged and the more general terms of VASCULITIS or ANGIITIS are then applied.

Buerger's disease (thromboangiitis obliterans)

In this very painful condition, the inflammation involves the small peripheral arteries of the legs and often the arms. Typically the victim is a young Jewish male (20–40 years) **heavy cigarette smoker.**

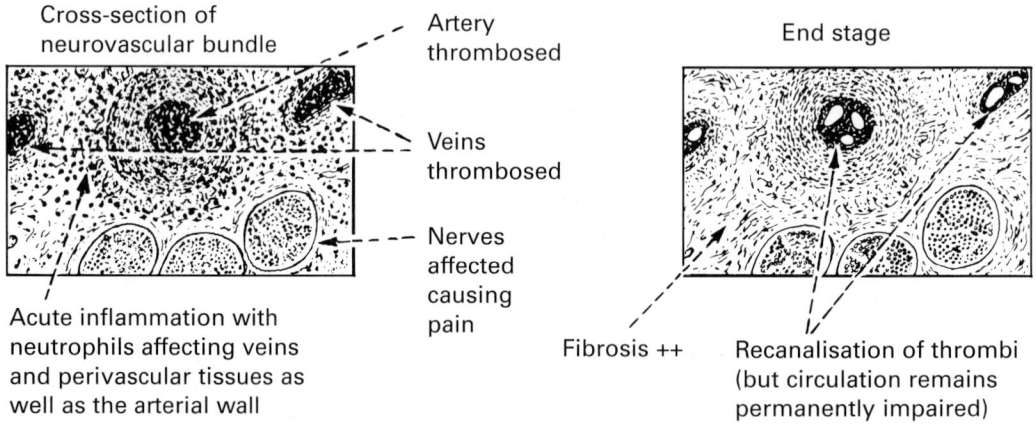

GANGRENE of the toes may follow as more vessels become involved.

DISEASES OF ARTERIES

Temporal arteritis (Giant-cell arteritis/cranial arteritis)

This disease of unknown aetiology affects elderly people (over 60 years). It may cause severe facial pain and headache and may be associated with ocular symptoms and cause blindness. In a significant number of old people, there are no symptoms.

Some cases occur along with polymyalgia rheumatica — a disease in which there are generalised muscle pains and systemic malaise. Commonly, branches of the external carotid arteries are affected, but sometimes other caudal arteries and even the aortic arch may also be involved.

The arterial wall is destroyed by an acute necrosis associated with neutrophil infiltration and usually thrombosis with partial organisation.

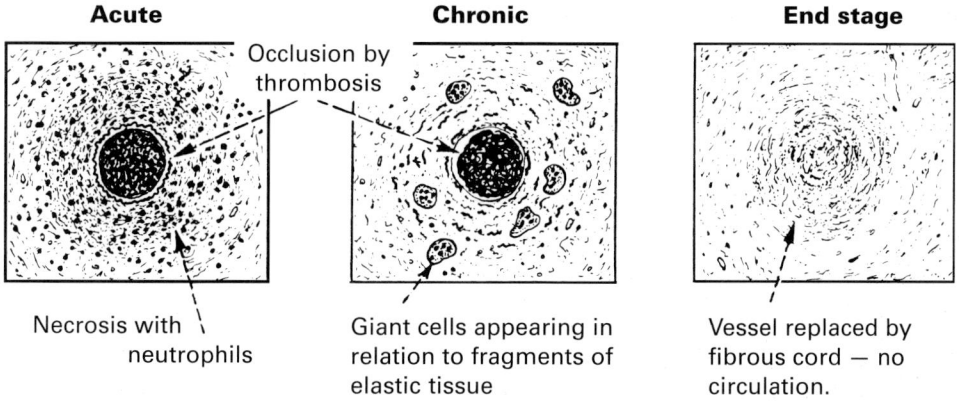

Takayashu's disease

In this rare disease, the typical victim is a young female (20–30 years). The patchy arteritis is more severe and affects the aorta and its primary branches, leading to ischaemia of BRAIN (cerebral arteries), EYES (ophthalmic arteries), FACE (carotid arteries), ARMS ('pulseless' disease), HEART (coronary orifices), KIDNEYS (causing HYPERTENSION) in varying combinations.

DEATH often follows these serious effects.

Miscellaneous vascular disorders

These include vasculitis associated with **rheumatoid arthritis**; **erythema nodosum** (inflammatory nodules in the subcutaneous fat); **Wegener's granulomatosis** and **Henoch-Schönlein** purpura.

The important vascular changes in **diabetes mellitus** are described on page 660.

ANEURYSM

A local enlargement of an artery is called an **aneurysm**. Although localised, it often reflects the presence of more widespread arterial disease.

MECHANISM of FORMATION

The two main forces concerned in the maintenance of the integrity of the shape of an artery are:

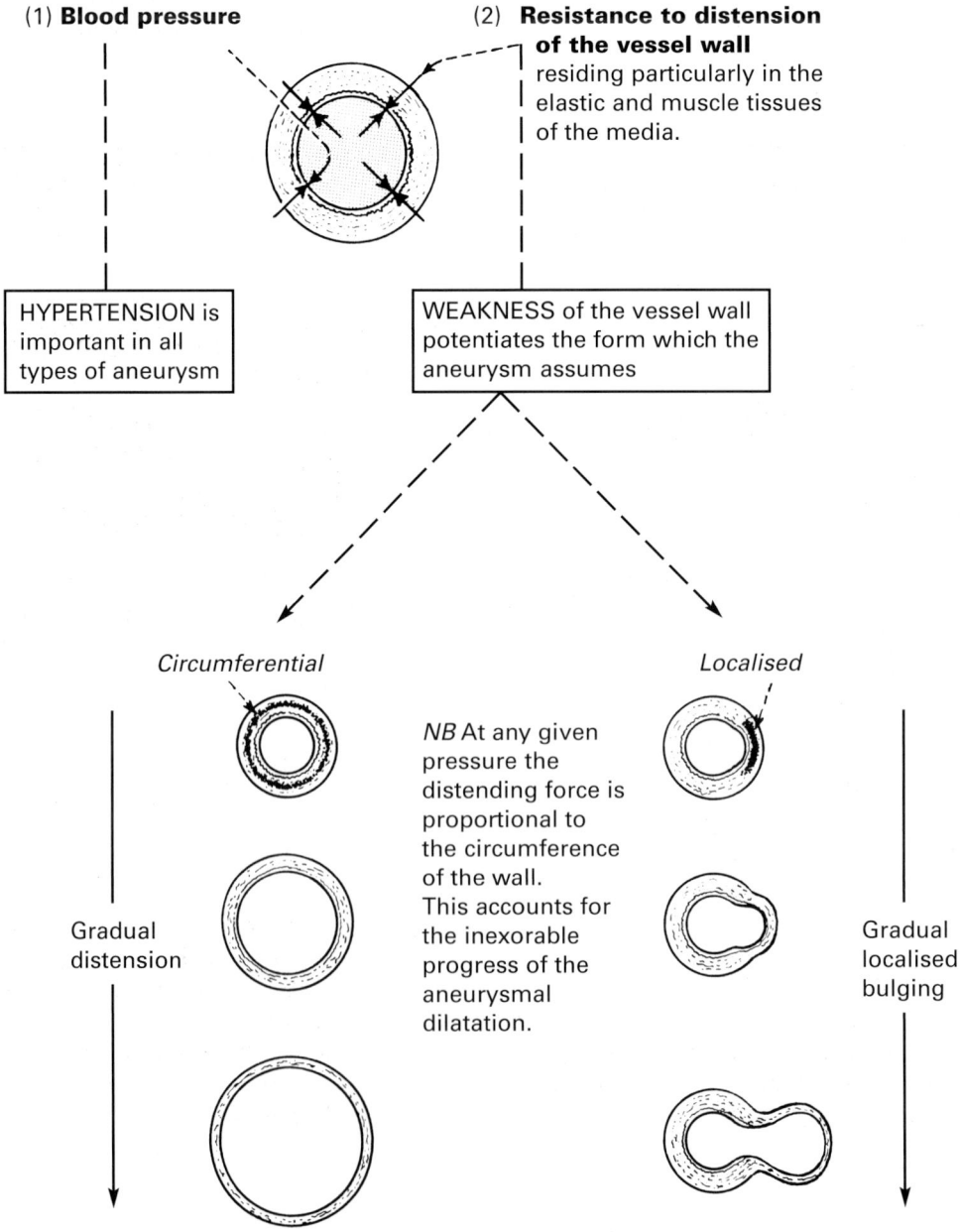

ANEURYSMS

TYPES of ANEURYSM

There are two main varieties:

(1) **Fusiform**

(2) **Saccular**

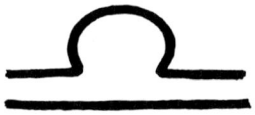

These are well illustrated in the aorta.

Fusiform aneurysm of abdominal aorta — usually due to atheroma; often below renal arteries and may also affect iliac arteries.

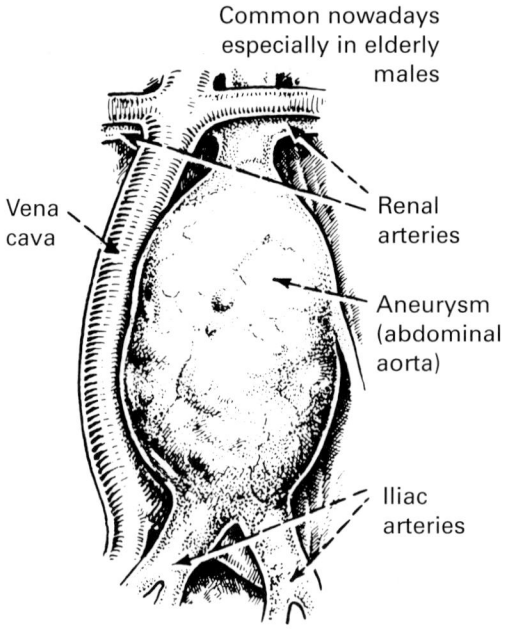

Complications

1. Local pressure effects — usually not serious.
2. Thrombosis with embolism to legs.
3. Fatal retroperitoneal or intraperitoneal haemorrhage.

Saccular aneurysm of aortic arch – now usually due to atheroma: in the past, syphilis.

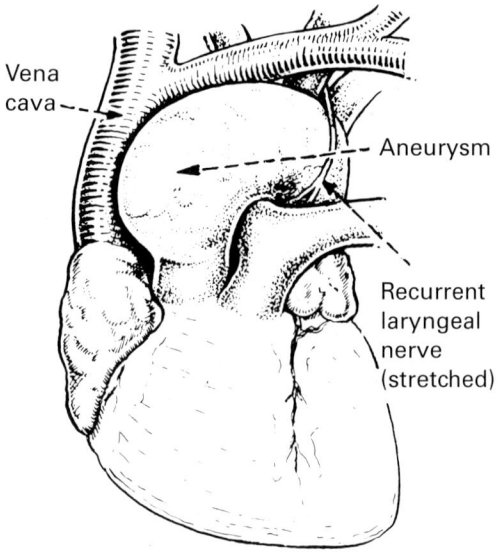

Complications

1. Pressure effects
   (a) on nerves, e.g. recurrent laryngeal nerve paralysis
   (b) on bones e.g. vertebral, sternal or rib erosion
   (c) on neighbouring viscera, e.g. oesophagus, heart, lungs.
2. Fatal haemorrhage.

VARICOSE VEINS

FACTORS WHICH INFLUENCE THE BASIC MECHANISM

(a) **Acting on the vein wall**

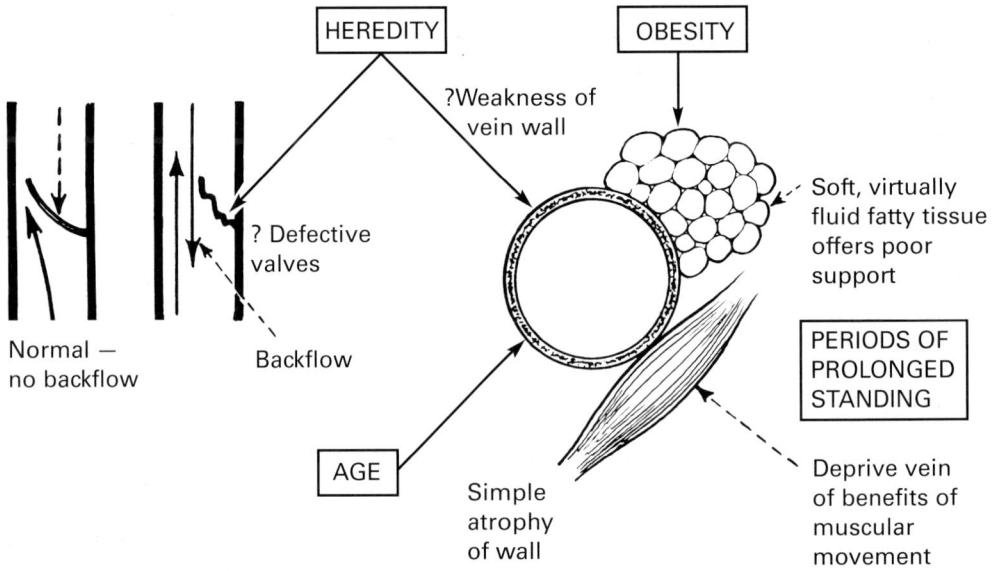

(b) **Increasing the intraluminal pressure**

1. Obstruction to venous flow
   — usually in the pelvis — by:
   Pregnancy
   Tumour
   Constipation with
   loaded colon
   Thrombosis in veins
   (also may destroy valves)
   Constrictions on limbs.

2. Special anatomical considerations.

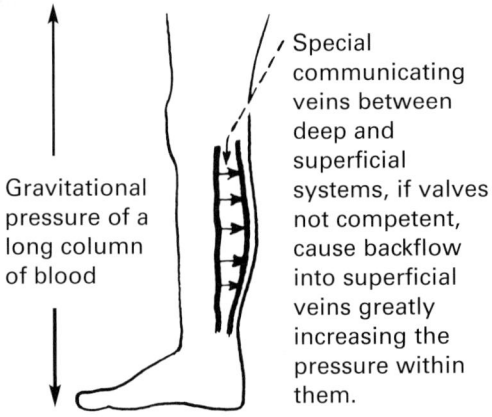

VARICOSE VEINS

Effects

1. Symptoms of leg fatigue and aching pains.
2. Trophic changes — varicose eczema with pigmentation due to haemosiderin deposition — may proceed to ULCERATION: very slow to heal.
3. Haemorrhage is a rare complication.
4. Thrombosis is a frequent complication.
   NB Superficial venous thrombosis is not usually associated with embolism; deep venous thrombosis is the dangerous condition.

VARICOSE VEINS IN SPECIAL SITES

Oesophageal varices

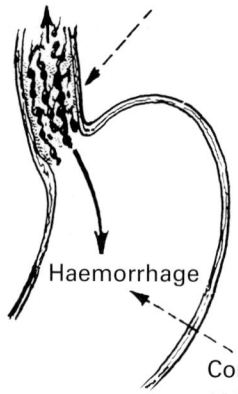

Usually due to portal venous obstruction when portal-systemic venous anastomoses open up.

Complicated by serious haemorrhage which may be fatal.

Varicocele

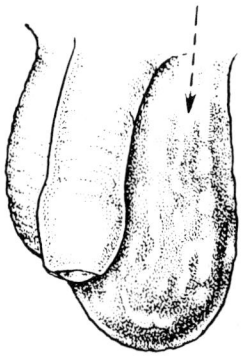

Affects the pampiniform plexus: feels like a 'bag of worms'. It may cause dull aching and, because the increased vascularity raises the scrotal temperature, the condition has been incriminated in some cases of infertility.

Haemorrhoids

Varices of the anorectal veins; usually associated with constipation.

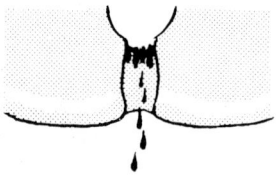

Complications are: 1. rectal bleeding.

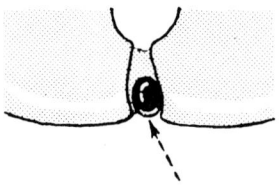

2. acute pain due to local haematoma (not a true haemorrhoid).

DISEASES OF LYMPHATICS

The lymphatic vessels participate in disease processes in two main ways:

1. They afford a natural route by which diseases can spread.
2. They may become obstructed, with serious results.

1. LYMPHATICS as a mechanism by which DISEASE SPREADS

Small lymphatics are thin-walled vessels which have a simple endothelial layer and readily allow entry of tumour cells, bacteria and foreign material often within phagocytes.

The mechanism is important in the spread of (a) infection and (b) tumours.

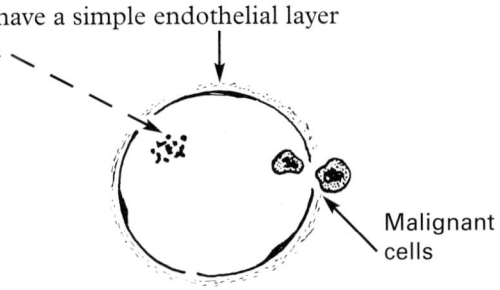

Acute lymphangitis

The lymphatics draining an area infected by pyogenic bacteria (especially streptococci) may themselves become acutely inflamed.

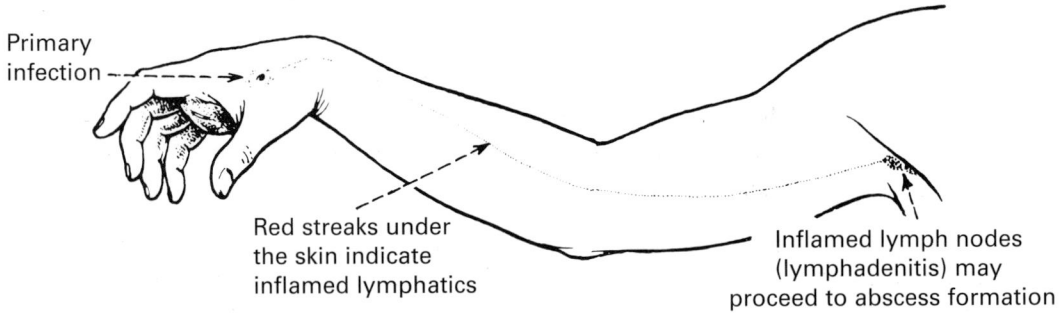

Chronic infections such as tuberculosis also spread by lymphatics (p.276).

Spread of tumours

This is an important route of spread of malignant tumours, especially carcinoma.

Disposal of particulate matter

This is well seen in the lungs where inhaled soot, especially in city dwellers, can be seen clearly indicating the lymphatic system under the pleura.

Soot (carbon) is relatively inert, but other dusts may initiate serious disease.

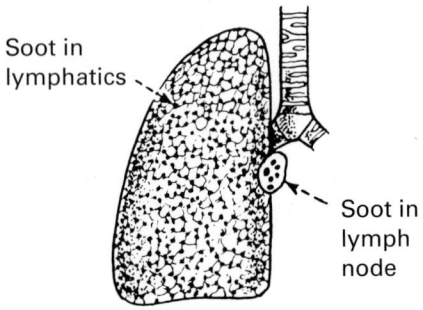

LYMPHATIC OBSTRUCTION

LYMPHATIC OBSTRUCTION

This is usually due to acquired disease but rarely there is a congenital deficiency of lymphatics (Milroy's syndrome).

The main causes of acquired obstruction are:

(a) **Tumour growth**

(i)
Obstruction by tumour permeation of lymphatics and/or destruction of lymph nodes, e.g. pelvic and groin nodes.

Limb swollen by brawny oedema

(ii)
Effects of treatment — scarring following surgery and radiotherapy.

Brawny oedema of arm

(b) **Blocking by parasites** — e.g. adult worms of filariasis in the tropics.

Effects of chronic lymphatic obstruction:
— accumulation of fluid in the tissues causes swelling of the affected part (lymphoedema).

Special varieties of lymphoedema

Peau d'orange — where the lymphatics of the skin are blocked by tumour.

Elephantiasis — where a limb and/or the scrotum is massively enlarged due to filarial lymphatic blockage.

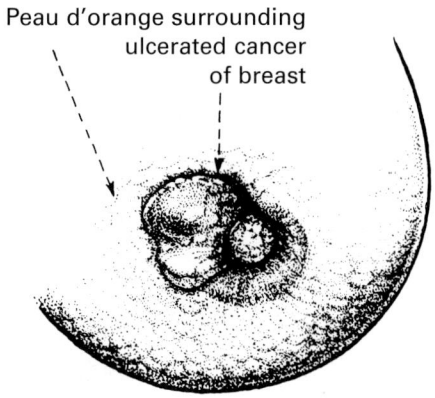

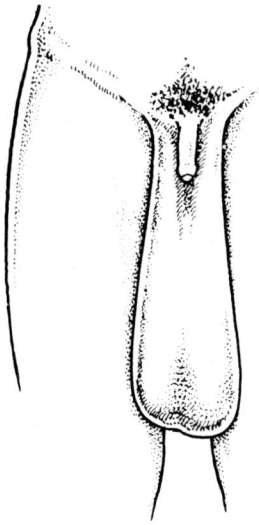

VASCULAR TUMOURS

Benign tumours of endothelial cells — ANGIOMAS — illustrate the difficulty in defining the borderline between the tumours (neoplasms) and hamartomas (developmental abnormalities). They are discussed on page 132.

Other varieties include:

1. PYOGENIC GRANULOMA – INFECTED ANGIOMA

There is debate as to whether this is a pre-existing angioma in which infection has supervened, or whether it is granulation tissue in which exuberant capillary growth is the main feature. It is a striking lesion appearing on the skin at a site subject to trauma and infection, e.g. around the finger nails, the nostrils or the tongue.

It not uncommonly occurs during pregnancy.

It grows over several days to form a small red nodular excrescence up to about 1 cm in diameter and is usually ulcerated.

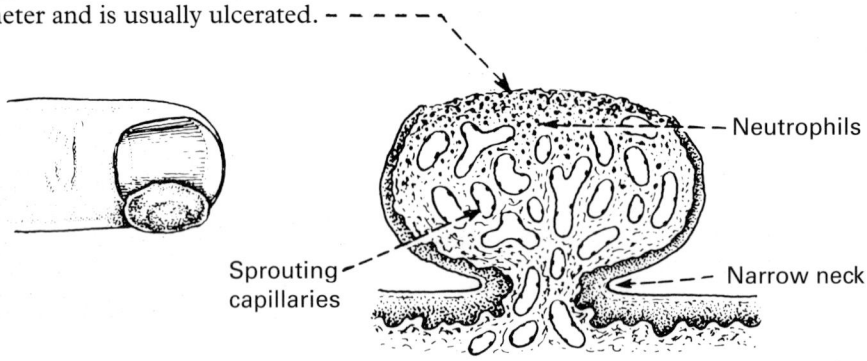

The lesion is entirely benign despite its rapid evolution and responds to simple removal.

2. TELANGIECTASIS

Small localised dilatations of small blood vessels. There are two main types: congenital and acquired.

(a) *Congenital.* In the rare hereditary haemorrhagic telangiectasis, the small lesions occur in the skin and mucous membranes and may be associated with bleeding (especially from the nose).

(b) *Acquired.* The small lesions, affecting the face and neck, are known as **spider naevi.**

The mechanism of their development is probably related to oestrogen excess, since they occur in pregnancy and in serious liver disease (oestrogen catabolism diminished) where they are an important diagnostic sign.

Telangiectasis may be seen in skin damaged by radiotherapy.

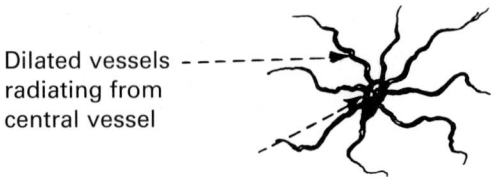

VASCULAR TUMOURS

3. **LYMPHANGIOMA**

Lymphangiomas are much rarer than haemangiomas and are usually without serious pathological significance.

Sometimes the abnormal lymphatic vessels become enormously distended and form fluctuant swellings with local pressure effects, e.g. 'cystic hygroma' of neck of babies and children.

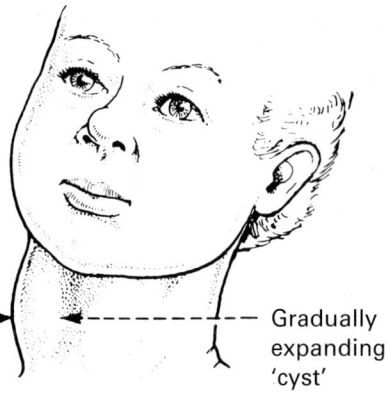

4. **GLOMANGIOMA** (glomus tumour) — arises from a specialised type of arteriolovenous junction which includes a rich neural component. A common site is the finger tip, perhaps under the nail: a very small but often excruciatingly *painful tumour.* Microscopically it consists of a complex of blood vessels lined by endothelium but cuffed by round clear cells with contractile properties (myoid cells). It is rich in nerve fibres.

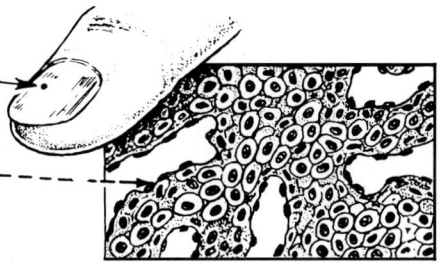

ANGIOSARCOMAS

These are uncommon malignant tumours of endothelial cells. They may affect the skin.

Lesions of the scalp occur in the elderly. They appear as spreading 'bruise-like' areas often with a central nodule. Chronic sun exposure is thought to be important.

Lesions often arise in the limbs in areas of lymphoedema e.g. in the past following irradiation and lymph node clearance for carcinoma of breast.

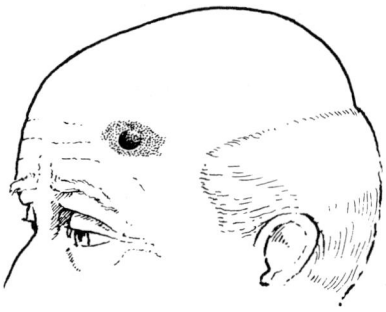

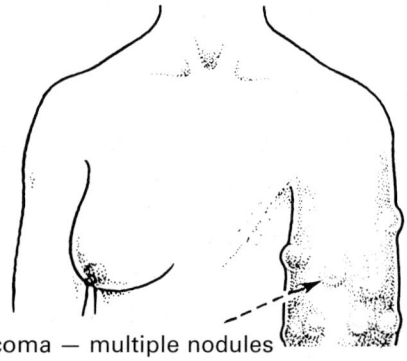

Angiosarcoma — multiple nodules

Angiosarcoma of the liver is associated with exposure to vinyl chloride monomer.

KAPOSI'S SARCOMA

This tumour has greatly increased in incidence in the wake of the spread of AIDS and HIV infection.

It is a tumour of endothelial cells possibly related to an oncovirus infection (e.g. Herpes virus type 8) occurring in immunocompromised patients.

It occurs in 3 main groups of patients.

(a) In IMMUNOSUPPRESSION – especially in AIDS but also in transplant patients.
(b) **Sporadic** (classic) – affecting elderly males (especially Askanazy Jews) living in the Mediterranean littoral.
(c) **Endemic** – mainly in central Africa, typically affecting young adults.

The disease presents as dark coloured (due to high blood content) **subcutaneous nodules** or plaques resembling bruises.

(a) The nodules may be **multiple** and fairly randomly distributed – this is seen particularly in AIDS cases.

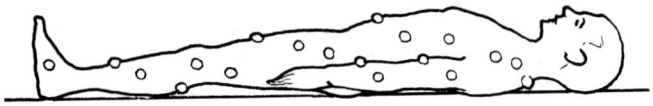

(b) In 'classic' Kaposi, the tumour begins as a **solitary** nodule particularly on the limbs.

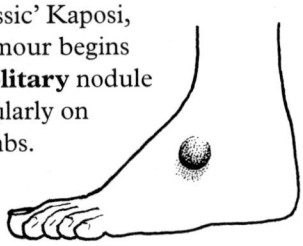

(c) In the African endemic Kaposi, lymph nodes are commonly affected.

The histological appearances are essentially non-descript: malignant spindle cells lining a network of sieve-like spaces with a high red cell content.

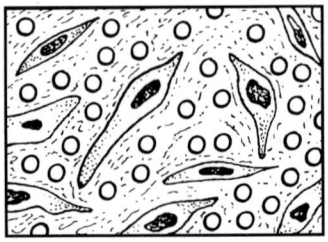

CHAPTER 8

RESPIRATORY SYSTEM

Upper Respiratory Tract 250
Rhinitis 251, 252
Acute Pharyngitis, Tracheitis and Laryngitis 253
Other Disorders of the Larynx 254
Tumours of the Upper Respiratory Tract 255
Lungs — Anatomy 256, 257
Respiration 258, 259
Acute Bronchitis 260
Bronchial Asthma 261
Chronic Obstructive Pulmonary Disease (COPD) 262
Emphysema 263–265
Bronchiectasis 266, 267
Pneumonia — Bronchopneumonia 268
Lobar Pneumonia 269
Legionnaire's Disease 270
Viral Pneumonias 271, 272
Pneumonia — Special Types 273
Lung Abscess 274
Tuberculosis (TB) 275
Spread of Tuberculosis 276
Pneumoconioses (Dust Diseases) 277, 278
Asbestosis 279
Fibrosing Alveolitis (Interstitial Pulmonary Fibrosis) 280
Lung Cancer 281–284
Other Tumours of the Bronchi and Lungs 285
Collapse of Lung 286
Diseases of the Pleura 287, 288

UPPER RESPIRATORY TRACT

ACUTE INFLAMMATIONS

Infections of the nose, nasal sinuses, pharynx and larynx are common. They are usually mild and self-limiting. Most cases are due to viral infection, but this is often followed by bacterial superinfection.

1. **Viral infection**
This phase is characterised by features of acute inflammation but without the exudation of neutrophils.

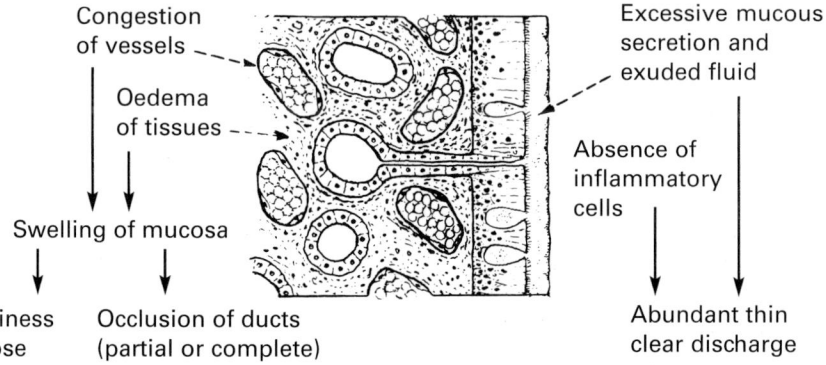

Viruses involved

A wide variety, of which the major types are:

(i) **rhinoviruses**
(ii) **coronaviruses** — responsible for more than half of cases of the common cold;
(iii) **myxoviruses** (e.g. influenza), **paramyxoviruses** (e.g. respiratory syncytial virus) can also invade the lower respiratory tract.

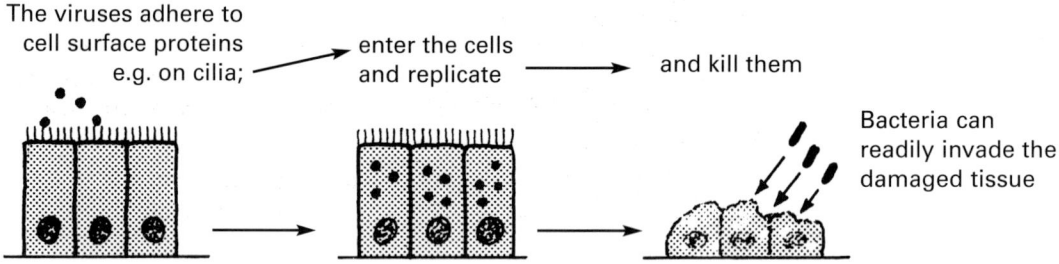

2. **Bacterial phase**
Many bacteria are commensal in the respiratory tract (e.g. *streptococcus mutans, haemophilus influenzae*) and can superinfect the damaged tissue, which then exhibits the typical features of acute inflammation including exudation of neutrophils.

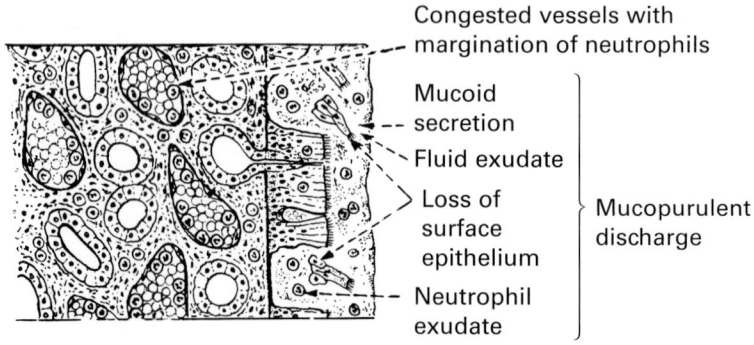

The wide variety of different viruses involved prevents protective immunity.

RHINITIS

COMMON COLD (Acute coryza)

This common respiratory inflammation usually involves the nose and adjacent structures.

The 2 phases, *viral* and *bacterial* are typically seen in this disease.

The drainage from the sinuses, especially the maxillary, is often blocked by swelling of the mucosa — giving rise to sinusitis.

The infection is spread by droplet spread of viruses by sneezing.

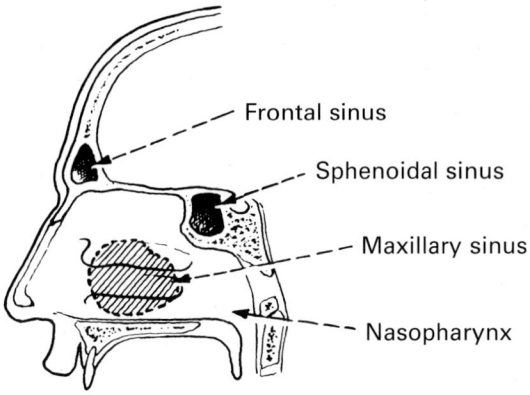

ALLERGIC RHINITIS 'Hay fever'

An allergic (immediate type hyper-sensitivity) type of inflammation (p. 103) is often seen. Patients develop immediate symptoms of sneezing, itching and water rhinorrhoea.

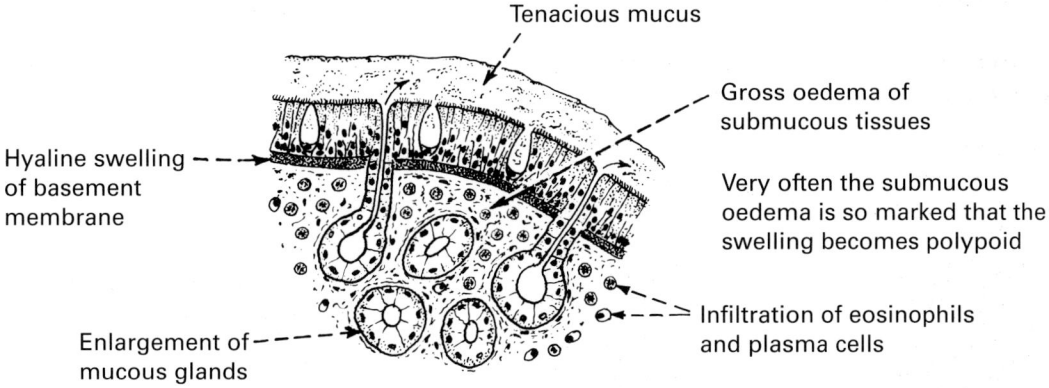

The repeated attacks frequently lead to chronic changes in the mucosa with polyp formation.

RHINITIS

NASAL POLYPS

These form particularly on the middle turbinate bones and within the maxillary sinuses.

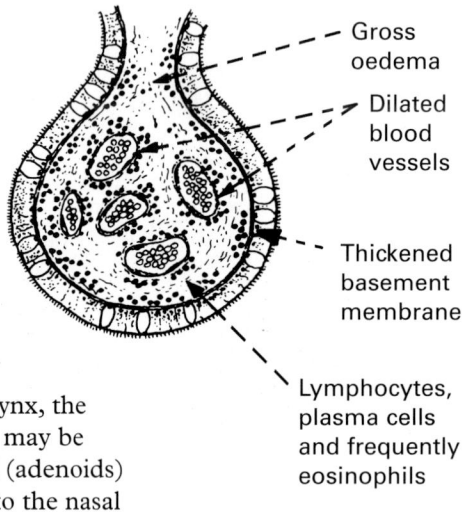

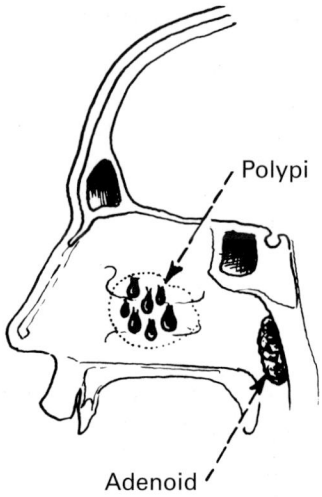

In the nasopharynx, the lymphoid tissue may be greatly enlarged (adenoids) and contribute to the nasal obstruction.

ALLERGIES

Seasonal allergy

This is due to pollens liberated from trees and grass.

Non-seasonal allergy

The main cause is the house dust mite, *Dermatophagoides pteronyssinus.* Allergy to pets is common e.g. cats — the allergens are usually salivary proteins from cat fur.

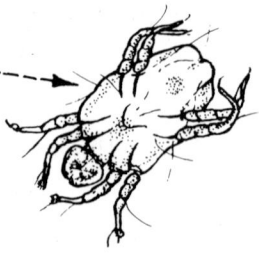

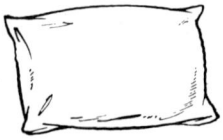

Feather pillow — invisible infestation

VASOMOTOR RHINITIS

This is a clinical diagnosis. The pathological changes are, to some extent, similar to those of allergic rhinitis, but the condition is more continuous, less spasmodic. Although the cause is unknown, viral infections in a polluted atmosphere (usually an urban setting) are thought to initiate the 'sensitivity' and non-specific stimuli such as bright light and smells precipitate an attack.

ACUTE PHARYNGITIS, TRACHEITIS and LARYNGITIS

ACUTE PHARYNGITIS and TRACHEITIS

Most sore throats are caused by **viruses** — including such as adenovirus and Epstein Barr virus.

Bacteria include *streptococcus pyogenes, haemophilus parainfluenzae* and *cornybacterium diphtheriae.*

Tonsillitis is a common acute inflammation, historically due to streptococcal infection but with the introduction of antibiotics viruses are the initiating infective agents in most cases.

Acute phase ⟶ may progress to (a) acute suppuration (quinsy)
or (b) CHRONIC TONSILLITIS

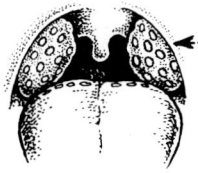

Swollen, red tonsils with purulent exudate at mouths of crypts.

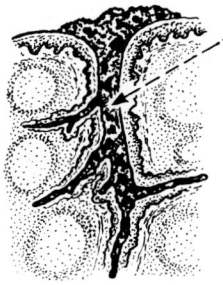

Dilated crypts containing inspissated exudate — harbouring bacteria and fungi.

Liability to relapse to acute inflammation.

Diphtheria, now uncommon in countries where vaccination is widespread, is a serious infection.

The formation of a pseudomembrane is striking.

Normal

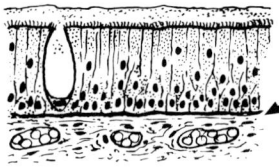

Basement membrane

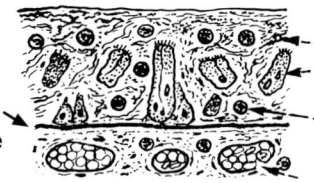

Membrane consisting of fibrin, necrotic epithelium and neutrophils and numerous bacteria

Congested vessels

This pseudomembrane may spread to block the larynx causing respiratory obstruction.

The EXOTOXIN of diphtheria is encoded by a bacteriophage (a virus which infects the bacterium). It can cause myocarditis (p. 213) and neuropathy (p. 590).

In **Acute epiglottitis**, typically due to *haemophilus influenzae*, there is severe inflammation and oedema. In young children, the larynx becomes obstructed necessitating tracheostomy and administration of antibiotics.

Acute laryngitis is often due to parainfluenza viruses. Acute *oedema of the glottis* is seen in some cases of anaphylaxis (p. 102) and angioneurotic oedema.

OTHER DISORDERS OF THE LARYNX

CHRONIC LARYNGITIS

Cigarette smoking, repeated attacks of infection and atmospheric pollution may lead to chronic inflammation of the larynx.

Two main changes are (a) changes in the lining epithelium and (b) increase in mucus secretion.

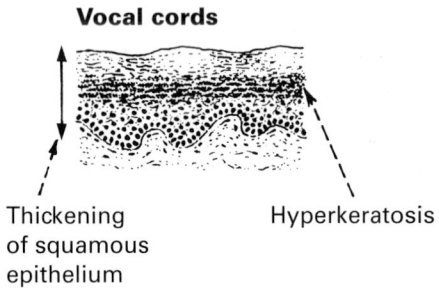

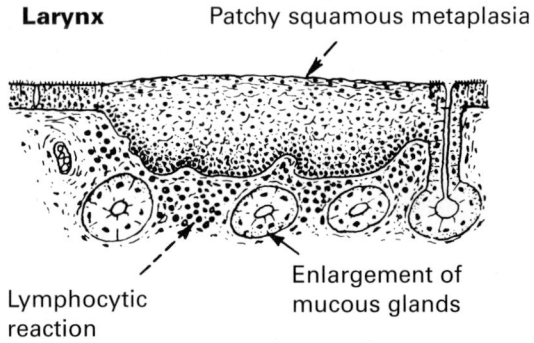

The following sequence of events tends to take place:

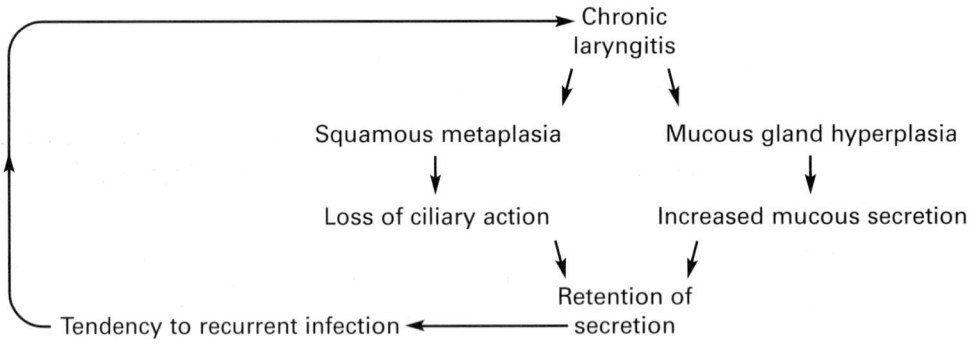

Tuberculosis — this can cause severe ulceration of the larynx and is usually secondary to pulmonary tuberculosis.

Vocal cord nodule (Singer's node)

This is found in singers and those who abuse their voice. Small smooth nodules may be seen on one or both vocal cords where the cords impact during phonation.

They consist of squamous epithelium overlying fibrin-rich and myxoid stroma.

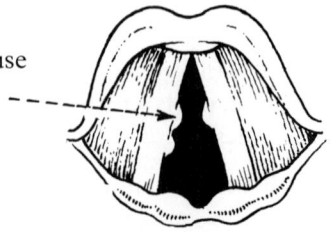

TUMOURS OF THE UPPER RESPIRATORY TRACT

BENIGN TUMOURS

(a) **Epithelial**

Papillomas may be single but are often multiple and due to infection by papilloma virus.

Squamous cell

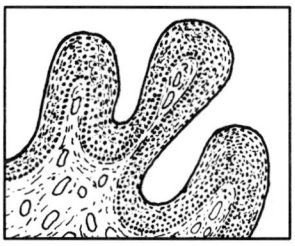

Transitional cell

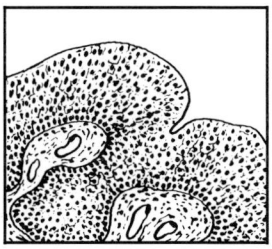

The abnormal epithelium grows down the glandular ducts and the name 'inverted papilloma' is applied. Such tumours often recur after incomplete removal.

(b) **Connective tissue**

Haemangiomas, especially of the nasal septum, can cause persistent nose bleeds. A special form, angiofibroma, affects male children and grows throughout childhood but typically regresses.

MALIGNANT TUMOURS

These are mainly squamous carcinomas and are commonly seen in the larynx. Intraepithelial neoplasia (carcinoma-in-situ) is a frequent precursor.

Smoking and asbestos exposure are aetiologically important. The rate of growth and spread is influenced by the site within the larynx.

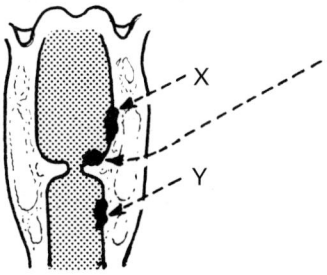

Tumours of the true cord tend to stay localised and have a better prognosis than supraglottic (X) and subglottic (Y) tumours — the looser surrounding tissues allow early local and cervical node spread.

Nasopharyngeal carcinoma is common in Eastern countries and is associated with Epstein-Barr Virus infection.

Adenocarcinoma of the nose is a rare tumour.

LUNGS – ANATOMY

ACINUS (PRIMARY LOBULE)

This is a sub-unit of pulmonary tissue consisting of respiratory bronchioles with associated alveolar ducts, atria and alveoli. Intercommunications exist between acini, and also between acini and terminal bronchioles. Thus disease can spread from acinus to acinus but, equally, functional deficiency in any part of one acinus can be compensated by by-pass mechanisms via these anastomotic channels.

SECONDARY LOBULE

This is the unit of pulmonary tissue served by a pre-terminal bronchiole. Self-contained and bounded by connective tissue septa, it has no anastomotic connections with other lobules.

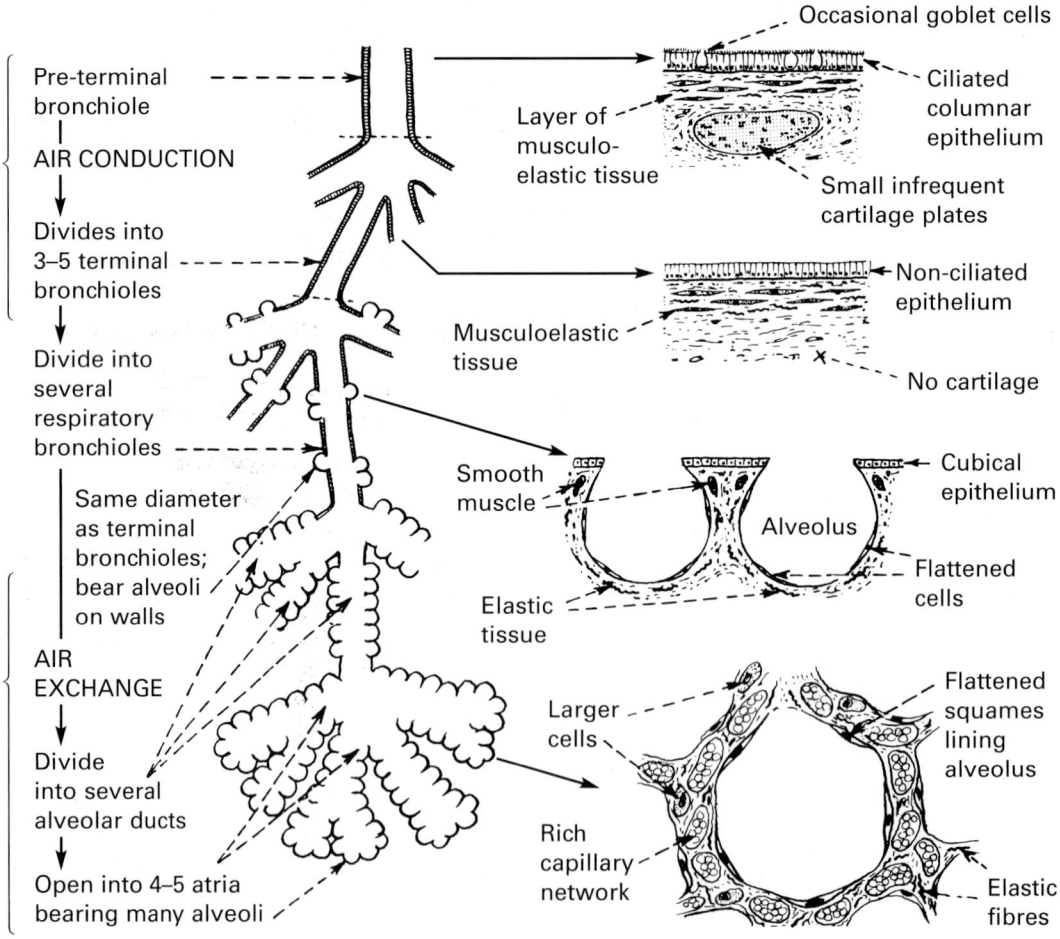

The total area for air exchange is very large (equivalent to a tennis court) allowing considerable reserve capacity.

LUNGS – ANATOMY

HISTOLOGY of the ALVEOLUS

Two types of cell (pneumocytes) line the alveoli:

Type 1
are flattened cells which cover >90% of the surface.

Type 2
These rounded granular cells secrete **surfactant** and undergo hyperplasia when Type 1 cells are injured.

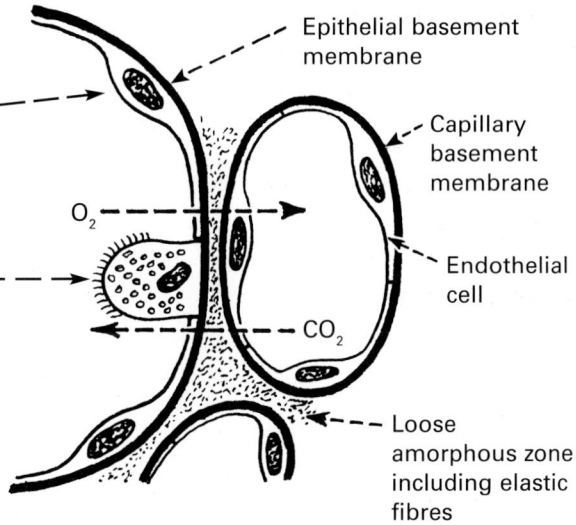

These relationships allow rapid diffusion of O_2 and CO_2

Macrophages and mast cells are also present in the alveoli.

PULMONARY VASCULATURE

Dual blood supply

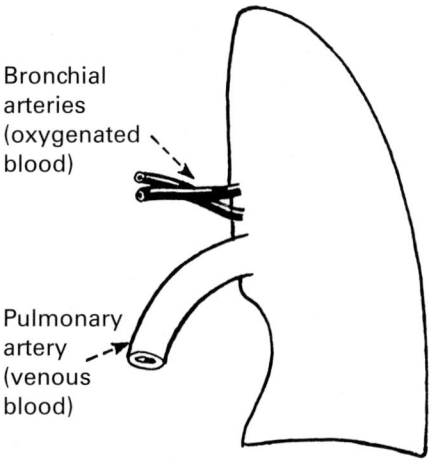

This dual supply is of importance when a pulmonary arterial branch is blocked.

Lymph drainage

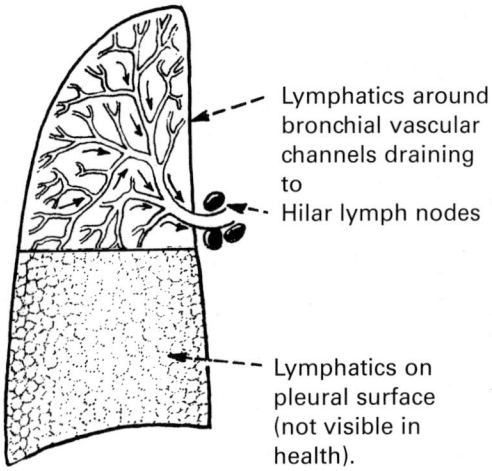

This fine network of lymphatics becomes visible when pigmented dust is inhaled over long periods.

RESPIRATION

The normal intake of air is around 7 litres per minute; of this, after allowing for non-functioning dead space (trachea, bronchi, etc.), approximately 5 litres per minute are available for alveolar ventilation. A definite flow of air is maintained as far as the terminal bronchiole. Beyond this point the actual flow ceases and gas exchange is effected by diffusion.

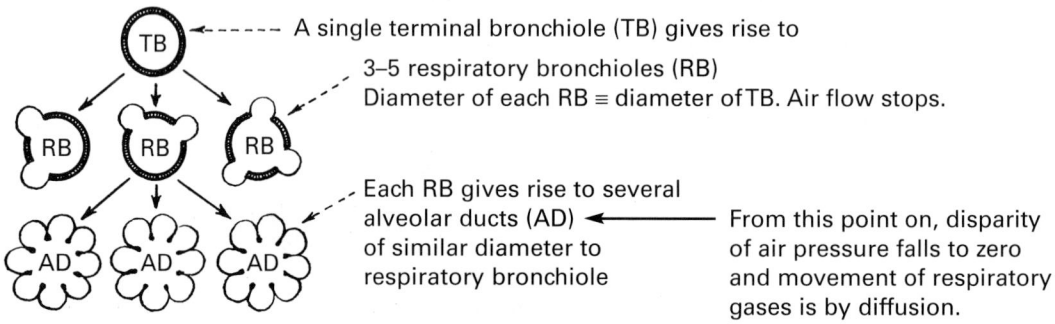

Three factors are involved in the maintenance of adequate respiration:

1. Adequate intake of air
2. Rapid diffusion along alveolar ducts and through alveolar walls
3. Adequate perfusion of pulmonary circulation

Interference with any of these factors will result in respiratory embarrassment (dyspnoea) and even respiratory failure.

Inadequate air supply to alveoli (hypoventilation)

This may be due to lesions and diseases which interfere with the mechanics of respiration, such as central nervous lesions affecting the respiratory centre, paralysis of muscles of respiration as in poliomyelitis, injuries and deformities of the thoracic skeleton (e.g. fracture of ribs, kyphosis) and pleural disease preventing lung expansion as in pleural effusion or pneumothorax.

The most common cause of hypoventilation is bronchial obstruction. This may be reversible due to bronchial spasm as in asthma or irreversible in chronic obstructive pulmonary disease (p. 262).

RESPIRATION

Impaired diffusion of gases (ventilation)
Three mechanisms may interfere with diffusion:

1. Reduction in the total alveolar surface available for diffusion, e.g. consolidated airless lobe in pneumonia, fibrosis of lung, tumour growth, advanced tuberculosis.
2. Increase in distance over which diffusion takes place as in emphysema.

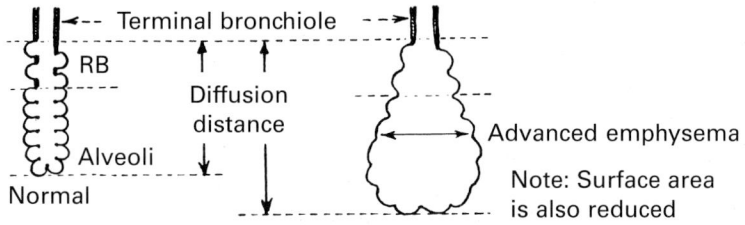

3. Increase in the thickness of the alveolar capillary membrane. Diffusion of gas across the membrane is so rapid this can be of little practical importance. CO_2 is more soluble than O_2 and diffusion through the alveolar wall is 20 times as rapid as O_2, therefore while blood O_2 progressively falls there is usually no retention of CO_2.

Altered pulmonary perfusion

Interference with the pulmonary circulation may occur in 4 main ways:

1. Occlusion of larger vessels by multiple emboli.
2. Slowing of the pulmonary circulation as in venous congestion due to left heart lesions or congenital left–right shunts.
3. Reduction in the pulmonary capillary bed by diffuse lung disease such as fibrosis, emphysema or extensive tuberculosis.
4. Pulmonary vascular spasm due to hypoxia. Permanent changes can occur in the vessels if the hypoxia is unrelieved.

Note: In addition to hypoxaemia, inadequate perfusion tends to cause retention of carbon dioxide.

In chronic lung disease, ventilation, diffusion and perfusion disorders are present in varying degrees.

Even in the normal lung there is imbalance between ventilation and perfusion

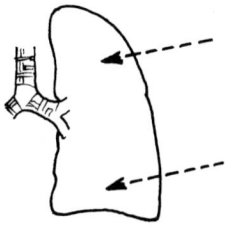

The upper area of the lung is better ventilated than perfused.

The base is better perfused

In many lung diseases this imbalance is increased. Admixture of well and poorly oxygenated blood results in hypoxaemia.

ACUTE BRONCHITIS

This is an inflammation of the large and medium bronchi. The condition may be serious if associated with pre-existing respiratory disease. Mucous and serous glands in the walls of the bronchi provide abundant mucoid secretion during the inflammation. Ciliated epithelia lining the bronchi aid passage of the exudate upward and help prevent spread down to the bronchioles.

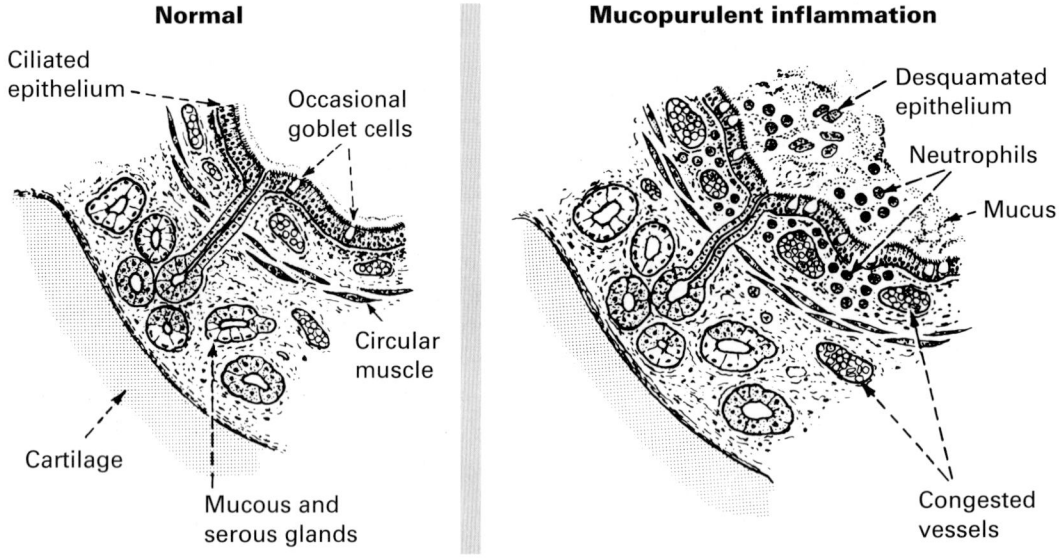

In most cases, the process is initiated by a viral or mycoplasmal infection. It is a common complication of influenza and measles. This initial phase is followed by bacterial invasion. *Streptococcus pneumoniae* and *Haemophilus influenzae* are commonest, but *Staphylococcus aureus* and *Streptococcus pyogenes* may be found, especially in infants.

The condition is usually mild, and spread to the bronchioles is unusual in healthy adults due to the effective ciliary action of the bronchial epithelium. Spread may occur however in debilitated people. Bronchiolitis and bronchopneumonia result and can prove fatal. Equally important is the serious effect of repeated attacks of acute infection in patients with CHRONIC BRONCHITIS (p. 262).

In **children:**

1. Whooping cough (due to *Borderella Pertussis*) may cause permanent damage due to the severity of the infection and the stress on the airways during the coughing and whooping attacks.

2. **Bronchiolitis** in the very young (<2 years), in the majority of cases, is due to *Respiratory Syncytial Virus* and the risk of progression to **bronchopneumonia** is high.

BRONCHIAL ASTHMA

In asthma, there are spasmodic attacks of reversible bronchial obstruction with wheezing and dyspnoea: and often a dry cough. The prevalence has markedly increased in recent years, possibly in part due to air pollution. There are 2 main patterns:

1. **Atopic asthma** (p. 103)
   - — typically starts in childhood.
   - — often a strong family history of asthma or atopic conditions (e.g. eczema).
   - — attacks provoked by IgE type I hypersensitivity reaction to inhaled allergens, e.g. pollen, cats, house mite dust.
2. **Non-atopic asthma**
   - — usually in middle age.
   - — usually no history of atopy: family history uncommon.
   - — no particular antigens incriminated.

Other varieties include occupational asthma and aspirin induced asthma.

The basic mechanism is as follows:

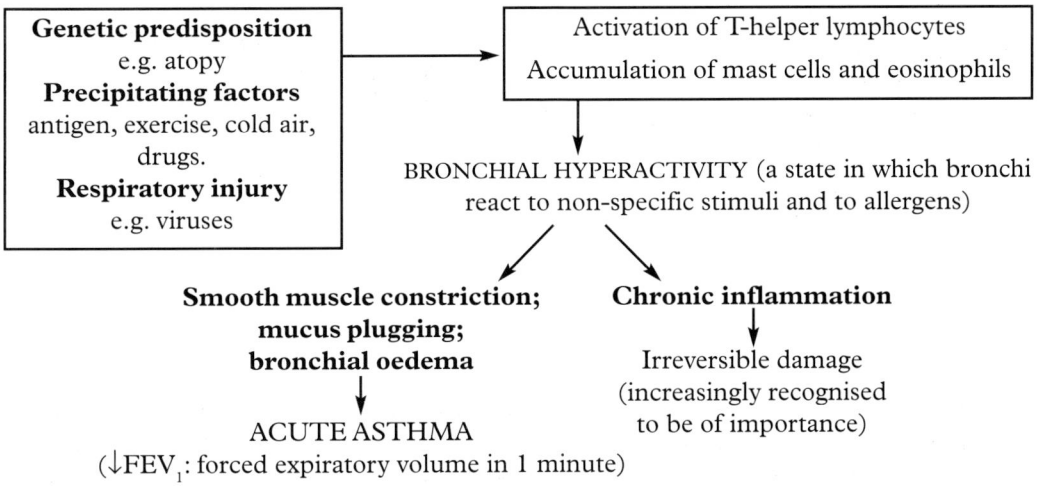

The **histological changes** are a combination of allergic reaction and muscular hypertrophy, the result of prolonged spasm.

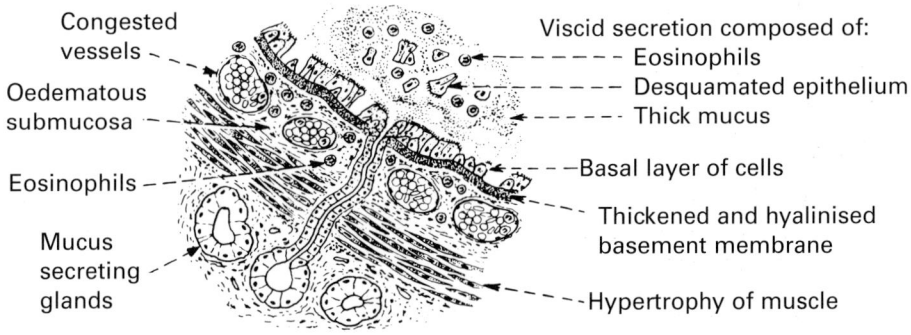

Sputum

In some cases the following may be seen:

1. *Curschmann's spirals* — appear as small white. granules in sputum.

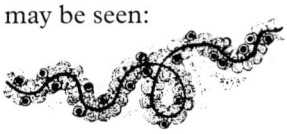

Charcot-Leyden crystals — in association with eosinophils.

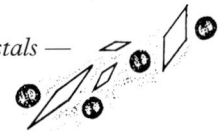

CHRONIC OBSTRUCTIVE PULMONARY DISEASE (COPD)

This term is applied to patients who have largely irreversible airways obstruction. It is a common disorder resulting in approximately 5% of male deaths in the U.K. It is associated with **chronic bronchitis** and **emphysema**, although the precise relationship of these conditions to airway obstruction remains incompletely understood.

Aetiology The main factors are:

1. SMOKING — by far the major risk factor and dose related.
2. α_1-antitrypsin deficiency. Reduced levels of this protease inhibitor correlate with lung damage, especially in smokers.
3. OCCUPATION, especially exposure to dusts, e.g. coal mining.

CHRONIC BRONCHITIS

The clinical definition is based on the presence of a productive cough lasting at least 3 months and occurring annually for at least 2 years.

Pathologically the following changes are seen:

The increase in thickness of the mucous gland layer is striking: at post-mortem the Reid index is measured — i.e. the ratio of the submucous layer (X) to the whole thickness (Y): a value greater than 1:2 is significant.

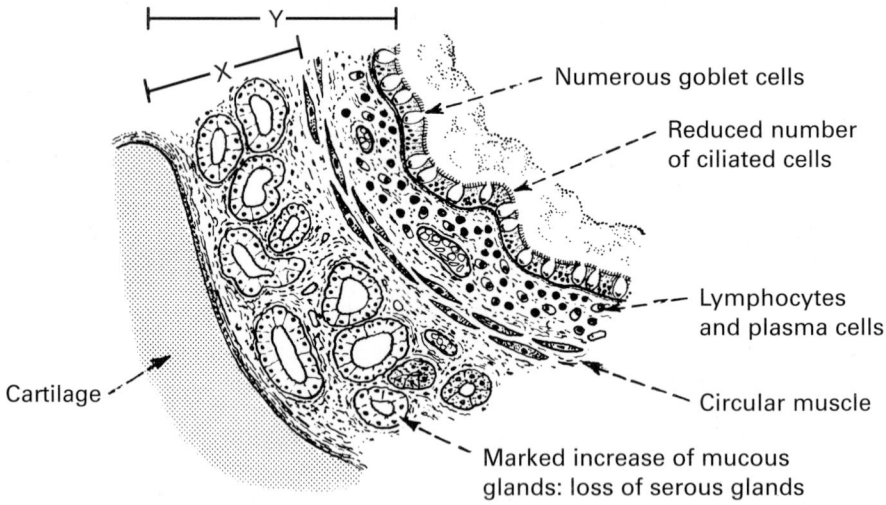

The effect of these changes is:

Increase in goblet cells
+
Increase in mucous glands
→ Large quantity of Viscid secretion ← Loss of ciliated epithelium

↓ EPISODES of ACUTE BRONCHITIS — these may precipitate respiratory failure and often cause death.

↓ COUGH and SPUTUM

EMPHYSEMA

This is defined as a permanent dilatation of air spaces distal to the terminal bronchiole due to destruction of their walls without fibrosis. It is an important component of COPD (p. 262) and has the same aetiological factors.

Changes seen on clinical examination:

Normal

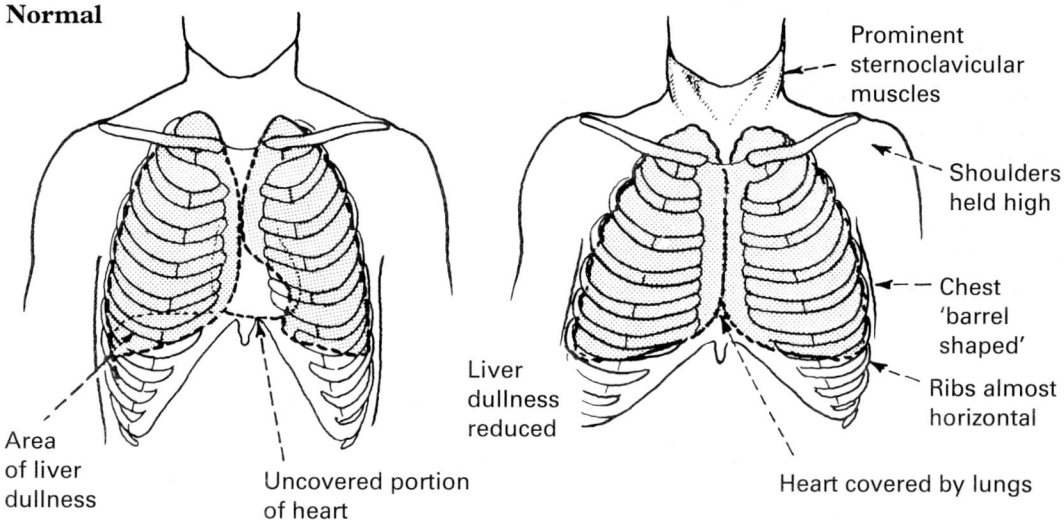

Anatomical changes due to increased use of accessory muscles of respiration and increased lung volume.

Pathological changes
At post-mortem the lungs are over-inflated

When removed the lung tends to collapse unless it is inflated with fixative and cut later.

External appearance

Cut surface

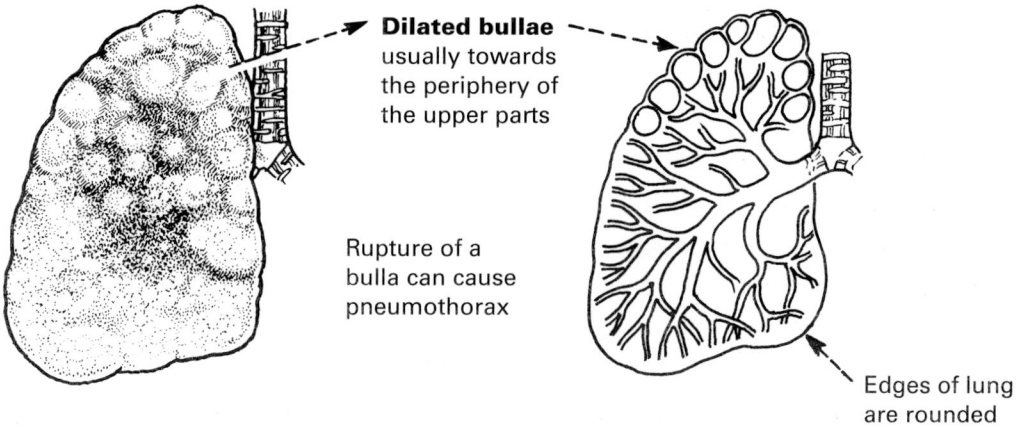

On the sectional lung 2 main patterns are seen.
1. **Panacinar emphysema** and 2. **Centriacinar (centrilobular) emphysema.**

EMPHYSEMA

PANACINAR EMPHYSEMA

The enlarged air spaces are distributed across the entire acinus.

Histological section

Naked eye cut surface | Normal lung | Panacinar emphysema

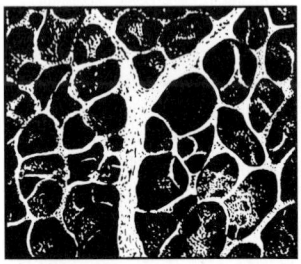

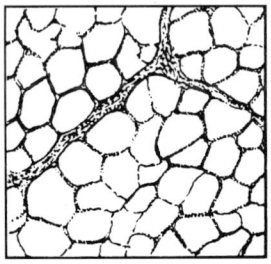

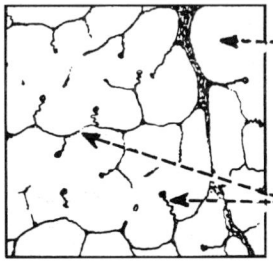

Distension of alveolar ducts

Alveolar walls thin, ruptured with retracted ends.

Special stains show loss of elastic tissue. The capillaries are stretched and thinned. The reduction in blood supply is probably a factor in leading to rupture of alveoli.

There is little evidence of bronchiolitis. The voluminous lungs produce characteristic radiological changes. The distension eventually spreads to involve the respiratory bronchiole, i.e. the whole acinus is affected — panacinar emphysema.

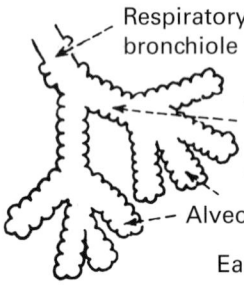

Normal

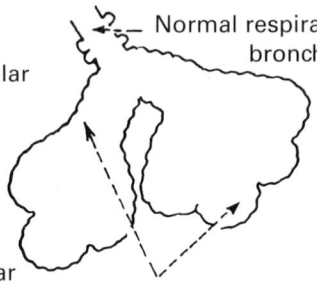

Early panacinar emphysema = Distended alveolar ducts and alveoli

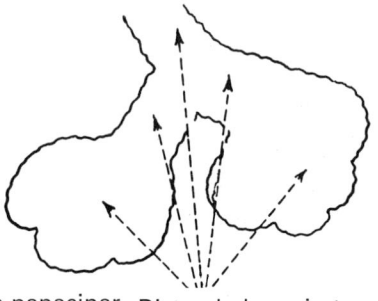

Late panacinar emphysema = Distended respiratory bronchiole, alveolar ducts and alveoli

CENTRILOBULAR EMPHYSEMA

In this form the dilated air spaces immediately surround and involve the respiratory bronchioles.

Naked eye appearance | Histological section

Normal alveoli

Dilated spaces around respiratory bronchioles

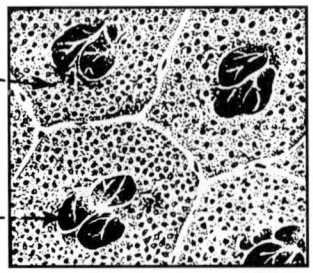

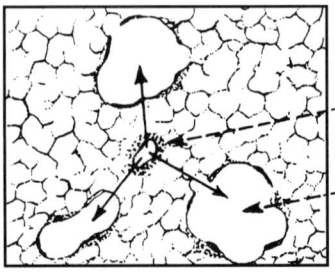

Narrowed terminal bronchiole showing chronic inflammation

Distended respiratory bronchioles

Chronic inflammation of the respiratory bronchioles is an important feature: eventually, in many cases, the distension extends to produce panacinar emphysema.

EMPHYSEMA

Aetiology

The essential cause is thought to be an imbalance between protease and anti-protease activity. The enzyme elastase is also important.

The imbalance may be due to:

(a) Reduced inhibitor e.g. α_1 antitrypsin (α_1AT) deficiency inherited as an autosomal dominant characteristic.

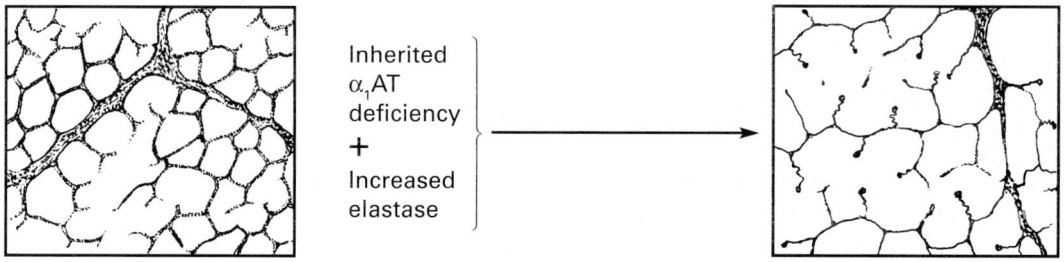

Normal lung

Gradual development of panacinar emphysema

(b) Excess enzyme production e.g. due to SMOKING

SMOKING → inflammation of bronchioles → ↑proteases → centrilobular emphysema

Emphysema is an important component of lung damage due to dust inhalation (*pneumoconiosis*) (see page 277).

Functional effects of Chronic Obstructive Pulmonary Disease (COPD)

Patients with COPD tend to fall into 2 groups depending on whether or not they tolerate hypoxia.

(a) PINK PUFFERS	(b) BLUE BLOATERS
Do NOT tolerate hypoxia.	Tolerate hypoxia.
Severe breathlessness.	Severe hypoxaemia and hypercapnia.
Hyperventilation.	Right ventricular hypertrophy.
Relatively normal blood gases.	Cor Pulmonale with peripheral oedema.
	Secondary polycythaemia.

Eventually many patients develop severe chronic respiratory failure and may die during an acute episode of bronchitis.

BRONCHIECTASIS

Bronchiectasis means a permanent dilatation of one or more bronchi.

Aetiology

There are 2 main subdivisions:

1. Obstructive bronchiectasis (secondary to bronchial obstruction).
   Dilatation occurs in bronchi distal to an obstruction e.g. a tumour, foreign body or enlarged lymph nodes.
2. Post-infective bronchiectasis.
   (a) Following childhood respiratory infection e.g. measles, adenovirus or whooping cough
   (b) In tuberculosis (often affecting the upper lobes).
   (c) Following repeated infection in cystic fibrosis (p. 380).

Pathology

The process affects bronchi distal to the 4th division (after which cartilage rings are absent. The dilatation takes 3 anatomical forms.

(1) **Cylindrical** i.e. of uniform calibre

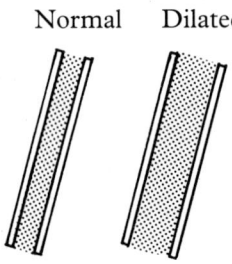

(2) **Fusiform** — the dilation is spindle shaped.

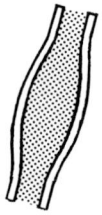

(3) **Saccular**

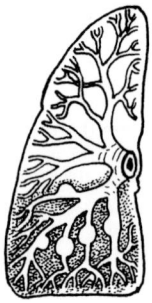

The lower lobes are typically affected, but in tuberculosis or cystic fibrosis the upper lobes alone can be affected.

The surrounding lung parenchyma is usually obliterated by fibrosis, infection or collapse.

Mechanism of formation

Childhood viral infection results in partial obstruction of bronchi by lymphoid aggregates

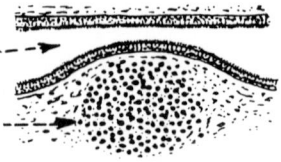

This obstruction leads to retention of secretion and to secondary infection.

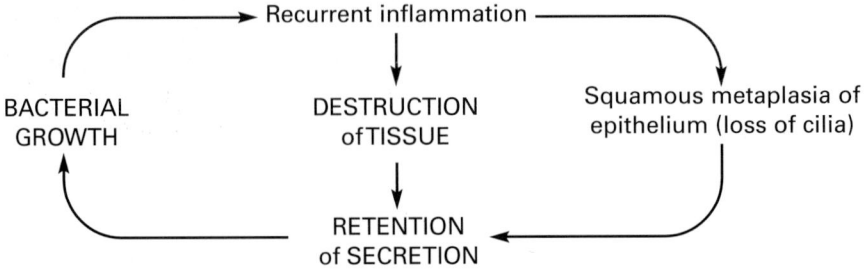

BRONCHIECTASIS

Effects

(1) Large quantities of secretion are retained in the bronchi and putrefactive bacteria produce a foul smell

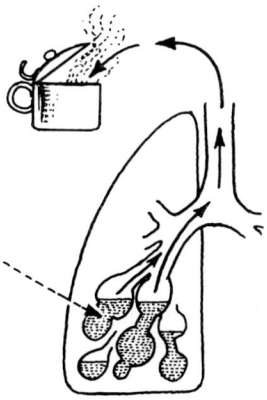

(2) Suppuration is common in the cavities and local complications arise, e.g. lung abscess bronchopleural fistula

empyema

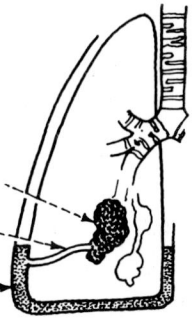

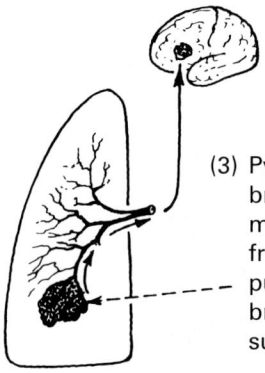

(3) Pyaemia giving rise to brain abscess or meningitis may result from involvement of a pulmonary vein branch by the suppurative process

(4) Clubbing of fingers (hypertrophic pulmonary osteoarthropathy)

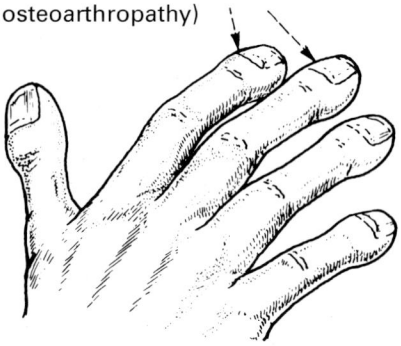

(5) Pulmonary hypertension (page 187)

progressing to

Right heart failure

(6) Development of amyloid disease, e.g. in kidney

Amyloid around glomerular capillaries and tubule basement membranes

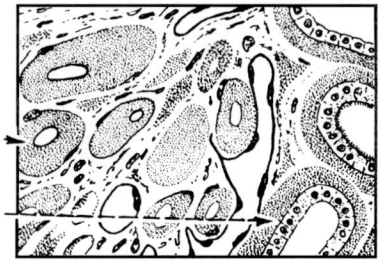

PNEUMONIA – BRONCHOPNEUMONIA

Pneumonia is an inflammatory process involving the alveolar tissue of the lungs. It is discussed under 3 main headings:

1. Bronchopneumonia
2. Lobar pneumonia
3. Miscellaneous pneumonias

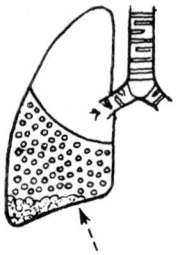

Bronchopneumonia — patchy consolidation.

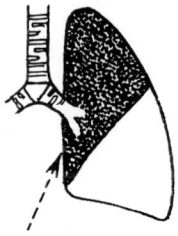

Lobar pneumonia — whole lobe affected.

1. BRONCHOPNEUMONIA

Bronchopneumonia caused by a variety of bacteria is the commonest form.
It may affect all ages, but it is particularly frequent in 4 circumstances:

(a) as a terminal event in a chronic debilitating disease.
(b) in infancy.
(c) in old age.
(d) as a manifestation of secondary infection in viral conditions e.g. influenza, measles.

Bronchopneumonia is primarily an inflammation spreading from terminal bronchioles to their related alveoli.

The lesions are initially focal, involving one or more lobules.

First red, then grey, they show a central bronchiole containing pus.

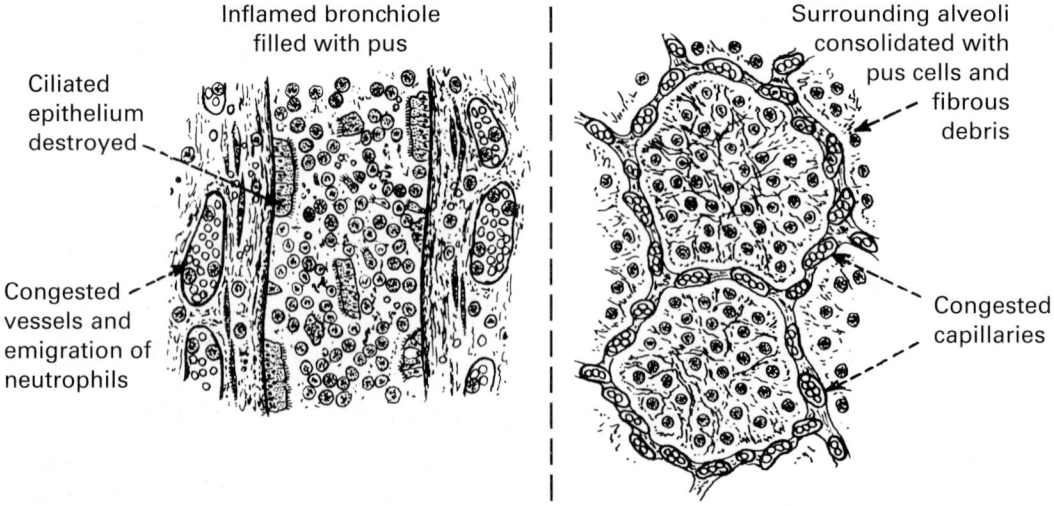

Possible sequels

1. Resolution — complete or partial (antibiotic and physiotherapy are important).
2. Patchy scarring.
3. Rarely, continuing sepsis with lung abscess formation.

LOBAR PNEUMONIA

2. LOBAR PNEUMONIA

As the name suggests, a complete lobe or even two lobes of a lung are affected, the most striking changes occurring in the alveoli. The disease is now rare in Western countries. It is seen typically in adults aged 20–50 years with males predominating and is caused by *Streptococcus pneumoniae*. Occasionally *Klebsiella pneumoniae* is the agent in the debilitated elderly, diabetics and alcoholics.

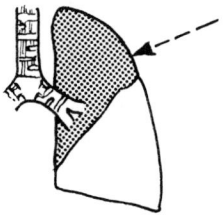

The whole affected lobe progresses uniformly through 4 distinct phases illustrating the classical progression of an acute inflammation: this has been so radically altered by antibiotic treatment that the following description is to some extent historical.

Clinically, the onset is acute with fever and often rigors. There is a dry cough and rusty sputum; dyspnoea and often chest pain due to pleurisy.

The **Pathology** is described in 4 phases merging sequentially: all the alveoli in the lobe are uniformly affected.

	Phase 1 CONGESTION	**Phase 2** RED HEPATISATION (consolidation)	**Phase 3** GREY HEPATISATION (consolidation)
Time	1–2 days	2–4 days	4–8 days
Gross appearance	Lungs are dark red and wet	Lungs are solid, RED and dry	Lungs are solid and GREY (due to high concentration of neutrophils)
Microscopic appearance	Congestion Fluid exudate	Fibrin strands Numerous red cells	Numerous neutrophils Dense fibrin strands

Phase 4 — RESOLUTION begins dramatically on day 8–10 and restoration to normal is rapid.

LEGIONNAIRE'S DISEASE

Previously confused with pneumococcal pneumonia, Legionnaire's disease occurs in small epidemics, is more common in males and is due to a tiny Gram-negative bacillus — *Legionella pneumophila*. The death rate can be high — up to 20%. Infection is associated with inhalation of aerosol from contaminated water storage systems.

Clinical features
Two phases are recognised:

Prodromal phase — vague flu-like illness lasting about 5 days.

Active phase
A dry cough develops. Vomiting and diarrhoea may be severe.
Patient becomes somnolent, confused and signs of consolidation appear.

Laboratory findings
Hyponatraemia. Lymphopenia. Neutrophils normal.
Signs of disseminated intravascular coagulation may develop.

Pathology
Both lungs are consolidated, dark red, heavy and oedematous. Fibrinous pleurisy or pleural effusion may be found.

Histology
Two stages are evident:

First stage

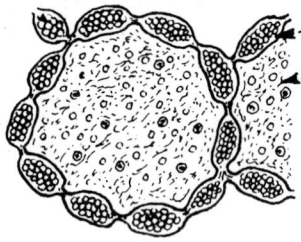

Second stage

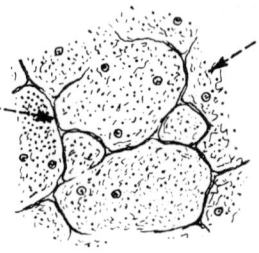

The exudate may organise, causing an increasing interstitial fibrosis with permanent loss of lung function.

VIRAL PNEUMONIAS

INFLUENZA

In most cases, influenzal infection is confined to the upper respiratory tract, but in debilitated persons and during epidemics, the whole respiratory tract is affected.

Trachea and bronchi

Intense inflammation with haemorrhage develops.

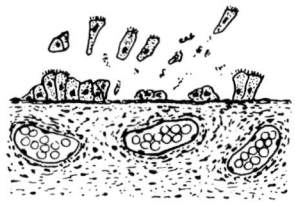

Initial necrotising changes — loss of epithelium

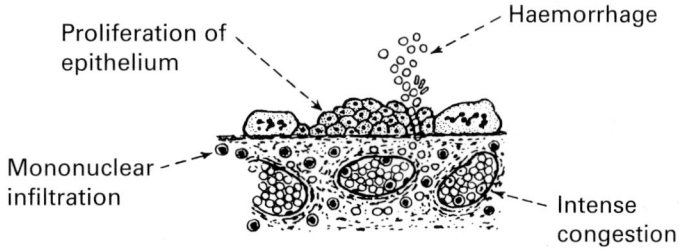

Reactive stage

Pneumonia changes

The lungs are bulky, purple red and exude blood-stained froth when cut. The microscopical changes vary from one part to another.

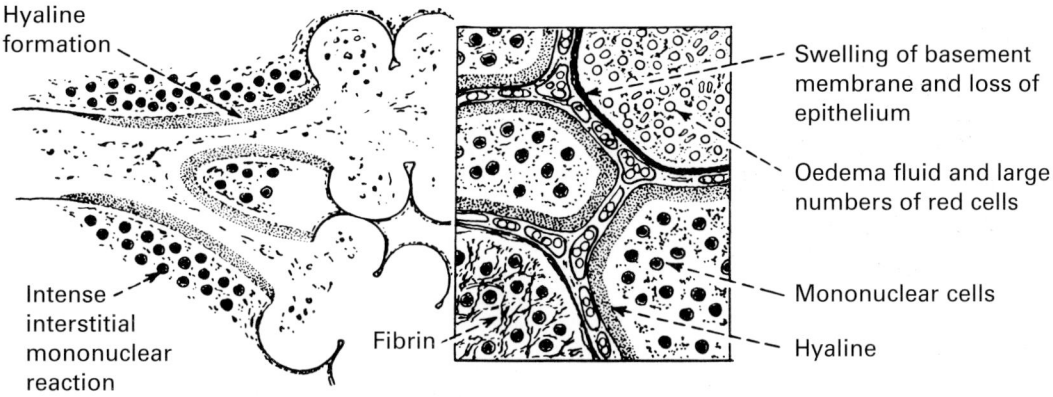

Infective agents

Of the three main types A, B and C, type A is the most virulent, and mutants of this type are responsible for most epidemics and the fatalities which occur.

Secondary infection is common, the bacteria most frequently involved being *Staphylococcus aureus*, *Haemophilus influenzae* and *Streptococcus pneumoniae*.

VIRAL PNEUMONIAS

There are a number of pneumonic conditions due to **viruses** and **virus-like agents** in which a common pattern of pathological change is observed.

1. **Necrotising bronchiolitis**

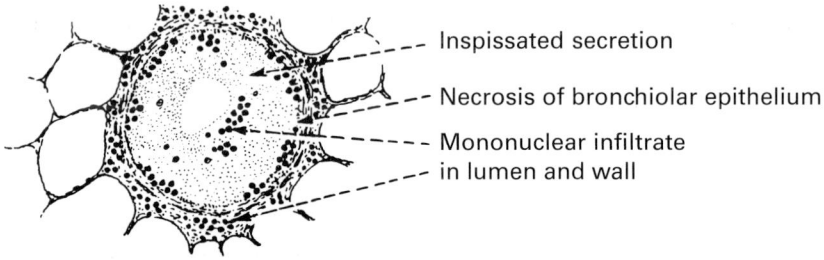

2. **Interstitial pneumonia**

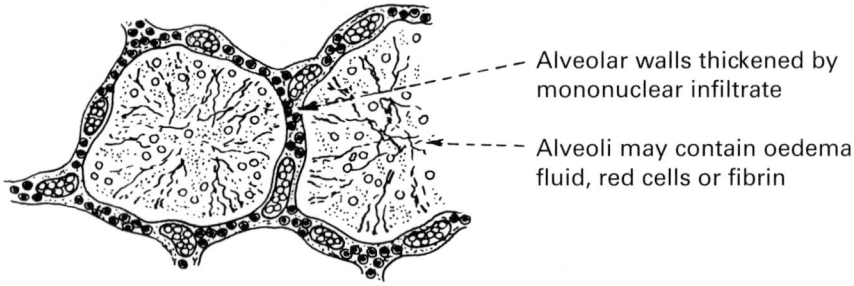

3. **Reactive changes**

The lining epithelial cells of bronchioles and alveoli are stimulated by the presence of the virus.

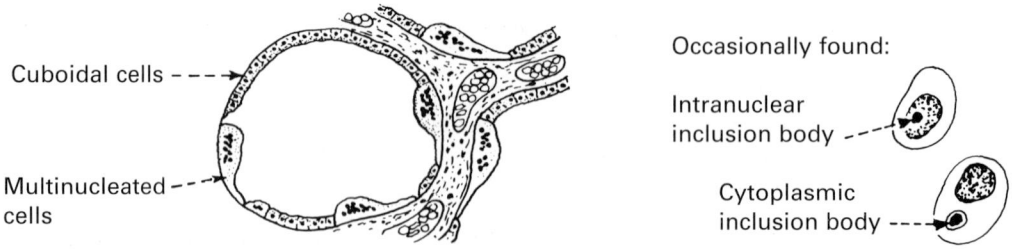

Variations in the basic pattern occur in different infections. Confluent consolidation is often found in psittacosis and ornithosis (viruses transmitted by birds) and in measles giant cell pneumonia. Interstitial pneumonia is produced by cytomegalovirus and in rickettsial infections such as Q fever and 'scrub typhus'. In mycoplasma pneumonia, inflammation spreads from the bronchioles into the lung parenchyma and may become chronic with fibrosis.

PNEUMONIA – SPECIAL TYPES

ASPIRATION PNEUMONIA

This is due to inhalation of food or infected material from the mouth or pharynx. It may occur during anaesthesia or coma or may complicate conditions associated with frequent regurgitation e.g. oesophageal obstructions, pyloric stenosis.

In adult cases the inhalation of acid gastric contents may cause an initial shock reaction: in other cases the onset is insidious.

Possible progression is as follows:

Inhalation of foreign material → Secondary infection → Bronchopneumonia lung abscess

Histologically 'foreign material', usually vegetable matter, may be seen evoking a foreign body giant cell reaction.

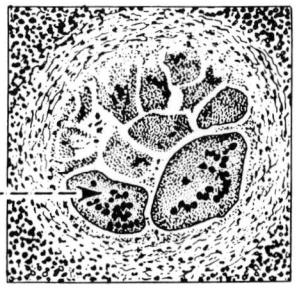

Lipid pneumonia

—The exogenous form is due to long-continued inhalation of small quantities of oily material usually derived from nasal medicaments: it is often clinically silent.

—The endogenous form is derived from tissue lipid debris distal to local bronchial obstruction.

Miscellaneous pneumonias

(1) Opportunistic infections are seen in therapeutically immunosuppressed patients and in AIDS cases.
The causative agents include:
Viruses — e.g. *Cytomegalovirus.*
Protozoa — e.g. *Pneumocystis carinii.*
Fungi — e.g. *Aspergillus fumigatus, Candida albicans, Cryptococcus neoformans.*

(2) The use of non-sterile equipment and material for intravenous injection by drug addicts may cause infected emboli with spread of the inflammation into adjacent lung tissue.

LUNG ABSCESS

This is now an uncommon condition due to prompt treatment of preceding infection. The usual causes are:

1. Inhalation of infected material from the larynx or pharynx.

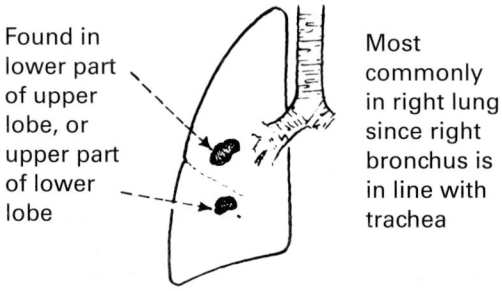

2. Obstruction of a bronchus by tumour growth or foreign body. Site depends on size of bronchus affected.

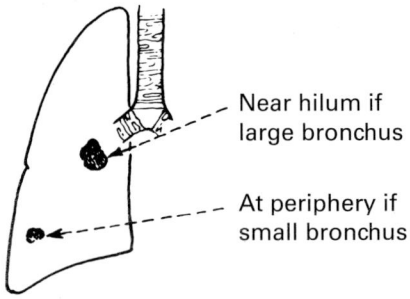

3. Infection of pre-existing cavities, e.g. in tuberculosis or bronchiectasis.
4. Pneumonia. Abscess is most likely to occur in debilitated persons with bronchopneumonia.

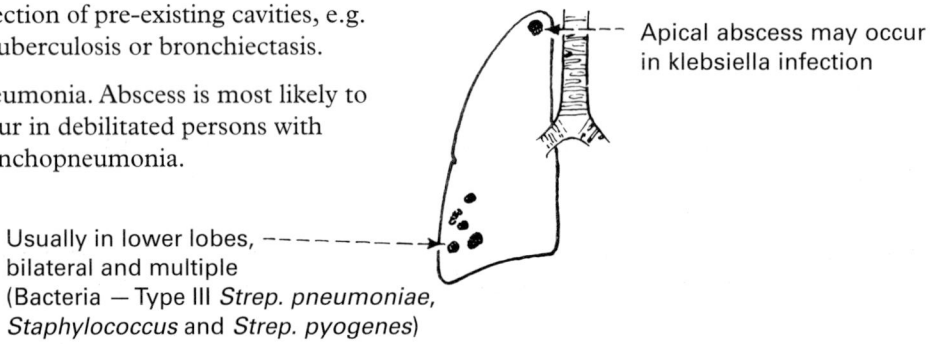

Rarer causes of abscess are: pyaemia, trauma to lung, extension from suppuration in mediastinum, spinal column or subphrenic region, and infection with *entamoeba histolytica*.

Sequelae of lung abscess

1. Small abscesses may heal.
2. Subpleural abscesses may extend to cause empyema.
3. Bronchopleural fistula resulting in pyopneumothorax is a further complication following on 2.
4. If a large pulmonary vessel is eroded, fatal haemorrhage can occur.
5. Rarely, blood spread leads to meningitis or cerebral abscess.

TUBERCULOSIS (TB)

The lungs are more commonly affected by TB than any other organ. The incidence of TB in developed countries is rising, partly due to AIDS. Drug resistant strains of Mycobacteria are an increasing problem.

There are 2 patterns of pulmonary tuberculosis — primary and secondary.

PRIMARY INFECTION

This occurs in patients, usually children, who have not been previously exposed to TB or vaccinated against it.

Infection is by inhalation.

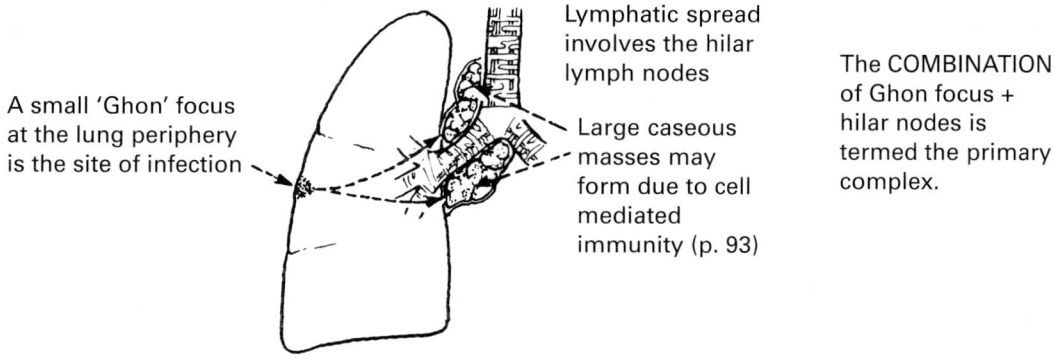

In most patients, the lesions undergo fibrosis or calcification and heal. Spread can, however, occur.

SECONDARY INFECTION

This is a recurrence of TB in later life — either reactivation or reinfection. The patients have immunity to TB and develop a cell mediated response leading to CASEATION.

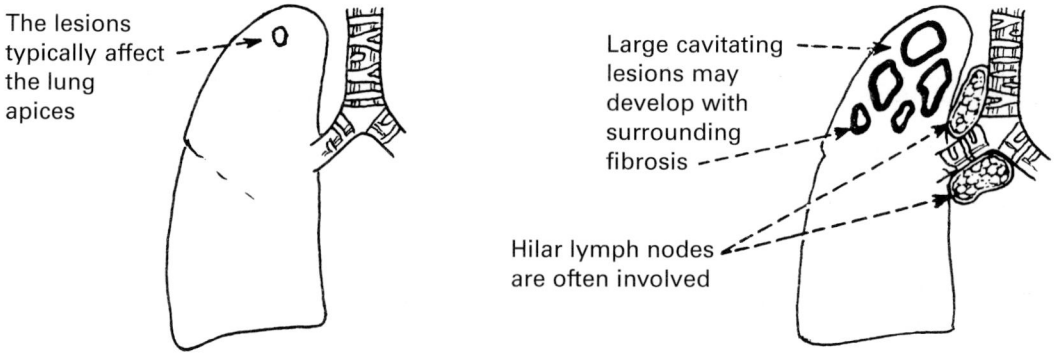

SPREAD OF TUBERCULOSIS

SPREAD OF TUBERCULOSIS

This is typically seen in secondary TB, but may also complicate primary infection.

The infection can spread by several pathways.

(a) **Direct spread** e.g. to pleura and pericardium.

(b) **By the bronchi.**
Tubercle bacilli may spread to the larynx or by the bronchi to give tuberculous bronchopneumonia ('Galloping consumption').

Consolidation is seen throughout large areas of lung parenchyma.
This occurs particularly in the immunosuppressed.

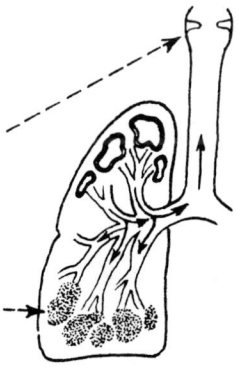

(c) **By the pulmonary veins.**
This may lead to isolated blood borne infection e.g. tuberculous meningitis (p. 570), renal TB and bone TB e.g. Pott's disease of the spine: or to miliary spread throughout the body.

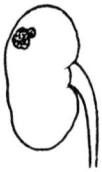

Kidney

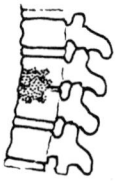

Spine

(d) **By the pulmonary arteries** (probably by lymphatics draining into the inferior vena cava).
In this, miliary spread occurs throughout the lung fields alone.

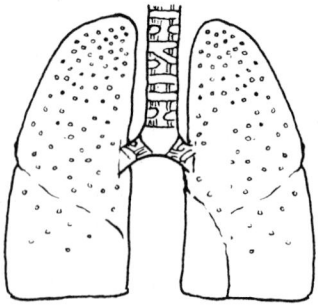

Miliary tubercles, approximately 1–2mm, are seen throughout the lung fields.

The clinical course of tuberculosis is variable and depends on the immune status of the individual, the response of the bacteria to drugs, and intercurrent disease.

The **histological** features are as described on page 72.

PNEUMOCONIOSES (DUST DISEASES)

The reaction to inhaled dust varies very considerably. Some dusts, e.g. pure carbon, are inert: others, e.g. silicates, cause severe lung disease.

Basic Pathology

1. *Inorganic dust* particles reaching the lungs are ingested by alveolar macrophages.

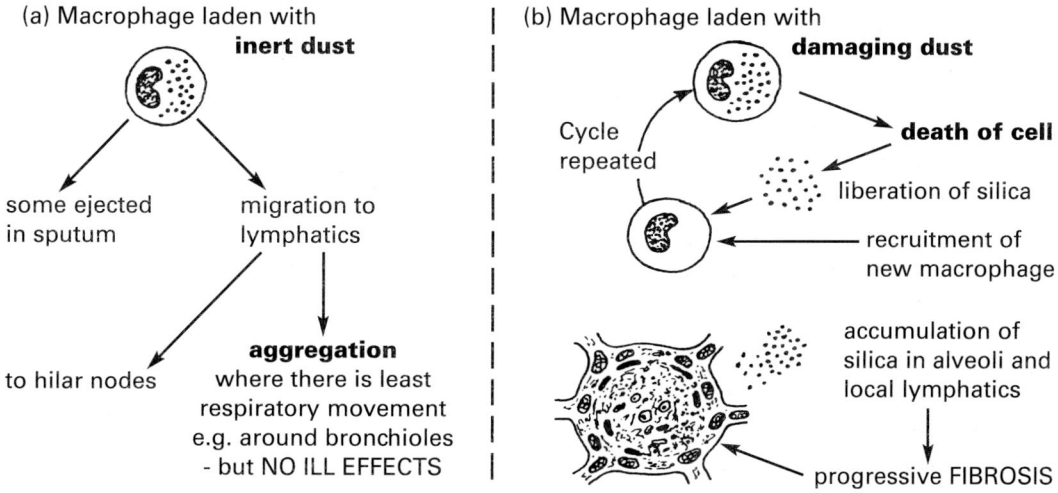

2. *Organic dust* particles which cause lung disease by a different mechanism include FUNGI encountered in many occupations, e.g. farmers, malt workers, bird fanciers.

   The basic pathology is an immunological sensitivity reaction and the term 'extrinsic allergic alveolitis' is used.

Inhalation of antigen → Antigen-antibody complex → Inflammation: repeated attacks → FIBROSIS

ANTHRACOSIS

Pure carbon is biologically inert and is deposited as in (a) above with no ill effects. Damage to the lung seen in coal-miners and in populations exposed to carbon polluted atmosphere is potentiated by the content of silicates and other pollutants.

Coal-miner's Pneumoconiosis

1. *Simple* aggregation of coal dust particles may progress with the formation of small dust nodules and mild centrilobular emphysema (p. 264) with MINIMAL FUNCTION LOSS.

2. In a few cases, Progressive Massive Fibrosis supervenes with SEVERE DISABILITY.

   The cause is unknown — theories include
   - silicates in dust:
   - concomitant tuberculosis:
   - sensitivity reaction.

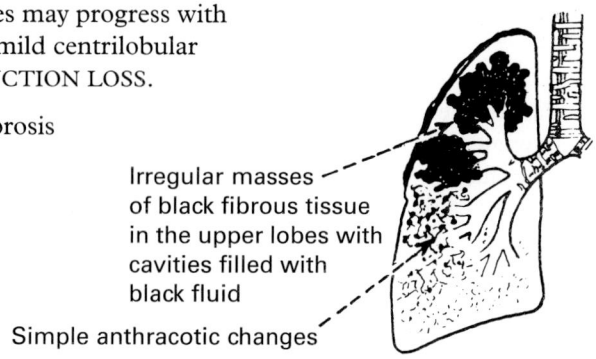

PNEUMOCONIOSES (DUST DISEASES)

The severe diseases caused by inorganic dust inhalation, usually occupationally, are described.

1. **Silicosis** — stone workers, sandblasters, miners.
2. **Asbestosis** — shipbuilding, insulation, electrical work.

The damage caused depends on:

(a) The type of dust e.g. soluble/insoluble.

(b) The shape of the particle e.g.

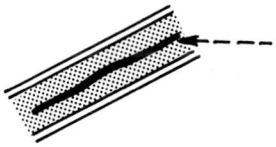

(c) The size of the particle — particles longer than 5μ are likely to be trapped in the nose and large airways.

(d) The amount of exposure — large amounts overwhelm the defence mechanisms (especially lung macrophages).

SILICOSIS

The lung lesions are slowly progressive over many years. Silicates are particularly damaging to lung macrophages.

Chronic exposure ⟶ Death of macrophages ⟶ Release of cytokines ⟶ Fibrosis

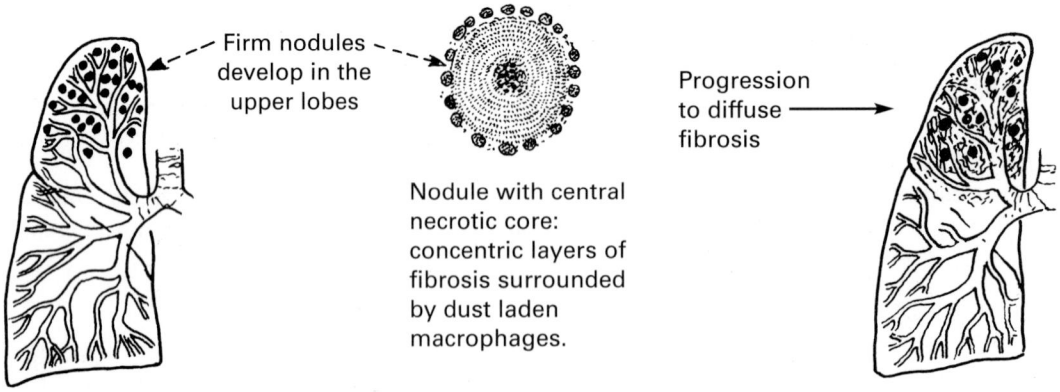

Patients develop increasing breathlessness and may die of respiratory failure and cor pulmonale.

The silicotic lung is particularly susceptible to **tuberculosis** and, historically, this was an important cause of death.

ASBESTOSIS

Asbestos is the generic name for a group of fibrous silicates widely used in heavy industry for insulation (particularly in shipbuilding).

The various types are popularly classified by colour — blue, brown, red asbestos: or by chemical names e.g. *crocidolite*.

Asbestosis results from chronic exposure.

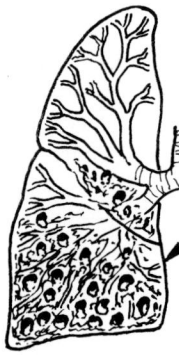

Diffuse fibrosis is most marked in lower lobes

↓

often progressing to honeycombing

Some asbestos fibres become encrusted with iron and protein

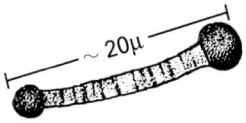

These ASBESTOS BODIES are present in SPUTUM and are diagnostic.

Other important complications are:

1. **Lung cancer**

   Asbestos workers have an increased risk of lung cancer, especially if they also smoke.
   Risk of cancer = risk due to smoking × risk due to asbestos.

2. **Pleural pathology**

   (a) **Pleural plaques**

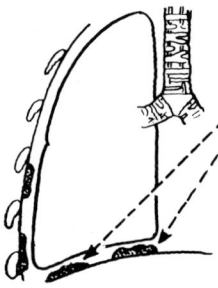

These are dense areas of hyaline fibrosis on the parietal pleura.

They cause no morbidity but are markers of exposure.

Rarely there is diffuse pleural fibrosis

   (b) **Mesothelioma** (Malignant tumour of the pleura)

   This can occur after short exposure particularly to blue asbestos (crocidolite).

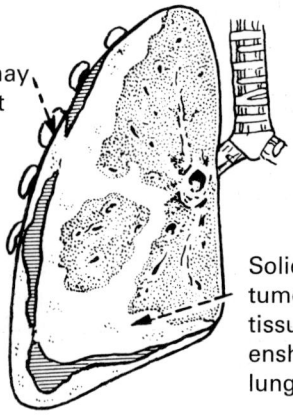

Growth may also affect parietal pleura

Solid white tumour tissue ensheathing lung.

Note: Mesothelioma may also affect the pericardium and peritoneum.

FIBROSING ALVEOLITIS (INTERSTITIAL PULMONARY FIBROSIS)

This group of disorders causes approximately 1500 deaths per year in the U.K. It mainly affects adults around 60 years of age. They present with dyspnoea, and often a dry cough. This progresses, usually over 4–5 years, to chronic respiratory failure and cor pulmonale.

In a significant number of cases where no cause is evident the term 'cryptogenic' is used. The many causes include:

Systemic diseases	**Drugs**	**Viral infection**	**Poisons**
e.g. Rheumatoid arthritis, Systemic lupus erythematosis, Systemic sclerosis.	e.g. Bleomycin, Amiodarone		e.g. Paraquat (very rapid progression)

Initiation of inflammation at alveolar (and bronchiolar) level (probably basically an auto-immune reaction).

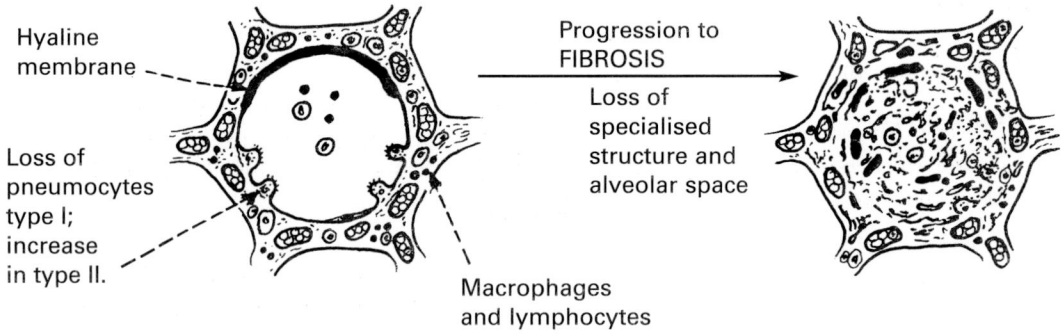

Progression to FIBROSIS of ALVEOLI → Restrictive lung defect

↓ increasing fibrosis

In the late stage the lung is described as 'HONEYCOMB', with numerous cysts particularly in the lower lobes.

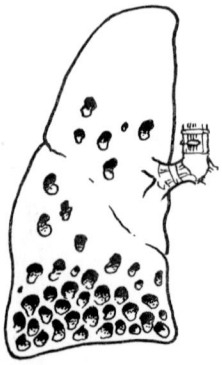

↓ Hypoxia → RESPIRATORY FAILURE

↓ Pulmonary hypertension

↓ Right ventricular hypertrophy (cor pulmonale)

↓ Right heart failure

Infection is a common terminal event, and there is an increased risk of lung cancer.

LUNG CANCER

Lung cancer (carcinoma of the bronchus) is the commonest form of cancer and one which is largely preventable. Approximately 35,000 patients die of lung cancer in the United Kingdom each year.

Gross Pathology

The tumour arises from the main bronchi or their large branches (central) or at the periphery of the lung (peripheral).

Most patients present with cough, haemoptysis or chest pain, but metastases may be the first sign.

The lung distal to the tumour may collapse or become consolidated (Retention pneumonia).

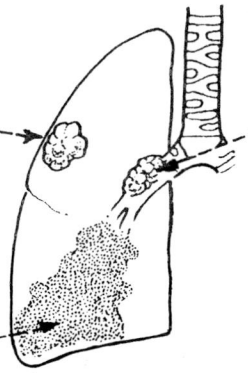

Central tumours arise from the bronchial mucosa and form a friable mass which often partly obstructs the bronchial lumen.

Tumour spread

(a) **LOCAL**

(ii) Pleural involvement often results in a haemorrhagic effusion.

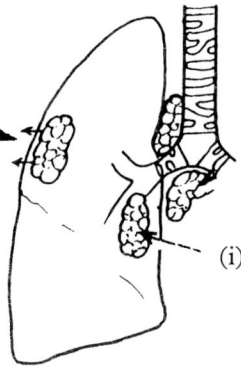

(iii) Hilar lymph nodes are often involved — with extension into mediastinal nodes.

(i) The tumour directly invades adjacent lung tissue. Invasion of a large blood vessel may lead to severe Haemorrhage (Haemoptysis).

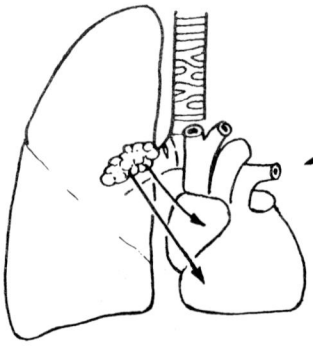

(iv) Direct spread to the pericardium may give pericardial effusion with subsequent involvement of the myocardium.

LUNG CANCER

LOCAL SPREAD (continued)

(v) Apical tumours (**Pancoast** tumour) can involve structures in the neck.

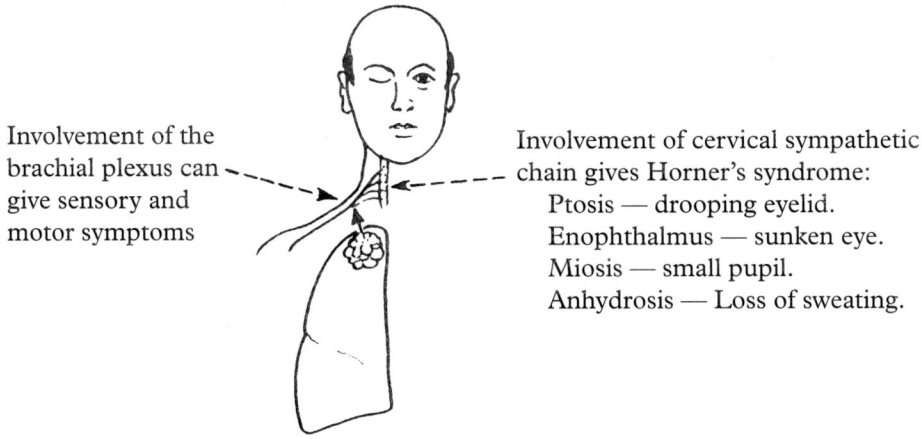

(iv) **Spread to the mediastinum**

(a) The superior vena cava can be obstructed — venous congestion in head and neck.

(b) Nerves may be involved —

Recurrent laryngeal ⟶ vocal cord paralysis.
Phrenic ⟶ paralysis of diaphragm.

(b) **DISTANT SPREAD**

Haematogenous spread is common, usually due to invasion of pulmonary veins. The common sites are: LIVER, BONE, BRAIN, ADRENAL (the last is usually asymptomatic but is found frequently at autopsy).

Lymphatic spread to cervical nodes and retrograde spread to the abdomen occurs.

NON-METASTATIC EFFECTS

These include:

1. ACTH secretion ⟶ Adrenal hyperplasia ⟶ Raised blood cortisol ⟶ Cushing's syndrome.
2. ADH secretion ⟶ Retention of water ⟶ Dilutional hyponatraemia
3. Parathyroid hormone related peptide (PTHrP) ⟶ Hypercalcaemia (p. 25).

Other syndromes include: encephalopathy, cerebellar degeneration, neuropathy, myopathy, Eaton Lambert syndrome, etc.

LUNG CANCER

HISTOLOGICAL TYPES

Four main types are recognised

1. Small cell anaplastic carcinoma (Oat cell) ..... 25%.
2. Squamous carcinoma ..... 35%.
3. Adenocarcinoma ..... 30%.
4. Large cell anaplastic ..... 10%.

The proportions vary between series.

The separation of small cell carcinoma from non-small cell variants is extremely important as the former tumour is treated by chemotherapy.

SMALL CELL LUNG CARCINOMA

This is the most aggressive form of lung cancer and metastasises early and widely. It does respond well, at least initially, to chemotherapy — some patients survive for up to 2 years.

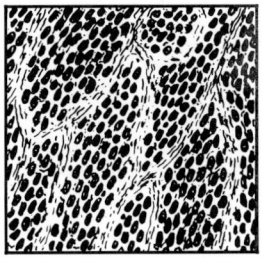

Almost no cytoplasm

Spindle-shaped dark nuclei; may appear to be rounded or oval. May be arranged in sheets, cords or small round aggregates.

On electron-microscopy, cells show neurosecretory granules.

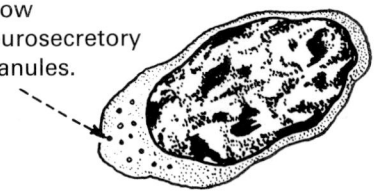

The tumour arises from neuro-endocrine cells and expresses markers such as synaptophysin. It is the form which most commonly has endocrine and other non-metastatic humoral effects.

SQUAMOUS CARCINOMA

These tend to arise centrally from major bronchi, within dysplastic squamous epithelium following squamous metaplasia.

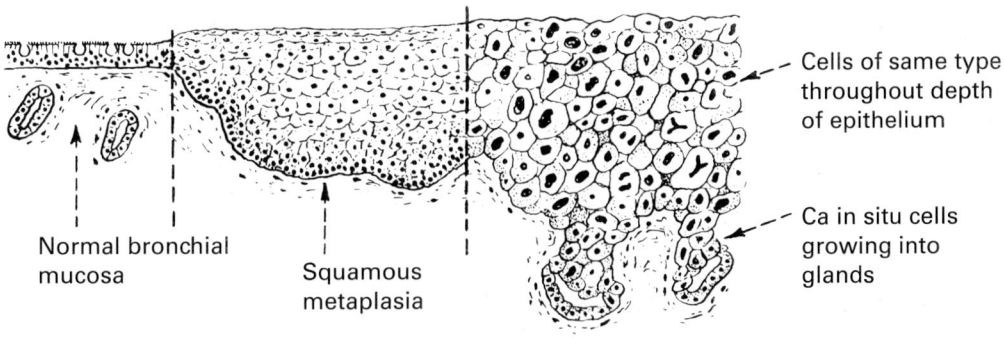

Although squamous carcinoma is often slow growing, there is often extensive destruction of local tissues. The affected bronchi are often blocked, leading to retention pneumonia or collapse.

LUNG CANCER

HISTOLOGICAL TYPES (continued)

ADENOCARCINOMA

This tumour is a common tumour in women and is seen in non-smokers, but is also associated with smoking. At least two-thirds arise in the periphery of the lung, sometimes in relation to scarring.

Two main patterns are seen:

(a) A well defined mass of malignant cells arranged in acini with a fibrous stroma.

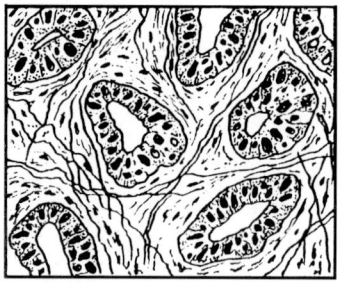

(b) Growth of tumour cells along the alveolar walls (so-called 'bronchioalveolar carcinoma')

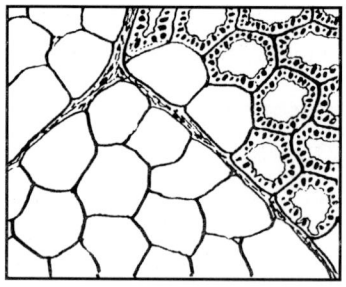

LARGE CELL ANAPLASTIC CARCINOMA

As the name suggests, this tumour consists of large malignant cells without any specific differentiation. The tumour usually arises centrally.

AETIOLOGY OF LUNG CANCER

The main factors are:

1. *Cigarette smoking* — This is by far the major cause, established by epidemiological and animal studies. Cigarette smoke contains carcinogens such as 3,4 benzpyrene and nitrosamines.

2. *Industrial and atmospheric pollution* — There is a large number of pollutant industrial processes e.g. asbestos workers, miners exposed to irradiation (e.g. radon, uranium) and metal smelters (e.g. chromium and nickel).

Lung cancer is more common in urban than in rural areas.

SECONDARY LUNG TUMOURS

It must always be remembered that many other cancers spread to the lungs both by blood and lymphatic routes.

OTHER TUMOURS OF THE BRONCHI AND LUNGS

Benign tumours of the bronchi and lung are unusual. There are 2 main types.

1. **SQUAMOUS PAPILLOMA**

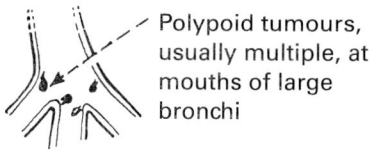

Papillomas are similar to the papillary tumours of the larynx. They occur in young people and on occasion may cause stridor due to partial obstruction. They are due to papilloma virus infection (types 6 and 11). Malignant change is exceptional.

2. **ADENOCHONDROMA**

These are uncommon hamartomas of the lung which consist of lobules of cartilage and cleft-like spaces lined by bronchial epithelium. Their importance is that they appear as 'coin lesions' on chest X-ray and may simulate primary or secondary tumours. They are completely benign.

CARCINOID TUMOURS

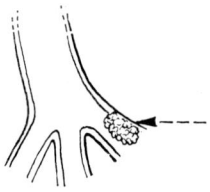

These tumours account for 1-2% of primary lung neoplasms. They often appear around the age of 50 years. Usually the tumour is situated in a primary bronchus or at the lung periphery. The tumour is a smooth surfaced yellow nodule.

Histologically these resemble carcinoid tumours of the appendix (see p. 331). A small proportion of these tumours metastasise to regional lymph nodes — all are potentially malignant.

Central tumours tend to block the bronchus pain which they arise.

Obstruction → Collapse of lung

Obstruction → Infection → Pneumonia, Bronchiectasis, Lung abscess

Atypical carcinoid tumours: This sub-group of tumours shows nuclear pleomorphism, mitotic activity and necrosis. Over half eventually metastasise.

Tumours of Bronchial glands

Both benign and low grade malignant tumours of the bronchial glands are occasionally seen. These present as obstructing lesions.

COLLAPSE OF LUNG

There are 2 basic causes of collapse of the lung.

(1) **Pressure** on the visceral pleura by fluid of air — this is discussed in more detail on page 288.

(2) **Bronchial obstruction** causing absorption collapse. The illustration shows collapse of a lung segment.

Absorption of air from alveoli

↓

COLLAPSED segment dark red in colour (haemoglobin not oxygenated)

The commonest causes are bronchial tumour and inhaled foreign body.

Sequel — if the obstruction is not relieved, infection ± fibrosis follows.

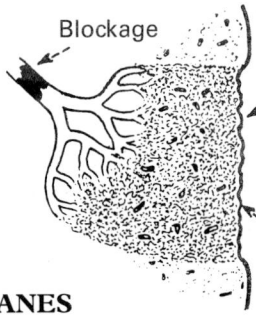

ATELECTASIS AND HYALINE MEMBRANES

Respiratory difficulties arising shortly after the birth of a baby are associated with pathological changes in the lungs.

Aetiology — there are 2 main factors

(1) *Premature birth* — (a) immaturity of lungs — deficiency of SURFACTANT (surfactant facilitates alveolar expansion and forms a protective layer between air and alveolar lining cells).

(b) immaturity of respiratory centre.

(2) *Cerebral damage* — respiration depressed.

Atelectasis means failure of the lungs to expand at birth.

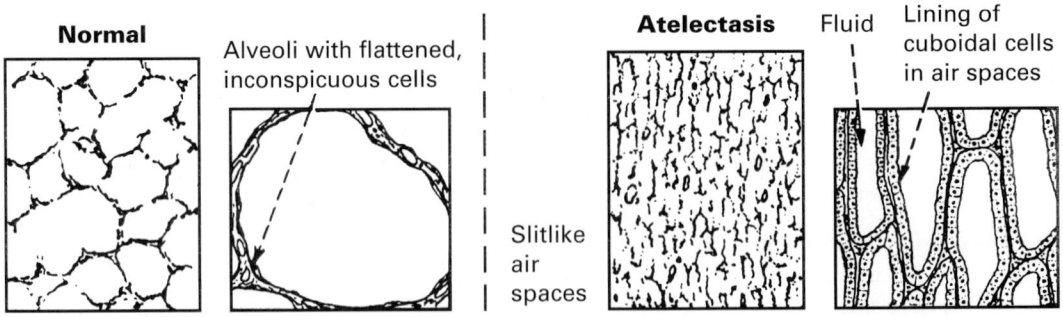

If respiration is not fully established, difficulties continue with the formation of HYALINE MEMBRANES due to the precipitation of protein along respiratory bronchioles and atrial ducts.

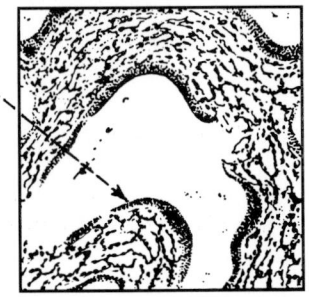

ADULT RESPIRATORY DISTRESS SYNDROME (ARDS)

The adult lung may show similar changes with hyaline membranes secondary to a wide variety of disorders: severe shock, inhalation of irritant gases and pure oxygen, paraquat ingestion and uraemia are examples.

The mechanism is illustrated under Shock lung (p. 173).

DISEASES OF THE PLEURA

INFLAMMATION (PLEURISY)

There are several causes.

(a) *Infection* — usually due to spread from pneumonia or tuberculosis.
— following penetrating injury e.g. stab wound.

(b) *Autoimmunity* - e.g. rheumatoid arthritis, systemic lupus erythematosus.

(c) *Overlying a pulmonary infarct* (p. 162).

FIBRINOUS PLEURISY

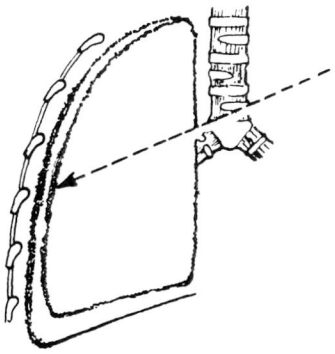

Fibrinous exudate on parietal and visceral layers → Pleural friction rub, pleuritic chest pain due to movement on respiration

The exudate is absorbed but organisation may lead to pleural adhesions.

If fluid accumulates in excess, there is a pleural effusion — pain and friction rub disappear as the inflamed layers are separated.

If infection of the pleura proceeds, an empyema (a collection of pus in the pleura) may form. This is now unusual.

PLEURAL EFFUSION

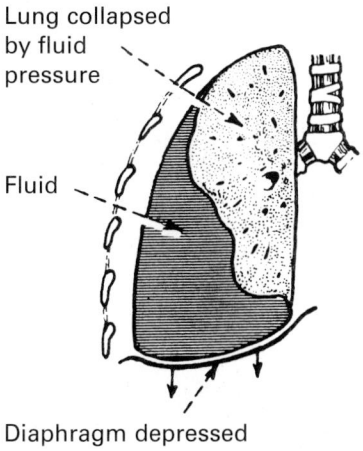

The accumulation of fluid within the pleura can be explained as a form of local oedema.

The composition of the fluid is related to the underlying cause.

TRANSUDATE	EXUDATE
e.g. in heart failure	e.g. in fibrinous pleurisy
— low protein content;	— high protein content;
— few inflammatory cells.	— numerous inflammatory cells.

Examination of the pleural fluid may show mesothelial cells, lymphocytes, macrophages, neutrophils and sometimes tumour cells.

DISEASES OF THE PLEURA

PNEUMOTHORAX

This is the accumulation of air in the pleural space. It may follow blunt trauma or penetrating wound e.g. stabbing. Older patients with emphysema may develop spontaneous pneumothorax. In young people this is usually due to rupture of small bullae.

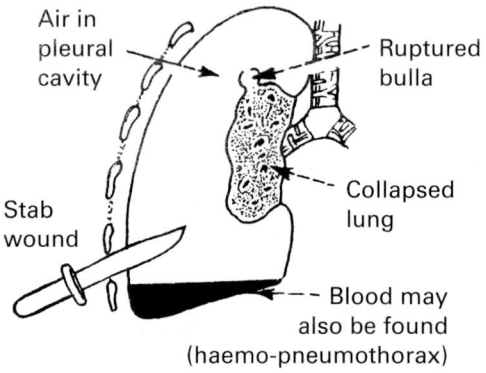

Patients complain of chest pain and breathlessness.

In a TENSION PNEUMOTHORAX there is a valve effect — Air continues to enter the pleura during inspiration but cannot exit during expiration.

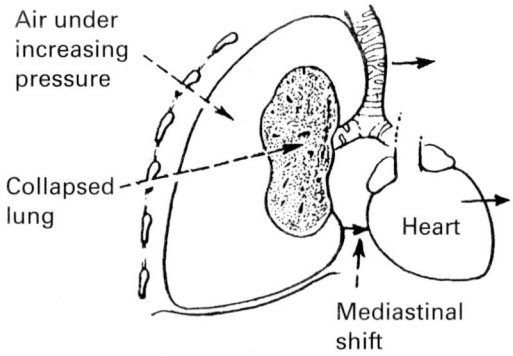

PLEURAL MALIGNANCY

Metastatic tumours affect the pleura in 2 ways.

(a) By LYMPHATIC spread — with numerous small nodules e.g. breast carcinoma.

(b) By DIRECT spread e.g. lung cancer.

There is usually a pleural effusion in which tumour cells can be found.

Malignant Mesothelioma

This primary pleural malignancy is usually due to asbestos exposure — often many years before.

The tumour may encase the entire lung and grow into the interlobar fissures

The tumour can metastasise to other sites, but most patients die due to the local respiratory effects.

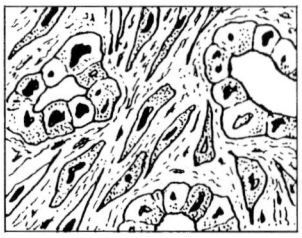

Histologically, the tumour shows a mixture of epithelial and sarcomatous tissues.

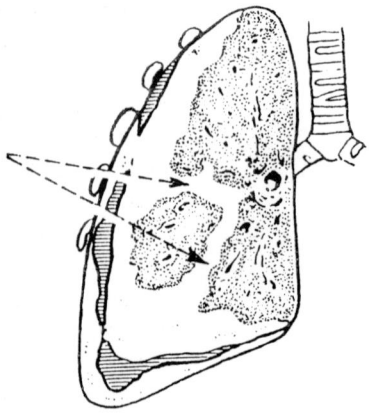

There is often a malignant pleural effusion.

CHAPTER 9

GASTROINTESTINAL TRACT

Mouth 290
Oral Cancer 291
Mouth 292
Dental Caries and Periodontal Disease 293
Diseases of the Salivary Glands 294
Salivary Glands — Tumours 295
Salivary Glands — Carcinomas 296
Oesophagus 297–300
Stomach 301
Gastritis 302–304
Peptic Ulceration 305, 306
Peptic Ulcer — Aetiology 307
Gastric Carcinoma 308–310
Small Intestine — Malabsorption 311
Malabsorption 312
Crohn's Disease 313
Ulcerative Colitis 314
Crohn's Disease and Ulcerative Colitis 315
Intestinal Infections 316, 317
Typhoid 318, 319
Bacillary Dysentery 320
Amoebic Dysentery 321
Tuberculous Enteritis and Pseudomembranous Colitis 322
Appendicitis 323
Appendicitis — Sequels 324
Diverticular Disease 325
Ischaemia and the Intestines 326
Intestinal Obstruction 327
Hernia 328
Hernia — Complications 329
Intussusception 330
Volvulus and Hirschsprung's Disease 331
Tumours of the Colon 332, 333
Carcinoma of the Colon 334, 335
Tumours of Small Intestine 336
Carcinoid Tumours 337
The Peritoneal Cavity 338, 339

THE MOUTH

INFLAMMATION

A wide variety of inflammatory conditions are seen.

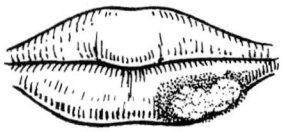

Blisters and inflammation

VIRAL INFECTIONS

Herpes simplex virus (usually type I) infects the mouth in young children — numerous vesicles and ulcers are seen. The virus can become latent in the trigeminal ganglion and repeated 'cold sores' occur on the lip in later life.

Coxsackie viruses can cause oral blistering (e.g. herpangina; hand, foot and mouth disease). Koplik's spots are a feature of measles.

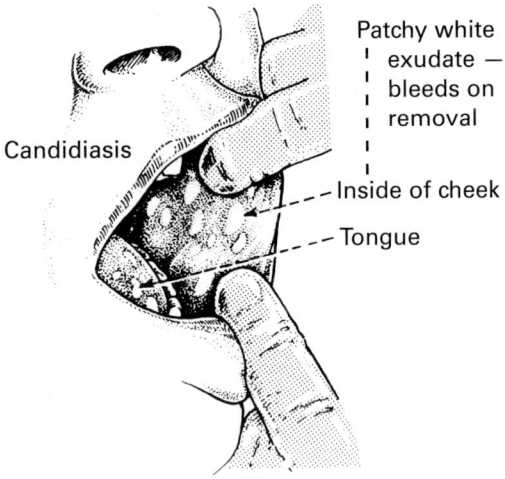

FUNGAL INFECTION

Candida albicans is an oral commensal in 20–40% of the population. Infection is seen in infants, in patients on broad spectrum antibiotics, steroid or cytotoxic therapy and also in the immunosuppressed and diabetics. Extensive oral candida is common in patients with AIDS.

BACTERIAL INFECTIONS

Acute ulcerative gingivitis and oropharyngitis (Vincent's angina) is due to coinfection with *fusibacterium fusiformis* and *Borrelia Vincenti.*

Syphilis, now uncommon in the West, can involve the mouth as a primary chancre, irregular lines of ulceration — snail track ulcers of the secondary stage, and as small gummas (tertiary).

Oral tuberculosis, usually due to coughed up bacilli from pulmonary TB, is now uncommon. Ulcers may occur on the tongue.

Aphthous ulcers

Around 30% of the population are troubled by these painful, usually small, ulcers on the cheek, tongue and gums. The aetiology is unknown; in some individuals they are provoked by stress or local trauma.

Dermatoses e.g. lichen planus — can affect the oral mucosa,

ORAL CANCER

Oral cancer accounts for 2% of cancers in the United Kingdom. There is wide geographical variation — commoner in S. East Asia. Males are at least twice as commonly affected as women — it is a disease of the elderly.

Aetiology

The major causes are:

1. Tobacco — especially pipe and cigar smoking. Chewing tobacco, sometimes mixed with betel nuts (in Eastern countries) is also implicated.
2. Alcohol, especially spirits.
3. Exposure to ultra-violet light (cancer of the lip).
4. Human papilloma virus (type 16) may be involved.

Pathology

Almost all cases are **squamous cell carcinomas**. The lip, tongue, floor of mouth, tonsil and fauces are affected in that order of frequency.

Ulcerated nodule often on the lower lip with raised edges.

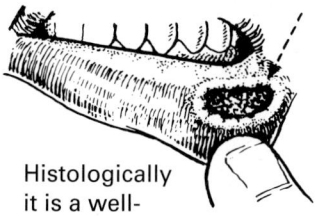

Histologically it is a well-differentiated keratinizing growth.

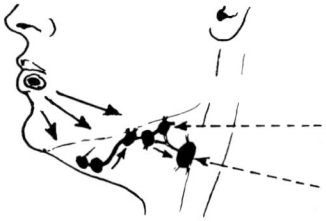

Growth is relatively slow but eventually dissemination to the submandibular nodes takes place and thence to the deeper cervical nodes

Tongue/Floor of mouth

Carcinoma of the tongue and other sites within the mouth is a more aggressive growth than tumours of the lips. Starting as a nodule in the buccal sulcus adjacent to the tongue, it quickly breaks down to form an irregular ulcer with ragged edges.

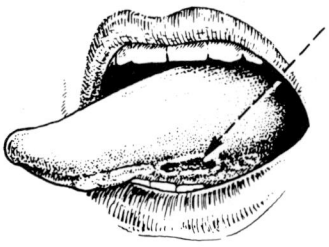

Local infiltration leads to fixation of the tongue. Spread may be extensive to floor of mouth, fauces, pharynx, and into the medullary cavity of the mandible via occlusal ridge gaps particularly in the edentulous patient.

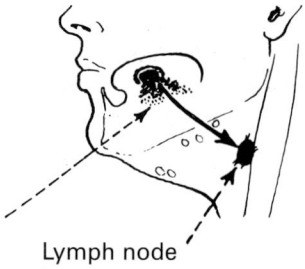

Lymph node involvement occurs early, usually to the deeper cervical nodes.

MOUTH

ERYTHROPLAKIA and LEUKOPLAKIA

Many oral cancers arise from dysplastic squamous epithelium.

Clinically, some appear as velvety red patches (erythroplakia)

Others are white patches (leukoplakia)

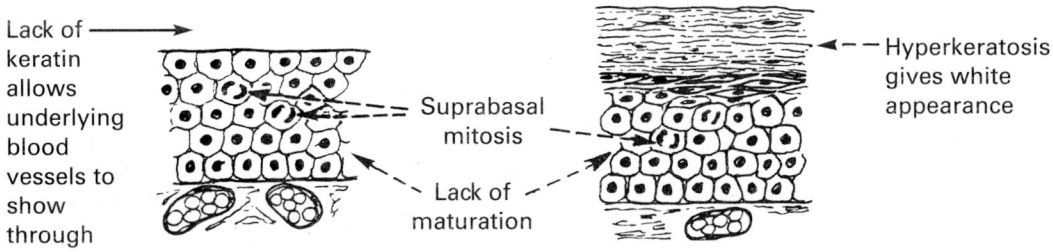

Not all examples of leukoplakia are premalignant; this is simply a descriptive term for a white patch.

It may also be due to: — chronic irritation (e.g. dentures)
— pipe smoking
— candida.

A distinctive form — 'hairy leukoplakia' — occurs on the lateral border of the tongue in patients with HIV/AIDS. It appears to be due to Epstein Barr virus infection, often with superimposed candida.

Pigmentations

Dark pigmentations of the gums are seen in chronic poisoning with heavy metals; lead (blue), bismuth (grey), mercury (purplish). Melanotic pigmentation of the mouth is seen in Addison's disease and the Peutz-Jeghers syndrome.

Benign Tumours

A variety of benign tumours are seen e.g. squamous papillomas. Haemangiomas (often on the lips or tongue) can interfere with swallowing and may bleed after biopsy.

Granular cell myoblastoma

This is a rare tumour and its importance lies in the fact that it may be mistaken for carcinoma of the tongue.

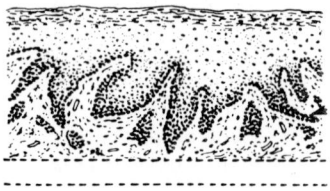

Overlying epithelium shows very irregular downgrowths — but it is not neoplastic (so-called pseudoepitheliomatous hyperplasia)

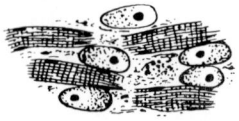

Large granular cells (thought to arise from Schwann cells or nerves) between and around muscle cells of tongue

Note: Epulis is a clinical term applied to swellings at the gum margin. Most of them are granulomas associated with chronic gingivitis. A few are true neoplasms.

DENTAL CARIES AND PERIODONTAL DISEASE

These two very common processes are primarily of importance to dentists but an understanding is also valuable for doctors.

DENTAL CARIES

This is the commonest disease of teeth.

Poor oral hygiene + high sugar intake lead to formation of plaque.

Plaque includes masses of bacteria e.g. Streptococcus mutans + sugar

Lactic acid and proteolytic enzymes

remove calcified parts of tooth (CARIES)

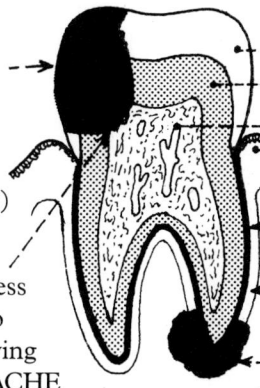

The process spreads to PULP giving TOOTHACHE

Further spread gives PERI-APICAL ABSCESS

PERIODONTAL DISEASE

This is the major cause of tooth loss in middle age. It is essentially due to gingivitis.

A pouch is formed between the gingiva and the neck of the tooth.

Bacteria e.g. bacteroides, fusobacterium, cause inflammatory reaction.

Inflammation spreads to the periodontal membrane.

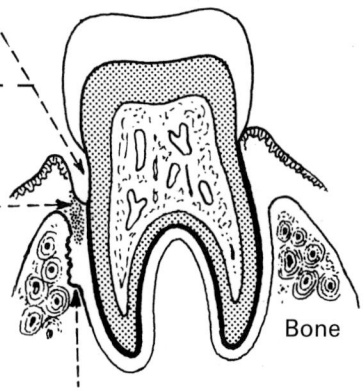

The supporting bone is resorbed

↓

Loosening of tooth

DISEASES OF SALIVARY GLANDS

INFLAMMATION

Simple bacterial infection of these glands is uncommon. It may occur during a prolonged illness, particularly if a calculus has formed in a duct.

More commonly acute inflammation is due to the virus of *mumps*, which produces acute swelling, particularly of the parotid glands, with oedema and mononuclear infiltration of the interstitial tissue. The testes and pancreas may also be inflamed and atrophy may follow.

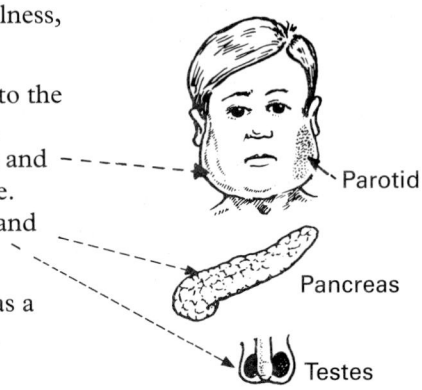

Chronic inflammation is rare. It may occur as a manifestation of sarcoidosis. The parotid gland becomes swollen and there may be an accompanying irido-cyclitis. This has given rise to the term 'uveo-parotid fever'. The parotid gland shows a chronic inflammatory reaction with granulomas typical of sarcoidosis.

Sjogren's syndrome

In this auto-immune condition there is a destruction of the gland tissue of the salivary, lacrimal and conjunctival glands by an infiltrate of lymphocytes (so-called lympho-epithelial lesions) and plasma cells. The duct epithelia often undergo reactive hyperplasia. It results in dryness of the mouth, caries due to lack of saliva, and ulceration of the conjunctiva caused by lack of secretion from the lacrimal and conjunctival glands. Polyarthritis is often present and the serum contains autoantibodies and rheumatoid factor.

Occasionally a B-cell lymphoma arises from the lymphoid proliferation.

Calculus formation

This can affect the submandibular or, less often, the parotid duct. Blockage of the duct leads to episodes of swelling after food and eventually to atrophy of the gland. Occasionally acute inflammation may be superimposed.

SALIVARY GLAND TUMOURS

The majority (80%) of tumours arise in the parotid gland and most in this site are benign.

The remaining 20% occur in the submandibular and minor salivary glands — in these sites 30–40% are malignant.

SALIVARY GLANDS – TUMOURS

PLEOMORPHIC SALIVARY ADENOMA (P.S.A.)

This is the commonest tumour of the salivary glands and most often occurs in the parotid. The term 'pleomorphic' applies not to the nuclei of the cells but to the different types of tissue found. These are derived from the epithelial and myoepithelial cells.

To the naked eye, the tumour appears rounded or lobulated and encapsulated.

Microscopically the cellular pleomorphism assumes several forms.

The **epithelial** elements form duct-like structures often with 2 cell layers

or

trabeculae

(Squamous differentiation may be seen)

The **myoepithelial** elements are seen as cellular clumps

or

may be separated by a myxoid ground substance

Cartilagenous metaplasia may also occur.

Although the tumour appears encapsulated, there are frequently small lobules which extend into the adjacent tissue.

If the tumour is 'shelled out' these lobules are left behind and cause local occurrence. For this reason superficial parotidectomy is usually performed, ensuring complete removal of the tumour.

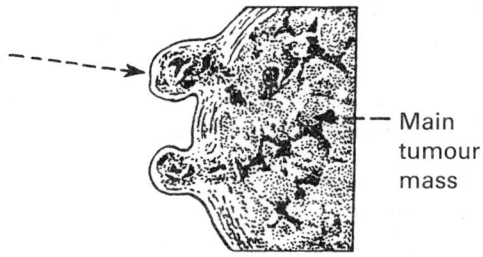

MALIGNANT CHANGE

Under 5% of these tumour become malignant, often after many years. Most of these are adenocarcinomas. CARCINOMA-IN-P.S.A. has a poor prognosis.

ADENOLYMPHOMA (Warthin's tumour)

This is a benign lesion, mainly in the parotid of elderly men. It consists of tall epithelial cells with eosinophilic cytoplasm (oncocytes) and a striking reactive lymphoid infiltrate.

SALIVARY GLANDS – CARCINOMAS

Adenocarcinomas of the salivary glands may arise *de novo* or from pre-existing P.S.A. They may affect major or minor glands. The prognosis is variable.

Three unusual subtypes are worth noting.

1. **Acinic cell carcinoma**
   Approximately 1/4 of all malignant parotid tumours are of this type. It grows slowly, recurs after removal and sometimes there is late extension to the regional lymph nodes and distant organs.

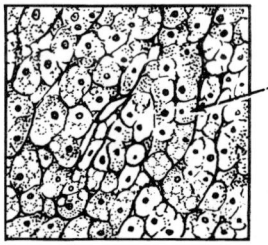

Closely aggregated cells containing secretory granules and sometimes glycogen.

2. **Adenoid cystic carcinoma**
   This usually occurs in minor salivary glands and accounts for 7% of salivary gland tumours. It extends by direct spread, but metastases can occur to lymph nodes, lungs and bones. There is a special tendency to spread along nerve sheaths.

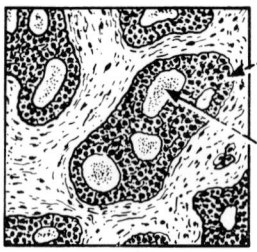

Cribriform pattern. Solid masses of epithelium enclosing small cystic spaces containing mucin. The cells resemble basal cells.

3. **Muco-epidermoid carcinoma**
   The malignancy of this type varies, but all tend to recur and infiltrate locally. More malignant growths metastasise to the lymph nodes and may invade the blood stream. They are generally found in the major salivary glands and form 3 or 4% of all tumours of these glands.

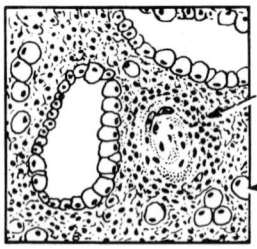

Squamoid cells

Mucus-secreting cells

OESOPHAGUS

The oesophagus is a muscular tube 25 cm long, which is lined by stratified squamous epithelium which is resistant to damage by heat, cold and mechanical trauma.

INFLAMMATION

Reflux oesophagitis

This is the commonest form of inflammation due to reflux of gastric acid into the lower oesophagus. It is a constant concomitant of hiatus hernia.

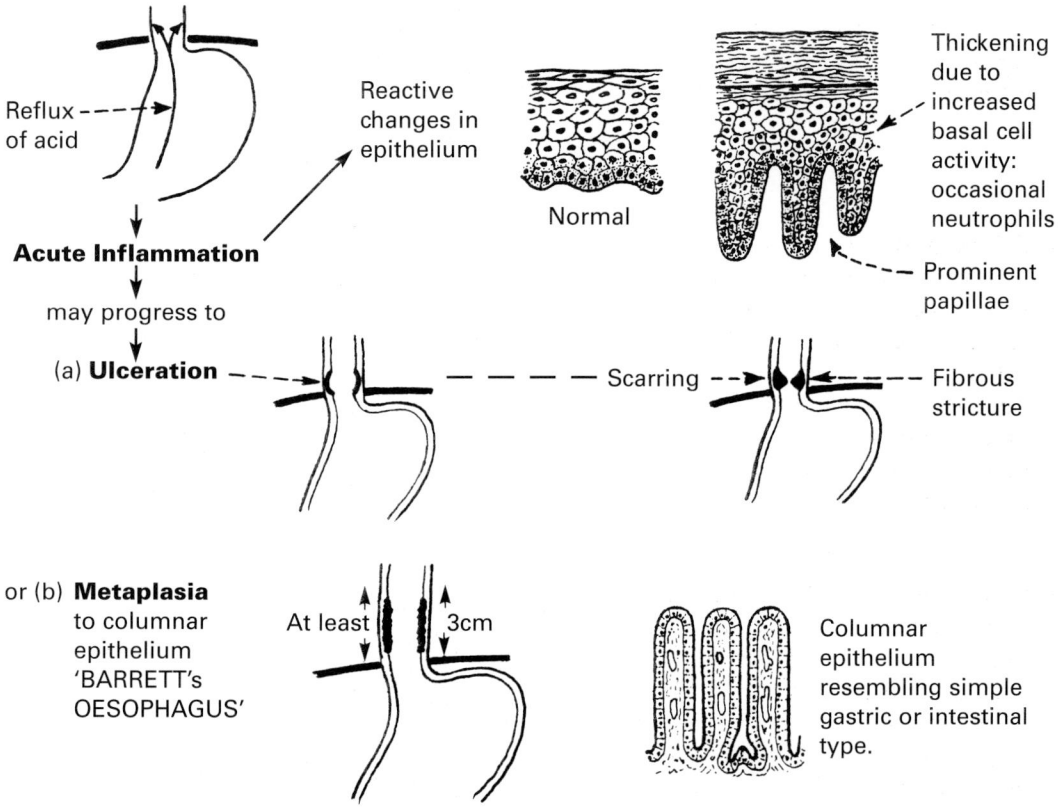

Note: This is an important premalignant lesion: the increased risk of CANCER developing is 30–40 fold.

METAPLASIA ⟶ DYSPLASIA (detected by endoscopy and biopsy) ⟶ ADENOCARCINOMA

Other forms of oesophagitis

(1) Infection by *Herpes Simplex Virus* and *Candida Albicans* occurs particularly in the immunosuppressed and AIDS.

(2) Ingestion of Caustic Poisons in strong concentrations causes wide-spread necrosis and sloughing of tissues. With weaker poisons the epithelium is destroyed and secondary infection with inflammation and scarring with stricture may follow.

OESOPHAGUS

HIATUS HERNIA

In hiatus hernia part of the stomach herniates into the thorax. This is common, particularly in the elderly, though often asymptomatic. Two forms are seen:

1. **Sliding hernia**
   — the distal oesophagus and proximal stomach slide proximally so the latter lies in the thorax.
   Most cases are of this type.

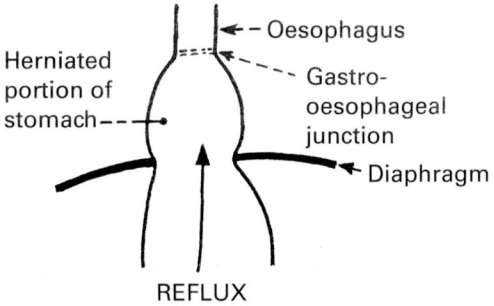

2. **Rolling hernia**
   — a loop of stomach rolls upwards and passes through the diaphragm alongside the oesophagogastric junction. Since this is preserved reflux is unusual.

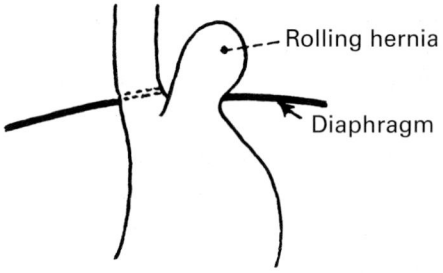

DIVERTICULA

These are relatively rare and are of 2 varieties.

1. **Pulsion type**
Involves pharynx (pharyngeal pouch). Sac is distended during swallowing of food. By pushing down behind oesophagus, it may compress this structure. Congenital weakness of the pharyngeal muscles is said to be an aetiological factor.

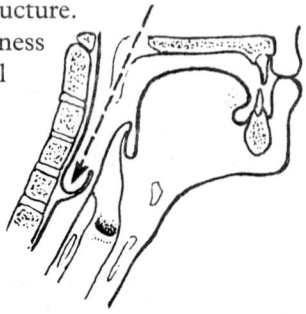

2. **Traction type**
This is due to traction of fibrous tissue produced by mediastinal inflammation, e.g. tuberculosis or silicosis of lymph nodes.

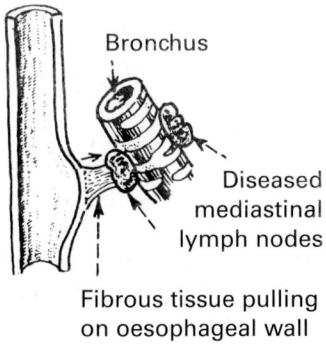

Rarely, there may be a congenital diverticulum at the level of the bifurcation of the trachea.

OESOPHAGUS

Obstruction usually leads to dysphagia — difficulty in swallowing. The causes form 2 main groups:

1. **Strictures** of the oesophageal wall due to:
   — inflammation caused by acid reflux or caustic ingestion.
   — carcinoma.
   — historically mucosal webs at the upper end were a feature of the Plummer-Vinson syndrome in chronic untreated iron deficiency anaemia.
2. **Functional** obstruction

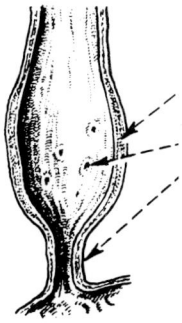

Achalasia of the oesophagus develops in young adults and may cause severe obstruction.
Above the obstruction the oesophagus is dilated, the muscle is hypertrophied and the mucosa may be ulcerated.
Narrowing occurs at the lower end.

It is due to a conduction failure in the peristaltic mechanism preventing opening of the cardiac sphincter. Reduced numbers of ganglion cells are found in the myenteric plexus.

(In South American trypanosomiasis the myenteric plexus may be destroyed and long-standing diabetic autonomic neuropathy may cause a similar problem.)

In **Systemic sclerosis**, replacement of muscle by fibrous tissue may seriously disturb oesophageal peristalsis.

OESOPHAGEAL VARICES

These are important lesions which occur secondarily to portal hypertension caused by cirrhosis of the liver (see p. 355).

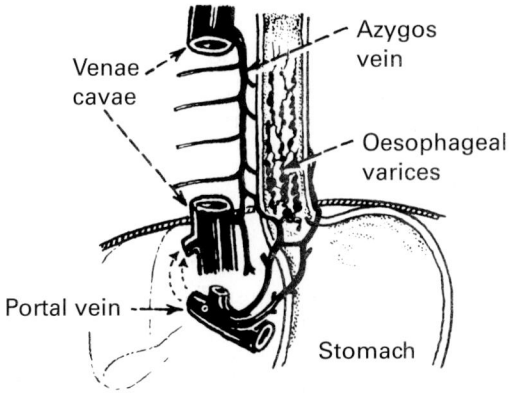

Fibrosis in the liver obstructs the flow of blood from the gastrointestinal tract in the portal system. Anastomotic channels connecting the portal and systemic venous systems open up and become distended. The most important are the oesophageal tributaries of the azygos vein which connect through the diaphragm with the portal system. They become varicose, and are easily traumatised by the passage of food, leading to haemorrhage which can be fatal.

Spontaneous rupture of the oesophagus is a rare condition of uncertain aetiology. Tears without rupture but causing haemorrhage and haematemesis may also occur (Mallory-Weiss syndrome).

Congenital abnormalities include stenosis and atresia with fistula formation.

OESOPHAGUS

TUMOURS

Benign tumours of the oesophagus are very rare. They are almost always of connective tissue origin (usually leiomyomas) and form polyps within the lumen, causing obstruction.

Carcinoma

This is the third most common malignant tumour of the digestive tract, carcinoma of large intestine and stomach taking precedence in that order.

It occurs at three levels:

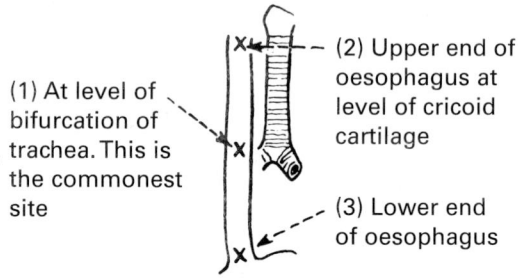

At the upper and middle third, SQUAMOUS CARCINOMA.
At the lower end, ADENOCARCINOMA (associated with Barrett's oesophagus).
The disease is more common in men by at least 2 to 1.
Two forms of growth are seen.

(1) Scirrhous encircling the tube and causing constriction

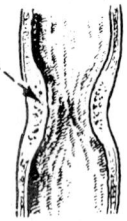

(2) Soft polypoidal growth filling lumen

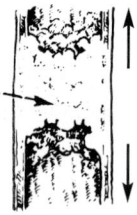

In both instances the growth tends to extend in a longitudinal manner in the submucosal lymphatics. This means that the surgeon has to remove the tumour with wide margins.

Spread

At the common site, near the tracheal bifurcation, spread may involve the trachea or a bronchus, ulcerating the wall and resulting in aspiration pneumonia. Tumours at other levels will involve the trachea or other mediastinal structures. Lymph node involvement is common. Death usually results from the oesophageal obstruction, but the patient may survive long enough for metastases to appear in other organs, e.g. liver.

Aetiological factors

The incidence shows a geographical variation, being common in China and Africa. The causes are unknown but smoking and dietetic factors including alcohol consumption are thought to be important. Post-cricoid carcinoma in women is a rare late complication of the dysphagia complicating iron deficiency anaemia.

STOMACH

The stomach is divided into five anatomical regions:

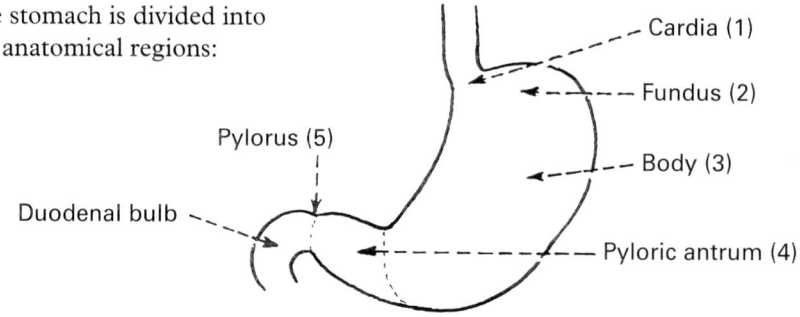

It has three secretory areas:

1. **Cardiac**

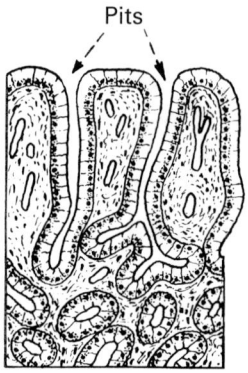

2. **Body and Fundus**
This is the main specialised secreting area.

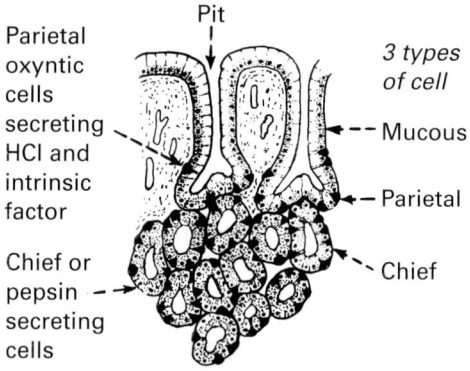

3. **Antrum and Pylorus**

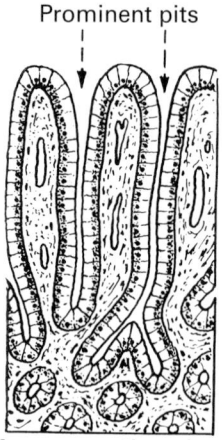

Note: (i) Mucus is secreted throughout the gastric mucosa: the specialised secretory cells are confined to the body and fundus.
(ii) There is a rapid turnover of the epithelial cells.

Vascular supply

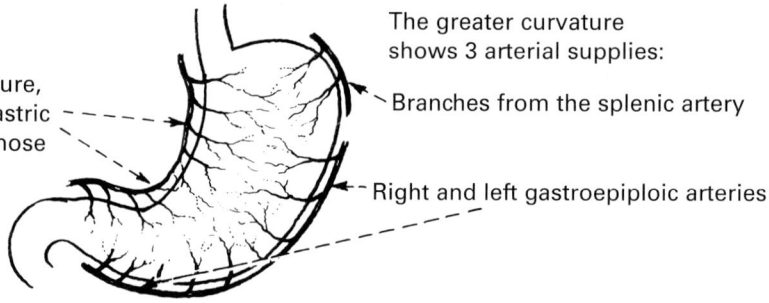

Along the lesser curvature, run the right and left gastric arteries, which anastomose directly.

The arteries anastomose freely in the muscular submucous and mucous coats, except along the lesser curvature of the pyloric antrum and including the first part of duodenum. In this area, there is little anastomosis between the terminal branches in the mucosa.

PEPTIC ULCERATION

SEQUELS and COMPLICATIONS

1. **Healing** is common, particularly when treated.

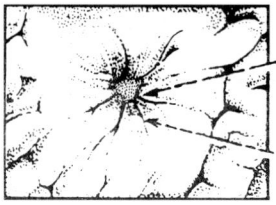

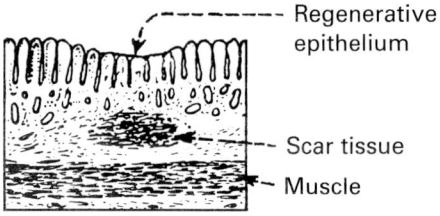

2. **Scarring** may lead to stricture formation.

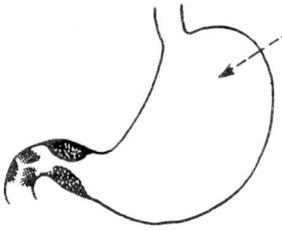

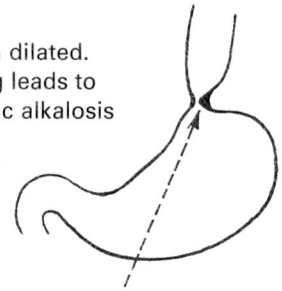

Lesions of duodenum or pylorus lead to gastric outlet obstruction.

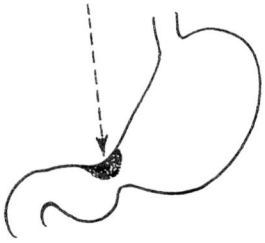

Lesions of the lesser curvature produce an 'hour glass' stomach.

3. **Perforation** of an ulcer causes **acute peritonitis**. This may be

Generalised or **Localised**

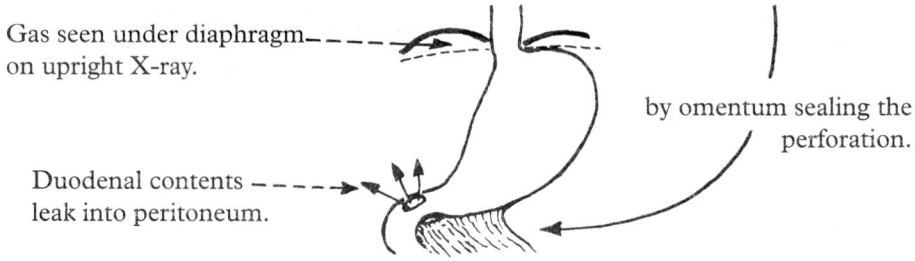

Note: Loculation of pus may occur e.g. subphrenic abscess.

HAEMORRHAGE

Minor haemorrhage is common but may not be apparent clinically.

Major haemorrhage can lead to haematemesis, to 'coffee ground' vomit or to melaena (tarry black stools).

It is no longer believed that there is a significant risk of malignant transformation of peptic ulcers.

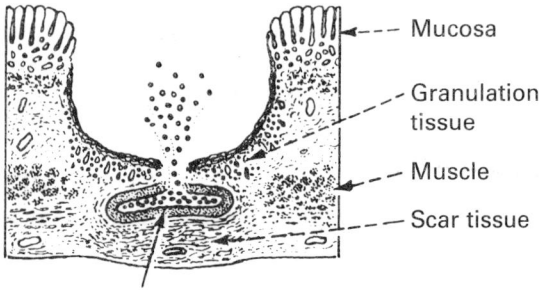

PEPTIC ULCER – AETIOLOGY

Normally gastric mucosal damage is prevented by a balance between the damaging agents and the mucosal defences.

Damaging agents
ACID (+ pepsin)

Mucosal defences
Surface mucus layer
+ bicarbonate
Epithelial cell integrity

Balanced

Peptic ulceration results from imbalance.

(a) INCREASED ACID (+ pepsin)
e.g. Zollinger Ellison syndrome

Normal defences

(b) Normal ACID (+ pepsin)

DECREASED DEFENCES

Although the mechanisms in gastric and duodenal ulcers differ in both, *HELICOBACTER PYLORI* infection is important.

Gastric ulcer

Colonisation of antrum by *H. pylori* (70%)

NSAIDs → REDUCED MUCOSAL DEFENCES

DUODENO-GASTRIC REFLUX (including bile; aggravated by smoking)

ACID (usually low or normal)

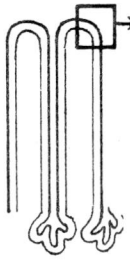

High magnification

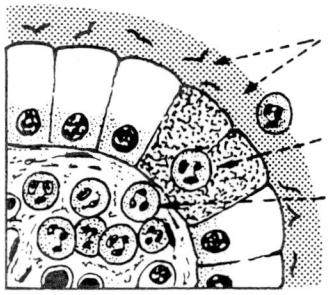

Duodenal ulcer (DU)

The main factors are **hyperacidity** and *H. pylori* infection (>95% of cases).

H. pylori → Gastric infection → Increased gastrin → **Hyperacidity** (genetic factors also important)

METAPLASIA

H. pylori infection of duodenum

+ and other factors, e.g. stress, smoking

ACID

DUODENITIS → ULCER

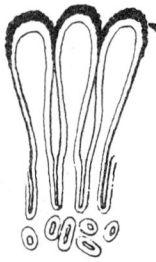

Focal metaplasia of tips of duodenal villi

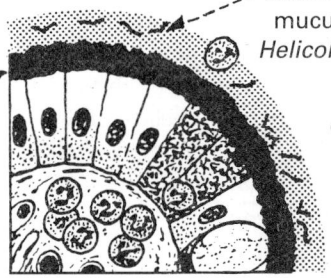

Cell damage
↓
Neutrophils
↓
Duodenitis

Note: DU is cured when *H. pylori* is eliminated and acid reduced.

GASTRIC CARCINOMA

This very important tumour is the second most common cancer worldwide, with an especially high incidence in Japan, Chile and Italy. Its incidence has fallen in the United Kingdom and the U.S.A.

The distribution within the stomach is:

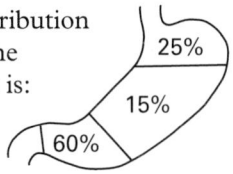

Morphologically, there are several types.

1. **EXOPHYTIC**

These exophytic tumours are commonly seen in the fundus.
Eventually the tumour spreads through the stomach wall to the serosa and is often ulcerated on the surface.

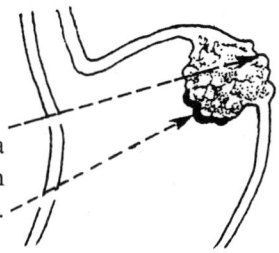

2. **ULCERATIVE**

These tumours, often in the antrum, produce large irregular ulcers with a rolled edge.
The rolled edge rather than the ulcer base should be biopsied.

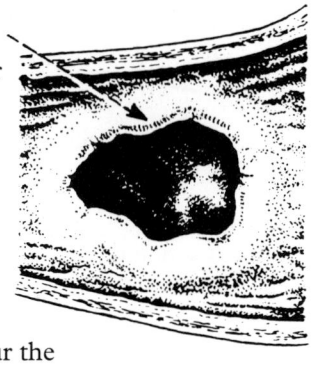

3. **DIFFUSE PATTERN**

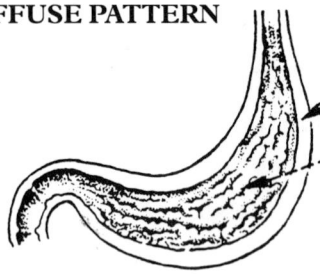

In this form of tumour the entire gastric wall is thickened.
Ulceration is usually minimal, but the mucosal folds are prominent.

This is sometimes knows as 'leather-bottle stomach' (linitis plastica).

Histologically, gastric cancers tend to fall into one of two types (Lauern classification),

(a) **Intestinal**

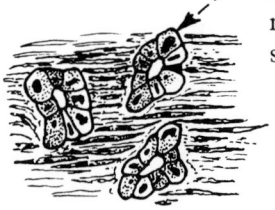

Malignant cells arranged in **acini** invade through the muscle of the stomach wall.

(b) **Diffuse**

Typically seen in linitis plastica. These tumours consist of **signet ring cells.**

Extracellular mucin may also be present.

Globules of mucin push the nucleus to one side.

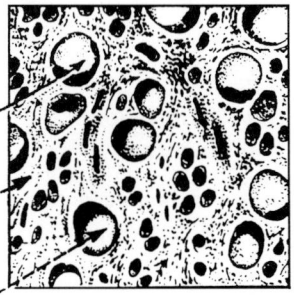

GASTRIC CARCINOMA

Gastric carcinomas are aggressive tumours with both local and distant spread.

LOCAL spread

To oesophagus

1.* Mucosal and **submucosal** lymphatic spread

to duodenum*

2. To draining lymph nodes

3. To adjacent viscera including liver

DISTANT spread

1. By lymphatics e.g. to supraclavicular node (Troisier's sign).

2. To lungs but usually late.

3. **Haematogenous to liver** (via portal vein)

4. Transcoelomic to ovaries (Krukenberg tumours)

**Note:* The duodenal mucosa is resistant to direct mucosal spread.

Staging is by the T.N.M. system (Tumour: nodes: metastases).

EARLY GASTRIC CANCER

Early gastric cancers are common in populations where there is screening e.g. Japan. The prognosis is far better than for deeply penetrating 'advanced' tumours.

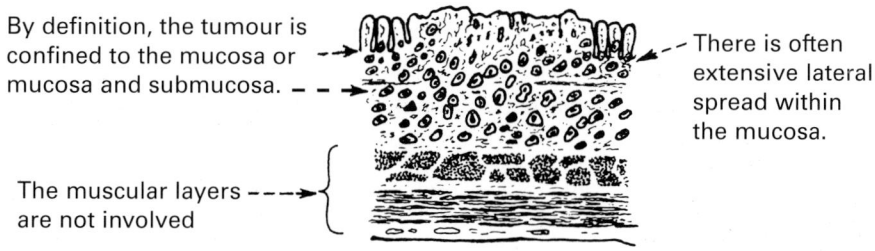

GASTRIC CARCINOMA

Aetiology

It has long been recognised that gastric cancer occurs in achlorhydric states, especially with chronic atrophic gastritis.

It is now clear that *Helicobacter pylori* is a major carcinogenic factor for these tumours arising in the distal stomach (but apparently not for those of the cardia).

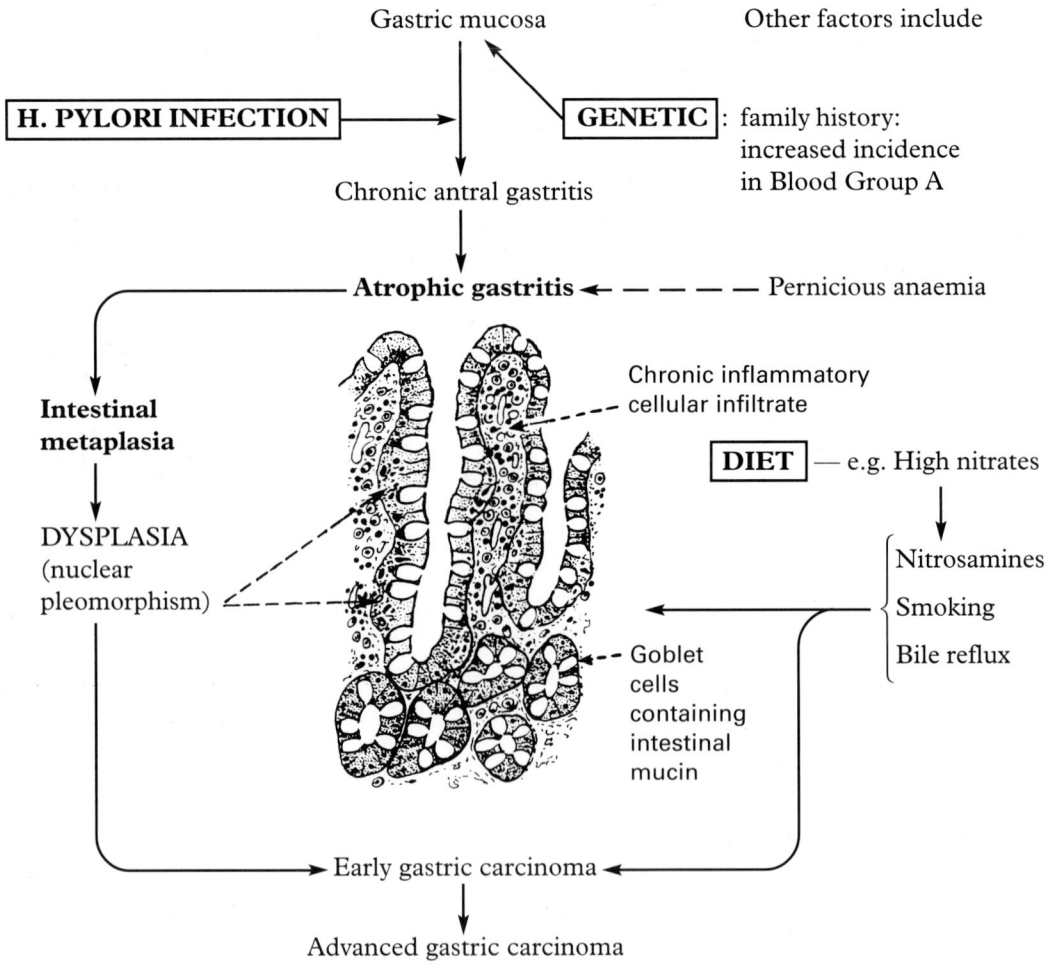

OTHER GASTRIC TUMOURS

Benign gastric polyps are often seen at endoscopy.

SMOOTH MUSCLE TUMOURS — both benign (leimyoma) and malignant (leiomyosarcoma) occur occasionally.

GASTRIC LYMPHOMAS account for 5% of gastric malignancy. They are usually 'B' cell lymphomas of MALT type (p. 447). They are strongly associated with *Helicobacter pylori* infection and some lymphomas respond to eradication of *H. pylori*.

SMALL INTESTINE – MALABSORPTION

The main function of the small intestine is digestion and absorption of food. **Malabsorption** may be due to disorders of the small bowel, pancreas and biliary tract.

COELIAC DISEASE

This important cause of malabsorption is due to sensitivity to gliadin, a component of the wheat protein **gluten**. The clinical features depend on the age at presentation.

Infancy — Failure to thrive, diarrhoea (steatorrhoea)
Childhood — Growth retardation, nutritional deficiencies of e.g. anaemia.
Adults — Anaemia, altered bowel habit, weight loss.

In coeliac disease there is partial or complete villous atrophy.

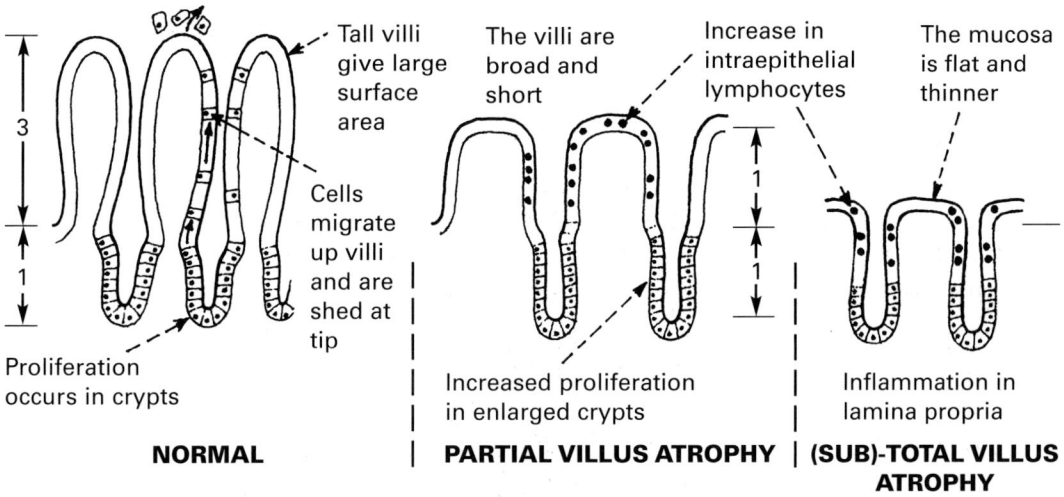

These changes are seen in biopsies of the jejunum (Crosbie capsule) and distal duodenum (by endoscope). The changes revert to normal if gluten is removed from the diet.

The basic mechanism is as follows:

Genetic predisposition
(e.g. HLA B8, DR3, DQ2 +ve)

Environmental trigger (unknown)

→ LOSS of ORAL TOLERANCE to GLUTEN → Auto-immune attack on S.I. → ↑ Loss of enterocytes → Crypt hyperplasia (regeneration) / VILLOUS ATROPHY → MALABSORPTION

Patients with coeliac disease also have increased prevalence of autoimmune diseases e.g. diabetes, autoimmune thyroiditis.

They are at increased risk of developing small bowel **lymphoma**.

MALABSORPTION

Other causes of malabsorption in the small bowel include:

1. **TROPICAL SPRUE**
This is a disease of unknown aetiology occurring in the tropics but largely excluding Africa. Villous atrophy is seen and patients develop steatorrhoea, weight loss and deficiency of B12 and Folate, leading to megaloblastic anaemia. Treatment with folic acid and antibiotics cause the disease to remit.

2. **GIARDIASIS**
An infection with the protozoan *Giardia lamblia*, giardiasis is associated with diarrhoea and malabsorption. Patients with hypogammaglobulinaemia are especially at risk.

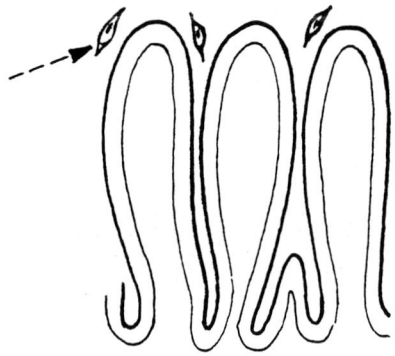

3. **WHIPPLE'S DISEASE**
In this rare condition, mainly of middle aged men, malabsorption, arthritis, lymphadenopathy and skin pigmentation are seen.

Large macrophages fill the lamina propria. They contain mucopolysaccharides (are periodic acid shift (PAS) positive). Electron microscopy shows numerous intracellular bacteria — now thought to be a gram-positive organism *Tropheryma Whippelii*. Antibiotics are curative.

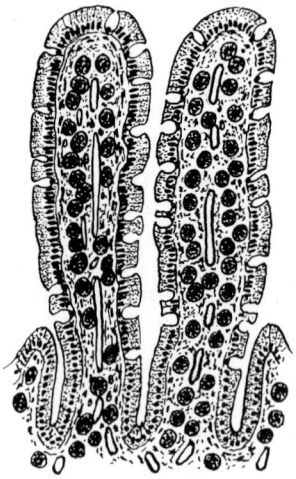

4. **CROHN's DISEASE**

5. After **SMALL BOWEL RESECTION**

6. **BIOCHEMICAL DISORDERS** e.g. disaccharidase deficiency, abetalipoproteinaemia

7. **BACTERIAL COLONISATION** of the small bowel e.g. Blind Loop Syndrome.

Pancreatic diseases e.g. cystic fibrosis (p. 380) and obstructive jaundice (p. 346) also cause malabsorption.

CROHN'S DISEASE

Crohn's disease and ulcerative colitis are two forms of **non-infective inflammatory bowel disease.** They have similarities and striking contrasts (p. 315).

CROHN'S DISEASE

Patients, usually young adults, present with diarrhoea, abdominal pain and weight loss. Although the disease can affect any part of the G.I. tract from the mouth to the anus, the great majority of lesions are seen in the distal **small bowel** and **colon.**

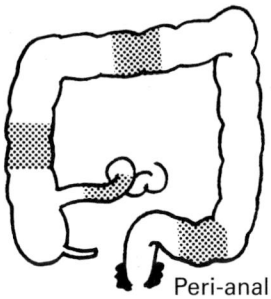

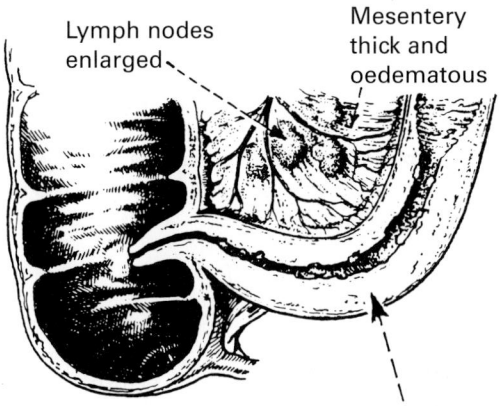

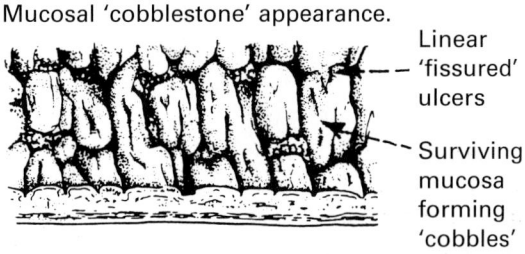

In its classic form, 'regional ileitis', the terminal ileum is thickened and the lumen narrowed and ulcerated.

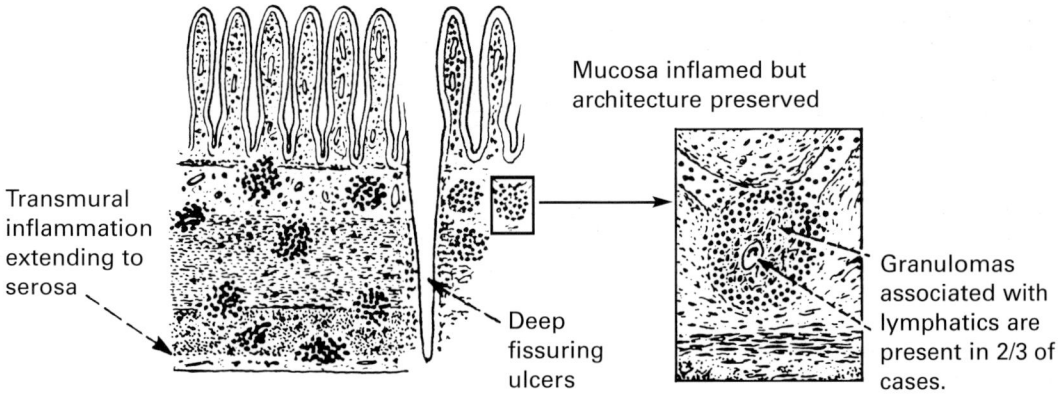

LOCAL COMPLICATIONS

Transmural inflammation ⟶ adhesions between viscera; fistulae to bowel, bladder, vagina.

Lumenal narrowing ⟶ intestinal obstruction.

Ileal involvement ⟶ malabsorption, especially of Vit B12.

Cancer ⟶ increased risk of colonic and **small intestinal** cancer, but not so great as the risk of colonic cancer in ulcerative colitis.

ULCERATIVE COLITIS

Clinical features

Patients, usually young adults, present with diarrhoea often bloody. The disease has a remitting/relapsing course. In severe cases weight loss and anaemia are common. The disease begins in the rectum and shows continuous spread proximally.

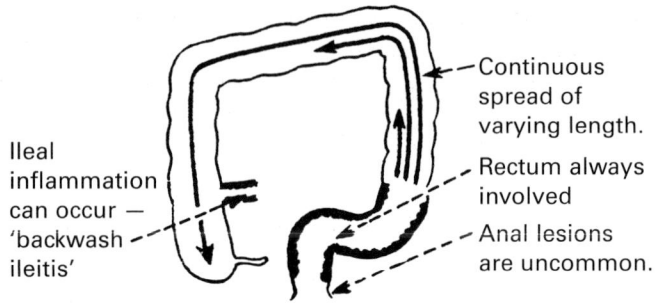

The whole colon is affected in 20% of cases

In the established disease the **gross appearances** are striking.

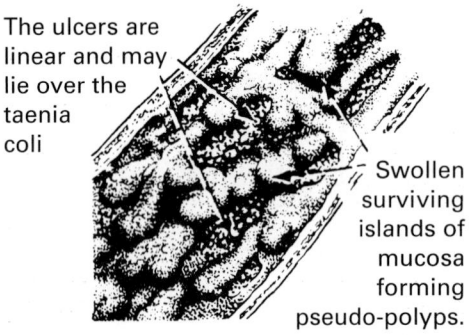

Microscopy shows the evolution.

Early phase

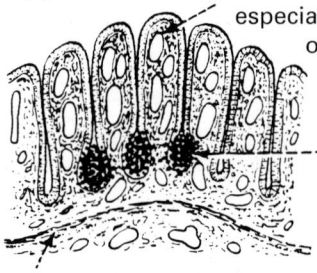

Established phase

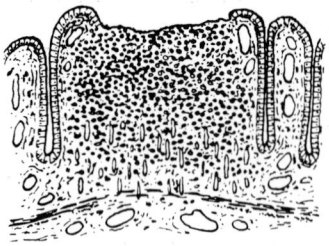

The inflammation is usually **confined to the mucosa**

Periods of remission occur when many of the ulcerated areas heal.

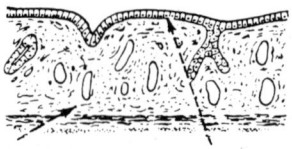

Ultimately the surface may be covered by a simple layer of mucus secreting epithelium without glands.

LOCAL COMPLICATIONS

Toxic megacolon: In a small number of patients inflammation is very severe and the colon becomes greatly dilated and thinned. There is a high risk of perforation with peritonitis.

Dysplasia and Colonic cancer: Patients with (a) early onset, (b) total colonic involvement and (c) long-lasting (10-20 years) have a greatly increased risk. These patients require colonoscopic surveillence with biopsy to look for dysplasia and cancer.

CROHN'S DISEASE AND ULCERATIVE COLITIS

The aetiology of these two conditions is uncertain. Both have mild familial tendency (approximately 10%). Infection by organisms unknown has been suggested for each. Granulomas in Crohn's disease suggest mycobacterial infection (M. pseudotuberculosis is a possible candidate). Food allergy and stress may be involved in ulcerative colitis. Ex-smokers and non-smokers have a higher risk of ulcerative colitis; the converse is true for Crohn's disease.

EXTRA-ARTICULAR COMPLICATIONS — both diseases.

1. Eye disorders — conjunctivitis and uveitis in <5%.
2. Joints — seronegative arthritis with spinal and peripheral joint involvement approximately 15% (p. 639).
3. Liver — sclerosing cholangitis and cholangocarcinoma may be seen in ulcerative colitis, but very rarely in Crohn's disease.
4. Erythema nodosum and pyoderma gangrenosa may be found in both.

Macroscopic differences in the pathology of U.C and C.D.

Ulcerative colitis	Crohn's disease
1. Lesions continuous — mucosal	Skip lesions — transmural
2. Rectum always involved	Rectum normal in 50%
3. Terminal ileum involved in <10% (backwash ileitis — mild)	Terminal ileum involved in 30%
4. Granular, ulcerated mucosa; no fissuring	Discretely ulcerated mucosa; cobblestone appearance; fissuring
5. Often intensely vascular	Vascularity seldom pronounced
6. Normal serosa	Serositis common
7. Muscular shortening of colon	Fibrous shortening; strictures common
8. Fistulas rare	Enterocutaneous or intestinal fistulas in 10%
9. Malignant change — well recognised	Malignant change — less common
10. Anal lesions, uncommon, 25%	Anal lesions in 75%; anal fistulae; ulceration or chronic fissure.

In about 10% of cases it may be impossible to distinguish between ulcerative colitis and Crohn's disease.

INTESTINAL INFECTIONS

Viruses, bacteria, protozoa and worms can all infect the gastrointestinal tract. There are 3 main patterns of infection:

1. Organisms remain within the lumen of the gut and release toxins which damage the surface epithelium e.g. cholera.
2. Organisms invade the wall of the gut, but remain localised to the gut wall e.g. bacillary dysentery.
3. Organisms invade the gut wall and spread systemically through the blood stream e.g. typhoid.

Acute diarrhoeal diseases

In these disorders, infection, mainly of the small bowel, produces little mucosal inflammation, but there is often profuse watery diarrhoea. In adults, this may be mild, but especially in infants dehydration can lead to death.

Responsible organisms include: *E. coli*, *Vibrio cholerae*, rotaviruses, *cryptosporidium parvum.*

Cholera is the classic example of the effects of toxin production.

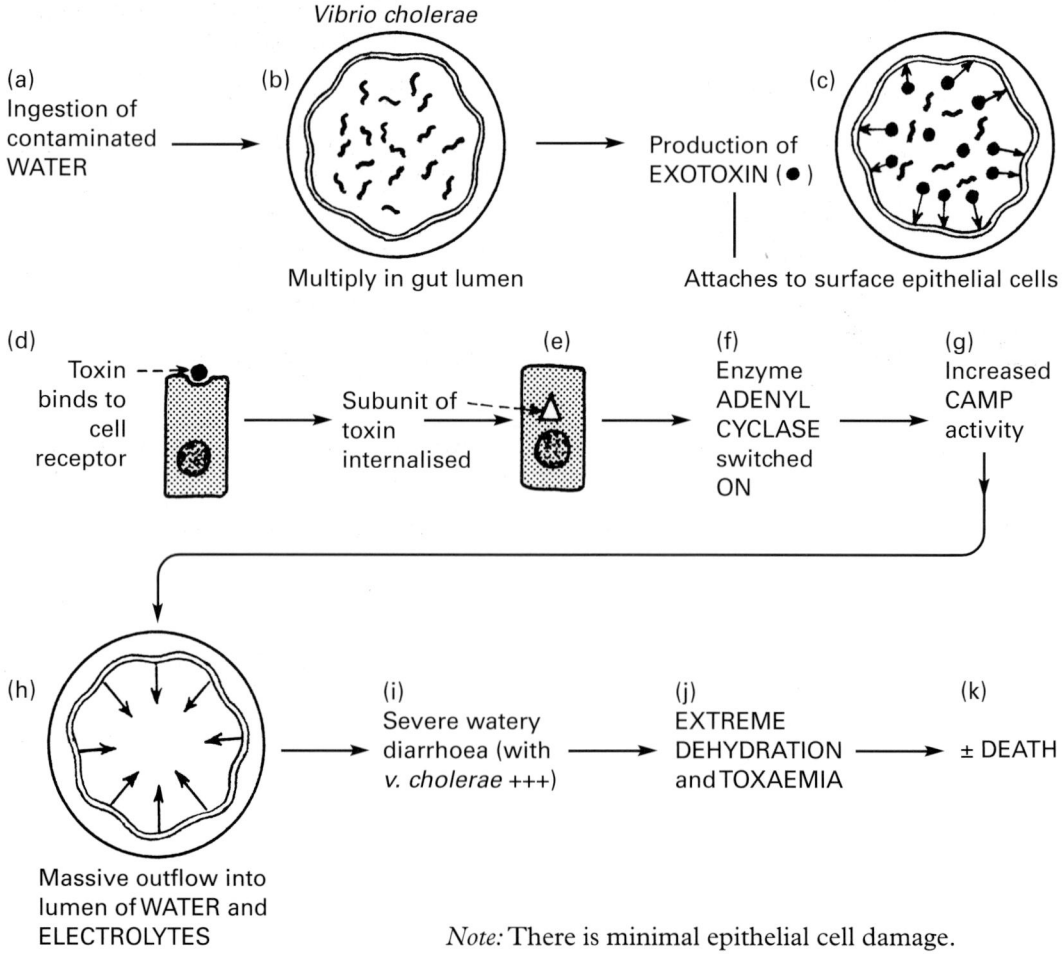

Note: There is minimal epithelial cell damage.

INTESTINAL INFECTIONS

INTESTINAL INFECTIONS (continued)

E. coli 0157 is a strain which produces exotoxin causing haemorrhagic colitis often complicated by renal failure in the elderly or the haemolytic uraemia syndrome in children. The contamination is on meat or meat products and outbreaks and sporadic cases occur worldwide.

Toxic enteritis (Food poisoning)

Many bacteria can elaborate enterotoxins in food before it is consumed: although cooking kills the bacteria the preformed toxin may be heat resistant. *Staphylococcus aureus* and *B. cereus* (in rice particularly) are good examples.

In **ROTAVIRUS infection**, seen especially in children under 5 years, the mechanism is different.

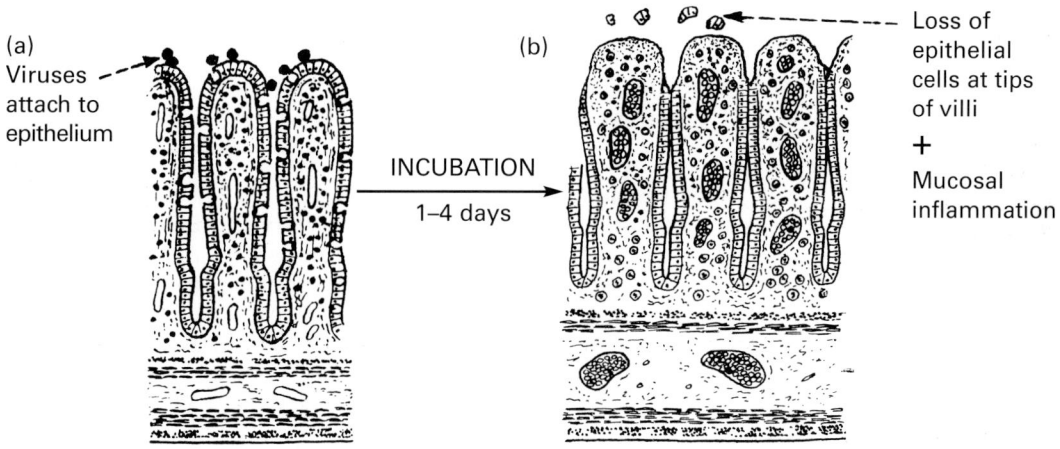

(c) LOSS OF ABSORPTION ⟶ (d) ACCUMULATION of FLUID IN LUMEN ⟶ (e) DIARRHOEA

Note: Recovery is usually rapid and complete, providing dehydration is treated.

TYPHOID

Salmonella infections

Salmonella infections vary from food poisoning, usually a mild inflammation with diarrhoea, to typhoid fever which if untreated is often fatal.

TYPHOID FEVER

Following ingestion of *S. typhi*, the disease process falls into three distinct phases.

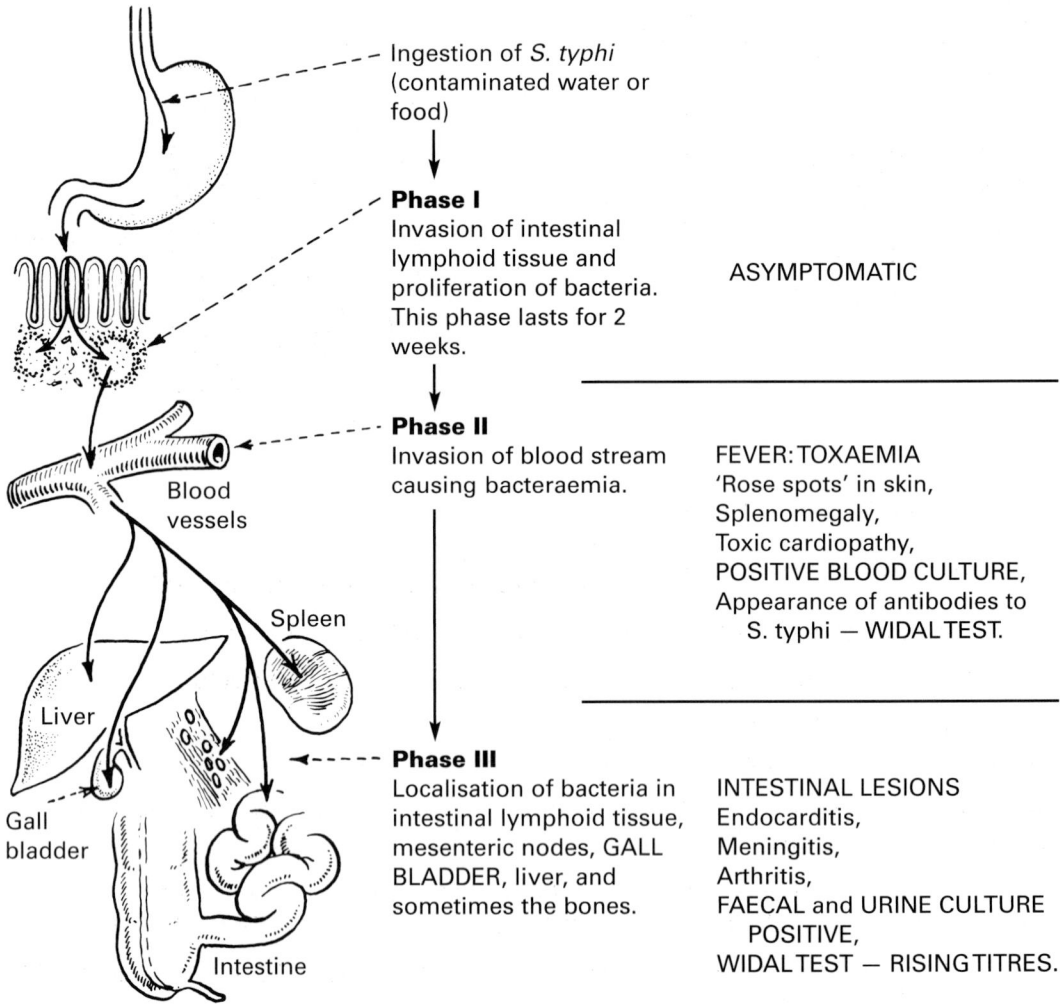

TYPHOID

TYPHOID (continued)

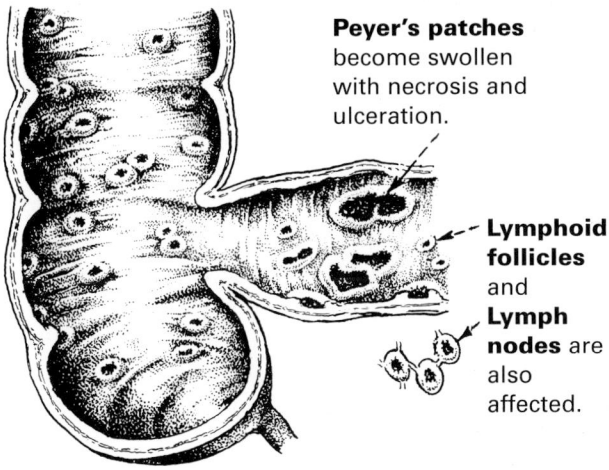

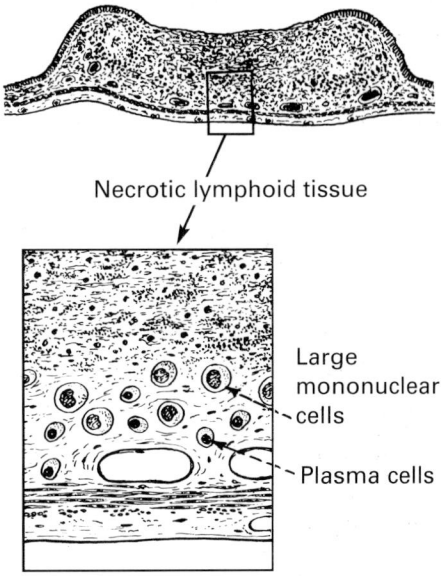

Sequelae

1. Healing is the usual outcome.
2. Deep intestinal ulceration — haemorrhage. / perforation and peritonitis (usually fatal).
3. Persistent infection (1–3%) — usually GALL BLADDER or urinary tract.

   These carriers appear healthy but are an important source of outbreaks.

PARATYPHOID FEVER

This disease is clinically indistinguishable from typhoid fever but is usually much less severe.

The pathological changes resemble those of typhoid fever but are commonly limited to a small portion of the bowel. Frequently there is an absence of ulceration.

Two serological types of the paratyphoid organism are recognised, A and B. Type B is a common cause of enteric fever in Europe. As in typhoid, patients often become 'carriers'.

Note: TAB vaccination, using antigens derived from *S. typhi* and *paratyphi A and B*, produces a very effective active immunity.

BACILLARY DYSENTERY

This is an acute inflammation of the large intestine, varying in severity according to the infecting agent.

The bacteria adhere to and *invade* the mucosa. They remain localised to the gut.

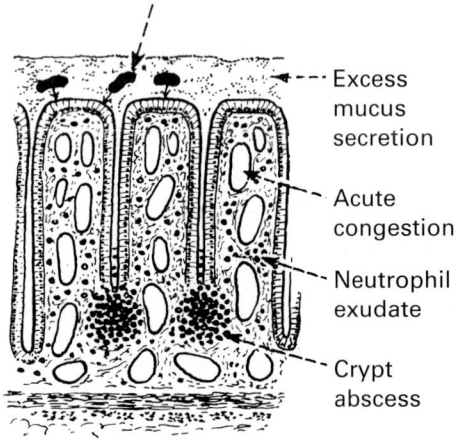

Shigella sonnei
Simple acute inflammation of colon.
Commonest form in the United Kingdom.

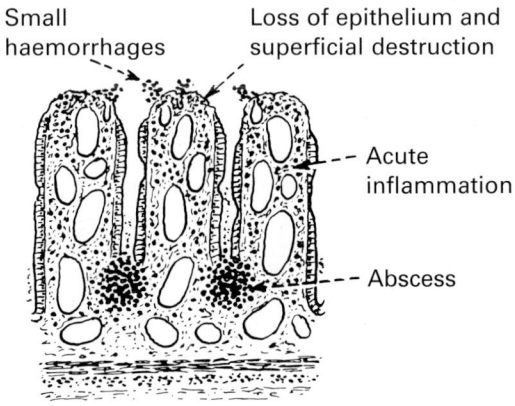

Shigella flexneri
Severe acute inflammation.

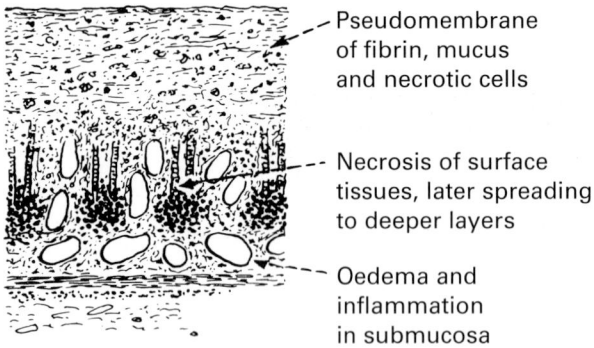

Shigella dysenteriae
Most severe type, occurs in tropics.

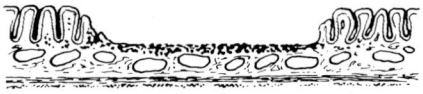

Irregular spreading ulcers with thin shredded margins are formed by shedding of necrotic material.

Clinical manifestations

There is acute diarrhoea with abdominal pain, tenesmus and the passage of blood-stained mucus. *S. dysenteriae* infections are often associated with severe toxaemia and sometimes a shock-like condition. Blood, mucus and neutrophils are found in the faeces, and in the early stages the bacilli can be isolated.

Healing by resolution with complete restoration of the mucosa is usual. Only in exceptional cases does relapse occur with consequent scarring.

AMOEBIC DYSENTERY

This is due to infection by *Entamoeba histolytica* in food and water. It is most often seen in tropical and subtropical countries.

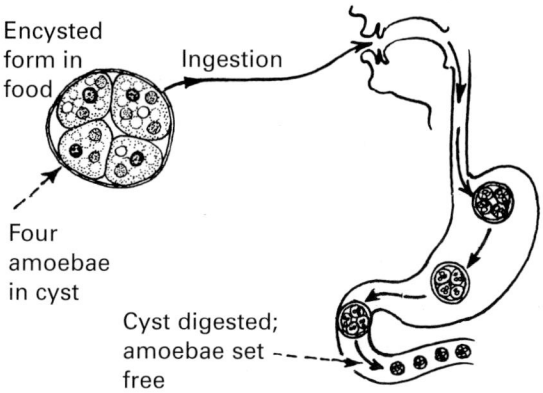

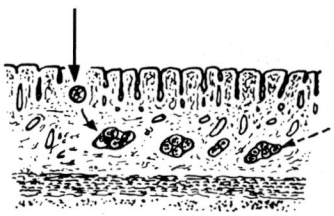

Vessels are congested but there is little inflammatory reaction.

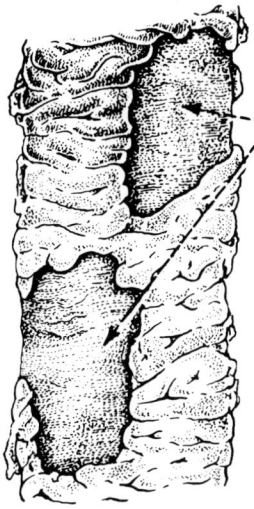

Ulcers form and coalesce, denuding larger areas with undermined ragged edges.

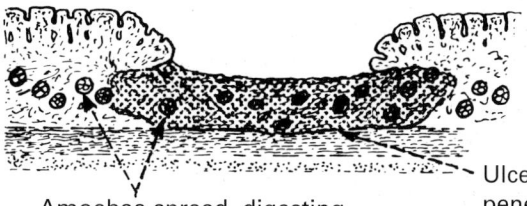

Amoebae spread, digesting submucosa and undermining the mucosa

Ulcer penetrates to muscle

Healing of the ulcers with fibrosis occurs. The disease persists with overgrowth of fibrous tissue, adhesions to various structures and fistulae may occur. Occasionally the amoebae may invade portal venous tributaries and cause amoebic abscess of the liver (p. 365).

Large numbers of motile amoebae can be found in the faeces during the acute phase of the disease. Later, in the chronic state, they are frequently in an encysted form. Mucus and blood are abundant, but unlike bacillary dysentery, there are few pus cells.

Note: Non-pathogenic amoebae can be found in the colon of healthy individuals.

TUBERCULOUS ENTERITIS and PSEUDOMEMBRANOUS COLITIS

1. **Primary tuberculous infection** usually follows ingestion of infected milk containing bovine tubercle bacilli and affects the small bowel. It is similar to primary tuberculosis of the lung — a small mucosal lesion and enlarged caseous lymph nodes. These usually heal with fibrosis and calcification.

2. **Secondary tuberculosis**
   This is due to swallowing tubercle bacilli from open pulmonary tuberculosis. The mucosal lesion is prominent and lymph nodes less affected. The lesions start in the Peyer's patches.

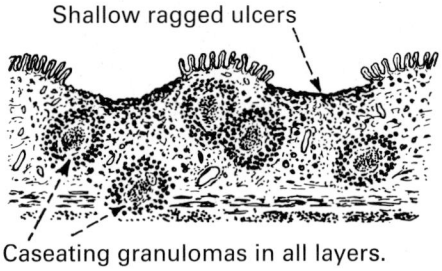

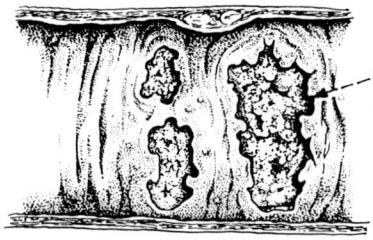

As in the lung, there is a good deal of fibrous granulation tissue surrounding the caseous lesions and the vessels undergo obliteration. For this reason, perforation and haemorrhage are uncommon. Adhesions to other loops of bowel are common and the caseating process may erode through the walls and cause fistula formation with short circuiting and resulting malabsorption. If the fibrous adhesions are dense, obstruction may arise.

PSEUDOMEMBRANOUS COLITIS

Varying lengths of colon show focal inflammation with the formation of surface yellow plaques (pseudomembranes). Most cases are associated with the use in elderly patients of antibiotics.

Microscopic

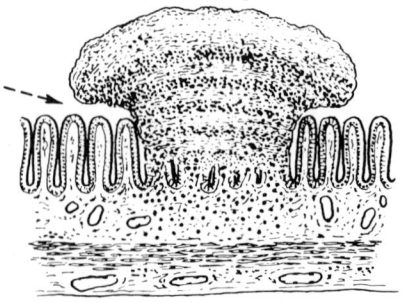

Naked eye appearance

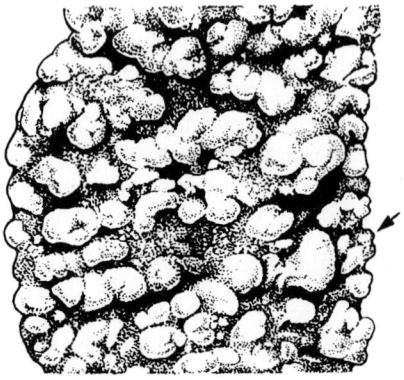

The lesions may coalesce forming typical adherent plaques over large areas, resulting in a fatal outcome. The lesions are caused by toxins from Clostridium difficile — an anaerobe normally present in small numbers which proliferate due to elimination of competing bacteria by the antibiotic. The toxin can be found in the stools.

APPENDICITIS

Acute appendicitis is a common cause of abdominal pain requiring surgery, particularly in the West where there is low roughage diet.

Appendicitis usually follows obstruction of the lumen with distal infection and ulceration. The usual causes are:

(a) Viral infection → reactive hyperplasia of lymphoid follicles. (Infection by *Yersinia enterocolitica* can have similar effects.)

(b) Inspissated faeces (faecoliths).

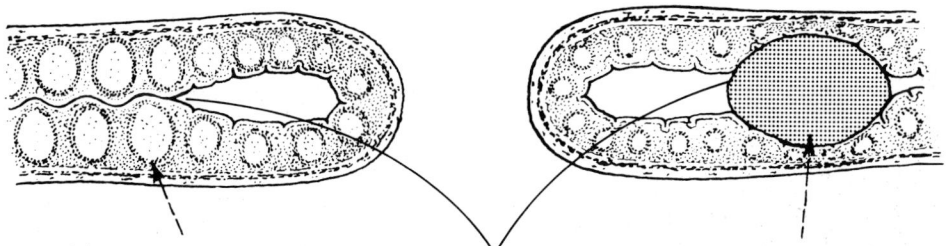

(a) Hyperplastic lymphoid follicles

(b) Faecolith

Obstruction of lumen

↓

Bacterial proliferation

↓

Inflammation and ulceration

The early pain of acute appendicitis is COLICKY and felt around the umbilicus — due to contraction against obstruction.

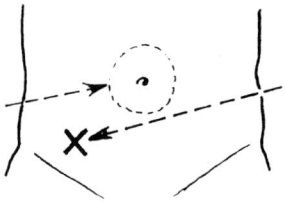

Later the pain localises in the RIGHT ILIAC FOSSA as the peritoneum becomes inflamed.

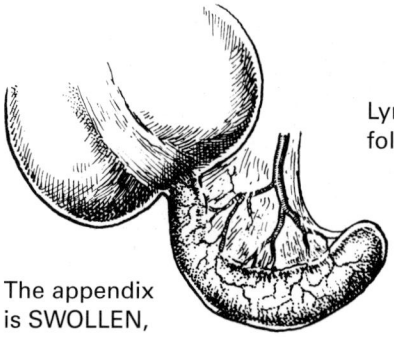

The appendix is SWOLLEN, CONGESTED and coated with a FIBRINOUS EXUDATE.

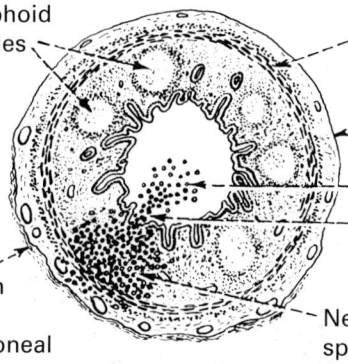

Lymphoid follicles

Muscle coats

Peritoneal surface

Neutrophil exudate in lumen

The acute inflammation often starts as a focus of mucosal ulceration

Fibrin on peritoneal surface

Neutrophil exudate spreads in submucosa and soon affects all layers

Cross-section

APPENDICITIS – SEQUELS

If untreated the appendicitis may become suppurative or gangrenous. The following complications are fortunately rare.

1. **General peritonitis** is the most important complication since it results in toxaemia and may be fatal. It is especially associated with gangrenous appendicitis but may complicate any type of acute appendicitis.

2. **Appendix abscess**
   This arises in the following way:

Abscess in appendix wall → Perforation + Fibrinous adhesions to adjacent structures (particularly the greater omentum) → Localised abscess in right iliac fossa

Further complications may arise due to spread of infection:

(a) Along the right paracolic gutter to produce a subphrenic abscess between the diaphragm and liver

(b) Into the pelvis to form abscesses around bladder and rectum. In the female the uterus and fallopian tube may be involved.

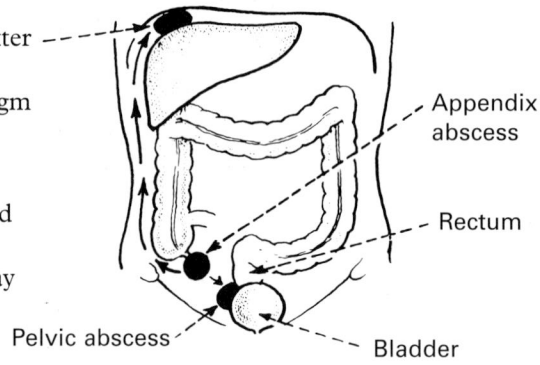

3. **Adhesions**
   Intestinal obstruction may result from constricting bands, or volvulus may be induced.

4. **Liver abscesses and portal pylephlebitis**
   These are now rare. They are due to spread of infection to the mesenteric veins resulting in septic embolism. Liver abscesses usually arise from infective emboli, but occasionally there may be a spreading suppurating thrombosis culminating in hepatic sepsis.

CHRONIC APPENDICITIS

In pathological terms, it is synonymous with fibrosis, which may be local or diffuse.

If the fibrosis causes complete obstruction of the lumen, continued mucus secretion may result in cystic dilatation — mucocele.

DIVERTICULAR DISEASE

Diverticula are common in the **sigmoid colon**, affecting at least 10% of adults in societies where the diet lacks fibre (low residue).

Reduced dietary fibre — low residue in distal colon → Induces muscular hypertrophy → Increased intralumenal pressure → Outpouching of mucosa

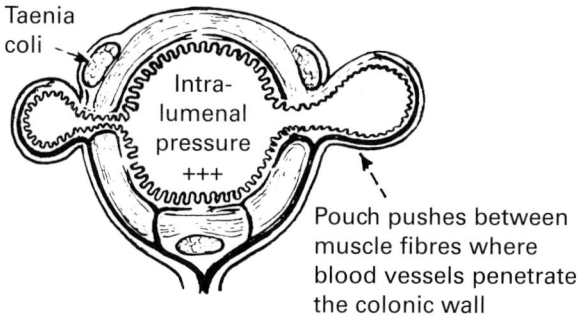

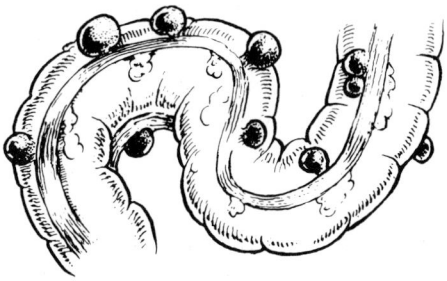

Complications

Diverticulitis is common

Inflammation and ulceration → abscess formation; fistulae (e.g. colo-vesical); haemorrhage

Repeated attacks
↓
Fibro-muscular thickening
↓
Stenosis

Note: This may simulate carcinoma

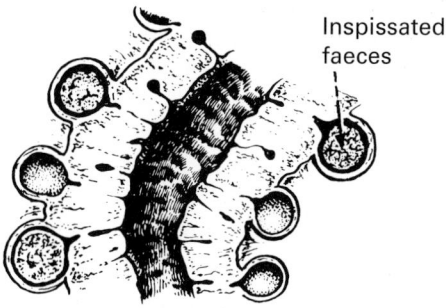

Inflammatory fibromuscular thickening

Other diverticula are also found in the caecum and small intestine: in the latter, colonisation by bacteria which utilise Vit B12 may lead to macrocytic anaemia.

Meckel's diverticulum of the small intestine is present in 2% of the population.

It is a remnant of the **vitello-intestinal duct** about 60 cm proximal to the ileo-caecal valve.

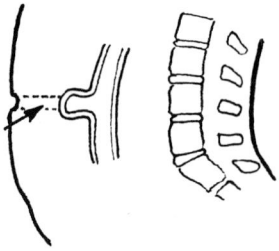

Complications are rare:

(1) The wide communication with the bowel precludes stasis and inflammation.

(2) Rarely ectopic gastric or pancreatic tissue cause local damage (p. 305).

ISCHAEMIA AND THE INTESTINES

ACUTE VASCULAR OCCLUSION

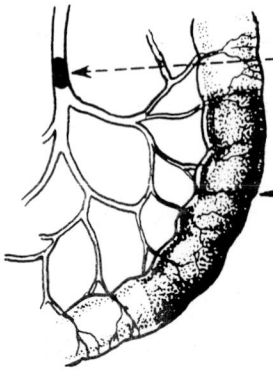

Occlusion of the superior mesenteric artery is usually due to thrombosis complicating atheroma, or embolism from the left side of the heart or aorta.

Infarction of a loop or much of the small bowel leads to abdominal pain. The infarcted bowel must be removed surgically. Many of these elderly patients die.

ISCHAEMIC COLITIS

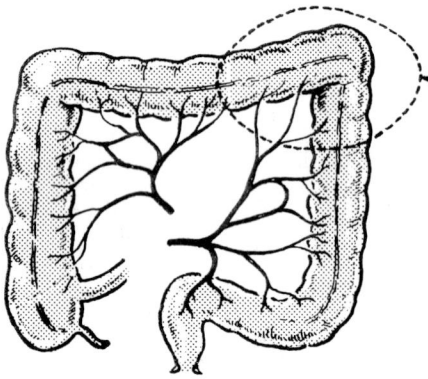

The colon is more vulnerable to chronic ischaemia than the small bowel.

Ischaemic colitis commonly affects the splenic flexure — the watershed zone. It often occurs in patients with arterial disease with hypotension e.g. due to shock or cardiac failure.

Milder ischaemia → mucosal ulceration
↓
healing with stricture

Severe ischaemia → gangrene of bowel

Intestinal ischaemia may also be due to arteritis (p. 231), as a side effect of radiation therapy. Drug induced ulcers, e.g. potassium tablets and non-steroidal anti-inflammatory drugs, appear to be due to local ischaemia.

NEONATAL NECROTISING ENTEROCOLITIS

This lesion occurs in premature babies in their first week.

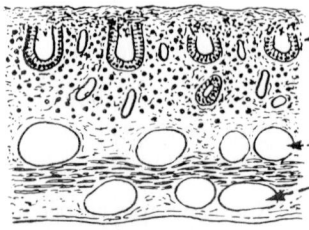

Necrosis and inflammation occur in bowel wall.

Gas bubbles in the submucosa and muscle give a characteristic X-ray appearance.

Bowel ischaemia appears to be the initial event, but there is then bacterial superinfection, especially by gas forming organisms.

INTESTINAL OBSTRUCTION

Intestinal obstruction can be caused by:

(a) Intralumenal blockage — e.g. gallstone ileus (p. 372).
(b) Lesions of the bowel wall — e.g. tumours, inflammatory strictures, intussusception.
(c) External compression — e.g. hernias, volvulus.

The patient may present with colicky abdominal pain, vomiting and failure to pass flatus or faeces.

Acute obstruction

Immediately following the obstruction there is a period of very active peristalsis

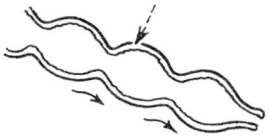

This is followed by immobility and distension

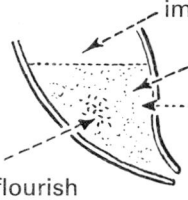

Increased secretion

Decreased absorption

Bacteria tend to flourish

Subacute obstruction

As the condition develops gradually, hypertrophy of the muscle is seen proximal to the obstruction.

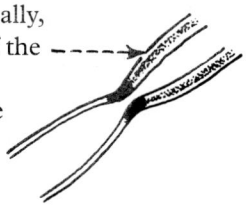

Later, obstruction increases and muscle hypertrophy cannot compensate.

Dilatation of the bowel follows with accumulation of gas and fluid.

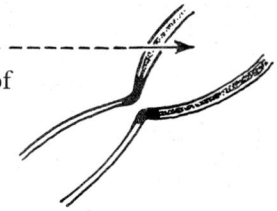

This gross distension has several effects:

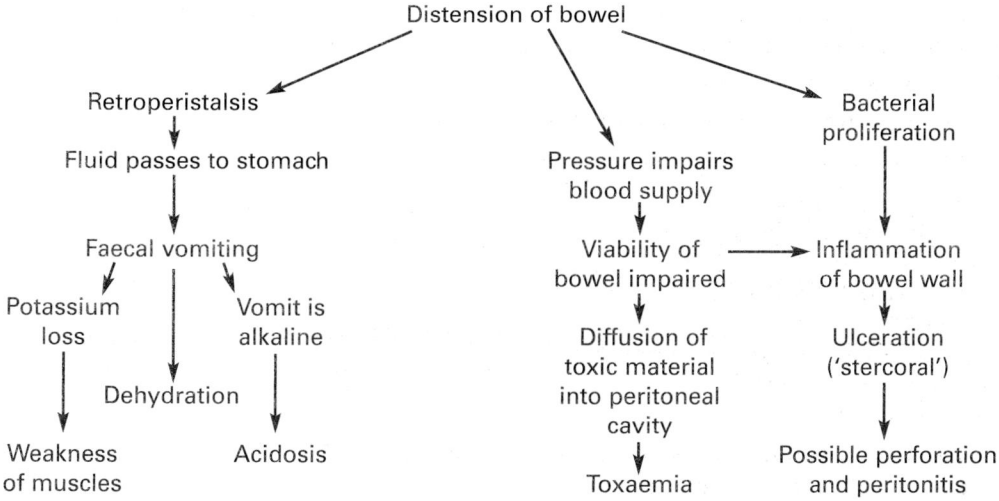

HERNIA

HERNIA

This means the protrusion of peritoneum through an aperture.

When the hernial swelling appears on the surface of the body, it is termed 'external'; those which do not present on the body surface are 'internal'.

The main complication is protrusion of bowel through the aperture at:

1. Sites of potential weakness in the abdominal wall, e.g. inguinal canal, femoral canal, umbilicus, diaphragm. There may be congenital weakness in some individuals at these sites. In these cases a pouch of peritoneum protrudes through the aperture.
2. Normal peritoneal extensions, e.g. the foramen of Winslow leading to the lesser sac, jejunoduodenal fossa.
3. The abdominal wall following operation due to stretching of scar tissue.

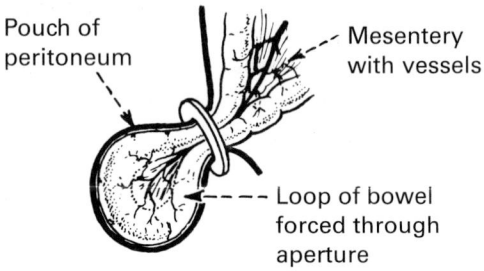

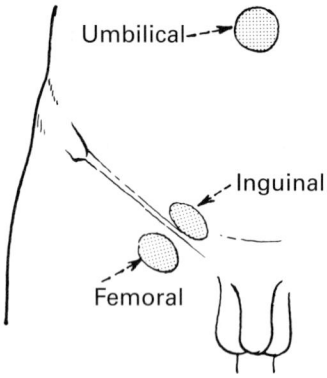

Inguinal hernia

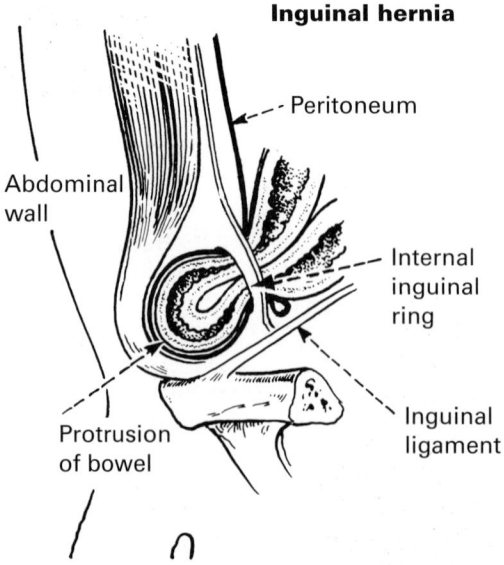

Cross-section viewed from above shows:

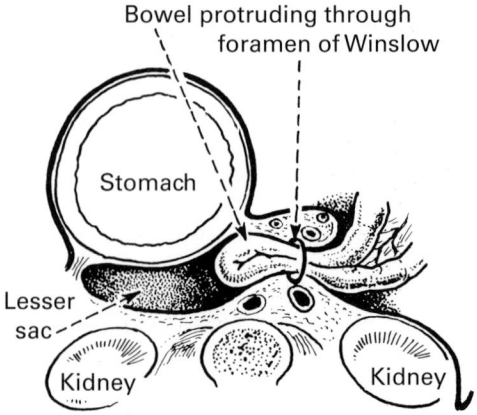

HERNIA — COMPLICATIONS

Complications of hernia

Initially, when the herniated portion of bowel is small it can be pushed back into the abdominal cavity — *reducible.*

Increased intra-abdominal pressure, e.g. during muscular exertion, coughing or straining due to constipation, helps to induce the herniation, tends to make it progressive, and secondary changes occur.

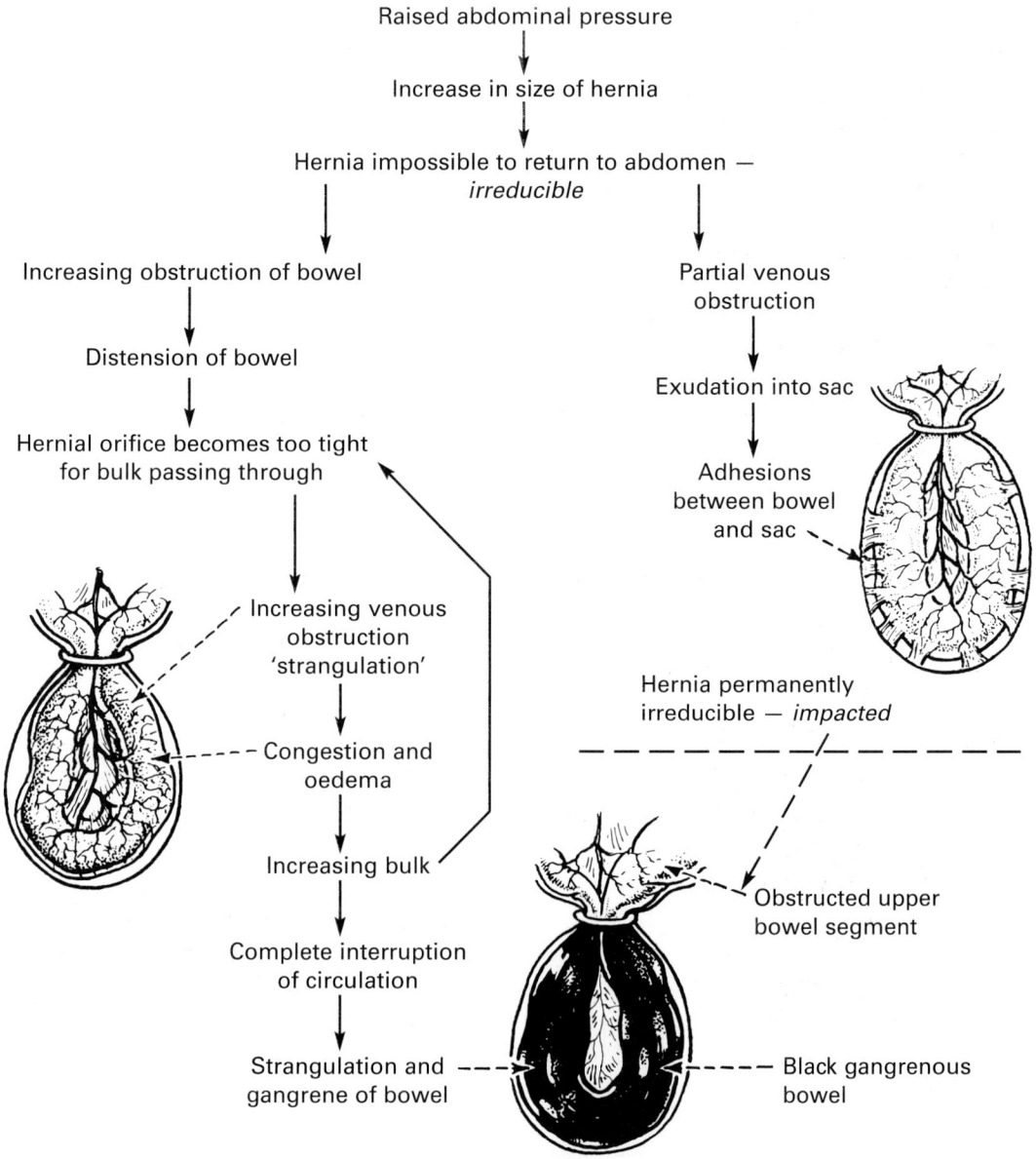

INTUSSUSCEPTION

INTUSSUSCEPTION

This is a condition in which the bowel is invaginated into itself.

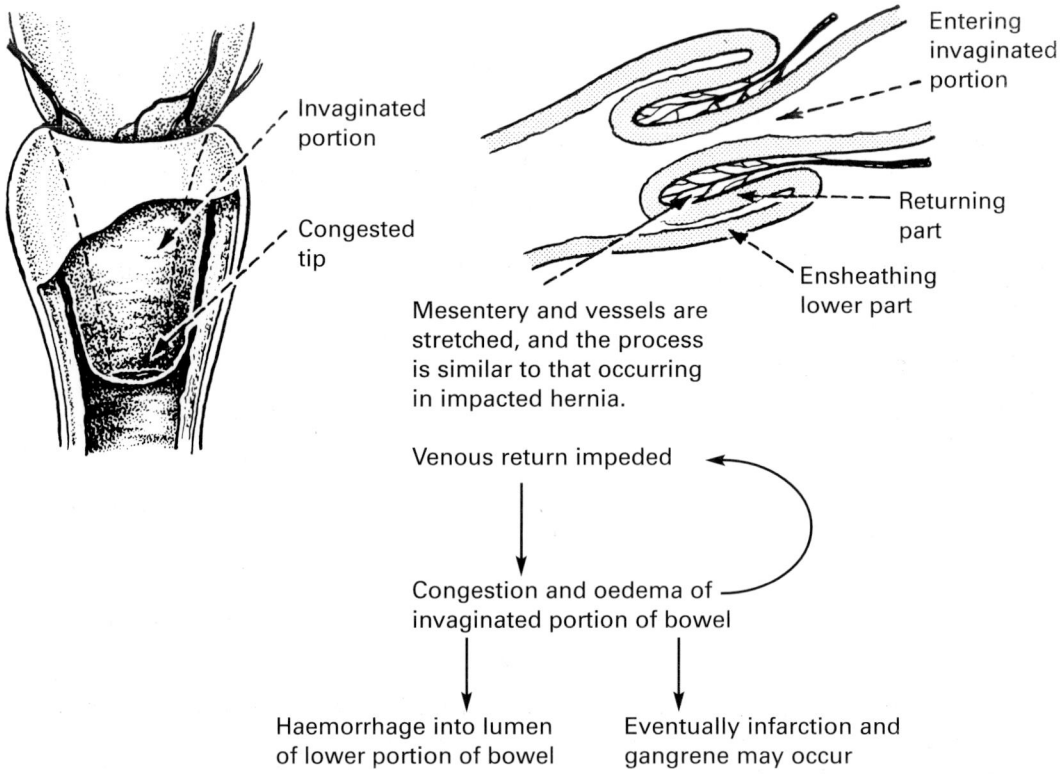

Sites

The commonest form is the ileocaecal type, the ileum being invaginated into the large intestine with the ileocaecal valve forming the apex. Less commonly, a portion of ileum may pass through the ileocaecal valve. Other sites are occasionally affected, e.g. small intestine or parts of colon.

Clinical manifestations

The patient presents with the signs and symptoms of acute obstruction, a mass in the abdomen and blood is passed per rectum.

Aetiology

It is thought that most cases arise as a result of a swelling in the intestinal wall which is pushed distally by peristalsis, dragging the wall of the bowel with it. Most cases arise in childhood due to swelling of lymphoid tissue produced by virus infection.

Polypoidal tumours of the intestine may cause intussusception in adults.

Very occasionally, adhesions develop between the peritoneal surfaces of the invaginated portion of bowel and the external sheathing portion. The gangrenous invaginated portion may separate and the lesion heal spontaneously.

VOLVULUS AND HIRSCHSPRUNG'S DISEASE

VOLVULUS

As the name suggests, this is a rotation or revolving of the bowel. It affects bowel with a long mesentery. Another factor is the closeness of the ends of the affected loop.

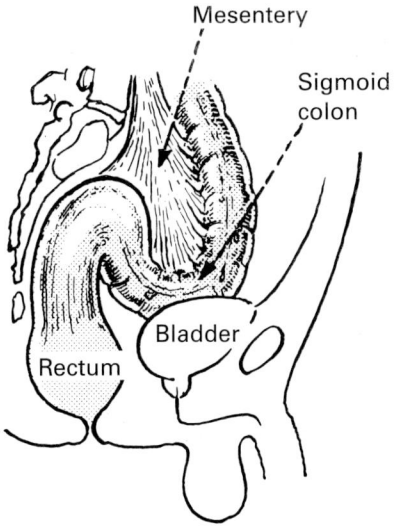

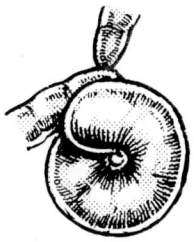

The sigmoid colon has this anatomical arrangement and is the common site of volvulus. Less commonly, the small intestine is affected.

The subsequent changes are the same as in intussusception.

Twisting of the loop around its own axis

↓ Acute obstruction

↓ Venous return interrupted

↓ Congestion and oedema

↓ Infarction and gangrene with peritonitis and shock

Aetiology

In the case of the sigmoid colon, constipation causing loading of the loop in an individual with an abnormally long mesocolon is probably the initiating factor.

Volvulus of the small intestine usually occurs in children. Commonly the mesentery is distorted by disease, e.g. tuberculous nodes.

Very occasionally two loops of bowel may become wrapped round each other.

HIRSCHSPRUNG'S DISEASE

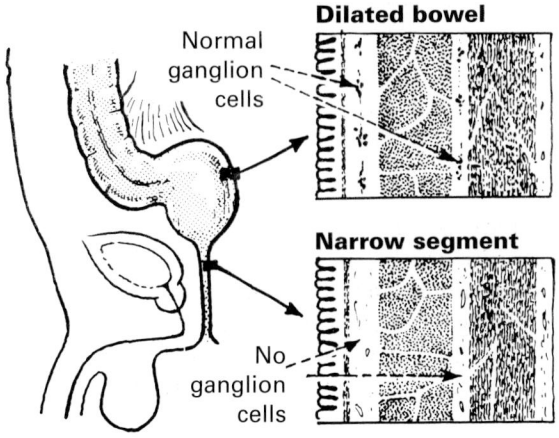

Hirschsprung's disease is a rare cause of chronic intestinal obstruction. It is due to a congenital absence of ganglion cells in the parasympathetic Auerbach and Meissner complexes of the rectum.

The aganglionic rectal segment and anus remain contracted due to unopposed action of the sympathetic nervous system, the bowel above becoming grossly distended and hypertrophied.

TUMOURS OF THE COLON

The main tumours of the colon are epithelial — adenomas and carcinomas.

Adenomas — These are important because they may lead on to carcinoma. (Adenoma — carcinoma sequence, p. 143)

TUBULAR ADENOMA

The majority of tubular adenomas occur in the rectum and sigmoid colon. In the beginning it is a sessile swelling but soon becomes pedunculated.

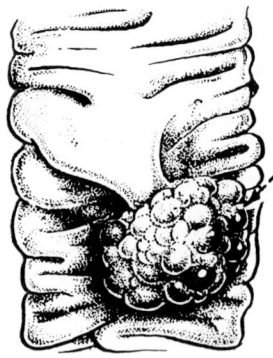

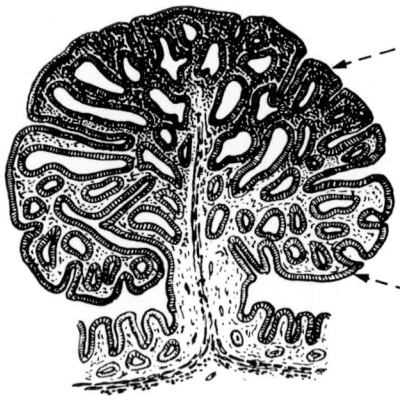

They are common in the older age groups and are frequently multiple.

VILLOUS ADENOMA

Villous adenomas are most commonly found in the rectum. They form a sessile mass which may be quite large and have a delicate frond-like structure.

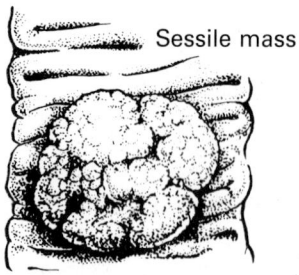

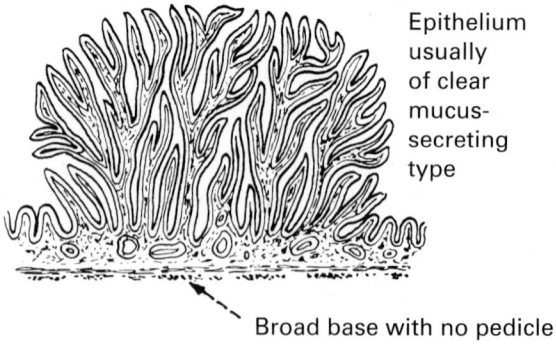

These often present with rectal bleeding.

Very rarely, there is an excessive production of mucus and fluid which may lead to marked loss of potassium, causing muscular weakness.

Many polypi are of mixed variety — part adenomatous, part villous. Both show a tendency to malignant change. If the tumour is of sessile variety invasion of the deeper tissues is immediate. In the pedunculated varieties, invasion of the intestinal wall is delayed — the stalk is first invaded.

TUMOURS OF THE COLON

ADENOMATOSIS COLI

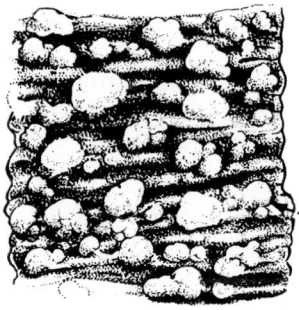

This is an inherited condition (autosomal dominant: 50% of children affected) due to mutation of the APC gene, a tumour suppressor gene on chromosome 5.

Adenomatous polyps are found throughout the entire colon, appearing in late childhood. Carcinoma almost always occurs by the 3rd or 4th decade if colectomy is not carried out.

Tumours may also be seen in the stomach and small bowel.

Other Colonic Polyps

The following are not true neoplasms.

(1) METAPLASTIC POLYPS

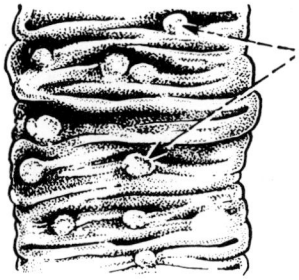

These are usually multiple and present as a small sessile nodule showing unusual feathery metaplastic change in the epithelium. They are found in later life but seldom become malignant.

(2) JUVENILE POLYPS

These are globular protrusions of the rectal mucous membrane in children. They are usually ulcerated and inflamed but probably represent a developmental abnormality. They are occasionally multiple. There is a small risk of malignancy.

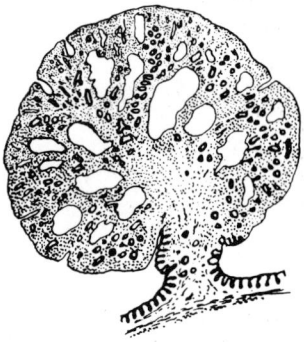

(3) **Inflammatory polyps** associated with chronic inflammatory bowel disease are described on page 314.

CARCINOMA OF THE COLON

This common malignancy accounts for about 10% of cancers in the Western World. Tumours in the right and left side tend to present differently.

RIGHT COLON

Lumen wide
+
Liquid faeces
↓
NO OBSTRUCTION

Tumours present late

Blood loss → Anaemia

Abdominal mass

Liver metastases

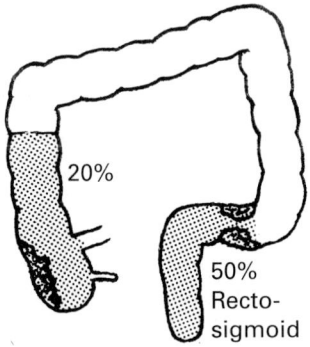

LEFT COLON

Lumen narrow
+
Solid faeces
+
Stenosing tumour
↓
ALTERED BOWEL HABIT
or
OBSTRUCTION
or
RECTAL BLEEDING

Types of growth

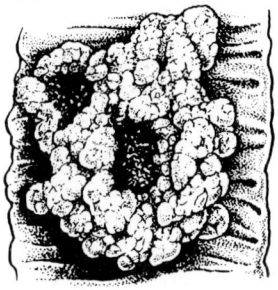

Polypoid carcinoma
— mainly in right side
e.g. caecum

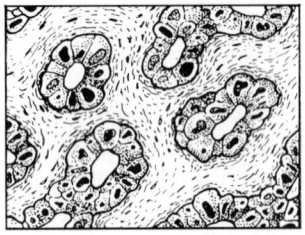

Most tumours are adenocarcinomas

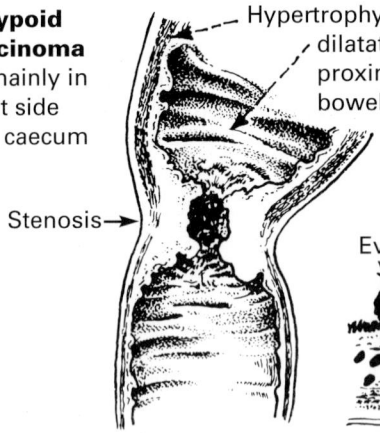

Stenosing carcinoma
— mainly in left side
e.g. recto-sigmoid

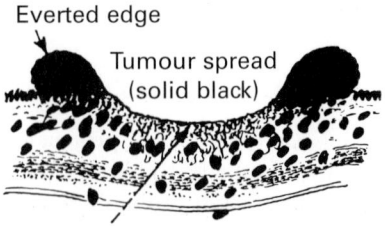

Aetiology

There are genetic and environmental factors.

(a) **Environmental:** Diets rich in animal fat and protein, especially low residue diets.

(b) **Genetic:** e.g. adenomatosis coli.
Hereditary non-polyposis colorectal cancer syndrome
MOST CASES ARE SPORADIC.

(c) **Pre-existing lesions**
1. Adenomatous polyps including adenomatosis coli.
2. Inflammatory bowel disease (especially ulcerative colitis).

CARCINOMA OF THE COLON

SPREAD and STAGING (Dukes' staging)

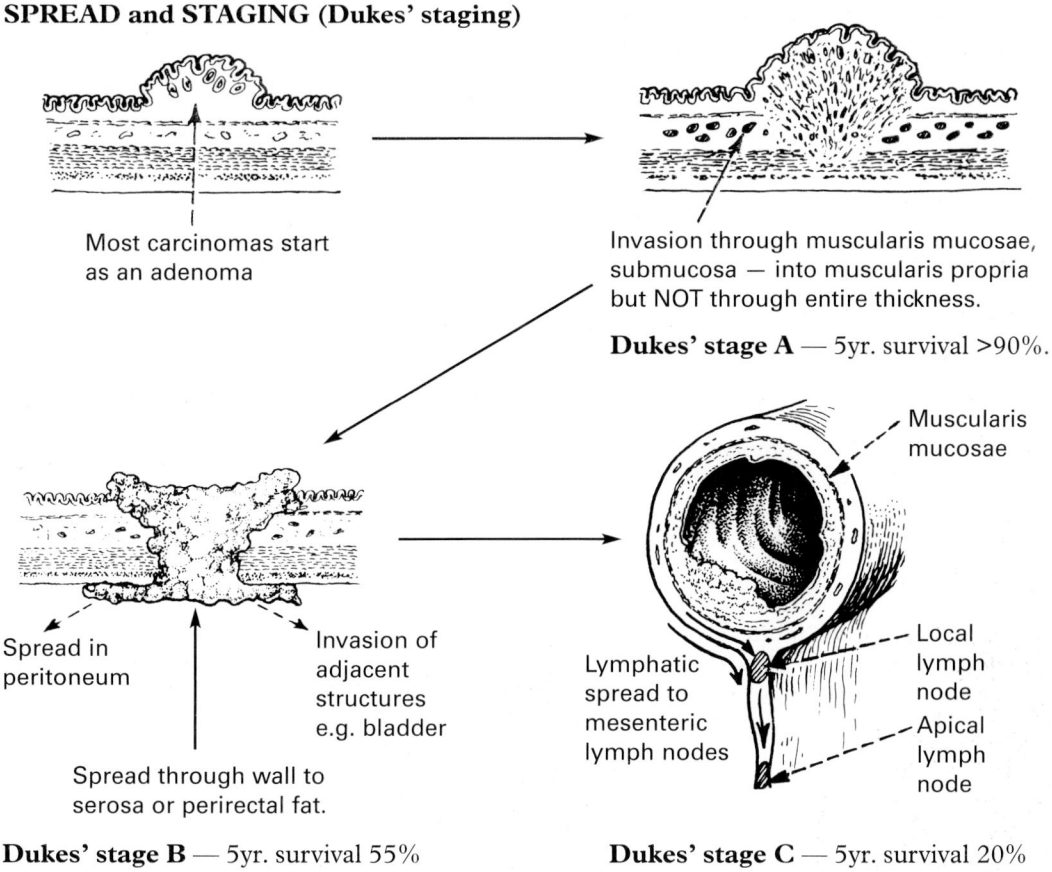

Blood borne metastases to the liver usually occur later.

Carcinoembryonic antigen (CEA)
This is a glycoprotein normally produced by fetal endodermal tissues. It is also formed by a number of cancers, among them a proportion of colonic carcinomas, and appears in the blood. It cannot be used as a diagnostic test since it is found in non-neoplastic lesions such as inflammation of the bowel. After treatment, however, changes in the blood concentration of CEA may be used as an indication of recurrence of tumour growth.

Other tumours
Carcinoid tumour (p. 337), lymphoma and connective tissue tumours e.g. leiomyomas and haemangiomas are occasionally found.

TUMOURS OF SMALL INTESTINE

BENIGN TUMOURS: adenomas, leiomyomas and lipomas are rare, but may cause intussusception (p. 330).

Hamartomatous polyps, consisting of glands and muscle, occur in the Peutz-Jeghers syndrome, an autosomal dominant condition. Melanotic pigmentation of the lips and mouth is also seen.

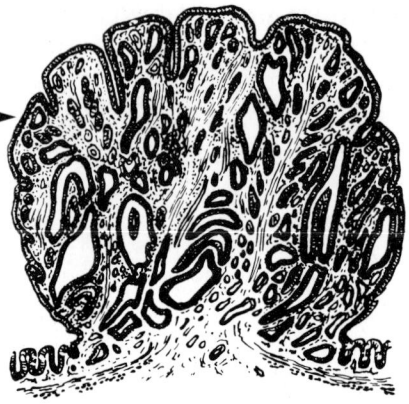

CARCINOMA: adenocarcinoma is 50 times rarer in the small intestine than in the colon. About 40–50% occur in the duodenum, mainly around the ampulla of Vater. These present with obstructive jaundice. Tumours in the jejunum resemble those of the colon and may obstruct the lumen. An increased risk of carcinoma is seen in patients with Crohn's disease, coeliac disease and Peutz-Jeghers syndrome.

LYMPHOMA: these are non-Hodgkin's lymphomas of 'B' or 'T' cell type.

(a) **Enteropathy associated T-cell lymphoma.** These are seen in middle aged patients who often have had coeliac disease for many years.

(b) **B-cell lymphomas are usually of MALT type.** They are usually of low grade and usually solitary.

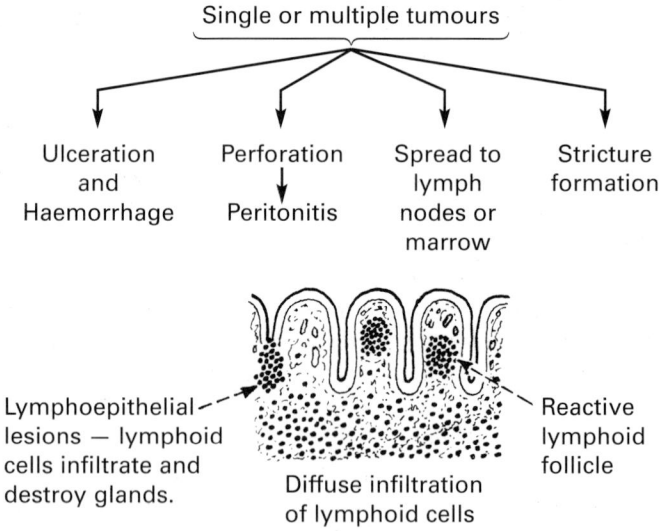

(c) **Mediterranean lymphoma (α chain disease)**
? Infective origin (some cases respond to antibiotics).

↓

Diffuse proliferation of lympho-plasmacytic cells (initially polyclonal)

↓ MALABSORPTION

↓ PROGRESSION TO MONOCLONAL B CELL LYMPHOMA

↓ PRODUCTION OF EXCESS IgA

CONNECTIVE TISSUE TUMOURS

Malignant intestinal stromal tumours of smooth muscle or neural type may present with bleeding, obstruction, or an abdominal mass. They often metastasise to the liver.

CARCINOID TUMOURS

These tumours arise from **endocrine** cells and can occur in the gut and lung. They are commonest in the appendix and small bowel.

APPENDICEAL CARCINOIDS

These may be incidental findings at appendicectomy or may cause appendicitis.

SMALL BOWEL CARCINOIDS

These are commonest in the ileum.

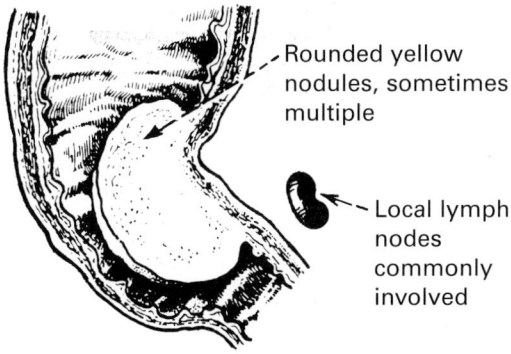

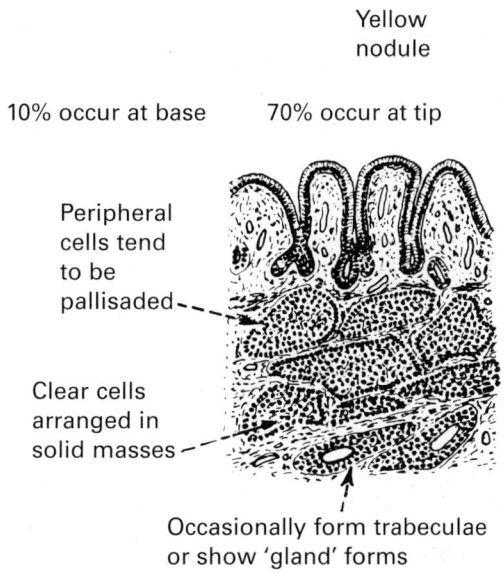

The cells can bind and reduce silver compounds and are known as 'ARGENTAFFIN CELLS'. They contain neurosecretory granules (E.M.) and express endocrine markers, e.g. chromogranin.

CARCINOID SYNDROME

These tumours may secrete a variety of neuroendocrine and paraendocrine substances, in many cases without any apparent clinical functional effects.

However, ileal carcinoids tend to produce two important peptides:

(1) Kallikrein, leading to excessive BRADYKININ production and

(2) 5-hydroxytryptamine (5HT) (serotonin).

These are normally destroyed in the liver and lungs: when metastatic deposits are present in the liver the active agents enter the general circulation and produce the CARCINOID SYNDROME, characterised by episodic flushing, diarrhoea and right heart failure.

Excess 5HT: Kallikrein (+ Bradykinin)

- Hypertrophy of intestinal muscle → fibrosis → 'Obstructive' symptoms diarrhoea
- Vasodilation → Episodes of flushing
- Fibrin formation → Deposition on valves of right heart → Organisation → Fibrosis → STENOSIS (Pulmonic and tricuspid valves)

THE PERITONEAL CAVITY

PERITONITIS

Acute Peritonitis usually follows inflammation of a viscus,

e.g. 1. Appendicitis, cholecystitis, pancreatitis.
2. Perforation e.g. duodenal ulcer, ruptured diverticulum.
3. Ischaemia — vascular occlusion, volvulus, intussusception.

Patients on chronic ambulatory peritoneal dialysis (CAPD) are prone to episodes of peritonitis.

Primary Peritonitis

In the absence of visceral inflammation, primary peritonitis may occur in children with the nephrotic syndrome (pneumococcus) or in adults with cirrhosis (usually coliforms).

Peritonitis can be

LOCALISED
e.g. appendix abscess

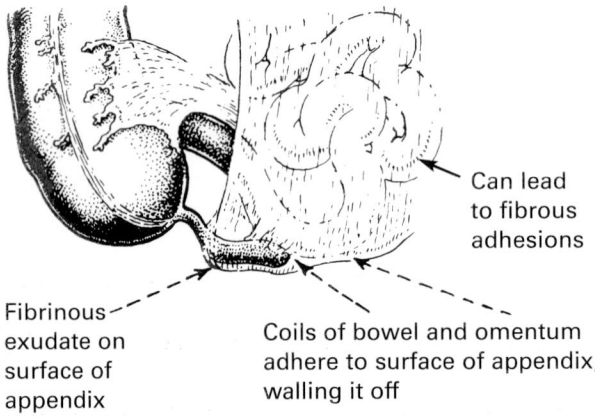

GENERALISED

Bacteria → Endotoxin release
Exudation → Hypovolaemia
→ SHOCK (mainly endotoxic)

Consequences of peritonitis.

(a) Shock ⟶ death.

(b) Recovery.

(c) Adhesions due to organisation of exudate ⟶ intestinal obstruction.

(d) Localised collections e.g. pus.

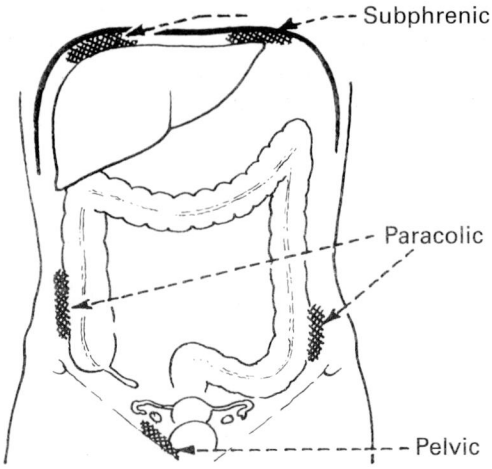

THE PERITONEAL CAVITY

Chronic peritonitis

The most common type of chronic inflammation involving the peritoneum is that resulting from non-resolution of acute peritonitis.

A form of sclerosing peritonitis may complicate long term peritoneal dialysis.

Tuberculosis of the peritoneum is uncommon in Western civilisation, but frequent in underdeveloped countries. It commonly takes one of the following forms:

1. **Serous effusion.** Small grey tubercles are usually scattered over the peritoneal surface. In addition, the omentum is more extensively involved with the formation of a large fibrous mass in the upper abdomen.
2. **Caseation.** This can vary in extent, from isolated small masses to diffuse caseation involving most of the cavity.
3. **Adhesive peritonitis.** The cavity may be reduced to small pockets containing serous fluid. The source of infection may be caseous lymph nodes, tuberculous salpingitis or tuberculous ulcer of the intestine.

Ascites

Accumulation of serous fluid can occur:

1. As part of a general oedema from any cause such as cardiac or renal failure.
2. Portal venous obstruction as in hepatic cirrhosis, portal thrombosis or compression of the portal vein by tumour growth.
3. Tumours of the ovary.
4. Tumours of the peritoneum.

Tumours

Secondary tumours are common, due to spread of carcinoma from the stomach, ovary and large intestine.

Eventually loops of bowel are stuck together by tumour and adhesions resulting in 'frozen abdomen'.

Pseudomyxoma peritonei is seen when mucin secreting tumours e.g. of ovary or appendix spread widely throughout the peritoneum.

Primary tumours are rare. Mesothelioma is the most important. It is related to the inhalation of asbestos and the pathology is similar to that of mesothelioma of the pleura; large white plaques of solid growth.

CHAPTER 10

LIVER, GALL BLADDER AND PANCREAS

Liver — Anatomy 342, 343
Anatomy — Hepatic Lesions 344, 345
Jaundice 346
Viral Hepatitis 347–349
Hepatitis B Infection 350
Viral Hepatitis 351
Chronic Hepatitis 352
Alcoholic Liver Disease 353
Alcoholic Hepatitis 354
Cirrhosis 355–357
Hepatocellular Failure 358–360
Portal Hypertension 361
Metabolic Disorders of the Liver 362
Infections and Infestations 363–366
Tumours of Liver 367
Primary Carcinoma of Liver 368
Primary Liver Cell Tumours 369
Gallbladder and Bile Duct 370
Gallstones 371, 372
Gallstones — Aetiology 373
Pancreas 374
Acute Pancreatitis 375–377
Chronic Pancreatitis 378, 379
Cystic Fibrosis of Pancreas (Mucoviscidosis) 380
Tumours of Pancreas 381

LIVER – ANATOMY

Conventionally the liver was considered to be composed of regular lobules, each arranged around a 'central vein' with portal tracts at the periphery.

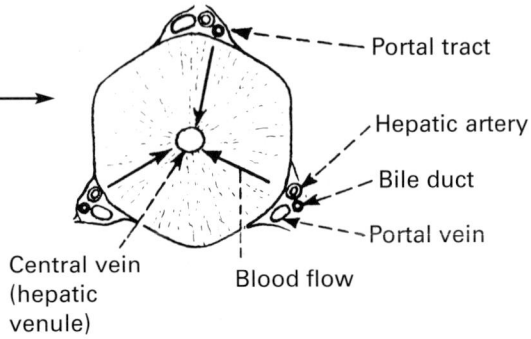

Histologically, it is evident that this is not quite true. The liver in section often has this appearance.

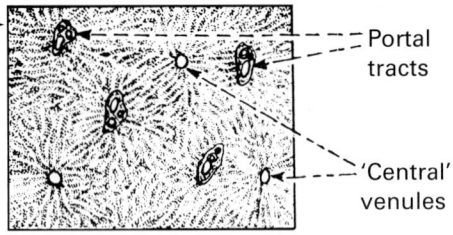

The portal tracts and hepatic venules appear to be distributed in a slightly haphazard manner.

Instead, the acinar concept is now used.

The smallest unit is the simple acinus of varying shape.

The portal venule and hepatic arteriole both send terminal branches into the acinus (2/3 of the blood supply is portal and 1/3 arterial). They join to form a common trunk which will then contain partially oxygenated blood, and this percolates through the sinusoids to several 'terminal hepatic venules' (as in diagram).

In terms of oxygen supply and other nutrients, 3 zones exist.

Zone 1, with the best supply
Zone 2, with a reasonable supply
Zone 3, with the poorest supply which makes it most vulnerable to hypoxia.

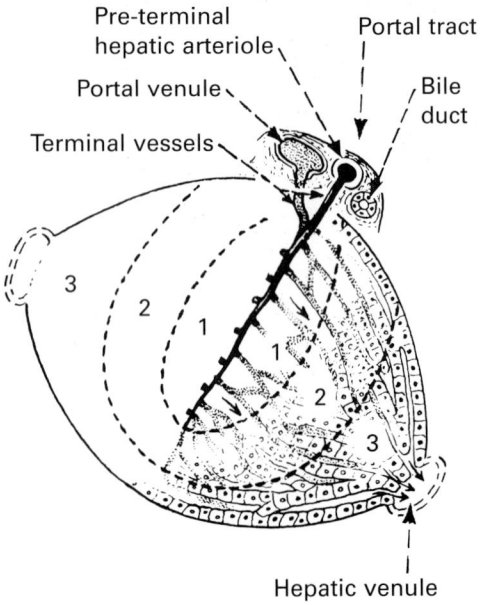

In Zone 1, glycogen synthesis and glycogenolysis take place. It is also the main area of protein metabolism and formation of plasma proteins. Conjugation of certain drugs takes place.

Zone 3 is associated with glycogen storage, lipid and pigment formation and metabolism of certain drugs and chemicals. Zone 2 shares functions with the other zones.

LIVER – ANATOMY

A complex acinus consists of at least three simple acini organised around the terminal branches of a pre-terminal portal venule, hepatic arteriole and bile duct. The blood circulates through the parenchyma and drains into two or three hepatic venules.

Zones 1, 2 and 3 form roughly concentric layers, zone 1 being the core of the complex acinus. Zone 3 is the outer layer at the periphery of the circulation and, at certain points, can come quite close to the pre-terminal vessels.

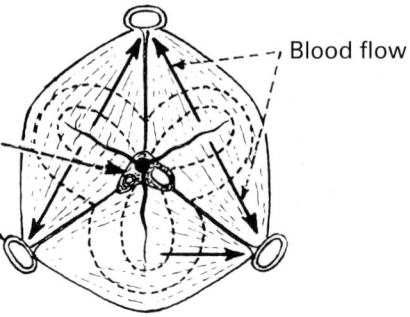

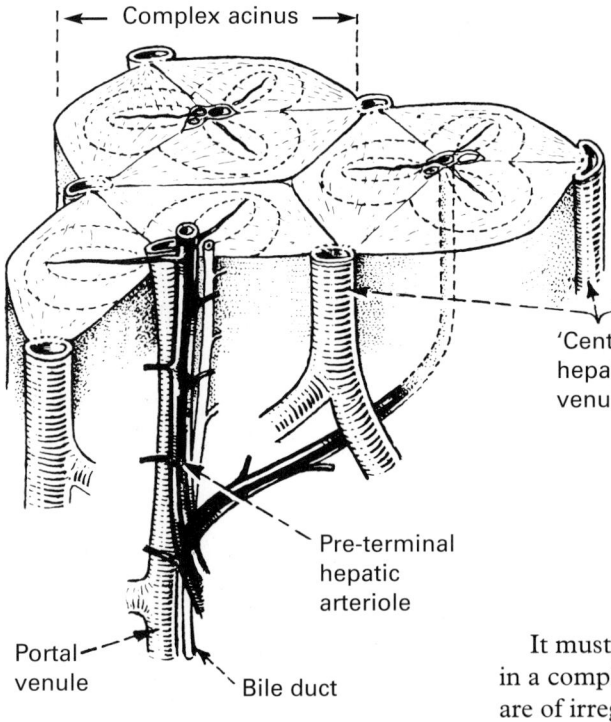

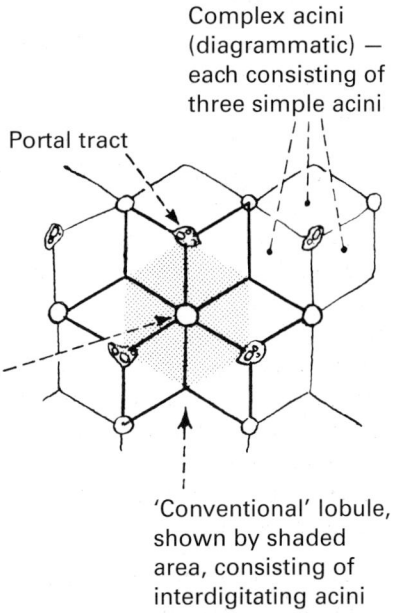

It must be realised that the acini interdigitate in a complex way so that masses of hepatic cells are of irregular shape and the apparent regularity shown in the diagram is merely schematic. This explains the difficulty in recognising the functional units in histological sections.

ANATOMY – HEPATIC LESIONS

The site of hepatic lesions is determined mainly by the microcirculation. Factors involved are:

1. PO_2 of blood
2. Enzyme functions of the zones
3. Filtration function.

LIVER NECROSIS

In this text the modern description of the liver anatomy is used, providing an explanation of lesions in functional terms. The older lobular nomenclature is shown in brackets.

Perivenular necrosis (Centrilobular necrosis)

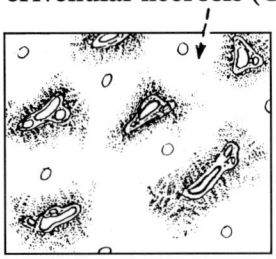

This form is a feature of many apparently unrelated conditions. It is brought about by damage in zone 3 of interdigitating acini (A in diagram). Thus it is a feature of shock due to circulatory collapse reducing the oxygen supply to zone 3. It also occurs in poisoning with chlorinated hydrocarbons (e.g. in chloroform) and drugs, e.g. paracetamol, substances metabolised in zone 3.

It is important to realise that zone 3, particularly, is continuous from one acinus to another, and in severe cases, the hepatic venules are linked together by necrotic tissues. Microscopically, therefore, the lesions appear irregular in distribution due to differing planes of section.

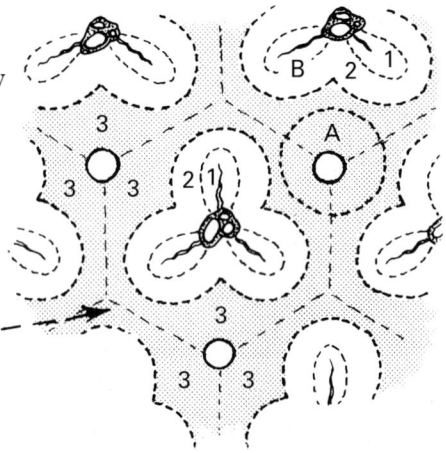

Mid-zonal necrosis

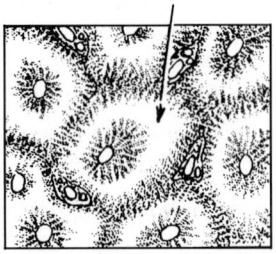

This is uncommon. It is seen in yellow fever and in acute peritonitis; probably the result of toxins affecting zones 2 and 1 (B in diagram).

Periportal necrosis (Peripheral necrosis)

This may represent damage in parts of zone 3 near the portal tracts, or changes in zone 1 due to its metabolism of drugs and chemicals; e.g. phosphorus poisoning causes marked fatty change in the peripheral parenchyma, followed by necrosis.

ANATOMY – HEPATIC LESIONS

Massive necrosis
This is an unusual lesion which can follow poisoning due to drugs, industrial chemicals or mushrooms. Rarely it is a complication of viral hepatitis.

Four factors may operate to bring about this necrosis:

1. **Personal sensitivity to the 'poison'.** This has been particularly observed in regard to drugs.
2. **Dosage.** The extent of necrosis is often related to the amount of poison ingested.
3. **Transfer of function.** If one zone becomes necrotic due to the formation of toxic substances when trying to metabolise a chemical, then the task of dealing with the chemical falls upon the adjacent zone. This occurs in paracetamol overdosage and poisoning by chloroform or carbon tetrachloride.

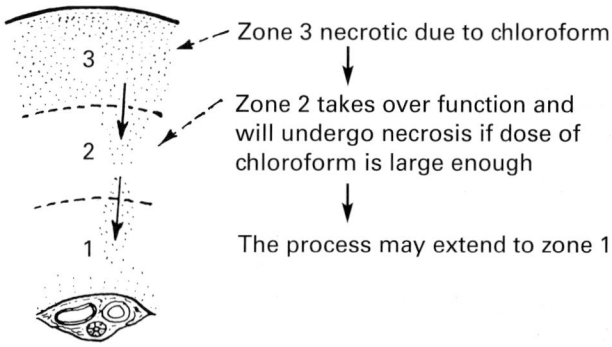

4. **Interference with circulation.** In any necrotic process, the local circulation of blood is bound to be upset, and this will tend to increase the damage which will spread in an increasingly haphazard manner if the cause is still operating.

The following substances are among the most important causing massive liver necrosis:
Drugs: monoamine oxidase inhibitors, paracetamol, halothane.
Industrial chemicals: carbon tetrachloride, tetrachlorethylene, chlorinated naphthalene and nitrobenzene compounds.

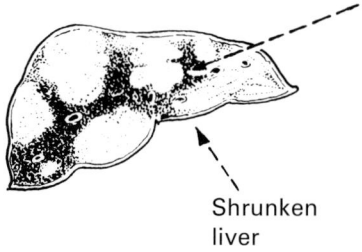

In the early stages, the liver is normal in size and is yellow. Soon the dead cells are removed, leaving collapsed dark red areas. Subsequently the surviving cells undergo hyperplasia resulting in a shrunken liver with nodules (multiple nodular hyperplasia) — a form of cirrhosis.

Early acute liver failure may prove fatal. Recovery leaves a liver with gross functional deficiency. The healing fibrotic process and complications inevitably follow.

JAUNDICE

If the serum bilirubin level exceeds 34 μmol/l, the patient becomes jaundiced.

Bilirubin is derived from the breakdown of effete red cells by the macrophage system, mainly in the spleen. It is conjugated to glucuronic acid in the liver and secreted in the bile.

Study of haemoglobin catabolism shows 3 main forms of jaundice:

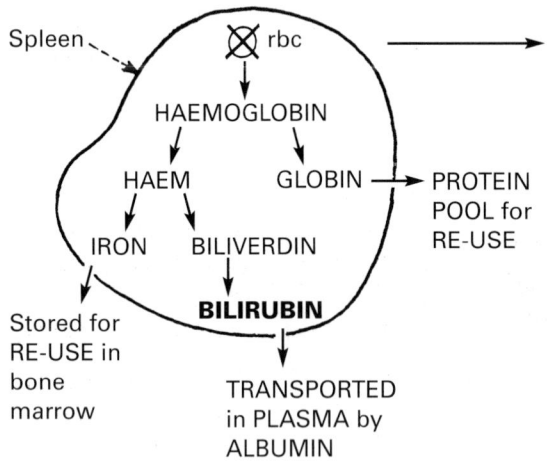

1. **PRE-HEPATIC JAUNDICE**
due to increased rbc destruction, e.g. haemolytic anaemia
↑ UNCONJUGATED BILIRUBIN
(bound to albumin; therefore does not appear in urine — so-called **ACHOLURIC JAUNDICE**).

In NEONATAL HAEMOLYTIC ANAEMIA bilirubin may damage the brain (kernicterus, p. 404).

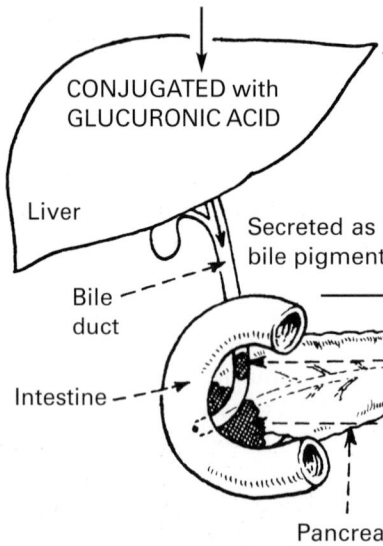

2. **HEPATOCELLULAR JAUNDICE**
e.g. in hepatitis.
Liver cell damage → failure to conjugate bilirubin. In addition, local cholestasis is often also seen.

3. **POST-HEPATIC (OBSTRUCTIVE JAUNDICE)** e.g.
Stone obstructing common bile duct
and
Carcinoma of head of pancreas.

FAILURE to EXCRETE CONJUGATED BILIRUBIN

→ reabsorbed → water soluble

→ excreted in urine.

FAILURE of BILE to REACH GUT → pale stools.

Intrahepatic cholestasis e.g. steroids and chlorpromazine can lead to cholestatic jaundice.

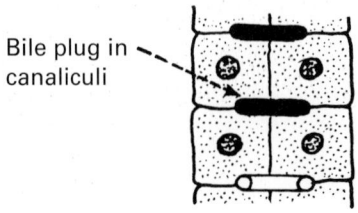

VIRAL HEPATITIS

ACUTE VIRAL HEPATITIS

Viral hepatitis is the most important form of hepatitis. It is seen worldwide. Viral hepatitis may be sporadic or epidemic, and, depending on the responsible virus, transmitted by the faeco-oral or parenteral route.

Clinical features

Many episodes of viral hepatitis are subclinical; mild symptomatic cases are characterised by nausea, fever and anorexia. Severe attacks are characterised by jaundice and hepatic failure, and may be fatal.

Pathological features

EARLY stage

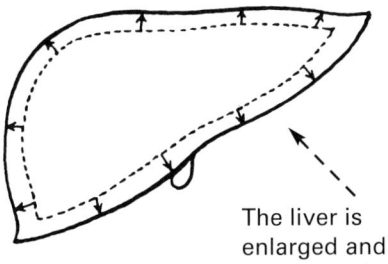

The liver is enlarged and congested (and often palpable)

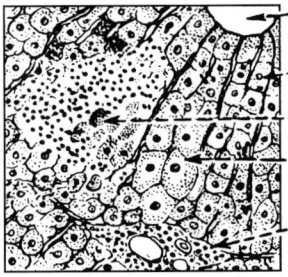

Hepatic venule

Normal cells

Councilman body (apoptotic cell)

Swollen hepatocytes

Lymphocytic infiltrate in portal tract and in parenchyma

Liver cell necrosis is always present. It is most marked in Zone 3 (p. 342).

Necrosis may be:

(a) focal (spotty) — scattered as single cells or
(b) more severe — forming areas of bridging between vessels (portal to hepatic venule) or
(c) panacinar: Necrosis of complete acini up to massive necrosis of a large part of the liver occasionally occurs. When it does, it is most marked in the left lobe.

LATER stage

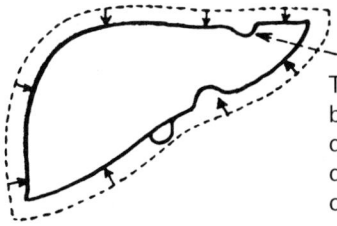

There may be focal depressions due to areas of collapse

Liver is smaller, yellow or greenish

There is evidence of healing with mitotic activity in the hepatocytes.

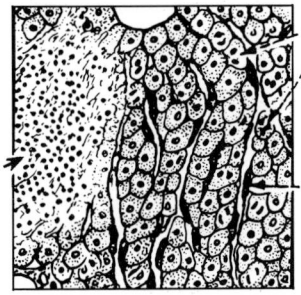

Binucleate and multinucleate hepatocytes

Lymphocytes, plasma cells, mononuclears and pigment; collapsed stroma

Pigmented hyperplastic Kupffer cells (contain bile and lipofuscin derived from dead hepatocytes).

VIRAL HEPATITIS

Biochemical changes

These changes result from liver damage

- Disruption of bile canaliculi/interference with excretion → Absorption of conjugated bile into blood (levels up to 300 μmol/l.)
- Necrosis of hepatocytes → Release of enzymes into blood → Transferase enzymes (ALT, AST) greatly increased
- Diminished production of special substances → Coagulation mechanisms upset → Prothrombin times increased

Clinical progress

1. In most cases, the disease is self-limiting and complete recovery occurs within 4-6 weeks.
2. Death may occur due to massive (panacinar) liver necrosis.
   (a) In the early pre-icteric stage within 10 days — fulminant hepatic failure.
   (b) In 2–3 weeks. The liver is reduced in size.

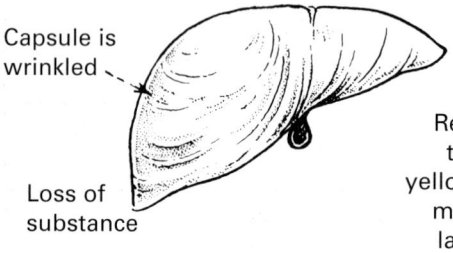

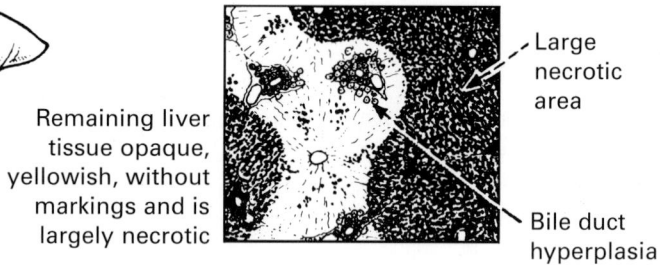

This condition was often termed 'acute yellow atrophy'.

(c) Several weeks later.
At this stage, regeneration is well advanced in places but function is inadequate and progressive failure occurs.

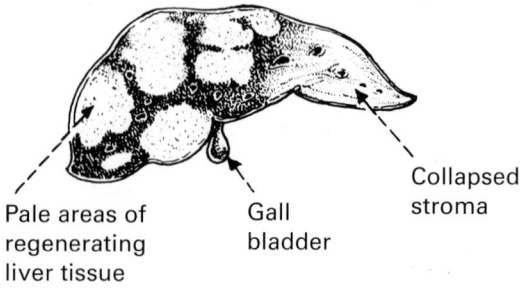

Some types of hepatitis may progress to
3. Chronic hepatitis (p. 352),
4. Cirrhosis,
5. Hepatocellular carcinoma may occur.

VIRAL HEPATITIS

At least 5 viruses cause liver damage without significantly damaging other tissues (hepatitis A,B,C,D and E). The features are summarised and then discussed individually.

VIRUS	H**A**V	H**B**V	H**C**V	H**D**V	H**E**V
TYPE	PICO**RNA** VIRUS	HEPA**DNA** VIRUS	RNA FLAVIVIRUS	DEFECTIVE RNA VIRUS	RNA VIRUS
SPREAD	Faeco-oral	Parenteral	Parenteral	Parenteral	Faeco-oral
INCUBATION PERIOD (days)	15–50	30–180	20–160	30–160	20–60
SEVERITY of HEPATITIS	Usually mild	Often severe	Usually mild	Severe	Often mild. Severe in pregnancy
CHRONICITY	No	Approx 5% of adults, 90% of children	Approx 50%	Coinfection 5% Superinfection 95% (p. 351)	No
CARRIER STATE	No	Yes	Yes	Yes	No
VACCINE	Yes	Yes	No	Protected by HBV vaccine if HBV-ve	No

Other viruses which can affect the liver, but also affect other tissues include:

Yellow fever;
Herpes viruses — Epstein Barr, Cytomegalovirus, Herpes simplex;
Coxsackie A and B;
Lassa fever.

HEPATITIS B INFECTION

The **hepatitis B virus** is a member of the HEPA DNA virus group. Infection is by the parenchymal route — mainly IV drug abuse, blood products and sexual transmission.

The virus has several components:

A core containing
(a) DNA — partly double stranded
(b) DNA polymerase
(c) Core antigen HBcAg
(d) e antigen HBeAg

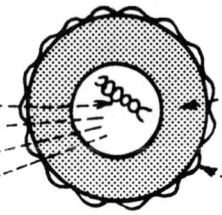

An **outer lipo-protein coat** (derived from the hepatocyte membrane) bearing Hepatitis B surface antigen (HBsAg)

42 μm diameter

The complete virion is known as the Dane particle. Spherical and tubular structures derived from the surface coat can also be found in the peripheral blood.

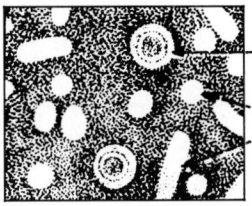

These antigens and antibodies to them are the basis for diagnosis of hepatitis B infection.

In **histological preparations**

HBsAg accumulates in the cytoplasm of cells — giving a 'ground glass' appearance.

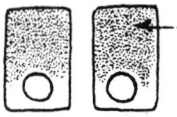

HBcAg is found in the nuclei.

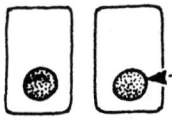

or can be stained by immunocytochemistry.

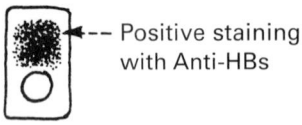

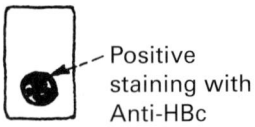

Serology: Antibodies to the various antigens appear in the blood.

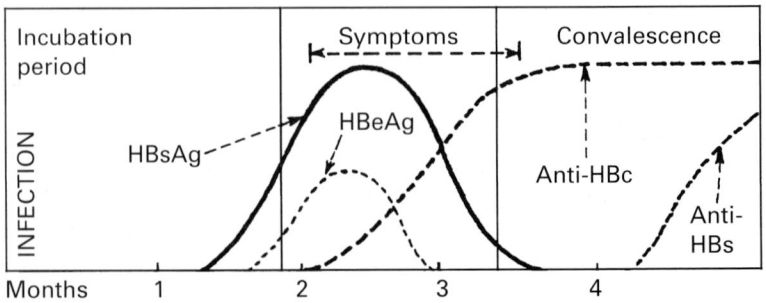

Six weeks after infection the surface antigen (HBsAg) appears in the blood, followed two weeks later by the e antigen (HBeAg), at the time of maximal viral replication.

VIRAL HEPATITIS

Outcome of Hepatitis B infection

In >90% of cases there is a vigorous immune reaction (cell mediated and humoral) to the virus resulting in elimination of the virus. In the remaining patients, the illness pursues one of several courses:

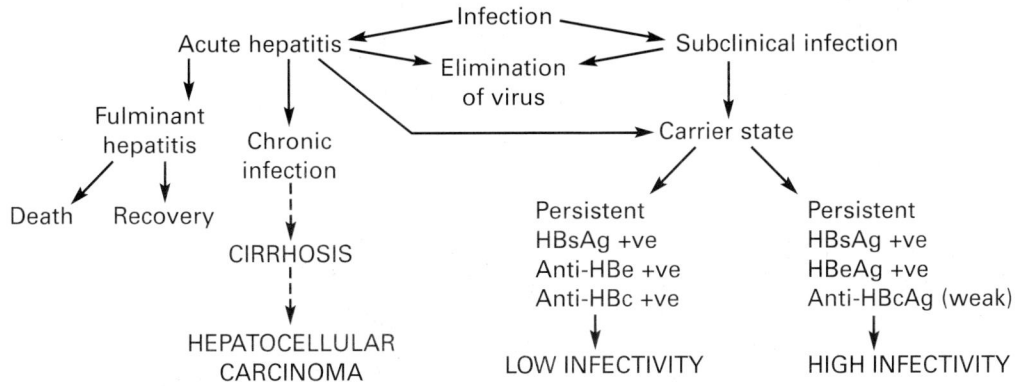

HEPATITIS D

This is a defective RNA virus which requires HB virus for its release and infectivity. There are 2 patterns of infection:

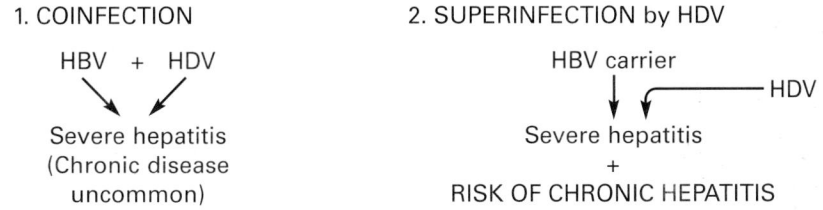

HEPATITIS C

This small RNA virus is transmitted parenterally and is seen in IV drug users or following infected blood transfusion. Acute hepatitis is mild and patients are rarely jaundiced. It is important because of the high risk of chronicity.

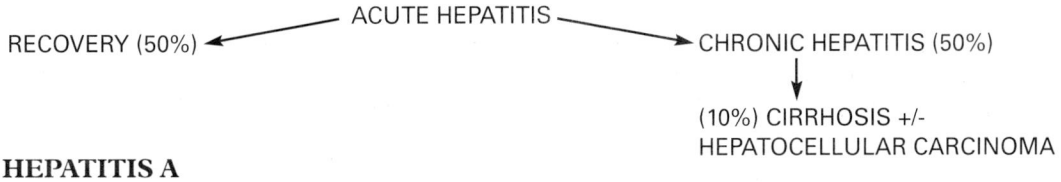

HEPATITIS A

This picornavirus is transmitted by the faeco-oral route, especially where hygiene is poor. Hepatitis is usually mild in children, but more severe in adults. IgM antibodies appear in the blood in the acute phase, and IgG during convalescence, thus conferring life long immunity. Chronic liver disease does not occur.

HEPATITIS E

This is most commonly seen in Africa and Asia. Although usually mild, it is particularly severe in pregnant women with a mortality of approximately 20%.

CHRONIC HEPATITIS

Inflammation of the liver which lasts for more than 6 months is regarded as chronic. (This definition excludes disorders such as alcoholic hepatitis.)

There are 4 main **causes:**

1. **Persistent viral infection** — hepatitis B, D and C.
2. **Autoimmune hepatitis.** This occurs especially in young women. In most cases antinuclear and anti-smooth muscle antibodies are present in the serum. Liver specific autoantibodies e.g. to a sialoglycoprotein receptor (ASGP-R) on periportal hepatocyte cell surfaces can also be found. These patients often have other autoimmune diseases e.g. thyroiditis. A smaller subgroup is defined by anti-Liver Kidney Microsomal antibodies (anti-LKM-1) and have a more aggressive disease.
3. **Drugs** — e.g. methyldopa, nitrofurantoin.
4. **In metabolic disorders** e.g. α_1 antitrypsin deficiency, Wilson's disease (p. 362).

Pathologically, these are similar conditions, although subtle differences exist. The severity of the inflammation varies — historically this was recognised by a division into 2 forms which are now recognised to be part of a spectrum.

CHRONIC PERSISTENT HEPATITIS

GOOD PROGNOSIS

CHRONIC ACTIVE HEPATITIS ----➤ RISK OF PROGRESSION TO CIRRHOSIS (p. 355)

POOR PROGNOSIS IF UNTREATED

Inflammation largely confined to portal tract

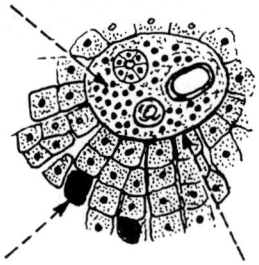

Occasional liver cell necrosis

'Limiting plate' preserved

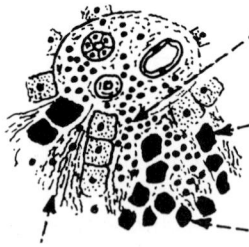

Inflammation spills into periportal liver

Liver cell necrosis 'interface hepatitis' (Piecemeal necrosis)

This may link portal tracts 'Bridging necrosis'

This is often accompanied by fibrosis

ALCOHOLIC LIVER DISEASE

Excess consumption of alcohol is associated with liver disease in three main forms.

EXCESS ALCOHOL INTAKE → FATTY LIVER (most individuals) → ALCOHOLIC HEPATITIS (20-40%) → ALCOHOLIC CIRRHOSIS (10-20%)

REVERSIBLE on WITHDRAWAL

ALCOHOLIC HEPATITIS: POSSIBLY REVERSIBLE or LIMITABLE

ALCOHOLIC CIRRHOSIS: IRREVERSIBLE (Prognosis improves with abstinence)

The progression from left to right does not occur in all patients: genetic predisposition, coexistant nutritional deficiencies, amount and duration of drinking and other factors determine the risk.

FATTY LIVER

This occurs in most heavy drinkers, even after a single episode of heavy intake. Fat accumulates in the hepatocytes due to abnormalities in the intermediate metabolism of lipids and carbohydrates.

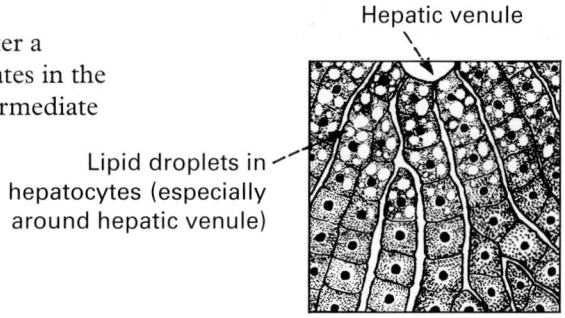

Alcohol metabolism

ETHANOL → Alcohol dehydrogenase → ACETALDEHYDE → Aldehyde dehydrogenase → ACETATE

ETHANOL → Microsomal ethanol oxidising system → Increases in heavy drinkers → Induction of CYTOCHROME (P450 2E1) — an alcohol specific enzyme

Alcohol dehydrogenase → H+ → NADH

Nicotinamide adenine dinucleotide NAD+ → NADH → DIMINISHED NAD+ → Abnormal LIPID METABOLISM → Increased TRIGLYCERIDE synthesis → ACCUMULATION of FAT within HEPATOCYTES

DIMINISHED NAD+ → Impaired CARBOHYDRATE METABOLISM → LACTIC ACIDOSIS

Impaired CARBOHYDRATE METABOLISM → Impaired GLYCONEOGENESIS → HYPOGLYCAEMIA

Note: Fatty liver usually resolves within 2-4 weeks of abstinence.

ALCOHOLIC HEPATITIS

Fatty change is reversible even when extensive. In 20–40% of heavy drinkers, alcoholic hepatitis is superimposed. This varies from asymptomatic hepatitis to a life threatening condition with nausea, vomiting, abdominal pain and jaundice. Signs of liver failure and portal hypertension may be found.

Histologically, the main features are seen around hepatic venules:

1. Liver cell swelling — Ballooning.
2. Accumulation of Mallory's hyaline — protein derived from intermediate filaments (mainly cytokeratin).
3. Liver cell necrosis.
4. Neutrophil polymorph reaction.
5. Pericellular fibrosis.

Acute Phase

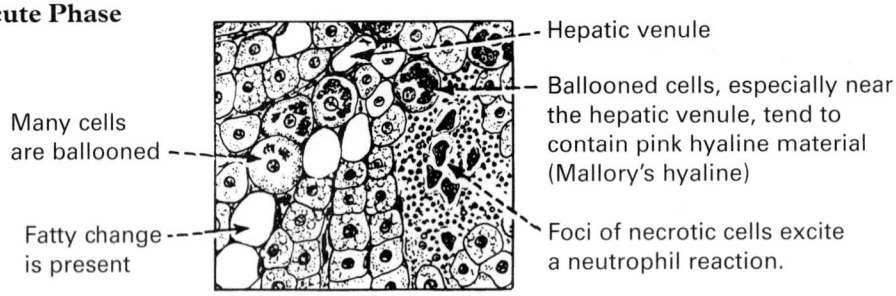

Progressing to pericellular fibrosis

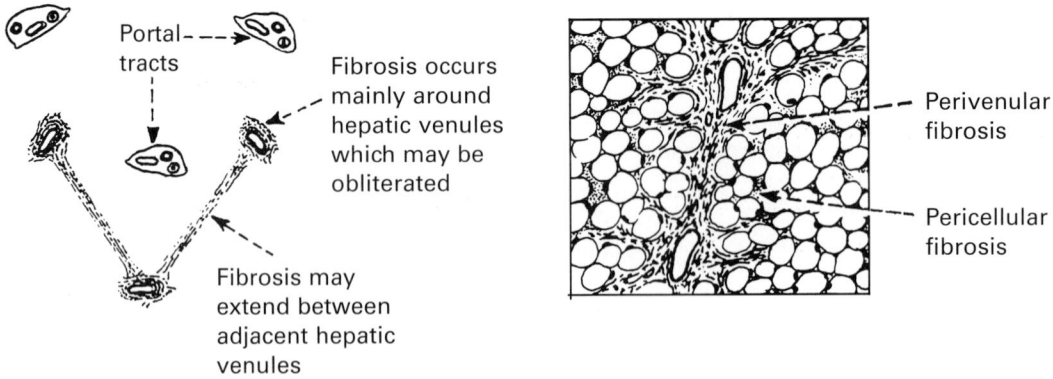

Alcoholic hepatitis is important as a cause of liver damage, and especially because of the high risk of progression to cirrhosis.

Non-alcoholic steatohepatitis (NASH) is a histologically similar form of hepatitis seen in non-drinkers. Diabetes mellitus, severe obesity, jejuno-ileal bypass for obesity and certain drugs appear to be responsible.

CIRRHOSIS

Cirrhosis is the end stage of many liver diseases. It is defined as:

A DIFFUSE process (i.e. the whole liver is affected) characterised by FIBROSIS and conversion of the liver architecture into abnormal NODULES.

Aetiology
There are very many causes including:

(i) Drugs and toxins e.g. alcohol, methotrexate, methyldopa.
(ii) Infections e.g. Hepatitis B and C.
(iii) Autoimmune diseases — chronic active hepatitis; primary biliary cirrhosis.
(iv) Metabolic conditions e.g. haemochromatosis, α_1 antitrypsin deficiency, Wilson's disease (excess accumulation of copper).
(v) Biliary obstruction e.g. gallstones, strictures, sclerosing cholangitis, cystic fibrosis.
(vi) Cryptogenic i.e. cause unknown.

The **mechanism** common to all cirrhoses is:

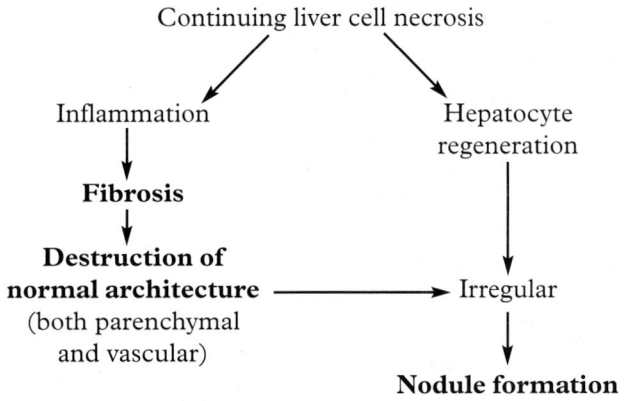

The **major complications** are:

1. Hepatocellular failure
2. Portal hypertension.
3. Hepatocellular carcinoma.

CIRRHOSIS

The initiating factor in the progression to cirrhosis is continuing hepatocellular damage. Its location within the acinus (p.342) and also its cause are reflected in the progression to irreversible damage.

The following contrasting diagrams illustrate this progression.

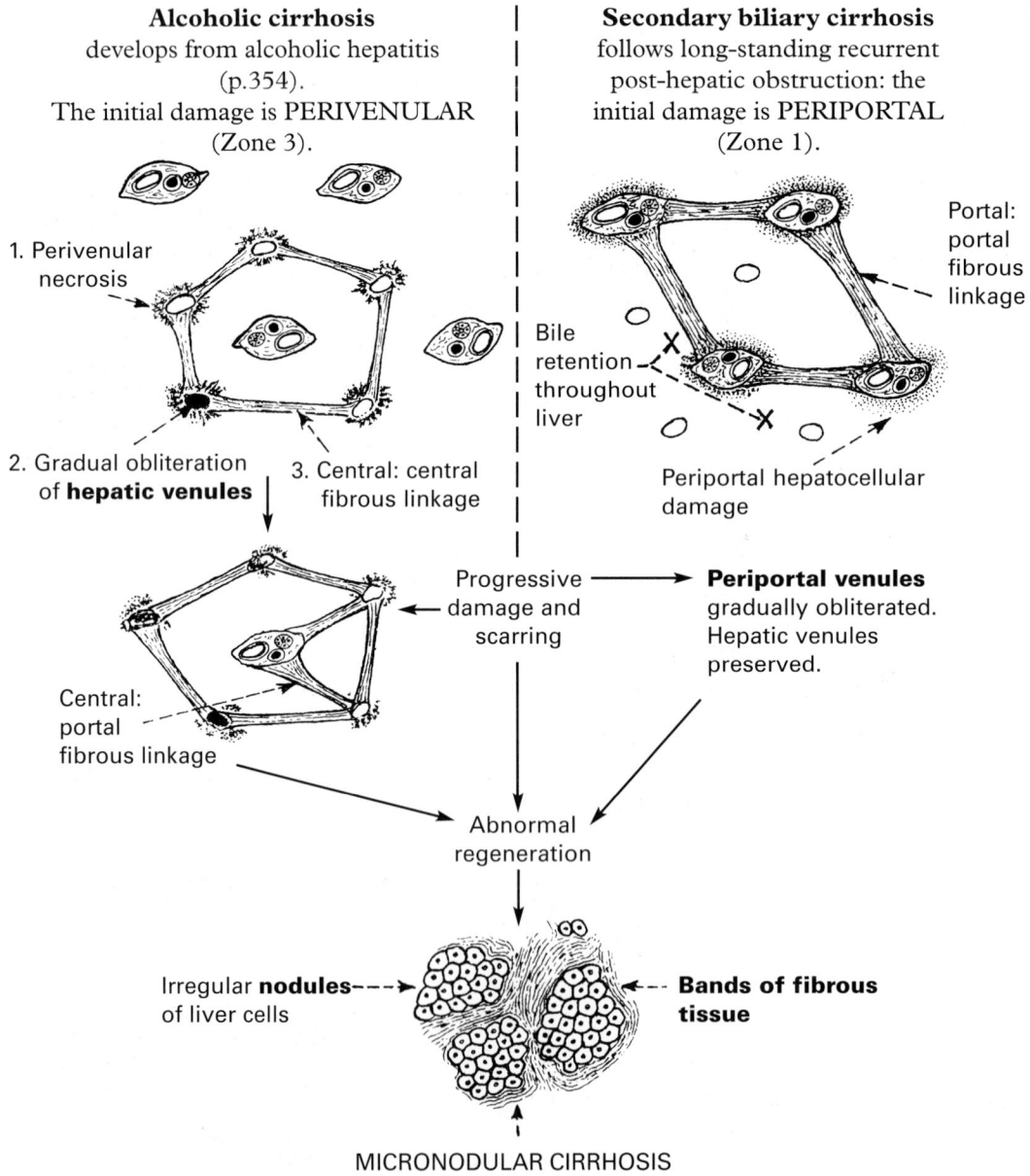

In **cirrhosis** progressing from **hepatitis D** the damage is more severe and widespread with more fibrous scarring and larger nodule formation — MACRONODULAR CIRRHOSIS.

CIRRHOSIS

PRIMARY BILIARY CIRRHOSIS (PBC)

This is a chronic disorder mainly affecting middle-aged women. Destruction of intra-hepatic bile ducts leads to scarring and eventually to cirrhosis. Patients typically present with fatigue, itching (from bile salt retention) or jaundice. Hyperlipidaemia is common.

Aetiology

This is an autoimmune disorder. Over 90% of patients have anti-mitochondrial antibodies in their serum. An overlap may be seen with autoimmune chronic hepatitis.

Pathology

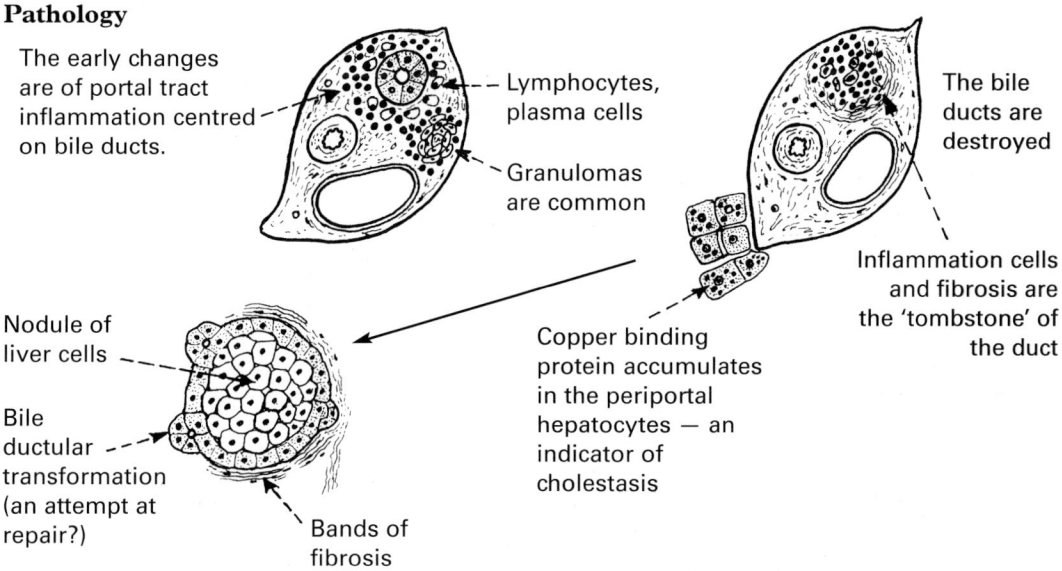

A few cases progress to secondary biliary cirrhosis after many years.

PRIMARY SCLEROSING CHOLANGITIS

This disease also attacks bile ducts, both intra- and extrahepatic. Men are usually affected and there is a strong association with ulcerative colitis.

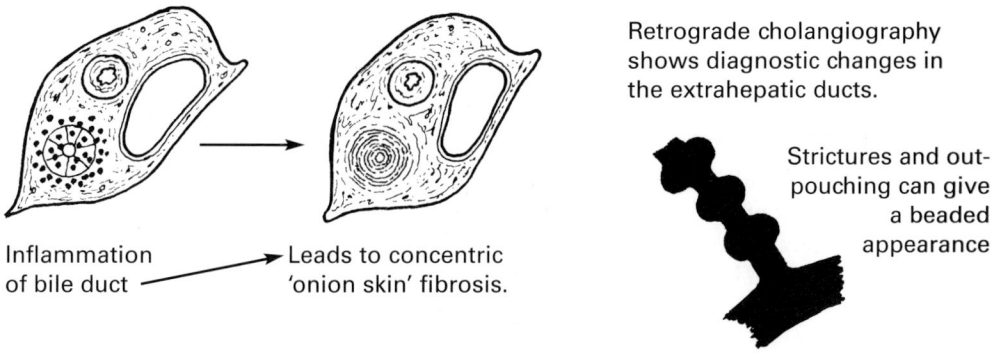

The late effects are similar to PBC. Liver failure and bile duct carcinoma are frequent complications.

HEPATOCELLULAR FAILURE

Failure of liver function can be:

1. Acute, with rapid onset (<8 weeks from onset of liver disease), e.g. in cases of massive necrosis due to poisoning (or, less commonly, acute hepatitis).
2. Chronic and sometimes recurring, of slow onset, e.g. in cirrhosis or chronic hepatitis — representing decompensation.

The mechanism is different in the 2 types.

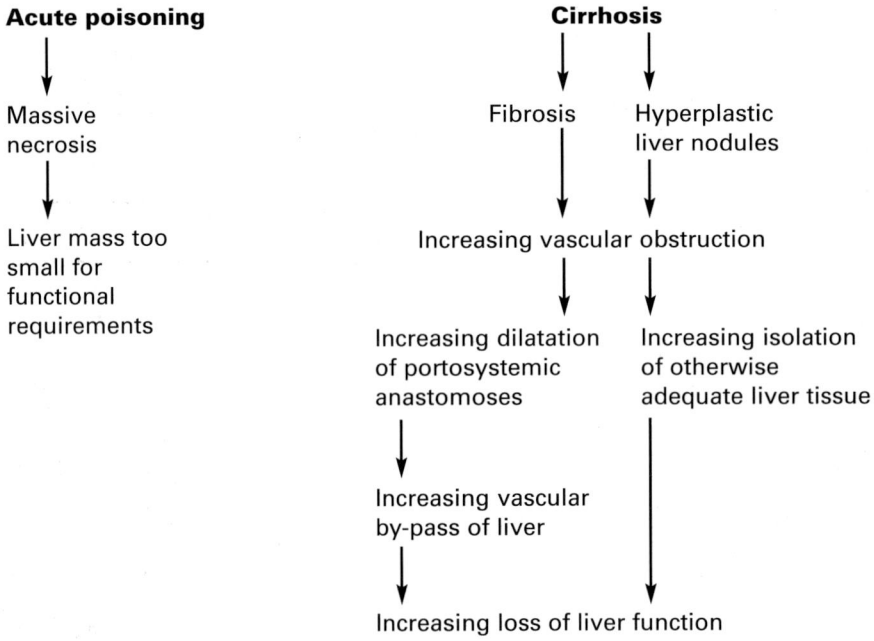

The **cardinal signs of hepatocellular failure are:**

1. Jaundice.
2. Hepatic encephalopathy.
3. Ascites.
4. Bleeding diathesis.

Other features include hypoglycaemia, acidosis and endocrine disturbances.

Jaundice

In acute liver failure, jaundice appears early and is related to the extent of liver damage. It arises as a result of lack of conjugation and excretion of bilirubin.

The time of appearance and type of jaundice in cases of chronic liver failure depend on the primary cause. In cases of biliary cirrhosis, the jaundice precedes other signs of liver failure and is of obstructive type, initially at least. Other forms of cirrhosis only give rise to jaundice at a late stage when it is of hepatic type, i.e. due to difficulties in bilirubin conjugation and excretion.

HEPATOCELLULAR FAILURE

HEPATIC ENCEPHALOPATHY

This term refers to the impaired mental state and neurological function due to liver failure. It takes the form of tremors, behavioural changes, convulsions, delirium, drowsiness and coma. In the acute form, severe symptoms such as convulsions, delirium and coma develop rapidly, while in chronic conditions milder changes are seen and coma is a late feature, unless a complication arises.

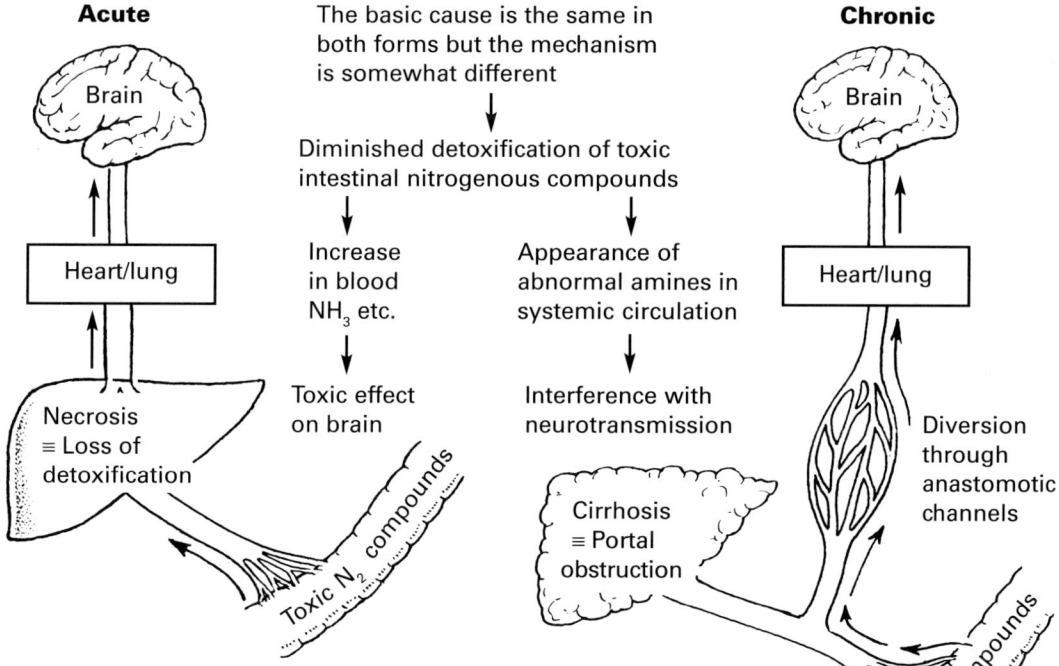

Despite the serious disturbances of function, pathological changes in the brain of fatal cases are surprisingly slight.

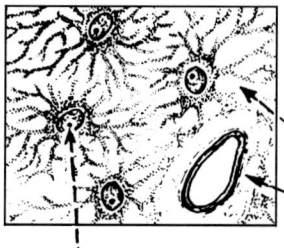

Interstitial oedema

Perivascular oedema

Protoplasmic astrocytes enlarged and increased in number. Nuclei large with prominent nucleoli.

Aggravated by breakdown products of blood e.g. from bleeding varices.

HEPATOCELLULAR FAILURE

HEPATOCELLULAR FAILURE (continued)

1. **ASCITES** is usually due to a combination of **portal hypertension** and **hepatocellular failure.**

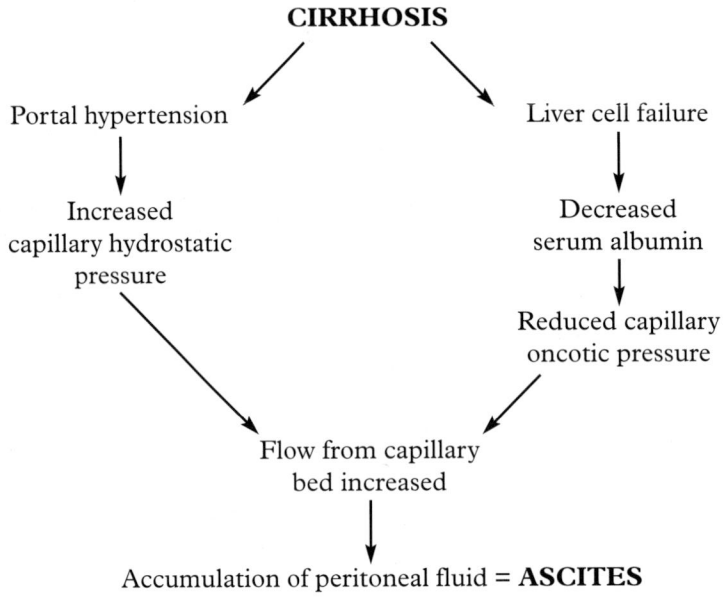

2. **ANAEMIA** usually of normocytic/normochromic type (p.420) is common — splenomegaly may cause hypersplenism and pancytopoenia (p.441)

3. **Metabolic disorders**
   (a) Reduced protein synthesis e.g. fibrinogen, prothrombin factors V, VII, IX, X ⟶ bleeding diathesis.
   (b) Reduced liver glycogen storage ⟶ hypoglycaemia.
   (c) Reduced elimination of endogenous oestrogen ⟶ gynaecomastia, testicular atrophy and spider naevi (small skin capillary telangiectasis).

4. **Hepato-renal failure** is an important complication of a major haemorrhage from oesophageal varices.

PORTAL HYPERTENSION

In cirrhosis of the liver, **portal hypertension** is important in addition to any hepatocellular deficiency.

Causes

By far, the most important cause is cirrhosis, but there are many others broadly classified as (1) pre-hepatic, (2) intra-hepatic and (3) post-hepatic.

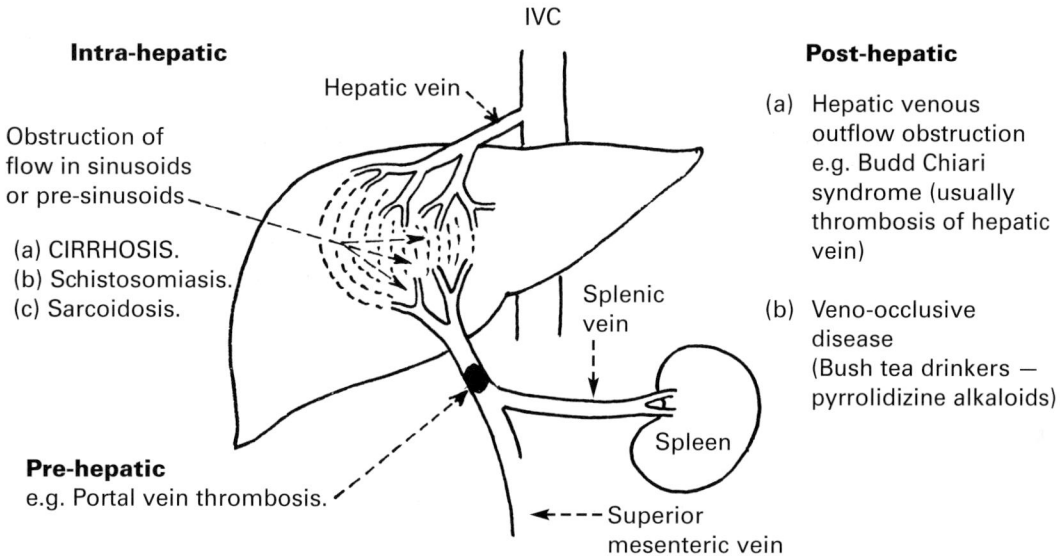

Effects

The main consequences are:

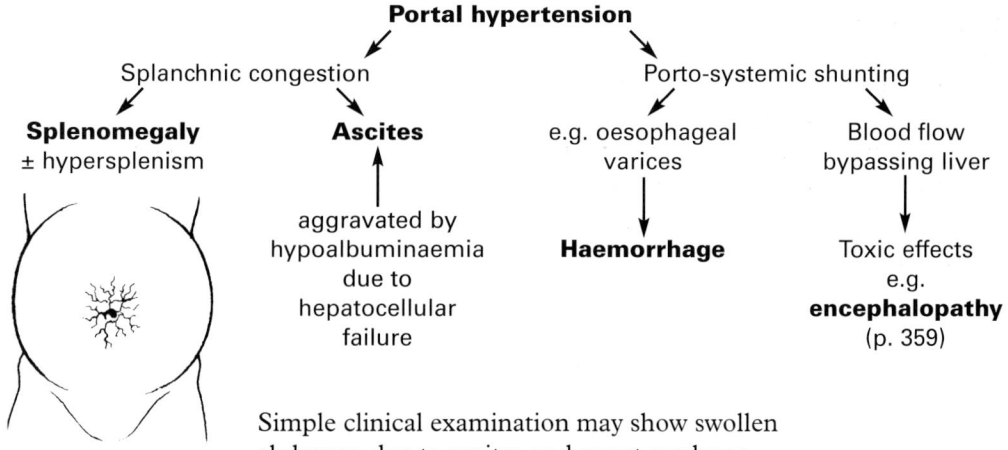

Simple clinical examination may show swollen abdomen due to ascites and caput medusae — engorged subcutaneous veins around the umbilicus.

METABOLIC DISORDERS AND THE LIVER

HAEMOCHROMATOSIS

This is due to a mutation on chromosome 6.
Heterozygotes absorb excess iron, but homozygotes develop the disease.

EXCESS ABSORBANCE OF IRON
↓
Deposition in parenchymal cells

Pancreatic islets	Myocardium	Liver
↓	↓	↓
DIABETES	CARDIAC FAILURE	Fibrosis
		↓
		CIRRHOSIS

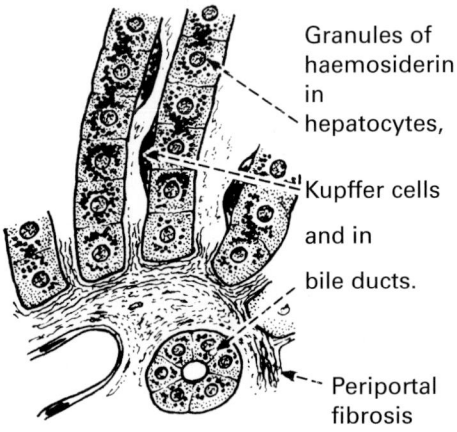

Note: In the skin, the iron is deposited mainly in the sweat glands: excessive melanin production in the epidermis explains the term 'bronzed diabetes' for these cases.

HAEMOSIDEROSIS — Excess dietary iron and repeated blood transfusions may overload the body iron stores but cause less liver damage.

WILSON'S DISEASE (HEPATO-LENTICULAR DEGENERATION)
A rare autosomal recessive condition (chromosome 13). This is characterised by accumulation of copper in the liver, brain (basal ganglia) and cornea (Kayser-Fleisher rings). Serum levels of caeruloplasmin (a copper binding protein) are reduced. The liver can show an acute hepatitis, chronic active hepatitis or cirrhosis.

α_1-ANTITRYPSIN DEFICIENCY

This enzyme is a protease inhibitor produced mainly by the liver. Reduced levels or activity of the enzyme (abnormal forms coded by allelic variants) may result in liver damage.

Liver disease is found in most **homozygotes** and presents as neonatal hepatitis, chronic active hepatitis or cirrhosis. Heterozygotes are rarely badly affected.

The abnormal enzyme is not secreted by liver cells and accumulates as globules in the periportal hepatocytes.

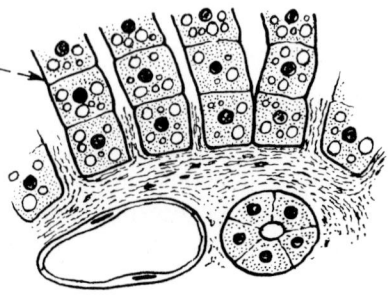

Note: α_1 antitrypsin deficiency is an important factor in the development of emphysema (p. 265).

INFECTIONS AND INFESTATIONS

PYOGENIC INFECTIONS

These are now much less common due to the efficient use of antibiotics. Abscess of the liver occurs mainly in two conditions:

1. **Ascending cholangitis**

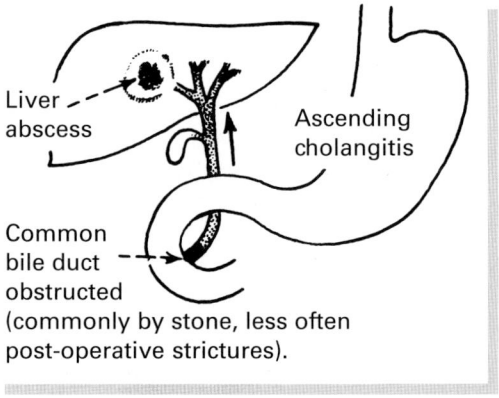

2. **Suppurative pylephlebitis**
   This arises from suppurative lesions in the abdominal cavity such as:

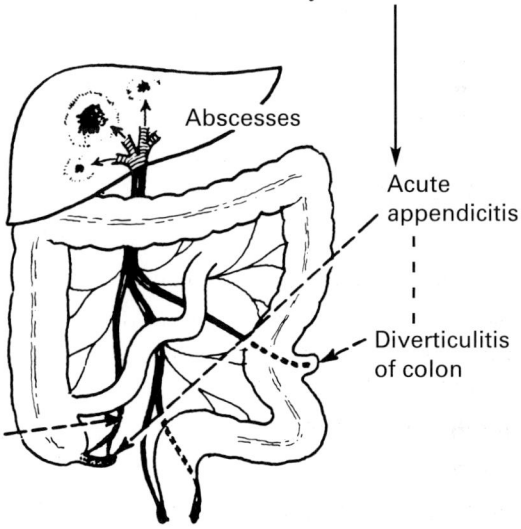

Inflammation
↓
Septic thrombosis of associated veins
↓
Septic emboli in portal veins or spreading pylephlebitis
↓
Liver abscess

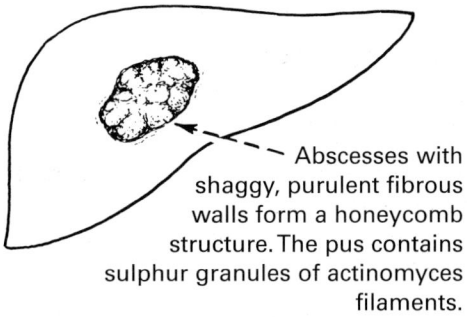

ACTINOMYCOSIS

The appendix is usually the site of the initial lesion. Spread to the liver is via the portal blood but may be direct. The liver lesion is characteristic of *Actinomyces israelii* infection.

TUBERCULOSIS

This is rare. Miliary tubercles may be seen in generalised infection.

HEPATIC GRANULOMAS (Tuberculoid reactions)

Giant cell granulomas are also common in sarcoidosis and may also occur in brucellosis, histoplasmosis and primary biliary cirrhosis, among many other causes.

INFECTIONS AND INFESTATIONS

SPIROCHAETAL INFECTIONS

Three spirochaetal infections can involve the liver.

1. **Leptospira icterohaemorrhagica (Weil's Disease)**

This organism is associated with the presence of rats and working in wet conditions. It is prevalent among workers in sewers and abbatoirs, miners, agricultural workers and sometimes soldiers on active service. The rat is a reservoir of infection, and rat excreta contain the organism. The disease is characterised by fever, jaundice, haemorrhages into and from various organs, e.g. lungs, kidneys, and renal damage. The liver lesion is characteristic. Death may occur from intrapulmonary haemorrhage or renal failure.

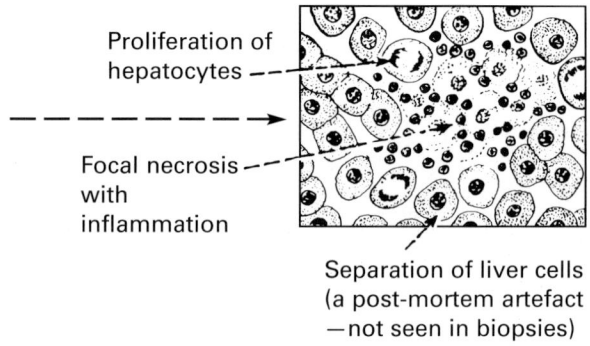

2. ***Treponema pallidum***

Syphilitic lesions of the liver are now uncommon in the U.K.

(a) *Congenital infection.* This usually produces a diffuse interstitial fibrosis which isolates individual liver cells and causes ischaemic atrophy. It is accompanied by a striking mononuclear infiltration and tiny areas of coagulative necrosis — miliary gummata. Spirochaetes are often plentiful.

(b) *Acquired infection.* Lesions can occur in the secondary and tertiary stages. In the secondary stage, a diffuse, inflammatory reaction with miliary gummata can occur. Large gummata may occur in tertiary syphilis. Gross scarring with distortion follows healing — hepar lobatum.

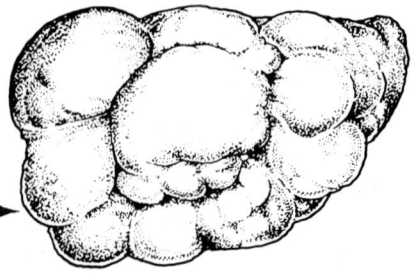

3. **Borrelia**

Borrelia occur in many parts of the world and several species exist e.g. B. recurrentis. They are transmitted by lice and ticks from animals acting as reservoirs, especially rodents. The infections produce peri-venular necrosis of the liver. Jaundice may be severe and liver failure can result in death.

INFECTIONS AND INFESTATIONS

PROTOZOAL DISEASES

Amoebic 'abscess'

This is a complication of amoebic dysentery due to *Entamoeba histolytica*. The 'abscess' is usually single, in the upper right lobe of liver. An irregular fibrous wall encloses what appears to be brownish pus. The 'pus' consists of necrotic liver cells, debris and red cells. Amoebae may be found in the inner wall. There are no pus cells. It may remain localised or track through the diaphragm into the lung, pleural or pericardial cavities.

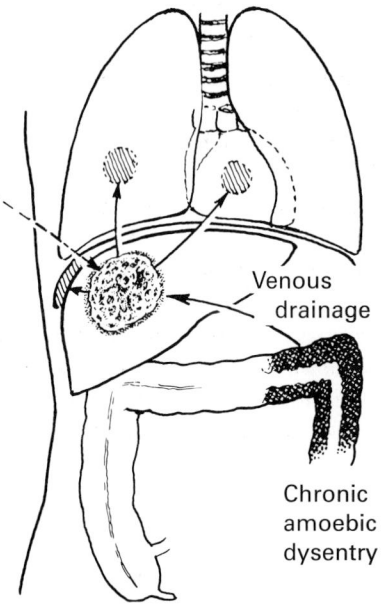

Malaria

On initial infection, the parasites develop within the hepatocytes but produce little damage. In chronic malaria, red cells containing parasites are engulfed by Kupffer cells which become hyperplastic and contain brown malarial pigment.
In benign tertian malaria, the parasite can survive for long periods within the liver cells (exoerythrocytic cycle).

Kala-azar (Visceral Leishmaniasis)

The liver is enlarged due to hyperplasia of the Kupffer cells which phagocytose many Leishman-Donovan bodies.

METAZOAL DISEASES Trematodes (flukes)

Schistosomiasis (Bilharzia)

S. mansoni is common in Egypt and other parts of Africa. *S. japonicum* is found in China, Japan and the Philippines. Both infections involve the liver.

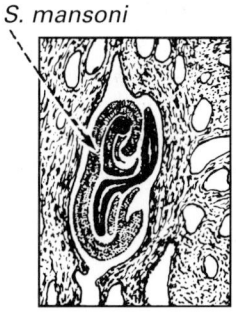

The schistosomes colonise the intestinal tract. They invade the intestinal veins; ova are released into the blood stream and embolise the portal venules of the liver. There is a focal granulomatous reaction which may lead to extensive portal fibrosis without cirrhosis. Portal hypertension can result with its associated complications.

INFECTIONS AND INFESTATIONS

METAZOAL DISEASES (continued)

Two other varieties of fluke disease exist — clonorchiasis (Chinese fish fluke) and fascioliasis (sheep fluke). Both produce an ascending cholangitis. Clonorchiasis can cause biliary obstruction and marked proliferation of bile ducts. Cholangiocarcinoma may develop. Infestation in both cases is due to eating raw or insufficiently cooked food.

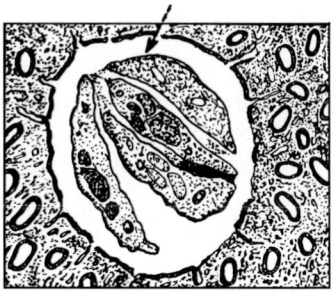

Hydatid disease

This is a cystic condition caused by the embryos of *Echinococcus granulosis*, a small tapeworm. The condition is commonest in sheep and may occur in humans in close contact with them. Cattle and pigs may also be affected. Adult worms are found in dogs fed on the infected tissues of sheep, cattle or pigs. Ova are excreted by the dogs and are ingested by other animals including man. The disease is commonest in Australia, New Zealand and South America.

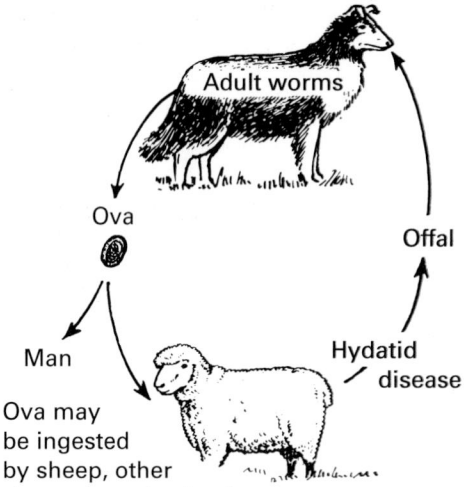

Digestion of the chitinous membrane by gastric juice liberates the embryos which invade the intestinal veins and reach the liver. Sometimes they pass into the systemic circulation and cysts form in the lungs, muscles, kidneys, spleen or brain.

The cyst may be very large, usually multilocular, due to budding of daughter cysts.

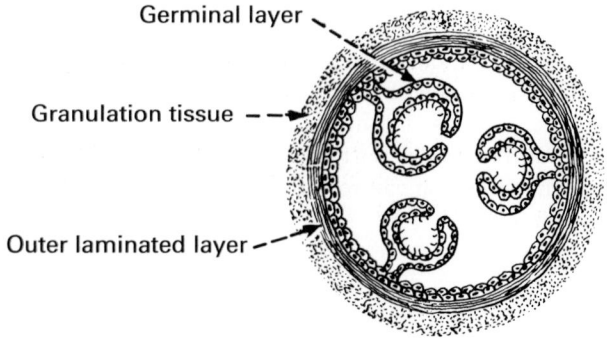

Patients show a hypersensitivity reaction to an intradermal injection of hydatid antigen (Casoni test: used in diagnosis.)

TUMOURS OF LIVER

PRIMARY BENIGN TUMOURS

Very few varieties are recognised.

1. **Cavernous haemangioma.** This is the commonest type. It forms a dark purple, sharply demarcated geometrical patch on the liver surface. It has the usual structure of a cavernous angioma (see p.132).
2. **Liver cell adenoma.** These small tumours are rare, but an increased incidence has been associated with the use of contraceptive and anabolic steroids. They consist of normal liver trabeculae without normal portal tracts. Intraperitoneal bleeding may occur.
3. **Bile duct adenoma.** These small tumours are uncommon — and are usually incidental findings at laparotomy. They consist of tiny bile duct structures set in loose connective tissue. Occasionally bile duct cystadenomas form large tumours.

SECONDARY TUMOURS

The liver is by far the most frequent site, of all organs, of secondary tumour deposits and they form the commonest type of liver tumour. Approximately 50% of all primary tumours in the portal area spread to the liver and 33% of all disseminated tumours, whatever the source, involve the liver. Apart from the gastrointestinal tract, the lung and breast are the most frequent sites of primary growth. Melanoma, leukaemic infiltration and involvement by lymphoma are also common.

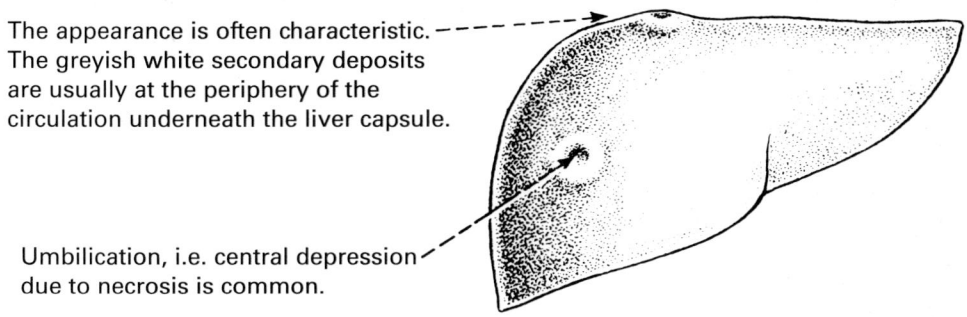

Variations in appearance are produced by haemorrhage, necrosis and the type of tumour, e.g. mucus-secreting carcinomas.

The secondary tumours grow rapidly and are frequently the main cause of death. An exception are the secondary deposits from a carcinoid tumour which grow slowly over a period of years (p.331).

PRIMARY CARCINOMA OF LIVER

HEPATOCELLULAR CARCINOMA (HCC)

This, the commonest primary malignancy of the liver, is unusual in Western Europe, but is very common in Africa and commonest in Mosambique: Males are particularly affected.

Three main types of growth are described:

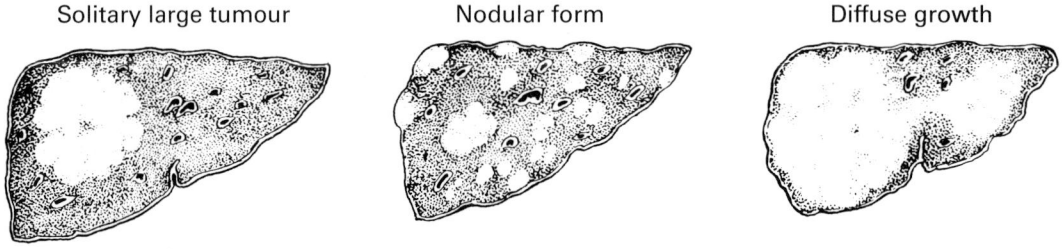

In all three 3 forms the liver is often cirrhotic (80%) (particularly in the West).
Histological structure: The cells grow in columns resembling normal liver.

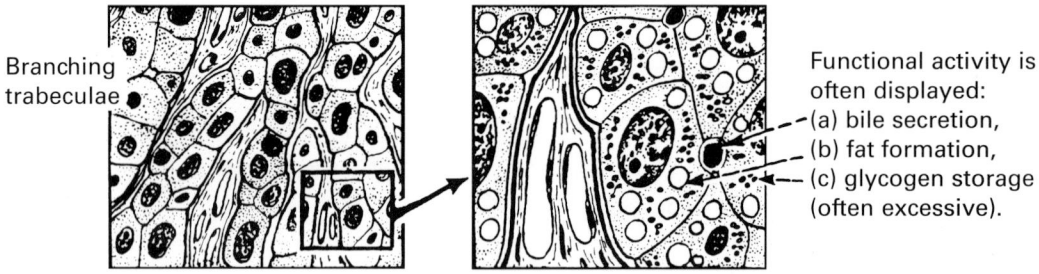

Some tumours are anaplastic with spindle and multi-nucleated giant cells. Others may show a part acinar structure.

Spread

In addition to diffuse growth within the liver, **invasion of hepatic veins** occurs early and there may be metastases to lung, bone and also the draining lymph nodes.

The proximate **cause of death** may be (i) liver failure, (ii) the complications of portal hypertension (especially in cirrhotic patients) and (iii) massive intraperitoneal haemorrhage.

Systemic manifestations include hypoglycaemia, hypercalcaemia and polycythaemia (due to production of erythropoietin).

Diagnosis

Liver biopsy is usually required. High levels of alpha-fetoprotein (normally produced in the fetal liver), >500 μg/ml are strong supportive evidence (not all tumours produce this protein).

Increased levels are also seen in:

1. Cases of testicular teratoma (p.539) or ovarian yolk sac tumour (p.523).
2. Liver damage (the levels are usually not so highly raised).

PRIMARY LIVER CELL TUMOURS

HEPATOCELLULAR CARCINOMA (HCC) (continued)

Aetiology

The aetiological agents vary in low and high incidence areas.

WESTERN EUROPE

ALCOHOLIC LIVER DISEASE

Also chronic active hepatitis including HBV + HCV haemochromatosis

S.E. ASIA and AFRICA

HEPATITIS BV (+C)

Aflatoxins (aspergillus flavus toxins)

In a minority of cases **no cirrhosis** is found

CIRRHOSIS

HEPATOCELLULAR CARCINOMA

FIBROLAMELLAR CARCINOMA

This uncommon variant (<5%) occurs especially in children and young adults. It is important because the prognosis is much better following surgical resection.

Histologically

Large polygonal tumour cells form trabeculae separated by fibrous stroma

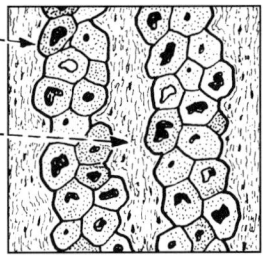

Other differences from conventional HCC are:

(1) Usually no cirrhosis
(2) AFP not raised
(3) Commoner in females
(4) Hepatitis B infection rare — aetiology uncertain.

CHOLANGIOCARCINOMA

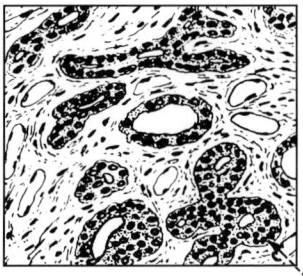

Cells resemble bile duct epithelium.

These tumours arise from bile ducts at both intra- and extrahepatic sites.

They are usually adenocarcinomas: some show excess mucus secretion and evoke a dense fibrous response.

Cirrhosis is rarely present.

There is an increased incidence in association with ulcerative colitis, and in the Far East there is a clear association with liver fluke (clonorchis) infestation.

GALLBLADDER AND BILE DUCT – ANATOMY

Anatomy

Liver

Hepatic ducts

Common bile duct

Gallbladder

Cystic duct (showing 'spiral valve')

COMMON BILE DUCT

Duodenum

Pancreatic duct

Ampulla of Vater

Histology
(Gallbladder)

1. The surface is lined by tall columnar cells.
2. Mucus secreting glands near the neck.
3. Longitudinal, circular and oblique muscle bundles.

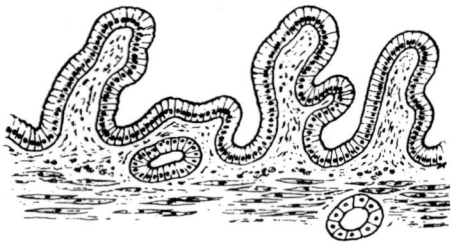

The function of the gallbladder is to concentrate and store bile.

GALLSTONES

Gallstones are the principle cause of gallbladder disease and its consequences.

There are 3 main types:

1. **Cholesterol stone** — is usually solitary, oval and up to 2–3cm in length.

Radiating glistening cholesterol crystals (pale yellow)

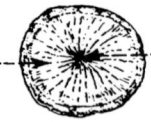

Often has a tiny dark central deposit

They are associated with excessive cholesterol in the bile.

2. **Bile pigment stones** — are always multiple and are usually due to chronic haemolysis with excess bilirubin production.

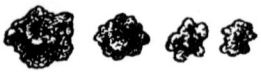

Rarely more than 1 cm in diameter, black and irregular.

3. **Mixed stones** account for 80% of all gallstones. They are always **multiple** and **faceted** due to contact with one another.

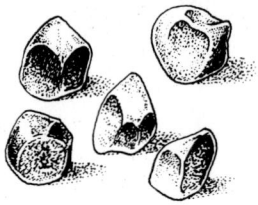

On section

Thin shell of calcium salts

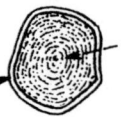

They have a laminated structure — layers of cholesterol, bile pigment and calcium salts.

GALLSTONES

Clinical manifestations and complications

Many subjects are asymptomatic or have only mild dyspepsia — most symptoms are attributable to the complications.

1. **ACUTE CHOLECYSTITIS**

Patients complain of acute onset of right hypochondrial pain and tenderness.

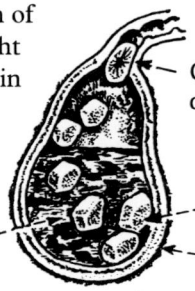

Progress

Mild cases → resolution.

Recurrent attacks → chronic cholecystitis.

Severe cases → perforation → peritonitis.

Severe cases → Empyema (distended bag of pus)

2. **CHRONIC CHOLECYSTITIS**

In the majority of cases the symptoms are of vague 'indigestion', intolerance of fatty foods and vague right hypochondrial pain: in some cases there is a history of acute attacks.

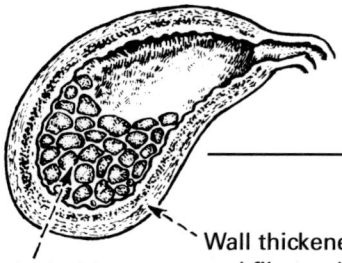

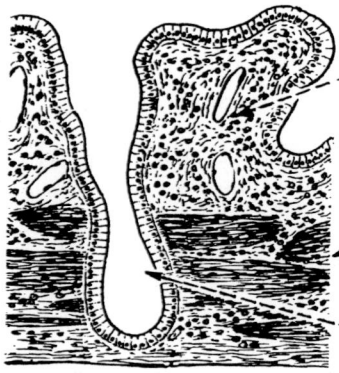

3. **MUCOCELE** — can occur when the cystic duct is blocked.

This occurs when there has been long-standing obstruction of the cystic duct.

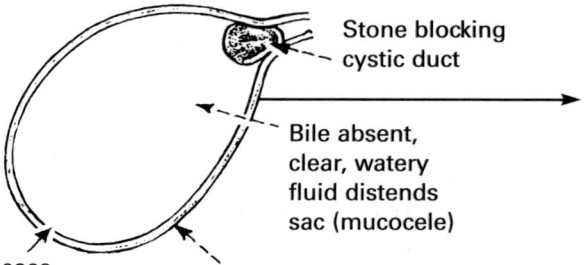

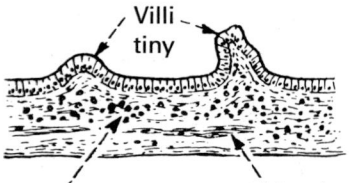

GALLSTONES

GALLSTONES (continued)

4. **COMMON DUCT GALLSTONES**

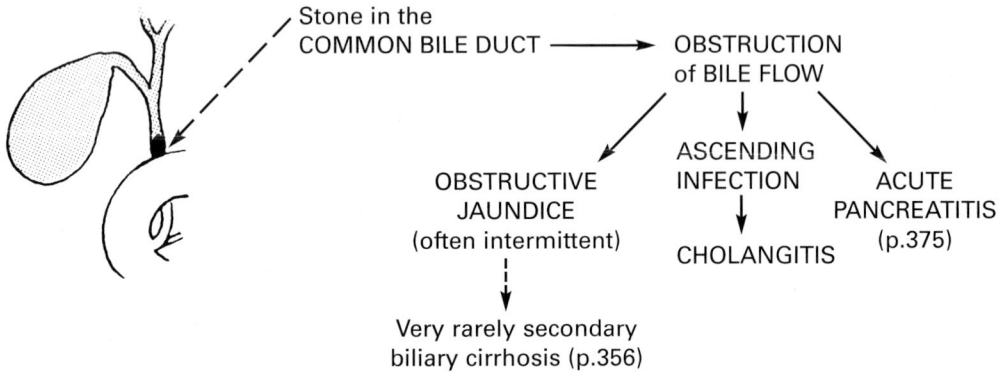

Note: In addition to jaundice, persistent skin itching, due to retention of bile salts, may occur.

5. **GALLSTONE ILEUS**
   Very rarely a stone may ulcerate through the gallbladder into the intestine and cause obstruction.

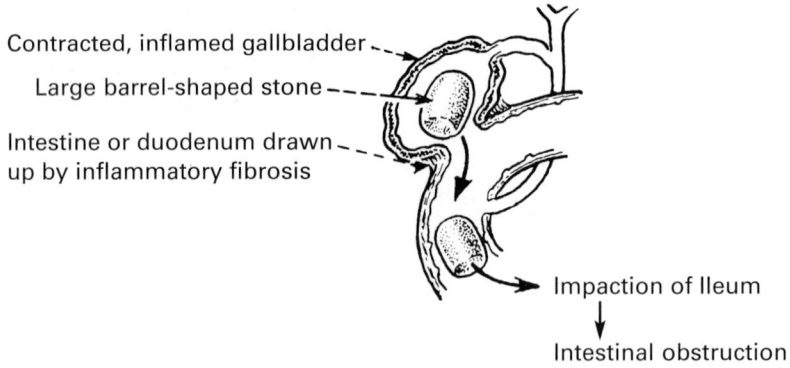

6. **CARCINOMA of the GALLBLADDER**
   This is uncommon, but almost always associated with gallstones.

   Most cases are adenocarcinomas which spread directly to the liver.

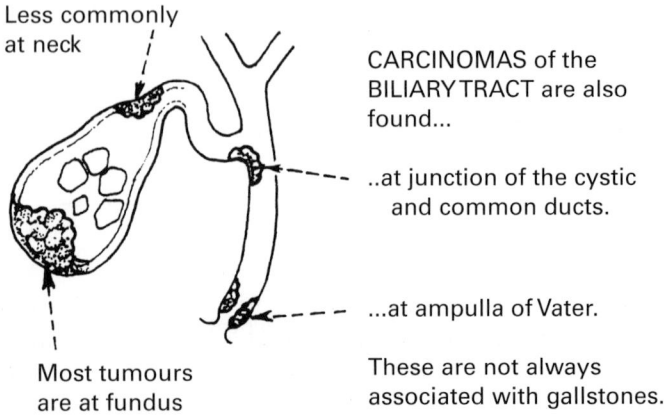

GALLSTONES – AETIOLOGY

Although gallstones are found in 10–20% of the population, the prevalence increasing with age, the exact mechanisms of their formation remain incompletely understood. Risk factors include (a) female gender, (b) obesity, (c) diabetes mellitus, (d) drugs such as the oral contraceptive and the cholesterol lowering drug clofibrate and (e) gastrointestinal disease e.g. Crohn's disease.

The principal constituents of bile are **cholesterol, phospholipids** and **bile acids** (cholic acid and chenodeoxycholic acid).

The **stability of cholesterol** depends on adequate amounts of bile acids. Micelles are formed.

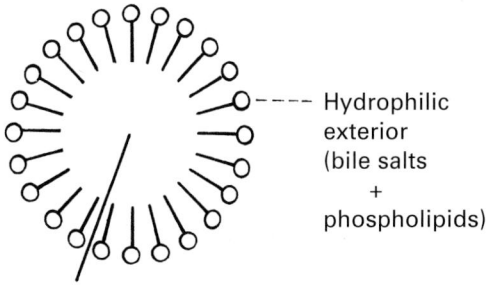

Cholesterol is held in the hydrophobic interior

Their **enterohepatic circulation** is essential to maintain adequate concentrations of bile salts.

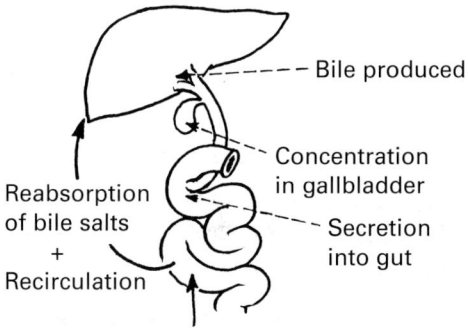

This can be interrupted by mucosal disease e.g. Crohn's disease

The ratio of cholesterol: bile salts is very important.

Increased biliary Cholesterol secretion
or
Increased cholesterol synthesis
or
Decreased bile acid (e.g. in Crohn's disease)

→ Ratio increased $\frac{\text{Cholesterol} \uparrow}{\text{Bile salts} \downarrow}$ → Precipitation of CHOLESTEROL → NUCLEATION (formation of tiny stones)

↓

Progressive accumulation of cholesterol and pigment

↓

ENLARGING STONES

Stones often lead to infection: it is likely that infection promotes further stone production.

These mechanisms are responsible for cholesterol and mixed stones. Pigment stones are seen in haemolytic anaemia, but also are seen in relation to infection e.g. of E.coli. The mechanisms are poorly understood.

PANCREAS

The exocrine glandular portion of the pancreas producing its digestive secretion which is delivered to the second part of the duodenum.

Anatomical variations occur in this region.

Commonly the pancreatic and bile ducts fuse as they enter the ampulla of Vater...

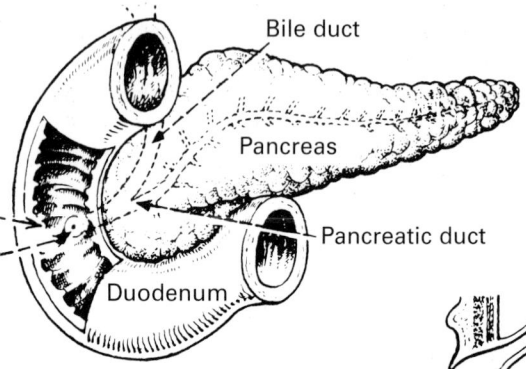

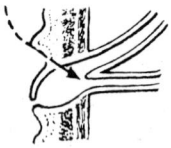

...but sometimes they enter the duodenum separately.

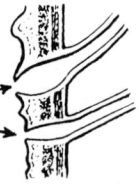

Microscopically, the exocrine tissue is similar to salivary glands.

In addition, foci of endocrine islet tissue occur throughout the pancreas (islets of Langerhans)

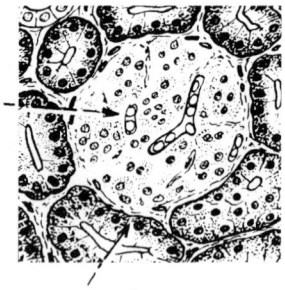

Exocrine secretory granules

Function: The exocrine pancreas produces an alkaline secretion containing digestive enzymes.
Sodium bicarbonate — gives a pH 7.5–8.0
Amylase — splits starches. Lipase — digests lipids.
Trypsinogen } converted to active proteolytic
Chymotrypsinogen } enzymes, trypsin, chymotrypsin.

The islet tissue produces insulin and glucagon (and other neuropeptides). Disorders of the islets e.g. diabetes, are discussed on page 657.

An understanding of the microcirculation is important. The gland has a lobular structure. The larger arteries, veins and ducts course in the fibrous septa between the *lobules.*

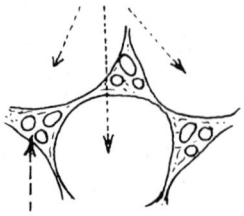

Interlobular artery, vein and duct

This diagram shows the circulation and duct system within the lobule (intralobular).

This watershed zone at the *periphery* of the lobule is susceptible when there is a circulatory perfusion deficit

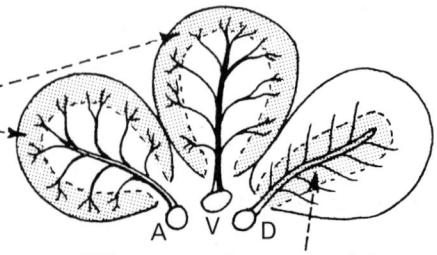

This zone at the centre of the lobule is susceptible if there is damage to the intralobular duct

ACUTE PANCREATITIS

There is evidence that mild pancreatitis is not uncommon but, in a significant number of cases, progression to a severe fatal disease occurs. Clinically, there is an acute abdominal emergency with pain and shock.

The essential pathological changes are due to tissue necrosis caused by the action of liberated enzymes on the pancreatic tissues. The severity of the lesion depends on the amount of enzyme set free, the distance it diffuses and the structures affected. The pancreatic damage occurs in two forms:

1. **Periductal necrosis** — in the centre of each affected lobule.

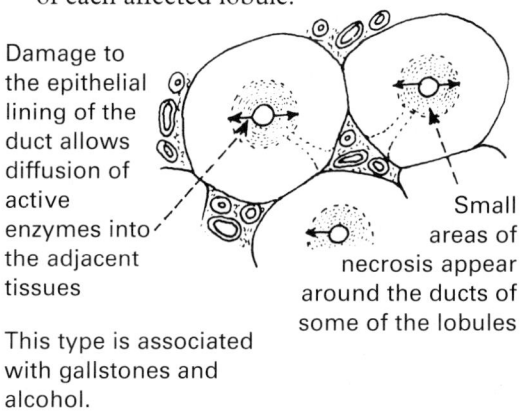

2. **Perilobular necrosis** — affecting the periphery of lobules.

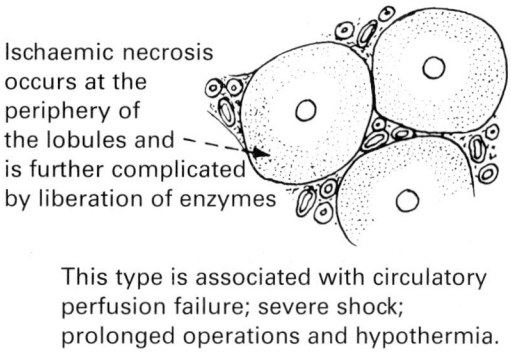

Both types of damage if not inhibited by antitrypsins and α_2 macroglobulins derived from the blood and pancreas itself will progress often very rapidly to the very severe form —

PANLOBULAR PANCREATITIS

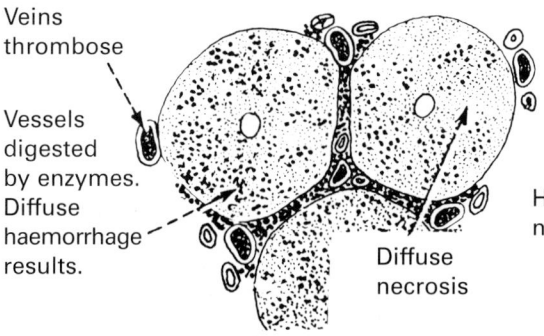

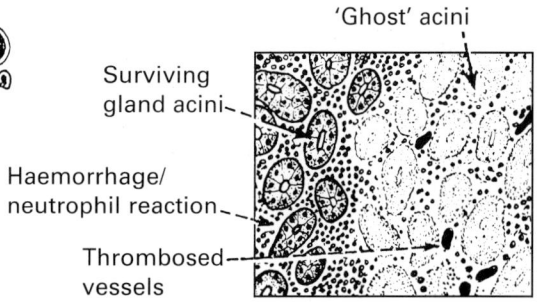

The initial damage is severe, and large quantities of enzymes are liberated, including trypsin, chymotrypsin, lipase, elastase and phospholipase. Locally, these set up a progressive pathological process.

ACUTE PANCREATITIS

SEVERE PANCREATITIS (continued)

Damage to pancreas
↓
Release of enzymes — especially activation of TRYPSIN
↓
Digestion of cell membranes
↓ ↓
Necrosis of gland tissue → Further release of enzymes
Necrosis of interstitial tissue → Thrombosis and necrosis of vessels
↓ ↓
Extension of pancreatic damage

The released enzymes spread beyond the exocrine tissues of the pancreas:

1. ***Via lymphatics to abdominal tissues*** especially the omentum and mesenteries

Naked eye appearance

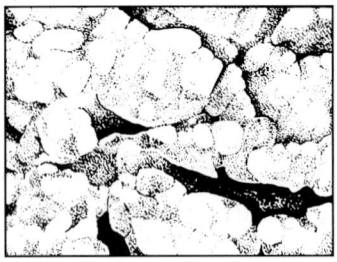

Opaque white patches of necrotic fatty tissue — due to phospholipase and proteolytic enzymes containing free fatty acids — lipase splits fat

2. ***Locally causing destruction of islet tissue*** — hyperglycaemia may occur.

3. ***Via blood stream.***

Enzymes and cytokines (e.g. TNFα)
↓ ↓ ↓ ↓
Clotting difficulties → Severe shock
Effusion of fluids in serous cavities and lungs → Severe shock
Lower blood pressure → Severe shock
Gastroduodenal haemorrhage → Severe shock

These effects are largely due to activation of thromboplastins and formation of vasoactive kinins. Hypoxia due to pulmonary oedema intensifies the shock.

Hypocalcaemia giving rise to tetany may occur due to deposition of calcium soaps in the necrotic fat cells of the omentum and peritoneum. Commonly hypocalcaemia merely reflects low serum albumin levels.

The appearance of amylase in the blood stream is used as a diagnostic test.

ACUTE PANCREATITIS

Aetiology
Two factors are important: (1) gallstones and (2) alcohol.

Gallstones
Between 40 and 60% of all cases of severe pancreatitis are associated with gallstones. Recurrent attacks are common, and in a recent study of known gallstone patients who developed pancreatitis, gallstones were found in the biliary tree or stools of 80%.

A likely mechanism postulated is of

Bile reflux
In most patients, the bile duct and pancreatic duct have a common entrance to the ampulla of Vater. Stones passing down the bile duct could, by blocking the ampulla, cause reflux of bile along the pancreatic duct.

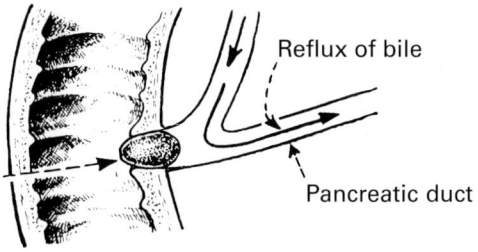

Note: Pancreatitis may occur in these patients whose common bile duct and pancreatic duct enter the ampulla separately (p.374).

Alcohol
Acute pancreatitis is common in alcoholics and the incidence of this association is directly related to the consumption of alcohol by the local population.

The causal relationship is obscure, but it is possible that in both gallstone and alcoholic pancreatitis there is a common pathogenic mechanism. Alcohol may cause ampullary spasm.

Other causes include:
Trauma, including surgery.
Viruses e.g. mumps, coxsackie B.
Hypercalcaemia e.g. in hyperparathyroidism.
Drugs e.g. steroids.

Complications
(i) Shock is common, leading to death in 10% of patients.
(ii) Recurrent attacks may lead to chronic pancreatitis.
(iii) Collections of fluid may be surrounded by fibrous tissue — pancreatic pseudocyst (p. 379).

CHRONIC PANCREATITIS

The true incidence of this condition is unknown but from post mortem evidence it appears to be quite common. Several types have been described, but the pathological changes are similar in all cases.

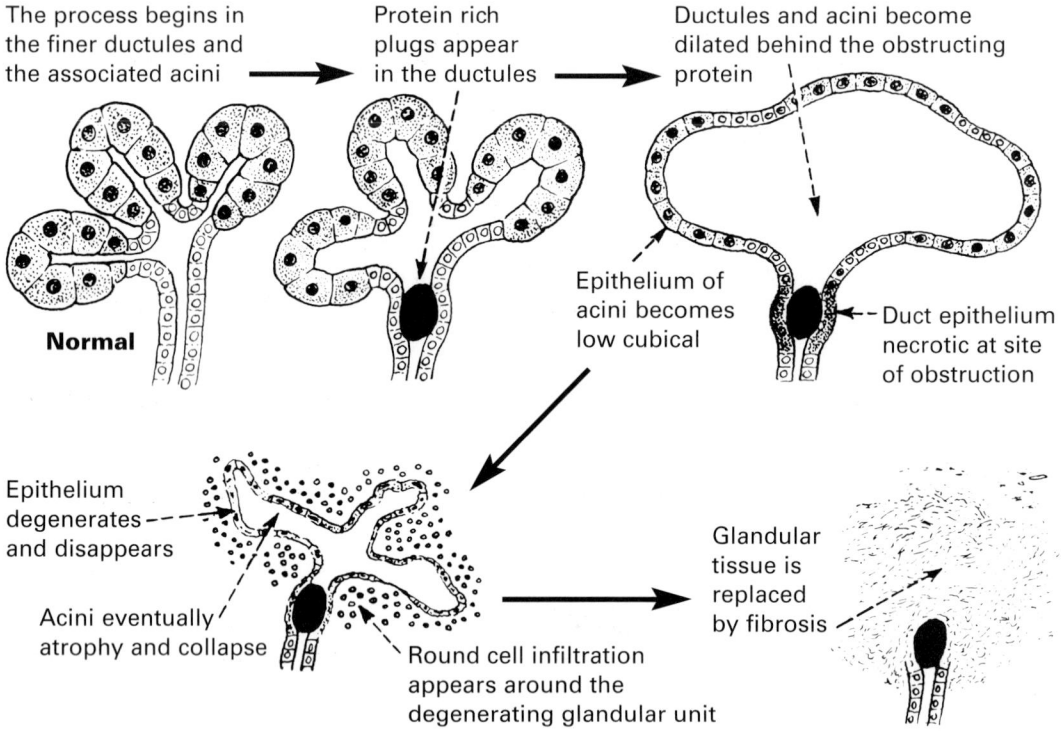

The change is focal. More and more protein plugs form, some in larger ducts. Obstruction of these may lead to production of cysts.

Ultimately, a large proportion of the exocrine tissue is destroyed.

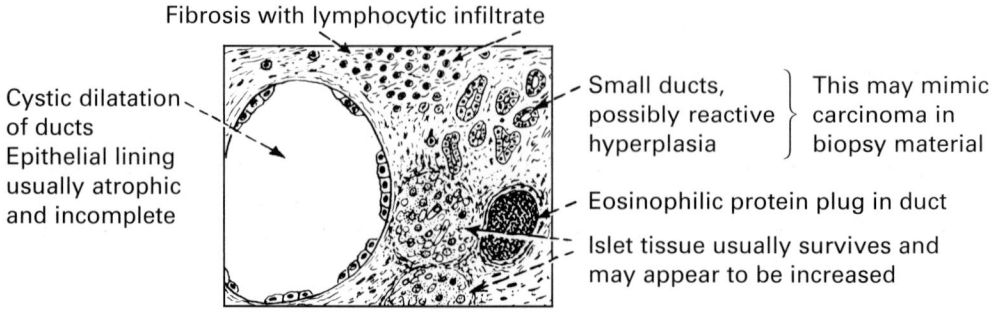

CHRONIC PANCREATITIS

With progress of the disease, two other developments take place:

1. *Calcification.* This occurs mainly in the protein plugs in the ducts, resulting in the formation of calculi.
2. *Rupture of the duct cysts into the surrounding tissues.* A granulation tissue reaction is set up with formation of a pseudocyst. The result depends on the site of the pseudocyst.

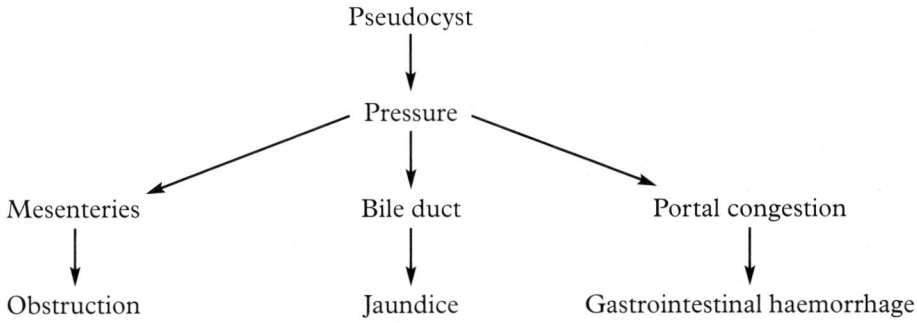

Rupture into the peritoneal cavity causes ascites, frequently haemorrhagic.

Progressive destruction of the parenchyma with fibrosis may ultimately convert the pancreatitis into a thin hard cord.

Effects

Patients typically complain of abdominal pain.

Apart from the complications due to cyst rupture, destruction of pancreatic tissue may lead to:

1. Insufficiency of exocrine secretion → steatorrhoea and wasting.
2. Diabetes mellitus. This is a rare complication due to destruction of islet tissue.

Aetiology

1. The main factor in 75% of cases in Western civilisation is alcohol. Patients have generally consumed more than 150 g daily over a long period of time.
2. In 1% of cases there is biliary disease.
3. Some cases may follow recurrent attacks of acute pancreatitis.
4. A peculiar type of chronic pancreatitis occurs in Africa and South East Asia. It is related to chronic malnutrition with particular deficiency of protein, from infancy. Extensive calcification of the pancreatic tissues occurs. It has been suggested that there is a genetic predisposition to the disease.

CYSTIC FIBROSIS OF THE PANCREAS (Mucoviscidosis)

This is a common autosomal recessive inherited disease due to genetic mutation on chromosome 7; a high percentage (about 4%) of the population are carriers.

The gene involved is called cystic fibrosis transmembrane conductance regulator (CFTR). Its essential function is the control of the transfer of chloride across cell membranes. Many mutations of the gene have been recorded, each being responsible for subtle variations in the evolution of the disorder.

All the exocrine secretory tissues are affected to a greater or lesser degree: the pathological results vary according to which organ is mainly affected — pancreas, bronchi, bowel, biliary tree, testis.

The essential change is as follows:

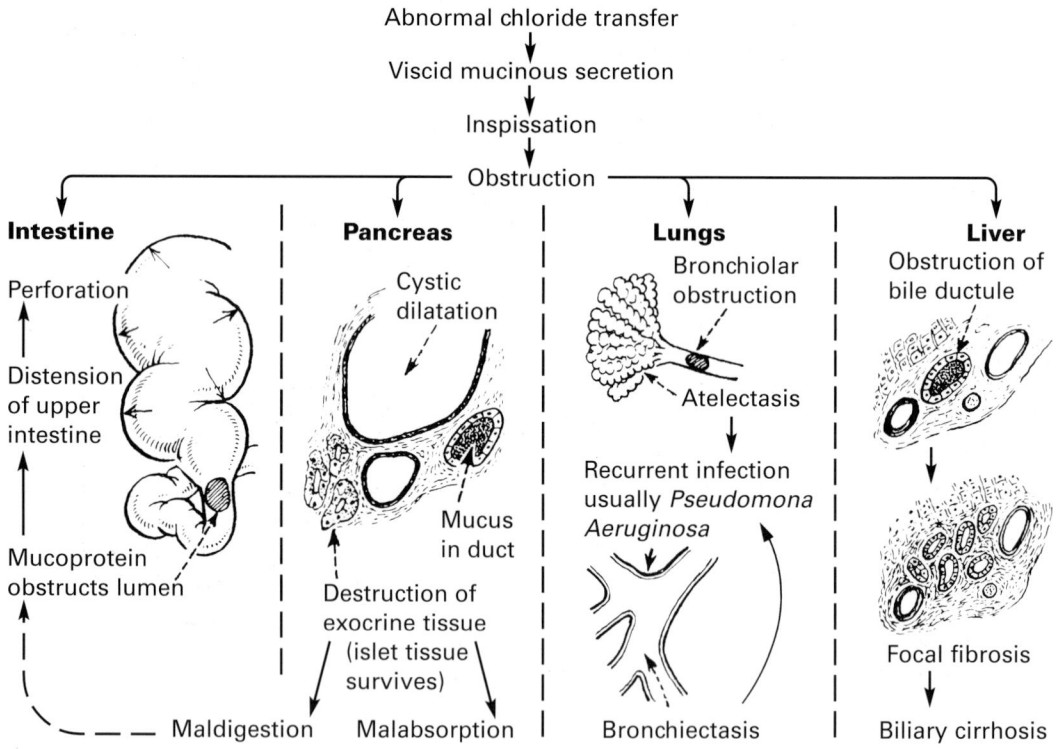

Clinical features

Neonatal

Intestinal obstruction (meconium ileus) may lead to intestinal perforation and fatal peritonitis.

Childhood:

There is failure to thrive due to maldigestion and malabsorption, and steatorrhea is common — all features of pancreatic insufficiency. If the lungs are affected, there is chronic respiratory difficulty with emphysema and bronchiectasis, usually proving fatal at an early age. Liver lesions are of late development.

There is increase of sodium chloride in the sweat of patients and their heterozygote siblings. This provides a diagnostic test which is now being replaced by genetic screening.

TUMOURS OF PANCREAS

Simple tumours of the pancreas are very rare. Occasionally cystadenomas, lipomas and fibromas occur. They may produce symptoms due to pressure on other structures.

CARCINOMA

This is by no means rare, particularly in Western countries and Japan.

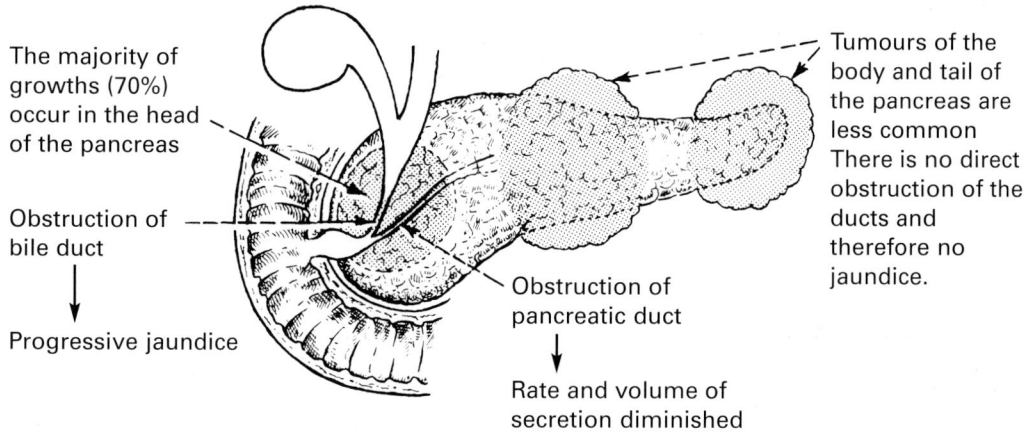

Regional and/or distant metastases are found in 85% of cases at the time of diagnosis and the 5 year survival rate is 1% — the lowest of all cancers.

The growth arises from the duct epithelium and in almost all cases it is an adenocarcinoma. Papillary cystadenocarcinoma, adenosquamous carcinoma and giant cell carcinoma are forms occasionally encountered.

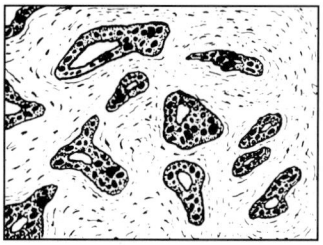

Tumours in the body and tail are commonly larger than tumours of the head, probably due to later diagnosis in the relative absence of symptoms. Thrombosis of unknown cause and at distant sites, e.g. femoral, is apt to occur when the tumour is in the body or tail.

Aetiology

1. Pancreatic carcinoma is most frequent in males in the 5th–7th decades.
2. There is a statistical association with alcohol, cigarette smoking and a diet high in fat and carbohydrate.
3. In the U.S.A., the incidence is higher in the black population and a similar situation is true of the Maoris in New Zealand.

Endocrine Tumours

Islet cell tumours are described on page 661.

CHAPTER 11

HAEMOPOIETIC AND LYMPHO-RETICULAR TISSUES

Haemopoiesis 384
Haematology — Laboratory Tests. 385, 386
Anaemia 387–390
Iron Deficiency Anaemia 391–394
The Megaloblastic Anaemias 395
Pernicious Anaemia (PA) 396–399
Folic Acid Deficiency 400
Acute Post-Haemorrhagic Anaemia .. 401
The Haemolytic Anaemias 402–405
Extrinsic Haemolytic Anaemias 406
Incompatible Blood Transfusion/ Haemolytic Disease of the Newborn. 407
Haemolytic Disease of the Newborn . 408
Extrinsic Haemolytic Anaemias 409–411
Extrinsic Haemolytic Anaemias — Malaria 412
Intrinsic Haemolytic Anaemias. 413, 414
Disorders of Haemoglobin Synthesis. 415
The Thalassaemias 416
Sickle Cell Disease 417
Anaemia of Chronic Disorders 418
Aplastic Anaemia 419
Anaemia — Morphological Classification 420
Polycythaemia 421
Neutrophil Granulocytes 422
Disorders of Neutrophils 423, 424
Platelets and Coagulation 425
Disorders of Platelets 426
The Coagulation Cascade 427
Acquired Defects of Coagulation 428
Inherited Defects of Coagulation 429
Disseminated Intravascular Coagulation 430
Thrombophilia —Thrombotic Disorders 431
The Lymphoid System 432
Lymphadenopathy 433
Lymphadenopathy — Infections 434
Lymphadenopathy 435
Lymphadenopathy — Non-Infective Causes 436
Spleen 437
Splenomegaly 438–441
Diseases of the Spleen — Miscellaneous 442
Thymus 443, 444
Neoplastic Lymphadenopathy 445
Non-Hodgkin's Lymphomas 446–449
Plasma Cell Tumours 450, 451
Non-Hodgkin's Lymphoma —T Cell 452
Hodgkin's Disease 453, 454
Leukaemias 455, 456
Acute Myeloblastic Leukaemia 457
Chronic Myeloid Leukaemia (CML) 458
Chronic Lymphocytic Leukaemia 459
Acute Lymphoblastic Leukaemia (ALL) 460
Myeloproliferative Disorders 461

HAEMOPOIESIS

The derivation of blood cells

In the **bone marrow** a **'pluripotent' stem cell** gives rise to **all blood cells.**

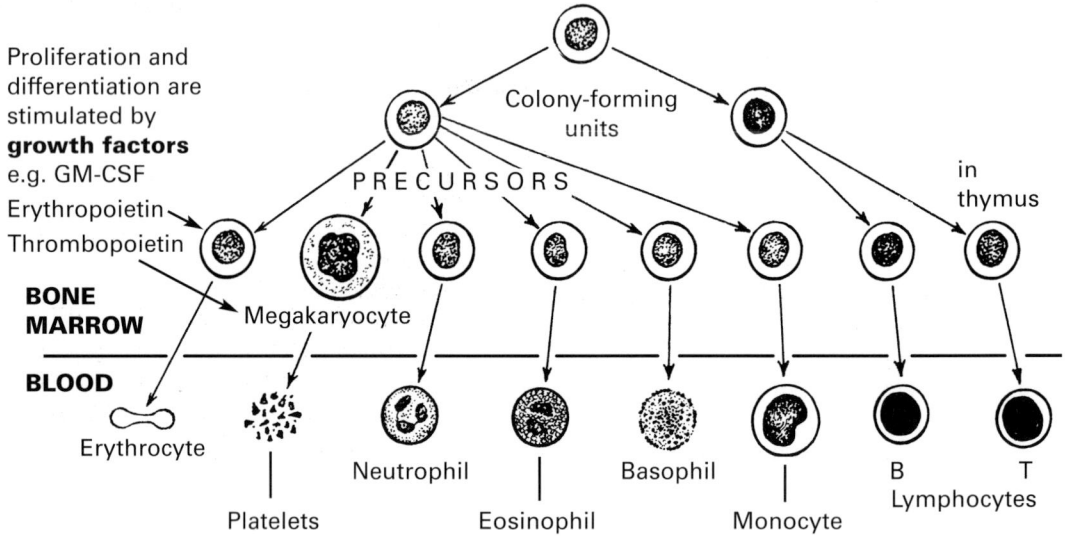

Haemopoiesis in bone marrow

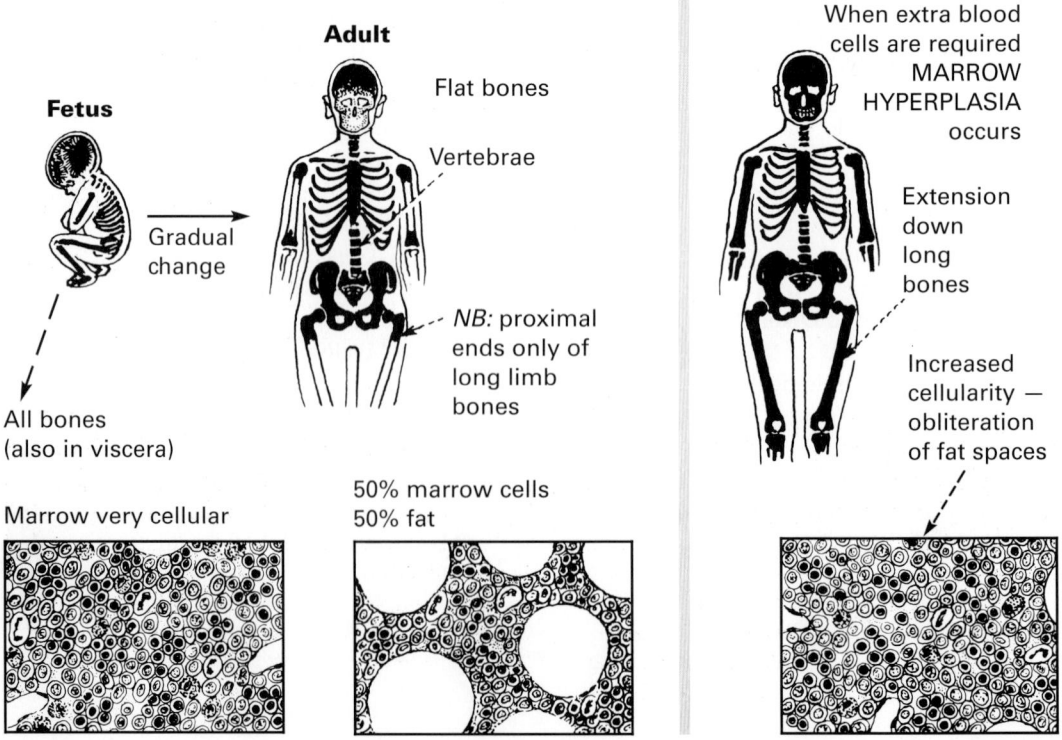

HAEMATOLOGY — LABORATORY TESTS

Investigation of blood diseases depends on examination of 1. PERIPHERAL BLOOD and 2. BONE MARROW.

1. PERIPHERAL BLOOD

Blood count: this is normally done by sophisticated electronic machines.

The main parameters are:

(i) **HAEMOGLOBIN (Hb) CONCENTRATION** (g/dl whole blood)
Normal values: Male 15.5±2.5: Female 14.0±2.5

(ii) **CELL COUNT**
Red Cell count: Males $5.5 \pm 1.0 \times 10^{12}$/l.
Females $4.8 \pm 1.0 \times 10^{12}$/l.
White Cell Count: $4–11 \times 10^9$/l.
Neutrophils — $2.0–7.5 \times 10^9$/l.
Lymphocytes — $1.5–4.0 \times 10^9$/l.
Monocytes — $0.2–0.8 \times 10^9$/l.
Eosinophils — $0.04–0.4 \times 10^9$/l.
Basophils — $0.01–0.1 \times 10^9$/l.
Platelets — $150–400 \times 10^9$/l.

(iii) **MEAN RED CELL VOLUME (MCV)**
Normal — 85±8 fl (femtolitres)

Also measured are:
MEAN CELL HAEMOGLOBIN
Normal = 29.5±2.5 picograms.
MEAN CELL HAEMOGLOBIN CONCENTRATION (MCHC)
Normal = 33±3 g/dl.

BLOOD FILM — stained by a Romanowski method.

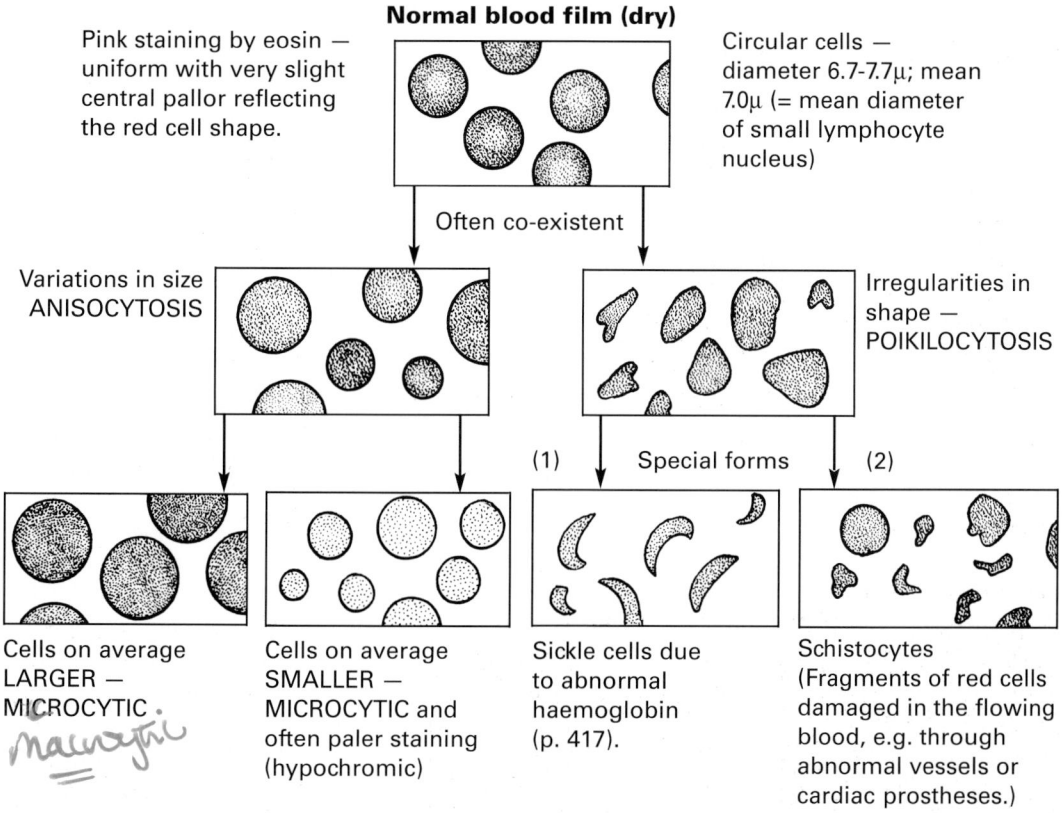

HAEMATOLOGY — LABORATORY TESTS

Another useful test is the measurement of the **PACKED CELL VOLUME (PCV).**

This is obtained by centrifuging anticoagulated whole blood in a haematocrit tube.

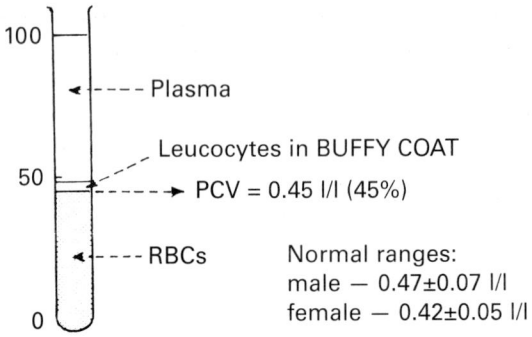

2. BONE MARROW EXAMINATION

Examination of bone marrow is important in explaining abnormalities of the peripheral blood.

In the past, aspiration of marrow from the sternum was commonly performed. Now the posterior iliac crest is used — it is safer and allows marrow to be **aspirated** and a **trephine** biopsy to be taken.

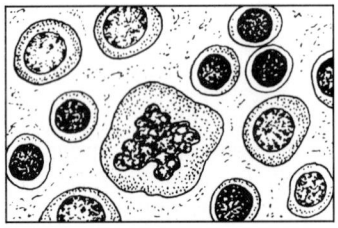

Film of aspirate allows detailed observation of **cell morphology.**

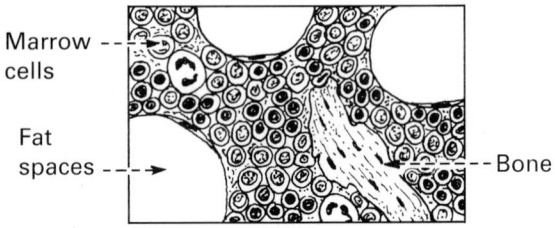

Histological preparation of trephine material allows assessment of **architecture.**

ERYTHROPOIESIS

Normal marrow erythropoiesis is said to be NORMOBLASTIC.

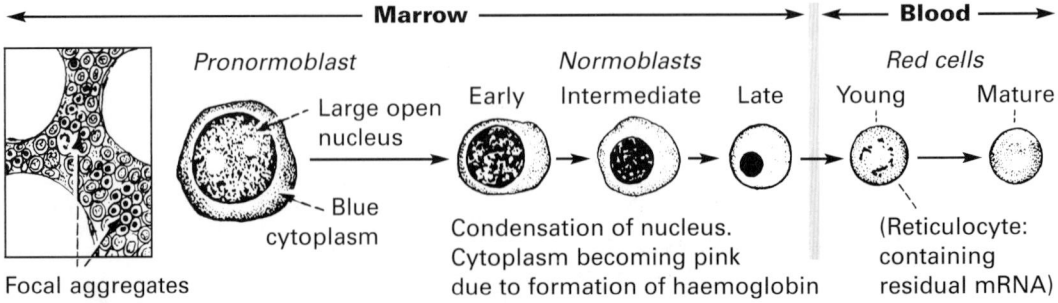

(1) Normal maturation involves condensation and ultimate discharge of the nucleus.
(2) Synthesis of haemoglobin in the cytoplasm.
(3) Diminution in cell size.

When the essential factors vit. B_{12} or folic acid are deficient, the red cell precursors show clear morphological changes — erythropoiesis is said to be MEGALOBLASTIC (p. 395).

ANAEMIA

The most important function of the red cell is the transport of oxygen bound to haemoglobin. The most common and important disorder associated with disease of the red cells is ANAEMIA, which is defined as a reduction below normal of the concentration of haemoglobin in the blood.

Anaemia in men — Hb < 13 g/dl: in women — < 12 g/dl.

Effect of anaemia

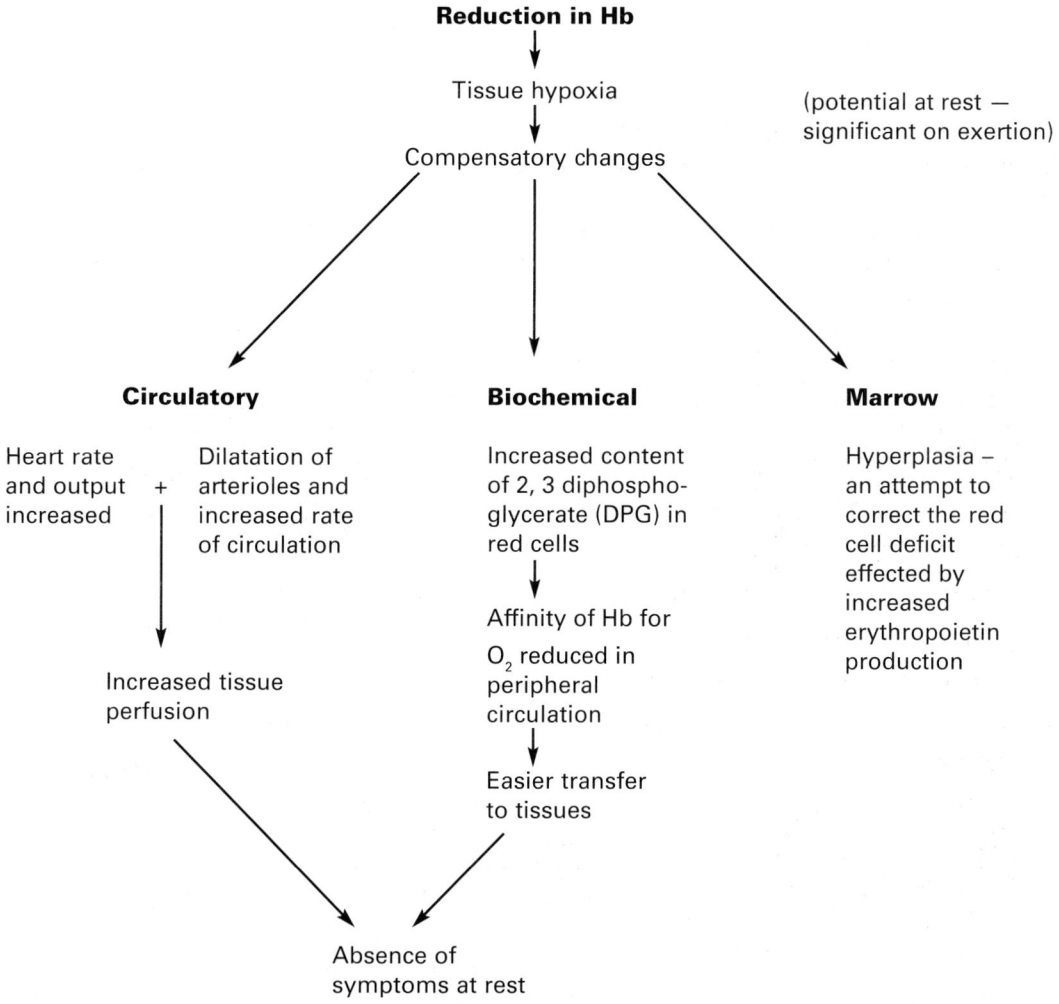

Clinical associations

1. Diminished exercise tolerance, i.e. dyspnoea on exertion.
2. Rapid, full, bounding pulse: decreased circulation time.

Note: Pallor is not a reliable sign of anaemia — it may be obscured by the circulatory changes.

ANAEMIA

The effects of anaemia are greatly influenced by its severity, duration and rate of development.

In moderate anaemias of slow evolution, symptoms such as dyspnoea only appear on exertion, and even when the haemoglobin falls as low as 6–7 g/dl, clinical indications may be slight.

Pathological complications of anaemia

1. Effects of degenerative arterial disease are aggravated, e.g. symptoms of ANGINA PECTORIS and lower limb CLAUDICATION are increased.
2. In severe anaemias effects are seen in organs.

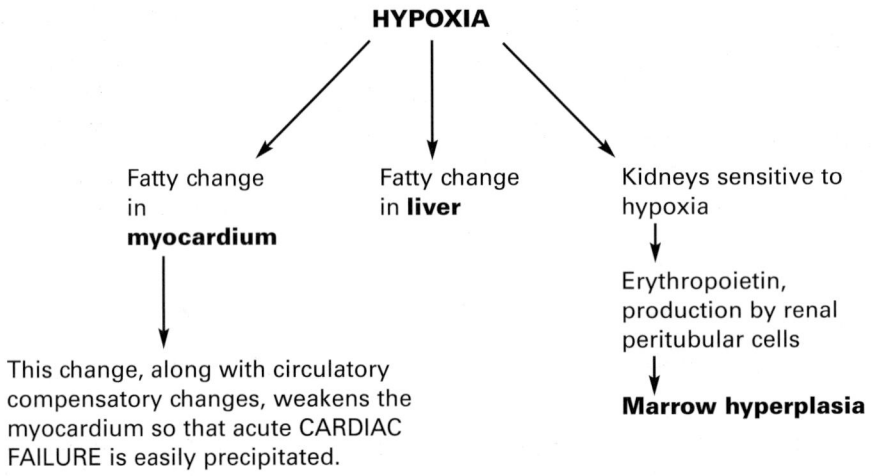

Note: Therefore blood transfusion used in the treatment of anaemia is given ***slowly*** and as ***packed cells*** to avoid fluid overload.

In very rapidly developing anaemias, the compensatory mechanisms cannot adjust adequately – the condition merges into SHOCK.

ANAEMIA

Aetiology

Although in the last analysis any anaemia is due to the failure of the bone marrow to produce sufficient red cells in any particular circumstance, an understanding of the role of various aetiological agents and of the **four main mechanisms** by which anaemia develops depends on a knowledge of the basic facts of the life cycle of the red blood cells.

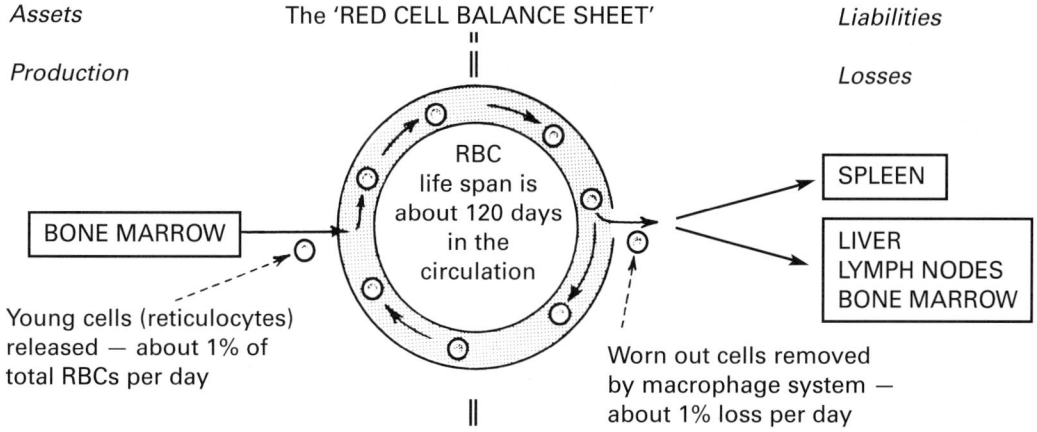

Mechanisms

(A) in the marrow

(i) Actual diminution in productive marrow (hypoplasia or aplasia) or marrow replacement by tumour.

↓

HYPOPLASTIC ANAEMIAS

(ii) Marrow unable to produce sufficient normal red cells, usually due to deficiency of an essential factor. e.g. iron: Vit B12.

↓

DYSHAEMOPOIETIC ANAEMIAS

(B) in the circulation

(iii) Excessive loss of RBCs due to acute haemorrhage.

↓

ACUTE POST-HAEMORRHAGIC ANAEMIA

(iv) Excessive destruction of RBCs by the macrophage system particularly in the spleen
(a) of normal RBCs e.g. in hypersplenism or auto-immunity,
(b) of abnormal cells e.g. hereditary spherocytosis.

↓

HAEMOLYTIC ANAEMIAS

Note: Many forms of anaemia have more than one component.

e.g. 1. The abnormal cells produced in the hypoplastic and dyshaemopoietic anaemias usually have a shortened life span so that a haemolytic element is superimposed.

2. The anaemia of chronic blood loss is almost wholly dyshaemopoietic in type due to the external loss of iron.

ANAEMIA

HYPOPLASTIC and APLASTIC ANAEMIAS

These are rare conditions and, as the names imply, are due to marrow failure with diminished numbers or absence of haemopoietic cells. Usually all three marrow cell lines are affected, resulting in *pancytopenia* in the peripheral blood.

Marrow failure of this type is dealt with in detail on page 419.

Marrow failure due to extensive tumour infiltration or fibrosis also occurs.

The anaemias associated with miscellaneous chronic diseases ('Secondary' anaemias) are dealt with on page 418.

DYSHAEMOPOIETIC ANAEMIAS

The usual cause of these anaemias is deficiency of an essential factor required for proper haemoglobin synthesis or erythroblast maturation and development. They are associated with a hypercellular marrow and are divided into two main groups:

(1) normoblastic and (2) megaloblastic, depending on the type of erythroblastic maturation in the marrow.

Deficiency of essential factor

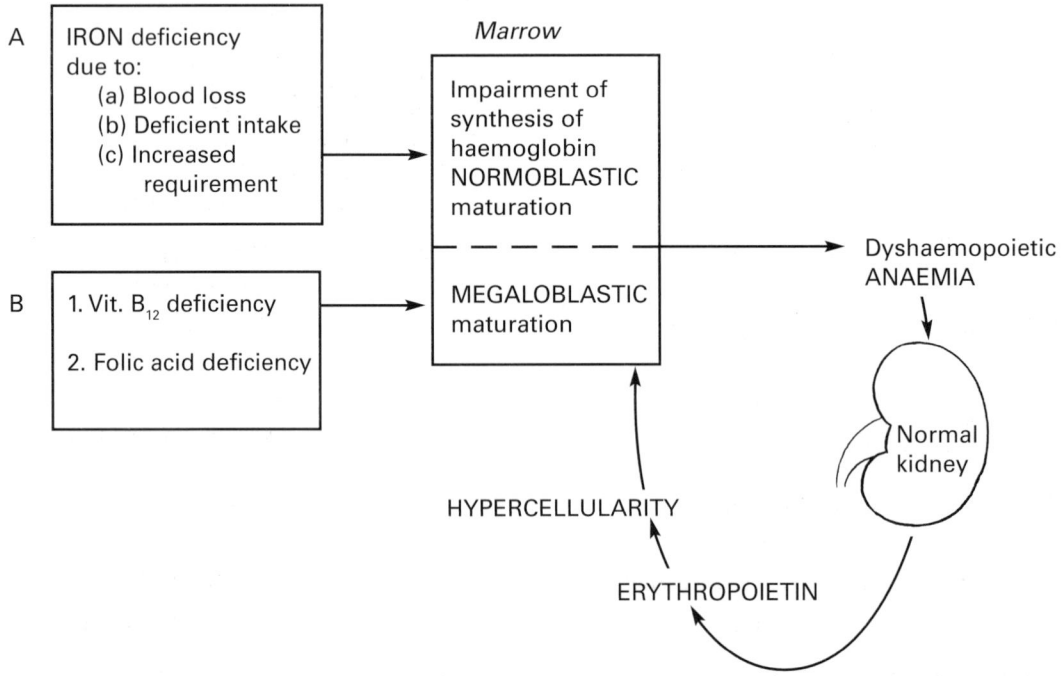

Note: In severe renal failure, deficiency of erythropoietin may contribute to anaemia.

IRON DEFICIENCY ANAEMIA

IRON DEFICIENCY ANAEMIA is the commonest anaemia on a world basis due to (a) poor nutrition, (b) intestinal parasites (esp. hookworm) causing bleeding and (c) multiple pregnancies.

In Western countries, in the adult male and post-menopausal women, iron deficiency anaemia is nearly always due to alimentary blood loss and reflects the incidence of the causative diseases, e.g. cancer, peptic ulceration, hiatus hernia, aspirin ingestion, etc.

Without IRON the haem moiety of the haemoglobin molecule cannot be synthesised.

IRON DEFICIENCY
↓
DEFECTIVE SYNTHESIS OF HAEMOGLOBIN
↓
ANAEMIA

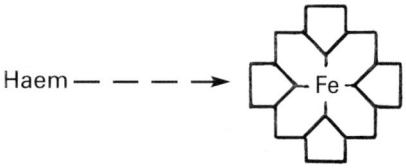

Changes in the blood are mainly in the red cells which become:

MICROCYTIC (cells smaller — mean diameter < 6.7μ)

HYPOCHROMIC (contain less haemoglobin ∴ less well stained).

Normal

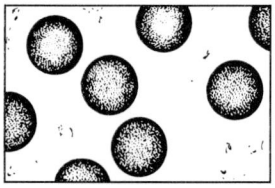

Fairly uniform red cells — size and shape (mean diameter 7.2μ)

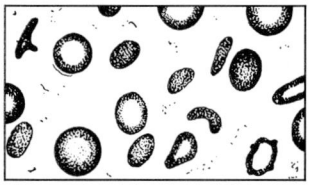

Definite central pallor — ring staining
Variation in size — anisocytosis
Variation in shape — poikilocytosis

MCV (fl) (mean cell volume) is ..... LOW (< 80)
(Normal: 80–92)

MCH (pg) (mean cell haemoglobin) is ..... LOW (< 27)
(Normal: 27–32)

MCHC (mean corpuscular haemoglobin concentration) is ..... LOW (30 g/dl)
derived from Hb and haematocrit PCV: $\frac{\text{Hb g/dl}}{\text{PCV l/l}}$ Normal mean: (34 g/dl)

Serum IRON (normal 10–30 μmol/l) is ..... LOW (< 7)
(0.7–1.8 mg/l)

Serum FERRITIN (normal 15–300 μg/l) is ..... LOW (< 10)

Serum IRON BINDING CAPACITY (45–70 μmol/l) is ..... RAISED (> 75)

Serum IRON SATURATION $\left(\frac{\text{IRON}}{\text{Binding capacity}} \times 100\right)$ [Normal16–60%] ..... LOW (10%)

The reticulocyte count is NORMAL except following episodes of haemorrhage. Usually there are no changes in the leucocytes and platelets.

The **bone marrow** is hypercellular and contains many small poorly haemoglobinised normoblasts; no stainable iron is present.

IRON DEFICIENCY ANAEMIA

IRON METABOLISM

Iron is normally conserved and is recycled so that absorption of iron from the diet, which occurs maximally in the duodenum and upper jejunum, is required to replace only the small inevitable losses. Since the diet contains iron in excess of requirements, the intestinal mucosal apoferritin mechanism exists to control absorption.

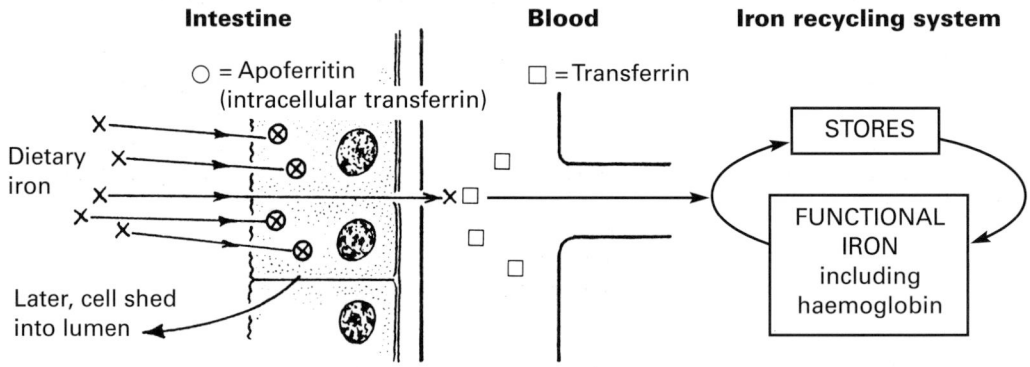

The iron (×) in the diet enters the mucosal cell and having combined with apoferritin (○) is retained in the cell as ferritin (⊗).

NB This bound iron is subsequently shed along with the cell into the lumen.

Iron unbound by apoferritin passes through the cell and is transported in the blood to join the iron recycling system.

Note: new haemoglobin formed in the bone marrow contains 95% iron from recycling system, 5% from diet.

The state of the iron stores controls the apoferritin (a form of intracellular transferrin) content of the intestinal mucosal cell by a feed-back mechanism, thus:

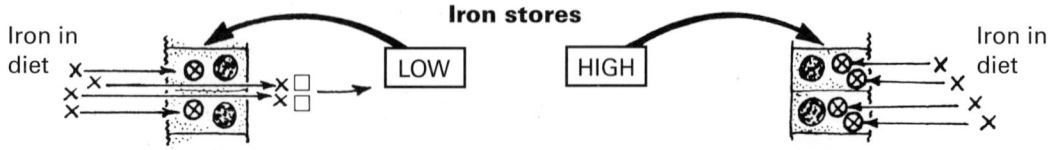

APOFERRITIN LOW
∴ Decreased binding (ferritin)
∴ *Increased absorption*

APOFERRITIN HIGH
∴ Increased binding
∴ *Decreased absorption*

ACUTE IRON OVERLOAD

If a large dose of medicinal iron preparations is taken (particularly by children in error) the absorption and transport mechanisms are overwhelmed and free iron radicles exert very toxic effects.

IRON DEFICIENCY ANAEMIA

The iron balance may be summarised as follows.

INPUT (Adult male)	BODY IRON Total 3-6g		OUTPUT
Average: 1 mg/day derived from foods (a) animal muscle (b) vegetables. The average diet contains 10–20 mg iron, of which about 10% is absorbed. In the adult female, the average daily input is about 2 mg.	(a) *Functional iron* in haemoglobin, myoglobin, enzyme systems, transferrin	80% at least	Average: 1 mg/day Skin desquamation and miscellaneous secretions *Menstruation* This extra loss of about 0.5 to 1 mg requires extra input in the female
	(b) *Storage iron* in liver, spleen, bone marrow as ferritin, haemosiderin	20% or less	

Anaemia results when this delicate balance is upset in one of three main ways.

1. *Increased output* This almost always is caused by blood loss — often small in amount and chronic (1 ml blood = 0.5 mg iron). In the female, uterine bleeding is a common cause, and in both sexes bleeding from the alimentary tract is important.
2. *Decreased input*
   (a) Poor diet (including diets containing substances antagonistic to iron absorption, e.g. phytates, phosphates)
   (b) Malabsorption — due to bowel disease e.g. coeliac disease, or post-surgical e.g. post-gastrectomy.
3. *Increased body requirement*
   (a) During rapid growth in childhood
   (b) In pregnancy.

Usually anaemia develops slowly (except in cases of serious haemorrhage).

(1) Iron deficiency → (2) Mobilisation of reserves (first haemosiderin then ferritin) → (3) Exhaustion of reserves → (4) Deficient synthesis of haemoglobin → (5) Anaemia

Increased absorption if available in diet may postpone (4)

IRON DEFICIENCY ANAEMIA

Associated changes

In addition to the pathological changes due to anaemia per se, the following conditions may be associated with iron deficiency anaemia.

(1) ***Angular cheilosis***
Atrophic glossitis

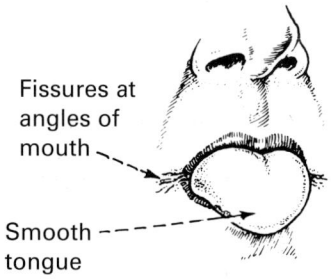

(2) ***Dysphagia*** — the Brown-Kelly-Paterson or Plummer-Vinson syndrome

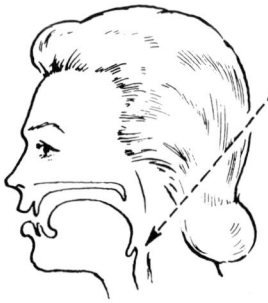

(3)

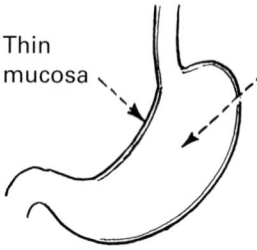

Hypochlorhydria
↓
Achlorhydria
} With gastritis and mucosal atrophy

This aggravates any malabsorption of iron

(4) ***Koilonychia***

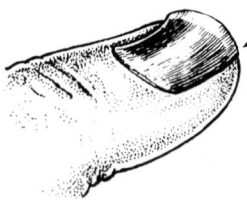

These associated changes are in part due to iron deficiency itself, but in many cases are probably the result of deficiencies of other factors in addition, e.g. vitamins and minerals.

THE MEGALOBLASTIC ANAEMIAS

These dyshaemopoietic anaemias are almost always caused by deficiency of either vitamin B_{12} or folic acid which are intracellular co-enzymes, particularly important for the synthesis of DNA.

The effects of deficiency occur in most organs of the body but are prominent where cell turnover is rapid, e.g. in the **marrow**.

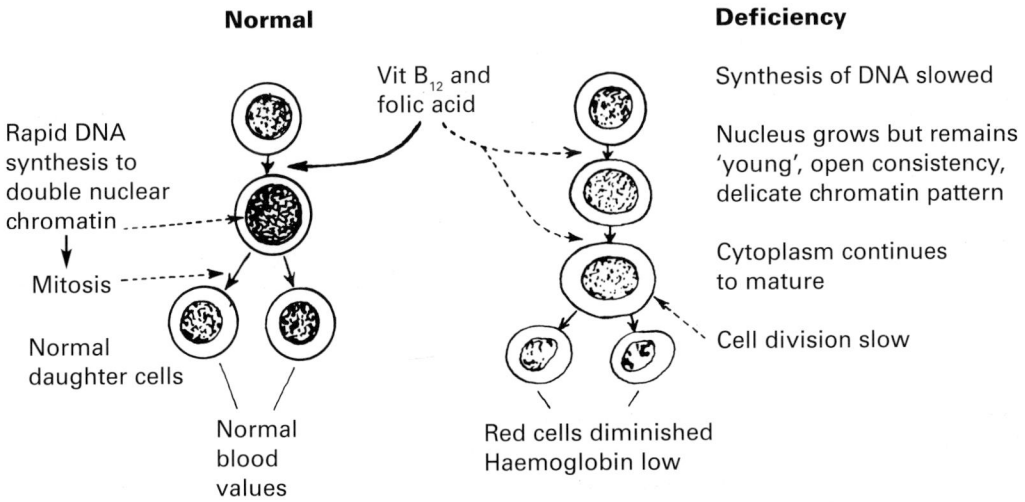

Results in organs particularly affected

1. MUCOUS MEMBRANES of alimentary tract and genitalia → Regenerative activity cannot balance surface cell losses → THINNING (atrophy) often with functional deficiencies

2. BONE MARROW blood cell precursors of all series affected → Many immature red cells are destroyed in the marrow. Red cells released into blood have a shortened life span. → Megaloblastic

   Increased growth factors cause increased cellularity. → Hypercellular

Note:

(a) Vit B_{12} (but not folic acid) has a separate function in the maintenance of the integrity of myelin. Therefore deficiency leads to neuropathies — particularly **subacute combined degeneration** (p. 399).

(b) The marrow and blood appearances are essentially similar in deficiency of vit B_{12} and folic acid from any cause. The classical disease of this type is **pernicious anaemia**.

PERNICIOUS ANAEMIA (PA)

This serious and severe anaemia was first described by the English physician Addison in the mid 19th century. At that time it was invariably fatal, but nowadays it can be treated with complete success. It is due to vitamin B_{12} deficiency and is always associated with achlorhydria and gastric mucosal atrophy.

Vitamin B_{12} metabolism and causes of deficiency:

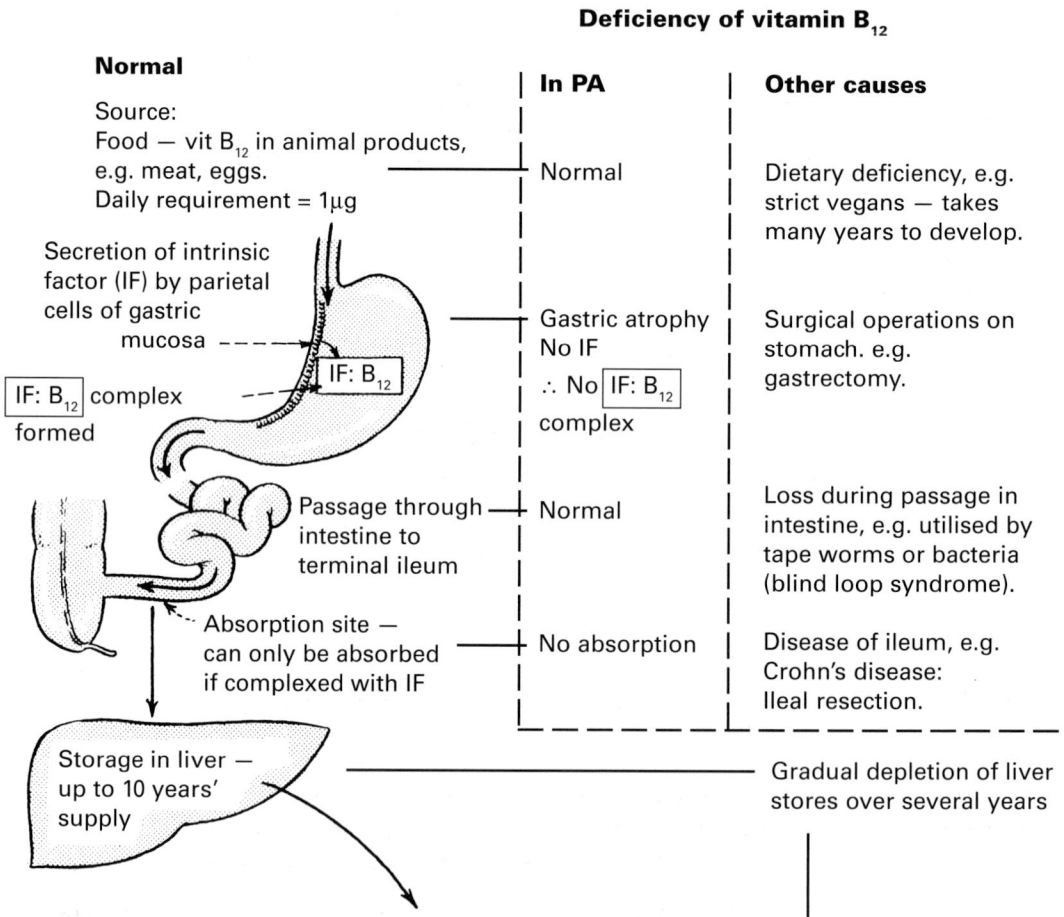

Released into blood stream bound to transcobalamin (T.C.) to act as important co-enzyme in several intercellular synthetic pathways but particularly of DNA.

Especially important to:

(1) Bone marrow . . . . . ANAEMIA (MEGALOBLASTIC)

(2) Nervous system . . . . . ± NERVE CHANGES

(3) Epithelial coverings . . . . ±TONGUE & VAGINA } ATROPHY

PERNICIOUS ANAEMIA (PA)

Blood changes

There is a pancytopenia, i.e. reduction in RBCs, granulocytes and platelets.

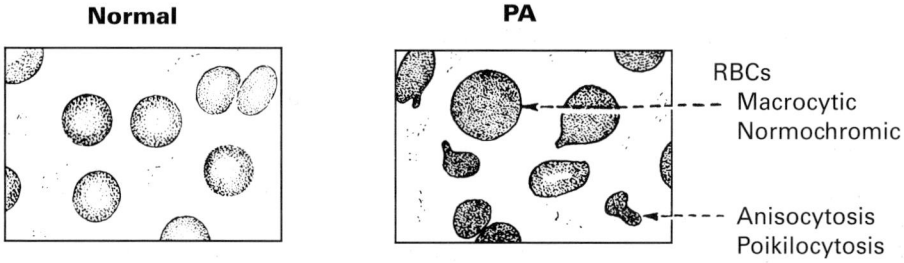

Special features

Seen specially in buffy coat preparations.

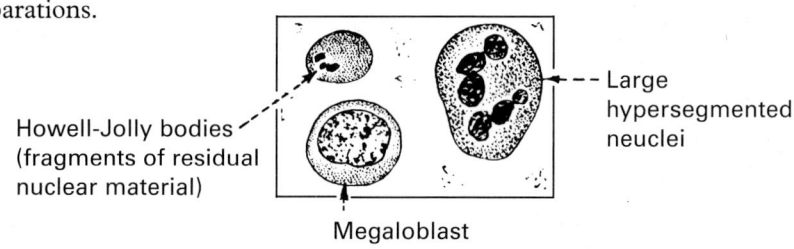

Absolute values

Red cell count ——— LOW (may be very low), e.g. 1.0 x 10^{12}/litre
Hb ——— LOW
PCV ——— LOW
MCV ——— HIGH, e.g. (average cell is larger than normal)*
MCH ——— HIGH (average cell contains more Hb than normal)*
MCHC ——— NORMAL (NB average cell contains normal Hb concentration)*

**Note:* Because the average cell is larger it contains more haemoglobin than normal but the haemoglobin concentration in the cell (as indicated by the MCHC) is normal.

Biochemical

Serum vit B_{12} ——— LOW < 120 (normal > 160 ng/l)
Serum bilirubin —— Slight increase — due to increased haemolysis of fragile cells.

PERNICIOUS ANAEMIA (PA)

Marrow changes

Hyperplasia — often complete cellularity in flat bones and extension down length of femur.

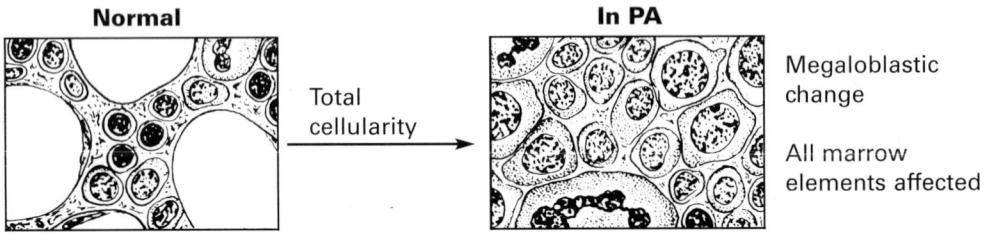

The gastric lesion — The extreme form of diffuse atrophic gastritis (see p. 303).

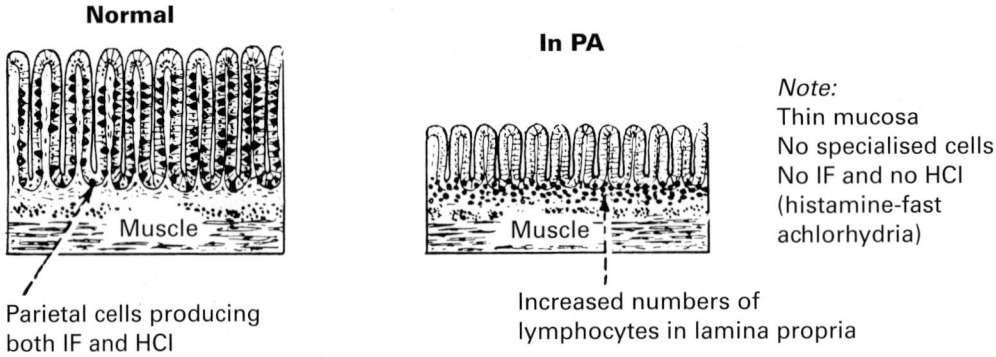

Mechanism of production of gastritis

PA is an autoimmune disease. The gastric atrophy is caused by an immune reaction against parietal cell cytoplasmic constituents and specifically by antibodies to intrinsic factor (IF).

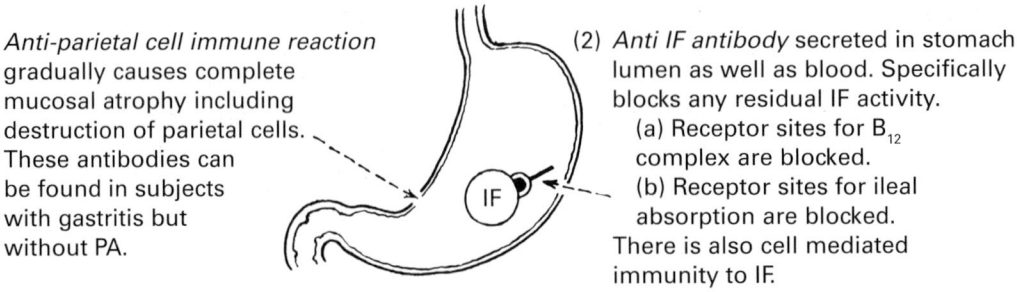

There is an increased familial incidence of PA and other organ specific autoimmune diseases, e.g. Hashimoto's thyroiditis.

PERNICIOUS ANAEMIA (PA)

Associated changes

1. *Nervous system*

(a) Subacute degeneration of spinal cord.

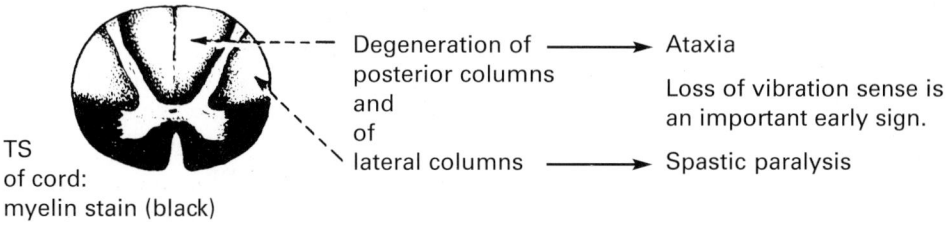

NB This serious degeneration may occur before clinical anaemia is present, and is aggravated by the administration of folic acid.

(b) Peripheral neuropathy — both sensory and motor loss.

2. *Epithelial surfaces*

Atrophy is common especially in the tongue and vagina — where senile atrophy is aggravated.

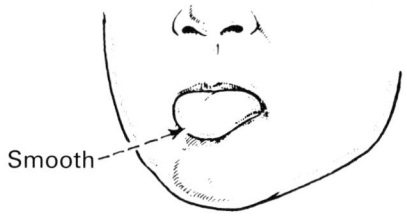

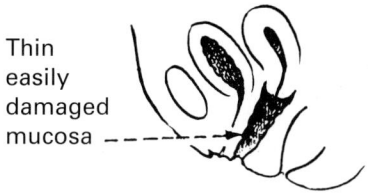

Vaginal smear

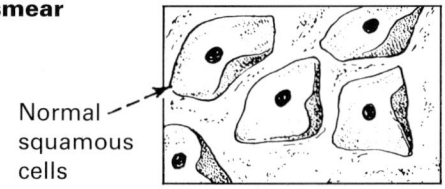

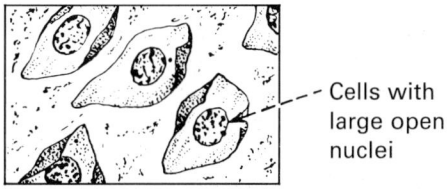

3. *Effects of long continued haemolysis*

The abnormal cells have a shortened life cycle.

(a) Mild/moderate splenic enlargement.

(b) Iron deposition in liver, kidney, spleen and marrow.

(c) Increased bilirubin in blood (mild jaundice).

FOLIC ACID DEFICIENCY

FOLIC ACID (Pteroyl-glutamic acid) DEFICIENCY

Normal metabolism

Source
Polyglutamines in green vegetables, cereals, meat, fish and eggs (not milk)

Minimum daily requirement
50 μg

Body reserves 50–100 days

Absorption
As mono-glutamate in jejunum

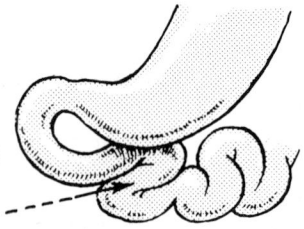

Utilisation
For DNA synthesis.
Vit B_{12} is necessary for synthesis of the active tetrahydrofolate form (FH_4)

Deficiency

Dietary
Anorexia, alcoholism, poverty (elderly), infants (late weaning)

Increased requirements
Pregnancy (fetal growth)
Infancy and childhood (rapid growth)
Haemolysis
Malignancy

Malabsorption
Coeliac disease: sprue
Surgical by-pass
Associated with dermatitis herpetiformis
Drugs (e.g. sulphasalazine)

Utilisation block
Drugs e.g. specific antagonists
e.g. in cancer chemotherapy, also anti-convulsants.

Note:

(1) Since the marrow and blood changes in folic acid and vitamin B_{12} deficiency are similar, the differential diagnosis has to be obtained by other laboratory tests — particularly the measurement of vit B_{12} in the serum and of folic acid in the serum and RBCs. Special tests of absorption of vit B_{12} (e.g. Schilling test) are available.

(2) Since the causes of vit B_{12} and folic acid deficiency are often non-specific and associated with malabsorption, other deficiencies (e.g. iron) may also occur at the same time.

(3) All megaloblastic anaemias are macrocytic, but *not all* macrocytic anaemias are megaloblastic.

(4) There is a strong association with folic acid deficiency in PREGNANCY with congenital neural tube defects.

ACUTE POST-HAEMORRHAGIC ANAEMIA

ACUTE POST-HAEMORRHAGIC ANAEMIA

The effects of severe acute haemorrhage are considered under two main headings:

1. The adaptive haemodynamic changes which are usually at least partly successful in maintaining perfusion of vital organs — see section on SHOCK (p.173).
2. The changes reflecting the body's reactions to restore the blood constituents.

The rate and volume of the blood loss are important influences on both types of effect. For example — in a young healthy adult male (assume blood volume = 5000 ml):

Blood loss ml	%vol.	**Duration**	**Effects of loss**	
500 e.g. Blood donation	10%	15 min	Nil or negligible	
1700	33%	3 hrs	Shock ↓ usually survival	**Aggravating factors** (a) pre-existing cardiac or debilitating disease (b) old age
2500	50%	3 hrs	Severe shock ↓ usually death	
2500	50%	36 hrs	Shock ↓ usually survival	

While the bleeding is continuing, the shock syndrome is predominant, and although the marrow begins to react to the anoxia, the full haematological effects — particularly the ANAEMIA — are not seen until the haemorrhage is controlled or stops and the plasma volume begins to be restored.

HAEMOLYTIC DISEASE OF THE NEWBORN

The basic mechanism is influenced by three important factors:

(a) The maternal immune response tends to be proportional to the number of fetal cells entering the circulation.

(b) The maternal immune response is boosted in successive Rh incompatible pregnancies — the highest maternal antibody titres are found in the latest of multiple pregnancies.

(c) Fetal/maternal ABO compatibility influences the Rh immune response.

e.g. ABO compatible		*ABO incompatible*	
Fetus	*Mother*	*Fetus*	*Mother*
Group O Rh+	Group O Rh-	Group A Rh+	Group O Rh-
Gradual elimination of fetal cells		Rapid destruction of fetal cells	
∴ *Maximum* immune response		∴ *Minimum* immune response	

Subsequent pregnancies: All Rh-positive fetuses conceived by a mother who has acquired anti-Rh antibodies either during previous pregnancies or by blood transfusion (in this case the first fetus also) are at risk.

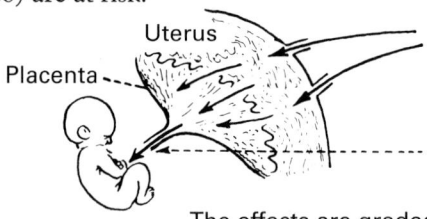

Maternal anti-Rh antibodies IgG type
↓
Pass placental barrier
↓
Enter fetal circulation and **destroy fetal red cells** (agglutination and haemolysis)

The effects are graded into three categories of severity:

(1) **Congenital haemolytic anaemia**
Usually mild anaemia and jaundice
↓
Usually self limited

(2) **Icterus gravis neonatorum**
Rapidly developing severe **anaemia** and **jaundice**
↓
± Brain damage due to kernicterus
Severe anoxia may cause death

(3) **Hydrops fetalis**
Stillbirth associated with severe anoxia in utero with cardiac failure and oedema
↓
Hepatosplenomegaly — due to extramedullary **haemopoiesis**

Film of cord blood

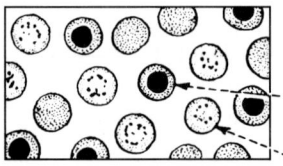

Very numerous nucleated red cells

Reticulocytes +++ (e.g. 30%)

Modern prophylaxis

Injection of anti-Rh antibody minimises immune response.

Anti-Rh (anti-D) usually obtained from male volunteers → Rh negative mothers immediately following delivery — Rh positive fetal cells in circulation → Agglutination and rapid elimination

Minimal or no immune response

EXTRINSIC HAEMOLYTIC ANAEMIAS

2. INFECTIONS

There are three mechanisms by which infections cause haemolysis:

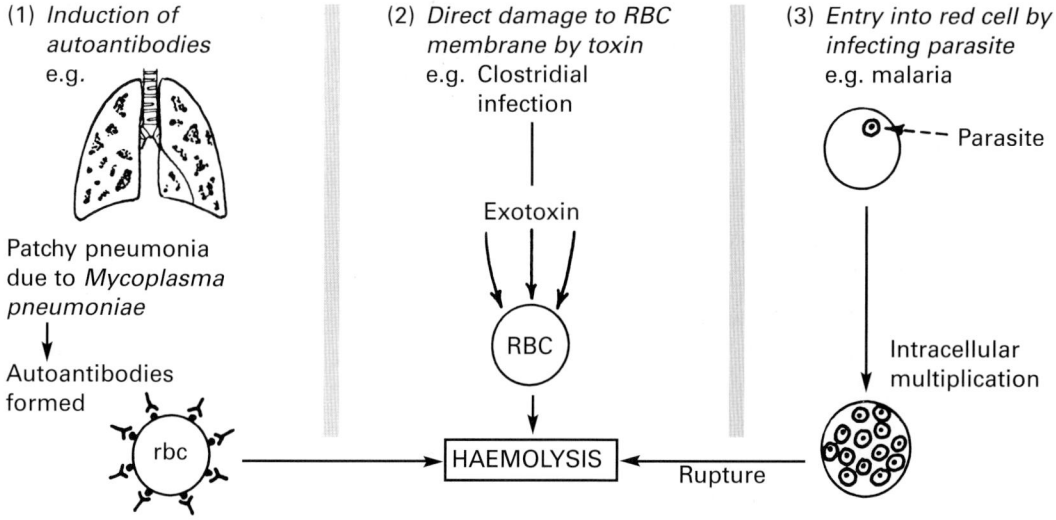

3. DRUGS AND CHEMICALS

The three main mechanisms by which drugs and chemicals cause haemolysis are:

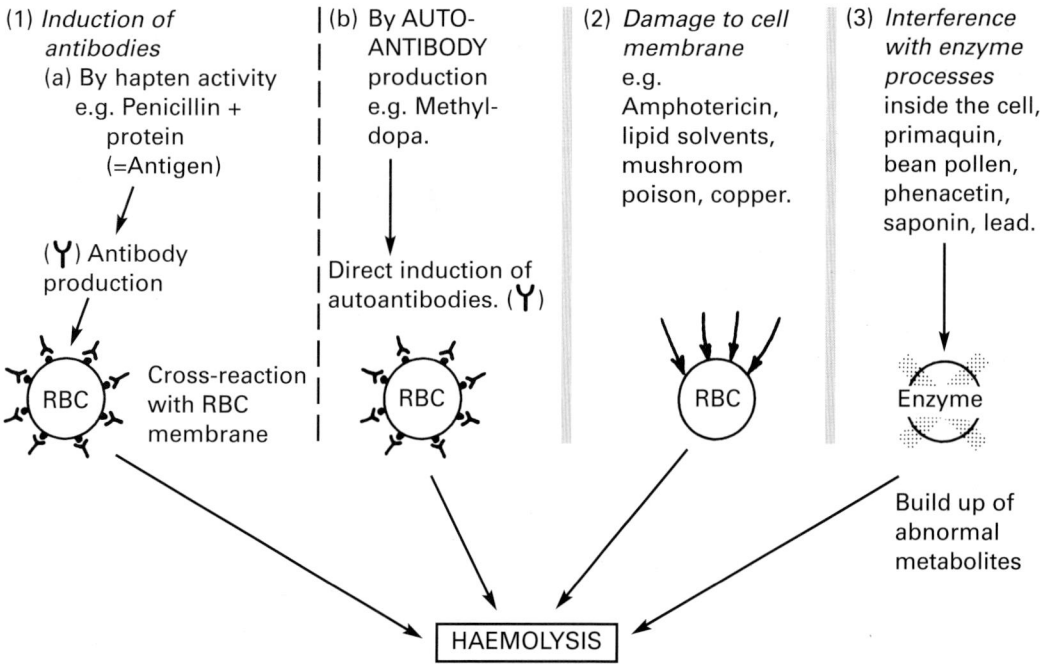

EXTRINSIC HAEMOLYTIC ANAEMIAS

4. MECHANICAL TRAUMA

The results of damage to red cells within the circulation are:

(1) Intravascular haemolysis

↓

Haemoglobinuria

(2) Formation of red cell fragments (schistocytes) seen in blood film as 'burr', 'triangle', 'helmet' cells

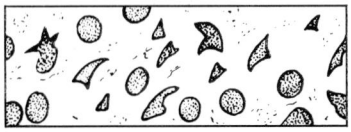

The main circumstances in which red cells are damaged are:

(a) In the **heart and great vessels**

When the blood flow is subjected to undue turbulence or jet effect. An important example nowadays is with prosthetic valves in left side of heart.

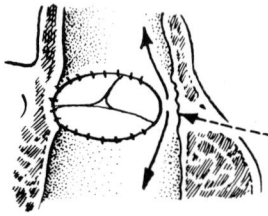

RBCs damaged by shearing stresses where valve seating is defective or through the valve itself.

Other examples are:
- Aortic stenosis and regurgitation
- Arterio-venous shunts.

Note that in this chronic situation, iron is lost in the urine so that *iron deficiency anaemia* is often superimposed.

(b) In the **microcirculation**

(i) When the blood flow in arterioles is impeded by strands of fibrin.

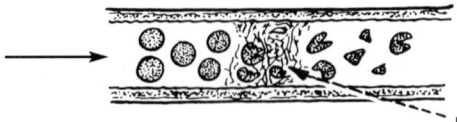

(1) Liberation of haemoglobin
(2) Emergence of fragments

RBCs being distorted and cut by fibrin sieve

This condition is called MICROANGIOPATHIC HAEMOLYTIC ANAEMIA and occurs in many disease states involving small blood vessels e.g. malignant hypertension and/or intravascular coagulation.

(ii) When blood vessels are subjected to direct trauma. This is seen classically in military recruits marching long distances in hard soled boots, when the blood vessels of the soles of the feet are squeezed with every step — **march haemoglobinuria**. The condition is also seen in karate exponents when the hand is repeatedly struck against hard objects.

The haemolysis is usually not severe enough to be of clinical significance, but haemoglobinuria may cause alarm.

EXTRINSIC HAEMOLYTIC ANAEMIAS

Other causes of haemolysis include:

1. **Hypersplenism**

In enlargement of the spleen from any cause, the sequestration of red cells is increased so that haemolytic anaemia may result.

Normal

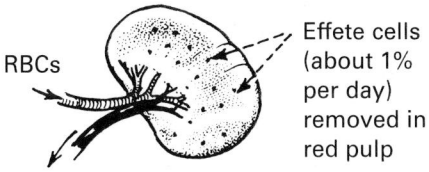

RBC life span 120 days

Hypersplenism

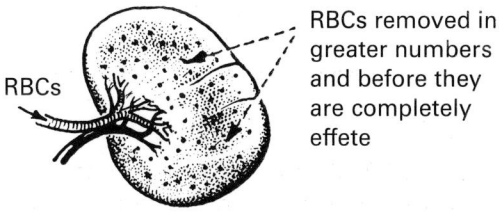

RBC life span reduced

2. **Burns**

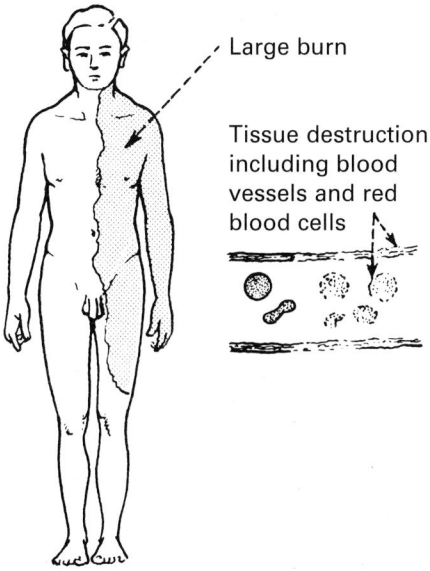

In severe burns haemolysis is an important component of the acute anaemia which develops.

3. **Inadvertent use of intravenous hypotonic solutions**

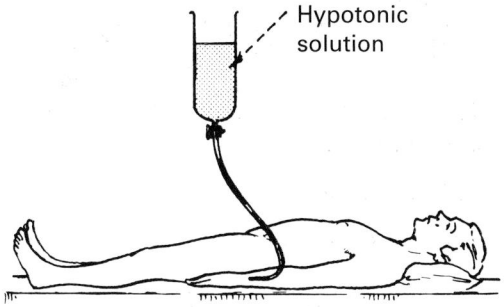

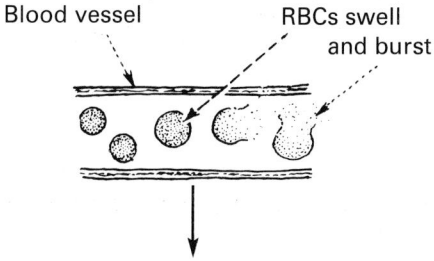

Intravascular haemolysis

This is a very rare accident but can have catastrophic consequences.

EXTRINSIC HAEMOLYTIC ANAEMIAS – MALARIA

Malaria is an endemic disease in many parts of Africa, Asia, Central and South America. Many millions of cases occur each year and the mortality is at least 1%. The disease is particularly severe in non-immune subjects from temperate climates; in endemic areas where the 'herd' immunity is high, a low grade chronic illness is common.

Female anopheline mosquitos act as intermediate hosts in the life cycle of the parasite, a protozoon (genus *Plasmodium*).

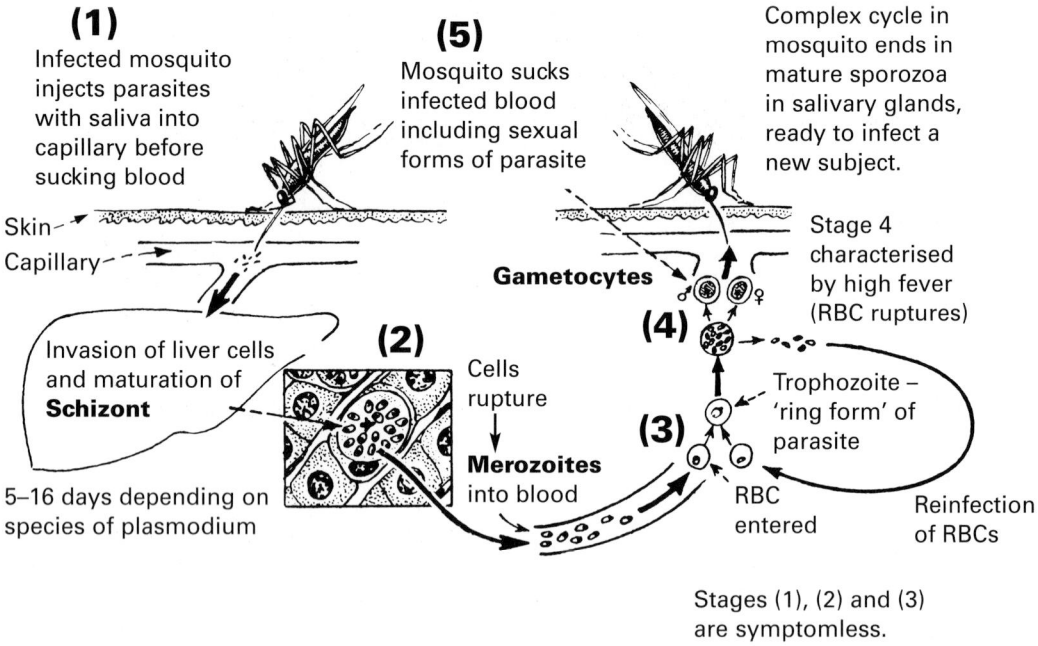

In some species, schizonts lie dormant in the liver; relapse may occur after long remissions.

Pathological changes

1. *Parasitism and destruction of red cells*
In a few severe cases, massive haemolysis leads to haemoglobinuria with kidney damage — **blackwater fever.**

Cerebral malaria is due to capillary blockage by parasitised RBC.

→ ANAEMIA (haemolytic)

→ Liberation of pigment and red cell debris → very marked macrophage activity
↓
SPLENOMEGALY
↑
Macrophage activity

2. *Immune responses:* humoral antibodies / cellular antibodies } + Macrophage activity

3. *Associations:*
(a) Recurrent attacks of malaria potentiate EB virus infection progressing to B-cell lymphoma
(b) The sickle cell gene protects against falciparum malaria

INTRINSIC HAEMOLYTIC ANAEMIAS

INTRINSIC DEFECTS —— Usually hereditary.

In (i) cell membrane (ii) enzymes (iii) molecular structure of haemoglobin (haemoglobinopathies).

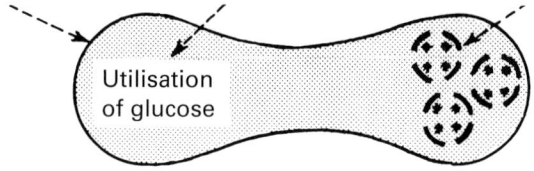

1. **Cell membrane defects**

(a) ***Hereditary spherocytosis:*** the majority of cases are familial (autosomal dominant).

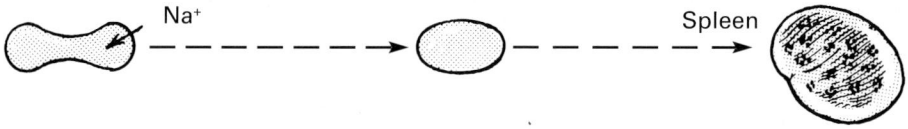

The primary defect is in the proteins which support the plasma membrane — SPECTRIN and ANKYRIN.

The cells assume a spherical shape due to instability of the plasma membrane.

Premature sequestration and destruction in splenic pulp. Splenomegaly is a constant association.

Note: Splenectomy is usually 'curative' but the red cell defect remains.

The severity of the haemolysis is variable; many cases are compensated and not anaemic, but crises are common. Intercurrent infections may precipitate increased red cell destruction with jaundice or temporary bone marrow hypoplasia with severe anaemia.

The laboratory diagnosis depends on:
(1) typical blood film with spherocytes,
(2) high reticulocyte count and
(3) increased osmotic fragility of RBCs.

(b) ***Hereditary elliptocytosis*** is similar to spherocytosis in many respects, but it is usually not severe enough to cause anaemia or jaundice. Haemolysis is usually mild.

(c) ***Hereditary abetalipoproteinaemia:*** a rare disease in which the red cell membranes are abnormal and the cells become spiky (acanthocytes).

(d) ***Paroxysmal nocturnal haemoglobinuria*** — a rare, acquired condition in which anchorage of proteins to the red cell membrane is abnormal. The cells are particularly susceptible to the action of complement (usually activated by the alternative pathway) at low pH. Intravascular haemolysis results.

INTRINSIC HAEMOLYTIC ANAEMIAS

INTRINSIC DEFECTS of the RED CELLS (continued)

2. Enzyme defects

Usually hereditary. Glucose is the source of energy with which the red cell metabolism is maintained. Glycolysis is effected by two classical enzyme pathways.

The following simplified diagram outlines the pathways and indicates only the main enzymes and substrates.

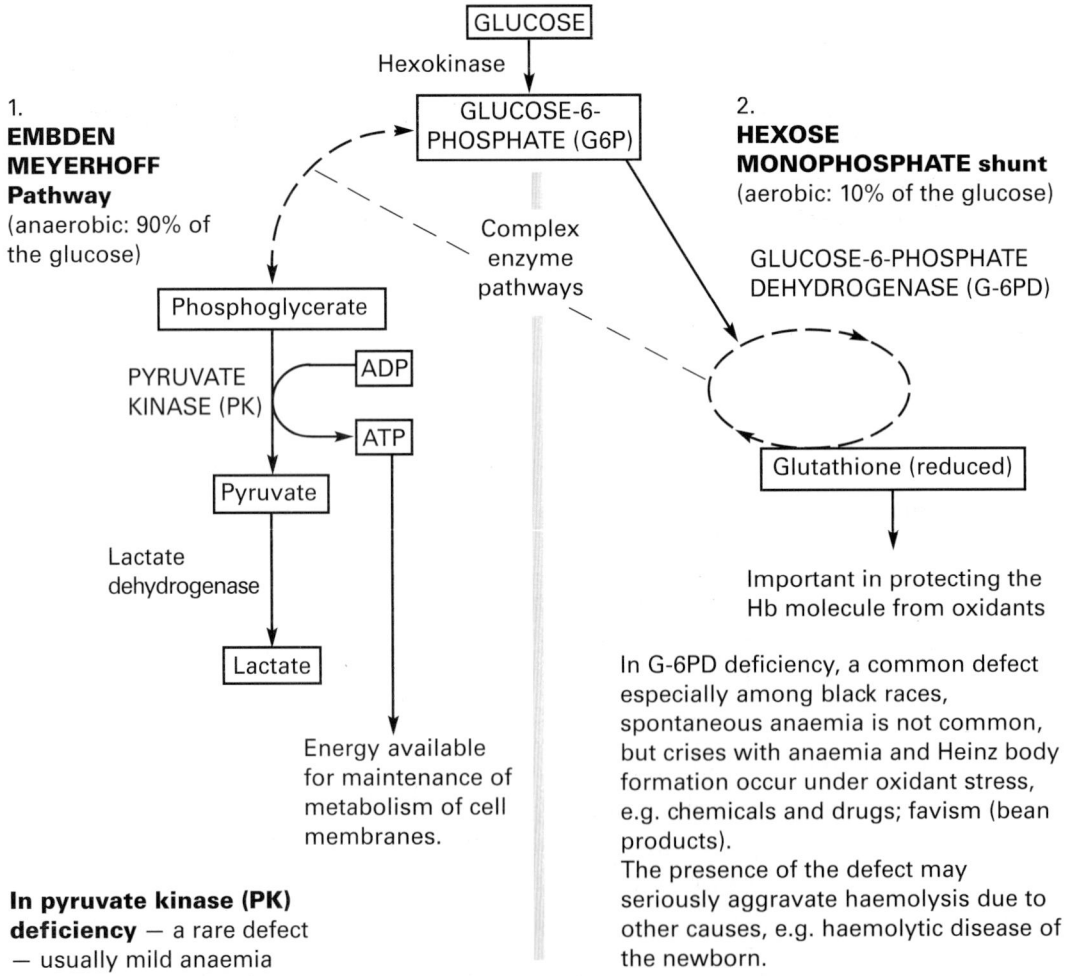

G-6PD deficiency shows X-linked inheritance so that in the male the defect is fully expressed, while in the female heterozygote there are two populations of red cells in the blood (1) normal cells and (2) defective cells.

In both these defects and in the rare defects of other enzymes in the pathways which have been described the expression of the abnormal gene is very variable from case to case.

DISORDERS OF HAEMOGLOBIN SYNTHESIS

3. Haemoglobinopathies

Varieties of normal haemoglobin are illustrated:

Normal haemoglobin molecule

4 subunits each consisting of a haem core with a polypeptide chain attached. The haem core is constant while the polypeptide chains occur in pairs.
4 different polypeptide chains occur normally.

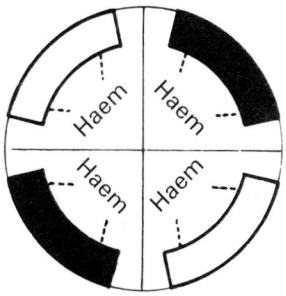

Mol. wt.= 68,000

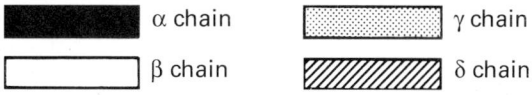

There are 3 types of normal haemoglobin.

97% adult Hb — 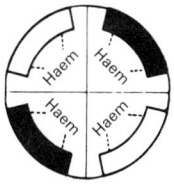 — Haemoglobin A = 2α + 2β chains

3% adult Hb — 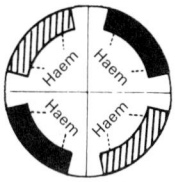 — Haemoglobin A_2 = 2α + 2δ chains

Fetal Hb — 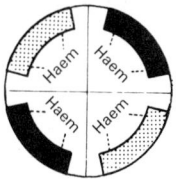 — Haemoglobin F = 2α + 2γ chains

Fetal haemoglobin is replaced by adult haemoglobin during the first year. Note that the α chain occurs in all normal haemoglobins.

Two copies of the α chain genes (αα/αα) are present on chromosome 16; β, γ and δ genes are found in a complex on chromosome 11. A number of globin-like genes are also present but are omitted for simplicity.

In the **thalassaemias** and **haemoglobinopathies** there are abnormalities in the production and structure of haemoglobin chains due to mutation of these genes.

THE THALASSAEMIAS

These are inherited disorders in which synthesis of globin chains is diminished or absent. They are common in the Mediterranean, Middle East and India.

α-thalassaemia — reduction of α chain synthesis.
β-thalassaemia — reduction in β chain synthesis.

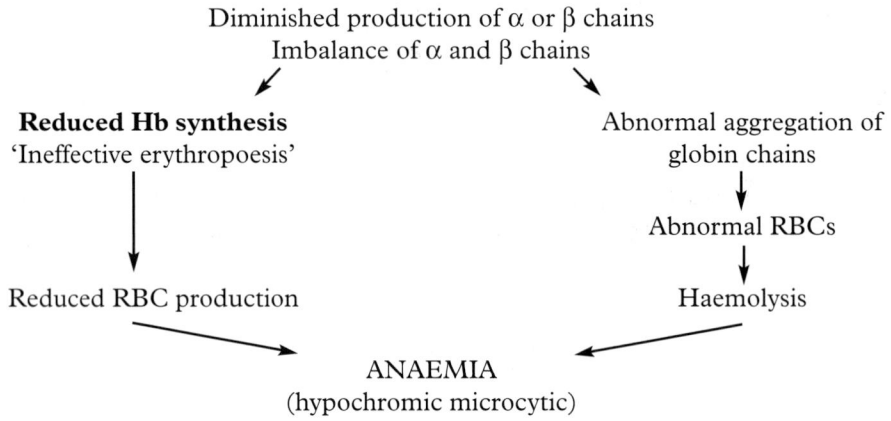

The severity of the disease depends on (i) the degree of globin chain abnormality and (ii) whether the patient is homozygous or heterozygous for the defect.

There are normally 4 α genes (αα/αα).
In the **α-thalassaemias** the genetic defects are illustrated as follows:

1. **Hb-Barts hydrops syndrome** (– –/– –)
   All 4 genes for the α chain are absent. Fetal Hb cannot be formed and the fetus dies *in utero.*
2. **Hb-H disease** (– α/– –): only one α gene is present. This leads to an excess of β chains which form tetramers called Hb-H.
   There is a moderate microcytic hypochromic anaemia with splenomegaly.

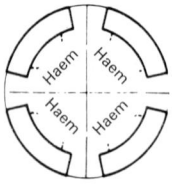

3. **α-thalassaemia** traits (– α/– α): even if two α genes are absent, the remaining two are active and the symptoms and anaemia are usually mild.

β-thalassaemia

β-thalassaemia major — two defective β genes.

The excess of α genes leads to severe anaemia with haemolysis. The marrow becomes hyperplastic and there is atrophy of bones. The main form of haemoglobin is HbF — which persists into adult life.

β-thalassaemia minor — one defective β gene.

The anaemia is mild. The red cells are microcytic and hypochromic and a mistaken diagnosis of iron deficiency anaemia can be made. These subjects act as carriers for β-thalassaemia major.

SICKLE CELL DISEASE

This disorder is very common in Central Africa but also occurs in the Mediterranean, Middle East and India. It affects the black population of USA and the Caribbean.

It is due to a mutation in the β chain of haemoglobin (the amino-acid glutamic acid is substituted by valine).

The effects are *mild* in heterozygotes (Hb AS) = **sickle cell trait**; they are *severe* in homozygotes (Hb SS) = **sickle cell anaemia**.

The effects are summarised as follows:

1. **At molecular level** HbS becomes less soluble in low levels of oxygen tension.

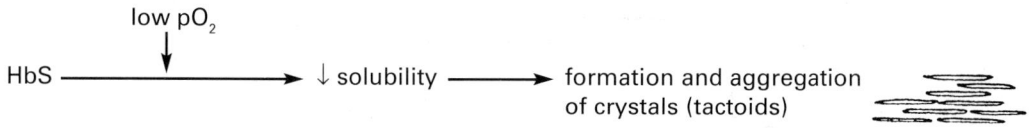

2. **In the red cell** this causes distortion (sickling).

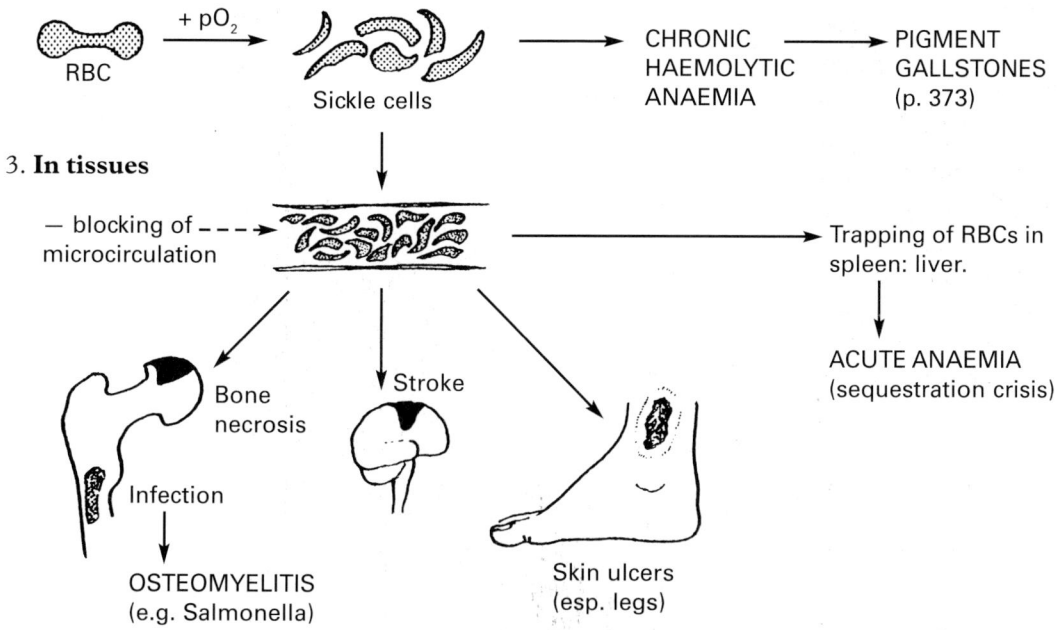

Acute sickle cell crises are often provoked by:

(1) infection, (2) cold, (3) low pO_2 e.g. flying in unpressurised aircraft.

In addition, infection, especially by **parvoviruses in childhood**, may provoke an **aplastic anaemia** crisis.

Note: HbS confers resistance to malaria: in terms of evolution this confers a survival benefit to those carrying the HbS gene.

ANAEMIA OF CHRONIC DISORDERS

This term describes the anaemias seen commonly in patients with chronic diseases e.g. (ia) Chronic inflammation e.g. rheumatoid arthritis, SLE (ib) Chronic infection e.g. T.B. (ii) Malignancy.

The anaemia is usually mild (Hb > 9 g/dl).

The mechanism is not well understood.

Postulated mechanism

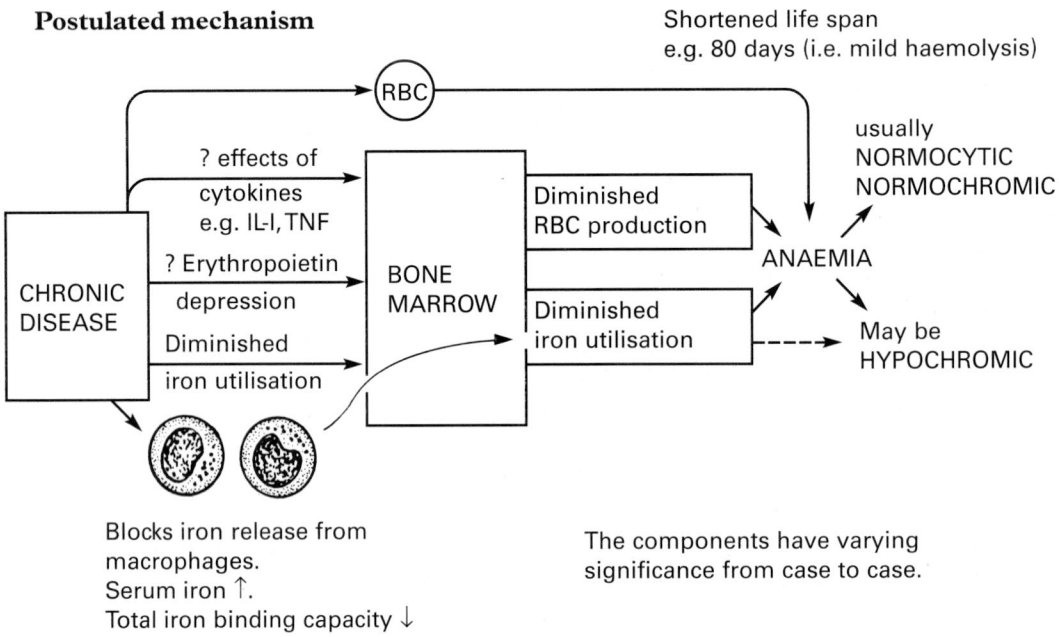

In addition, malignant tumour growth may cause anaemia by 2 more specific mechanisms.

(a) Chronic bleeding from the surface of an ulcerated tumour — especially from the alimentary tract ⟶ iron deficiency.

(b) Replacement of the bone marrow by malignant tumour.

Normocytic Normochromic Anaemias are also found in other systemic diseases.

e.g. (i) **Renal disease**
- ↓ erythropoietin ⟶ ↓ RBC production
- ↓ RBC survival — mechanism uncertain, varies with degree of **uraemia.**

(ii) **Liver failure** — additional factors are:

Liver
- Bleeding varices,
- Deficiency of coagulation factors,
- Hypersplenism,
- Alcoholic — other nutritional deficiencies.

(iii) **Endocrine disease** e.g.

hypopituitarism, hypothyroidism
- ↓ metabolism
- ↓ erythropoietin production.

APLASTIC ANAEMIA

In this disorder there is:

A reduction in bone marrow stem cells → Failure of production of mature cells → Pancytopenia (of varying severity)

↓

Bone marrow is hypoplastic →

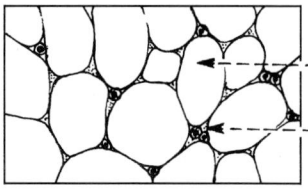

There are a number of different types

(a) **Idiopathic** — in 2/3 of cases no cause is found.
(b) **Drug induced** — this may be:
  (i) Predictable e.g. Cytotoxic chemotherapy.
  (ii) Idiosyncratic e.g. Chloramphenicol (1 in 25,000–60,000 affected).
  Phenylbutazone.
(c) **Virus induced** e.g. Hepatitis, Epstein Barr Virus.
(d) **Autoimmune.**
(e) **Inherited** e.g. Fanconi's anaemia — Autosomal recessive.

Treatment This consists of:

(a) Supportive therapy e.g. blood transfusion.
(b) Attempts to restore haemopoiesis e.g. bone marrow transplantation,
  — anabolic steroids,
  — immunosuppressive therapy,
  — withdrawal of causative drugs.

The sideroblastic anaemias

In these rare anaemias, failure of synthesis of the haem component of the haemoglobin molecule is indicated by the presence of a ring of iron granules around the normoblast nucleus.

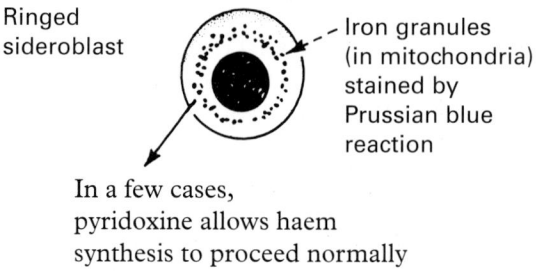

The condition arises secondarily in many of the chronic disease states mentioned on previous page, or as a result of drug treatment or chemical poisoning (e.g. lead). A few cases are 'primary' — possibly representing a form of myelodysplasia.

The anemia is usually *dimorphic*; i.e. showing hypochromic and macrocytic features combined.

ANAEMIA – MORPHOLOGICAL CLASSIFICATION

The initial investigation of any anaemia consists of an examination of blood (and/or marrow) films and determination of absolute values. A morphological classification is therefore very useful.

The three broad divisions which depend on the red cell size may be further subdivided in respect of haemoglobin content of the cell:

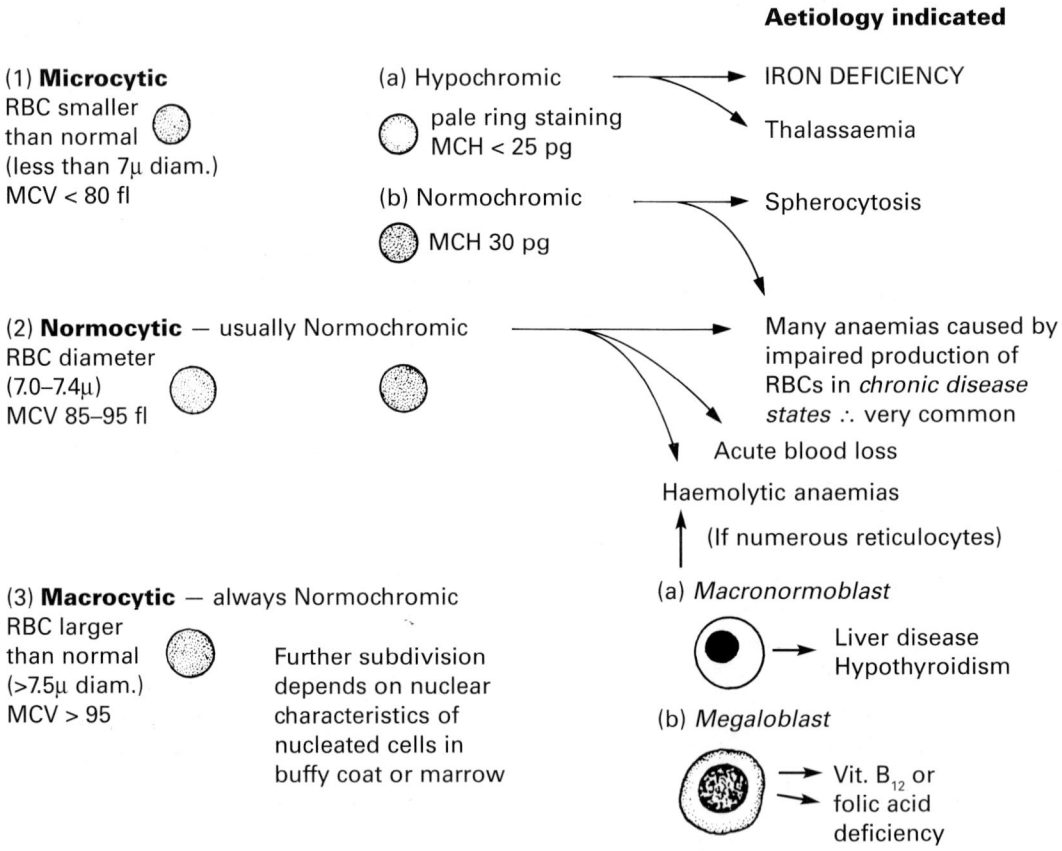

In some cases of anaemia, there are two distinct populations of abnormal red cells (e.g. microcytic/hypochromic and macrocytic/normochromic). These DIMORPHIC anaemias are usually caused by double deficiencies.

The logical use of these classifications in the investigation of anaemia:

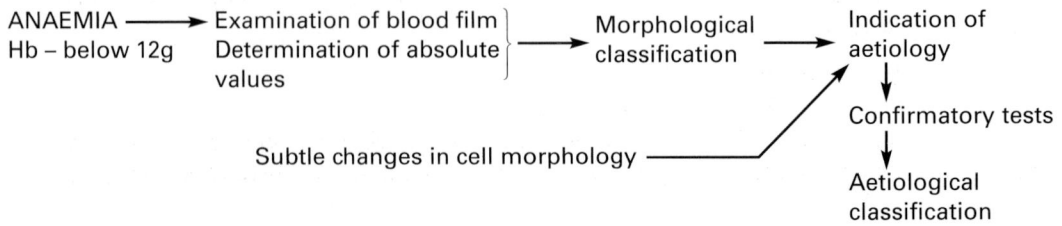

POLYCYTHAEMIA

POLYCYTHAEMIA

Polycythaemia (erythrocytosis) is defined as a sustained increase in red cell mass: the haematocrit is always elevated.

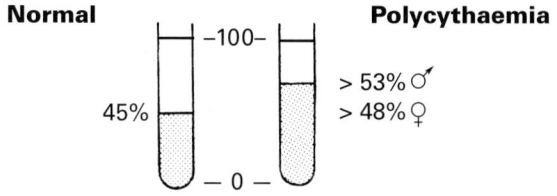

The red cell count is also raised

Note: **Relative Polycythaemia** is the result of fluid loss with a decrease in plasma volume. The apparent polycythaemia is due to the spurious raised haematocrit.

Aetiology

There are two main types
- 1. SECONDARY (reactive) — where a known abnormality causes the red cell increase.
- 2. PRIMARY (rare) — where the increase is autonomous.

SECONDARY POLYCYTHAEMIA

The red cell increase is the result of increased stimulation of marrow by erythropoietin. Two main groups of conditions are associated with this:

1. (Commonly) Conditions causing tissue HYPOXIA:
   - (a) Living at high altitudes
   - (b) Chronic cardiac disease especially R → L shunts
   - (c) Chronic respiratory disease
   - (d) Presence of abnormal haemoglobin causing defective release of O_2 to tissues — usually hereditary, sometimes due to drugs.

   → 'Appropriate' → ERYTHROPOIETIN production → MARROW HYPERPLASIA (RED CELLS) → POLYCYTHAEMIA — increase of red cells only

2. (Rarely) Renal tumours and ischaemia; occasionally tumours of other organs.

   → 'Inappropriate' → ERYTHROPOIETIN production → MARROW HYPERPLASIA (RED CELLS) → POLYCYTHAEMIA — increase of red cells only

PRIMARY POLYCYTHAEMIA *(Polycythaemia Rubra Vera)*

The red cell increase in this rare condition is autonomous. It may be associated with an increase in other marrow elements and is grouped within the myeloproliferative disorders. Splenomegaly is usually present.

Effects of polycythaemia

- (a) There is usually a distinctly florid complexion.
- (b) Increased blood viscosity causes: (i) hypertension and (ii) a tendency to thrombosis.
- (c) Increased marrow activity → increased uric acid metabolism → tendency to gout.

NEUTROPHIL GRANULOCYTES

NEUTROPHIL Neutrophil Granulocyte (Polymorphonuclear Leucocyte)
The essential function of these cells is protection against microbial infection by phagocytosis and killing. They are produced alongside red blood cells, platelets and monocytes from a common stem cell in the marrow.

Marrow Production – stained by a Romanowski method

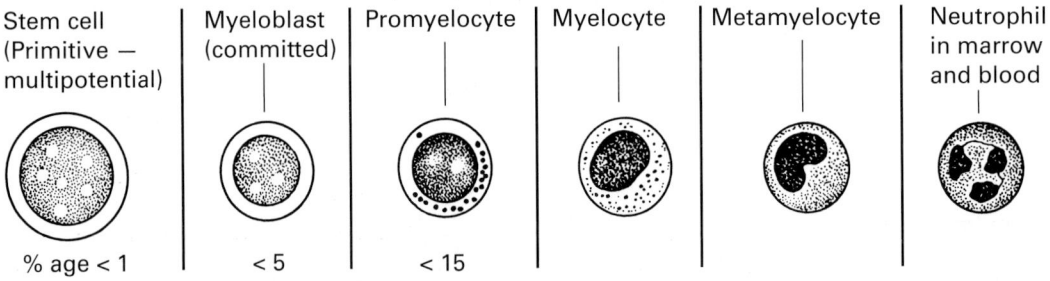

Note the nuclear changes progressing from large open nuclei and several nucleoli to the mature condensed multi-lobed state. The cytoplasmic maturation proceeds from a clear blue state to the acquisition of specific granules.

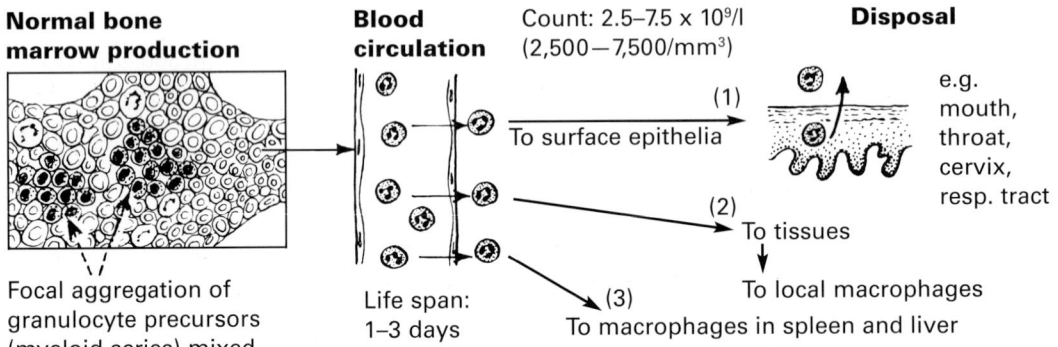

An increase in the number of circulating neutrophils reflects an increased activity in the tissues at the site of an acute inflammatory reaction.

Neutrophil activation

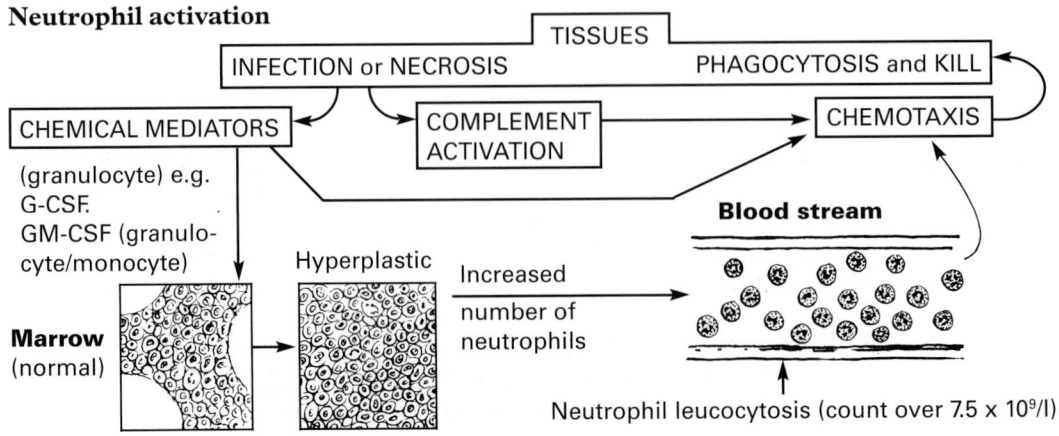

DISORDERS OF NEUTROPHILS

Neutrophil leucocytosis does not occur in: (a) some acute bacterial infections, e.g. typhoid fever, brucellosis, (b) many chronic bacterial infections, (c) most virus infections unless acute bacterial infection or necrosis occurs, (d) overwhelming infections with severe toxaemia.

In the **absence (agranulocytosis)** or **diminished numbers** of neutrophils — < 2.5 × 10/1 (2,500/mm^3) increased susceptibility to infection results.

There are 2 **main mechanisms** which often co-exist.

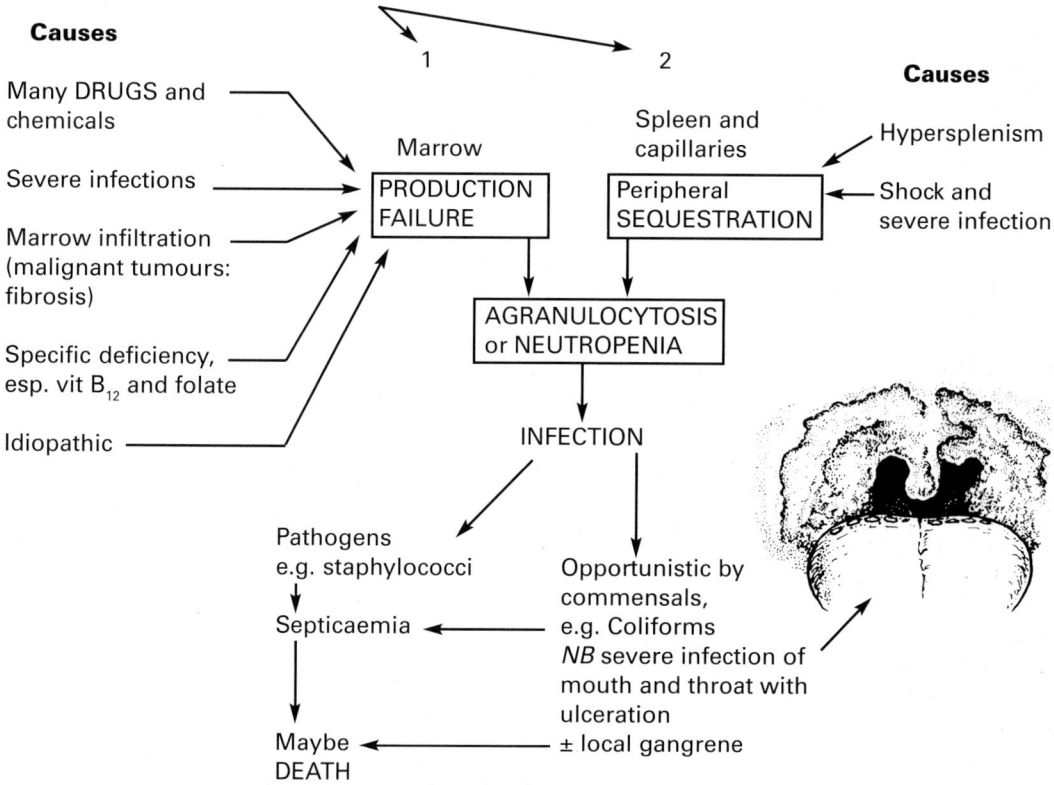

Drugs may act in the following ways:

1. By direct dose related toxic effect, e.g. modern chemotherapeutic agents.
2. By an immunological reaction, the drug acting as a **hapten**, e.g. amidopyrine.
3. By an idiosyncratic action in sensitive subjects small doses are effective, e.g. chloramphenicol (compare aplastic anaemia, page 419).

Marrow failure

Drugs and chemicals may affect the production of all three marrow cell types together or in various combinations.

DISORDERS OF NEUTROPHILS

Disorders of neutrophil function

Divided into 3 groups: (1) chemotaxis, (2) microbial phagocytosis and (3) microbial kill.

Chemotaxis and phagocytosis may be defective due to:

(a) an intrinsic defect of the neutrophils e.g. leucocyte adhesion deficiency — reduction of B_2 integrin expression.

(b) plasma deficiency of chemotactic factors and opsonins — seen especially when there are deficiencies in the complement cascade.

Microbial kill fails when there is an intracellular enzyme defect e.g. in *chronic granulomatous disease* (CGD) and the Chediak-Higashi syndrome where the neutrophils contain abnormal giant granules.

The normal sequence following phagocytocis is:

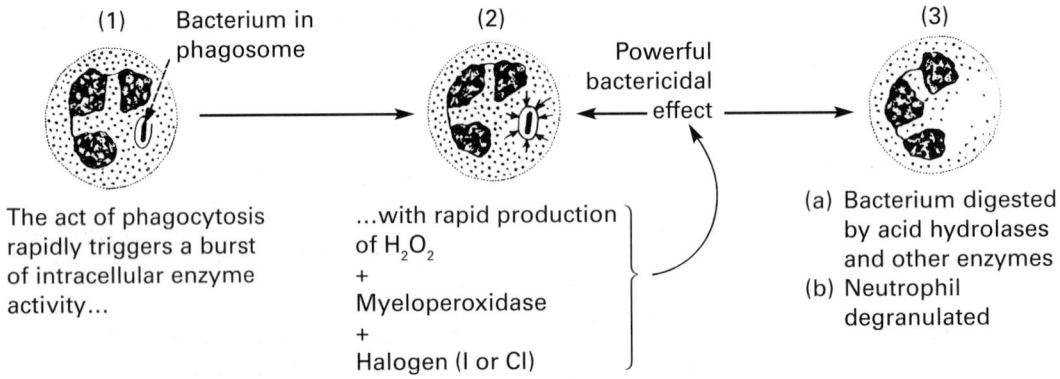

CHRONIC GRANULOMATOUS DISEASE (CGD)

It is a rare hereditary disorder in which the neutrophils have normal phagocytic function but are unable to kill certain bacteria. The disease is fully expressed only in males. It presents as multiple chronic abscesses and granulomas affecting skin, lungs, bones, spleen and liver.

The rapid production of H_2O_2 is defective (in the neutrophils and also in macrophages due to deficiency of NADPH-oxidase).

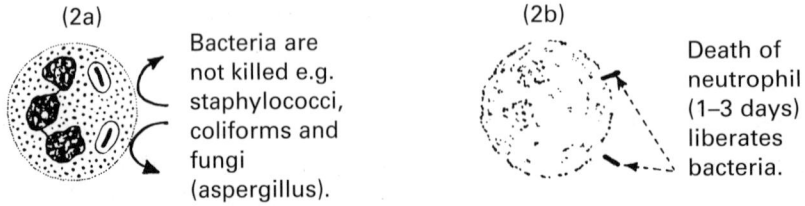

About 2/3 of cases are X-linked (fully expressed in males): the remainder are recessive. The neutrophils are unable to reduce nitroblue tetrazolium (used as a diagnostic slide test).

PLATELETS AND COAGULATION

These small, non-nucleated discs, derived from the cytoplasm of the bone marrow megakaryocytes, are released into the blood stream by a budding process.

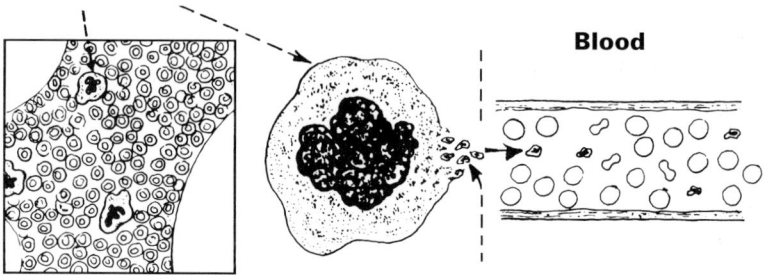

Count:
150–400×10^9/l
(150,000–400,000/mm^3)

Size: 1-3μ

Platelets contain adenosine diphosphate (ADP), vasoactive amines including serotonin (5HT) and histamine and phospholipid (platelet factor III).

Their main role is in preventing blood loss after injury.

e.g. skin wound.

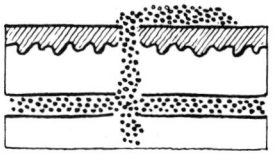

Free flow of blood

Rapid **activation** of **clotting mechanism**

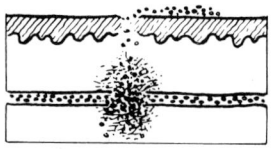

(a) Contraction of blood vessel

(b) **Aggregation of platelets** at site of endothelial damage — triggered by contact with collagen.

Release of ADP and thromboxane

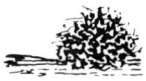

Further platelet aggregation and adherence.

Activation of clotting cascade

↓

Formation of fibrin network — reinforces platelet plug.

ABNORMALITIES OF COAGULATION

Blood may (a) CLOT INSUFFICIENTLY or (b) CLOT EXCESSIVELY

↓ ↓

HAEMORRHAGIC TENDENCY
- too few platelets (THROMBOCYTOPENIA)
  - excess destruction.
  - decreased formation.
- abnormal platelet function.
- deficiency of clotting factors.

THROMBOSIS
- too many platelets (THROMBOCYTOSIS).
- increased viscosity – e.g. in polycythaemia.
- due to deficiency of inhibitors of clotting factors.

DISORDERS OF PLATELETS

Disorders of the platelets include:
(a) deficiencies of number — thrombocytopenia — lead to bleeding tendency.
(b) defective function.

THROMBOCYTOPENIA

Although the normal platelet count ranges from 150–400 × 10^9/l, a risk of dangerous spontaneous haemorrhage is unusual unless the count falls below 30 × 10^9/1.

The causes of thrombocytopenia fall into two main groups:

1. Deficient marrow production	**2. Increased destruction**
Hypoplasia or aplasia } of marrow *Replacement* } of marrow (e.g. leukaemia, fibrosis)	Platelets damaged by *drugs, immune mechanisms*
Dyshaemopoiesis (e.g. Vit B_{12} deficiency)	Platelets sequestered in *hypersplenism* Platelets utilised in *coagulation disorders* (e.g. DIC)

Note: Marrow examination throws light on the possible mechanism.

In (1) megakaryocytes are reduced in number (except in vit. B_{12} deficiency)	In (2) megakaryocytes are increased and immature in an attempt to make good the platelet loss

PURPURA is the term used for disorders involving bleeding from capillaries, with the production of small petechial spots. Mild to moderate thrombocytopenia or defective platelet formation are the usual causes.

Two examples are illustrative:

1. **Idiopathic thrombocytopenic purpura** is due to **auto-immune** destruction of platelets.
   (a) **Acute:** mainly in children, provoked by viral infection: it is usually self-limiting in a few weeks.
   (b) **Chronic:** mainly in young women with an insidious onset and lasting many years: splenectomy is often required (the spleen is the major site of platelet destruction).
2. **Defective platelet function** has many forms — **von Willebrand's disease** (vWD) is the commonest.
   vWF is a large protein which potentiates the binding of platelets to subendothelial collagen and also acts as a carrier for coagulation factor VIII.

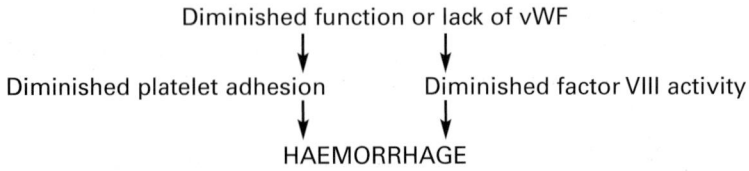

THROMBOCYTOSIS (increased platelet numbers) may occur in a mild form (with no clinical significance) as a concomitant of a variety of disorders.

Larger counts are seen as a concomitant of myeloproliferative disorders and are of serious clinical significance due to thrombosis.

THE COAGULATION CASCADE

The coagulation of blood is essentially the result of conversion of **FIBRINOGEN** to **FIBRIN,** but the chemical pathway leading to this final phase is a complicated cascade in which inert coagulation factors are serially activated. At each step augmentation takes place.

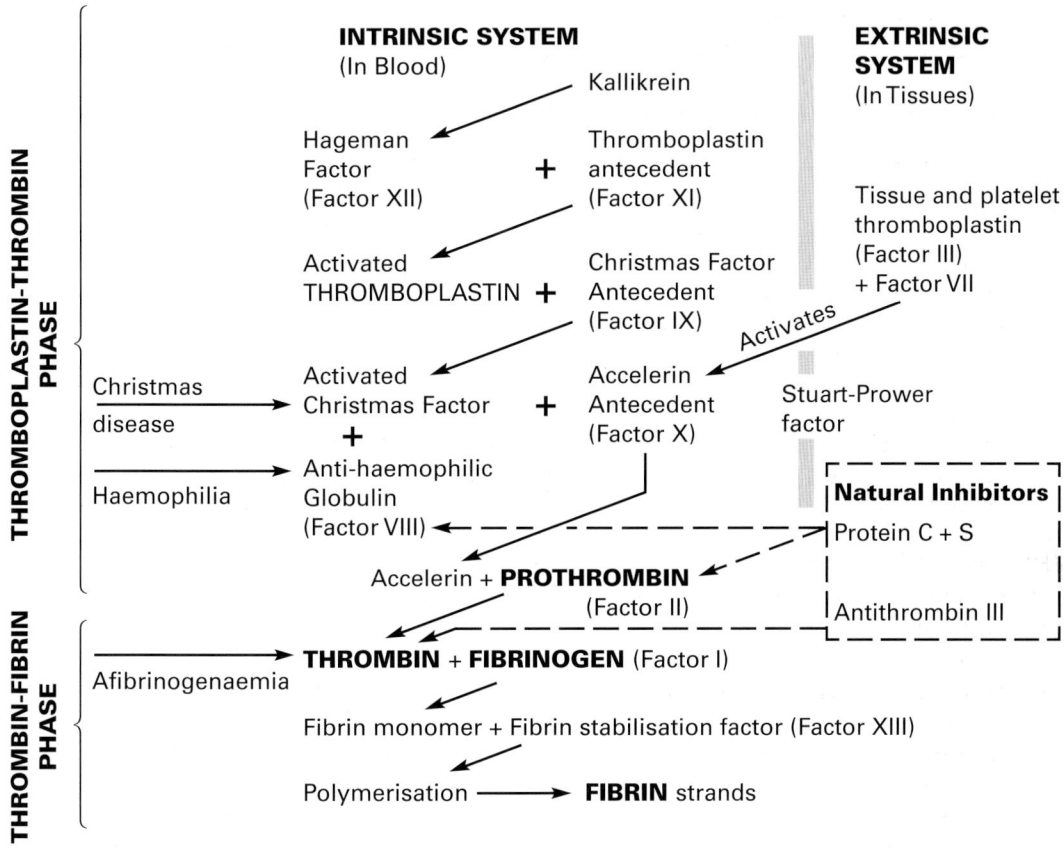

The system contains several feed-back loops (not illustrated) which can inhibit the cascade at various levels.

Anti-thrombin III and the protein C/protein S system are powerful inhibitors preventing uncontrollable coagulation.

Vitamin K is required for the production of prothrombin, Christmas factor and accelerin (also known as Stuart-Prower factor). CALCIUM ions and phospholipids (mainly derived from platelets) are essential for many of the steps in thrombin production. Once thrombin is formed, it appears to stimulate several of the preceding reactions and also the polymerisation of fibrin.

Fibrinolytic System — following fibrin deposition this is operative.

Plasminogen —(activated by tissue activator (or urokinase))→ **Plasmin** → Dissolution of FIBRIN → Degradation products

INHERITED DEFECTS OF COAGULATION

These are less common than acquired abnormalities, but are of considerable importance.

HAEMOPHILIA A

Haemophilia is due to deficiency of Factor VIII — an essential cofactor in the activation of Factor X in the intrinsic system.

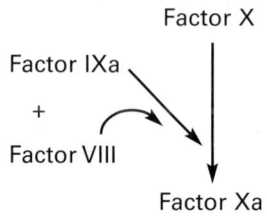

Factor VIII is encoded by a gene on the long arm of the X chromosome — haemophilia is inherited as an X-linked recessive, i.e. almost all patients are male. Their mothers are usually carriers, but about 30% of cases are due to new mutations. Around 1 in 5,000 is affected.

Clinical Features

The severity depends on the levels of Factor VIII.

		Level of Factor VIII
Severe:	Frequent spontaneous bleeding.	< 1 iu/dl (i.e. < 1% of normal).
Moderate:	Bleeding after minor trauma — rarely spontaneous.	1–5 iu/dl.
Mild:	Bleeding severe only after major trauma or surgery.	5–40 iu/dl.

Important sites of bleeding are:

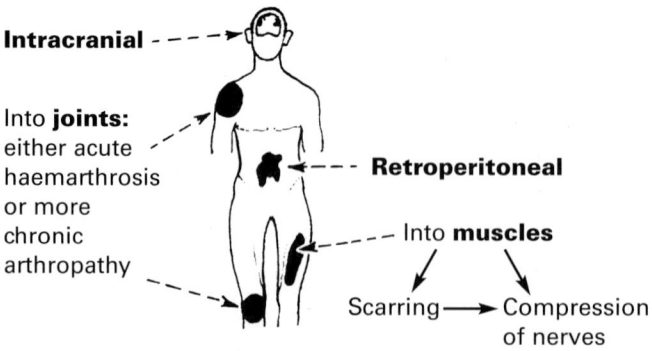

Note: In the past, the use of virus infected Factor VIII in treatment has caused HIV (AIDS) and Hepatitis C infection.

HAEMOPHILIA B (Christmas disease)

This is due to deficiency of Factor IX — also carried by a gene on X chromosome. The clinical features are similar, but the prevalence is lower (1 in 30,000 males).

Rarely deficiencies of other coagulation factors are seen e.g. fibrinogen, Factor XI and Factor V.

They are treated by infusion of the appropriate Factors.

ACQUIRED DEFECTS OF COAGULATION

This large and heterogeneous group of conditions includes:

VITAMIN K DEFICIENCY

Vitamin K, a fat soluble vitamin, is essential for synthesis of Factors II, VII, IX and X in the liver. Deficiency leads to spontaneous bleeding e.g. into skin and mucous membranes, and failure of blood clotting.

In **adults**, deficiency may be due to

(a) MALABSORPTION (particularly of fat)

(b) DIETARY DEFICIENCY — rare — Vitamin K is widely distributed e.g. in green vegetables, oils.

(c) INHIBITION — by COUMARIN anticoagulants e.g. WARFARIN.

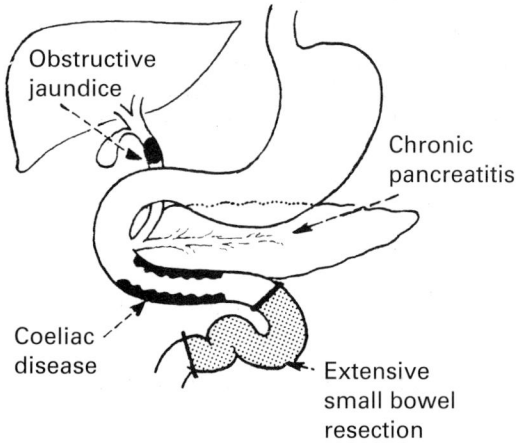

In **neonates**, vitamin K deficiency leads to bleeding — from GI tract (melaena neonatorum) and bruising. Breast milk contains little vitamin K — the disorder is uncommon in those receiving bottled milk. A severe deficiency may be seen in infants whose mothers took anticoagulants or anticonvulsants.

LIVER DISEASE

The bleeding tendency in these patients is multifactorial.

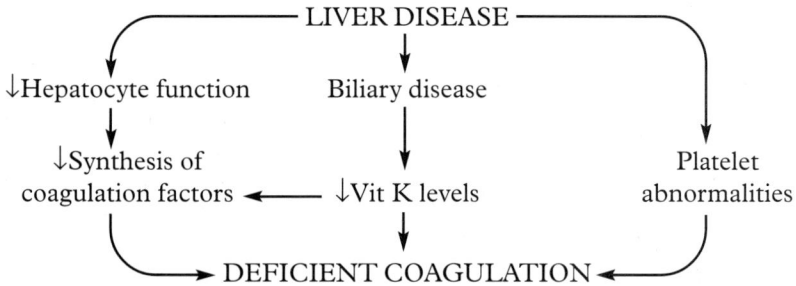

This complicates bleeding e.g. from OESOPHAGEAL varices.

'ACQUIRED HAEMOPHILIA'

Rarely, antibodies develop which block the effects of serum coagulation factors, especially Factor VIII. This may be idiopathic or follow auto-immune disease or drug treatment.

Disseminated Intravascular Coagulation (DIC) (see next page).

DISSEMINATED INTRAVASCULAR COAGULATION

In this disorder the coagulation system is activated, but the consumption of platelets and clotting factors which follows leads to a paradoxical bleeding tendency.

There are numerous **causes:**

(a) SEPTICAEMIA — especially gram negative septicaemia,
— in meningococcal infections.
(b) SHOCK e.g. following severe burns.
(c) OBSTETRIC DISORDERS e.g. abruptio placentae, amniotic embolism, eclampsia.
(d) MALIGNANCY — especially acute promyelocytic leukaemia and mucin secreting adenocarcinomas (e.g. of stomach).
(e) IMMUNOLOGICAL DISORDERS e.g. autoimmune diseases,
— incompatible blood transfusion.

The basic mechanism is as follows:

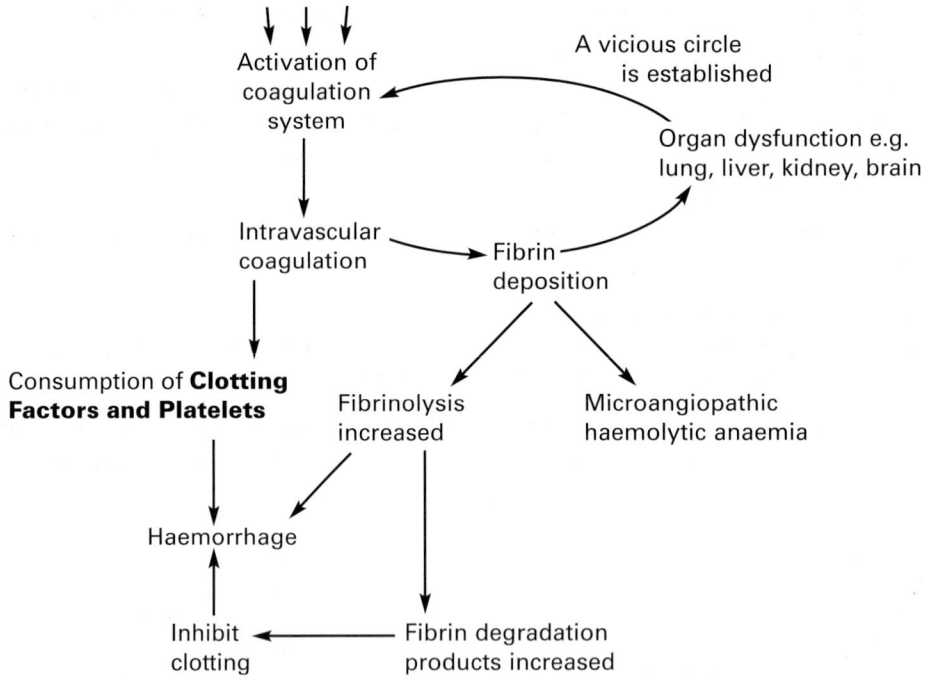

Patients frequently develop renal and hepatic failure and 'shock lung' [e.g. in the haemolytic uraemic syndrome (HUS) which is often associated with toxigenic E.Coli infection — especially E.Coli 0157 (see p. 317)].

THROMBOPHILIA – THROMBOTIC DISORDERS

The major types, causes and effects of thrombosis are discussed on pages 151–161.

Recently, a group of inherited disorders has been discovered where deficiency of NATURAL ANTICOAGULANTS leads to an increased risk of venous thrombosis. This may be deep venous thrombosis or visceral e.g mesenteric veins. There is also an increased risk of pulmonary embolism.

The main forms are:

(a) **ANTITHROMBIN DEFICIENCY**
Antithrombin, a member of the SERPIN group of **Ser**ine protease inhibitors, is synthesised in the liver. It blocks the action of F IXa, F Xa, F XIIa and thrombin. Deficiency is due to mutation of a gene on the long arm of chromosome 1 — the effects depend on the exact type of mutation. The prevalence is around 1 in 20,000.

Note: **Heparin**, the anticoagulant, acts by enhancing the action of antithrombin.

(b) **PROTEIN C DEFICIENCY**
This is a Vitamin K dependent protein, synthesised in the liver. Together with protein S it blocks the action of Factor Va and Factor VIIIa. Around 1 in 15–30,000 is affected. In addition to deep thrombosis, patients also get superficial thrombophlebitis.

(c) **PROTEIN S DEFICIENCY**
This protein is secreted by the liver, platelets and endothelial cells. Its function is to bind with protein C to inhibit Factors Va and VIIIa.

(d) **Activated Protein C Resistance**
This is an inherited disorder where a mutation affects the Factor V gene. The protein is resistant to the effects of protein C — simulating protein C deficiency.

The possible role of minor deficiencies of these genetic factors in the more common forms of thrombosis is not yet established. The well known risk factors for thrombosis are listed below.

Acquired risk factors for thrombosis include:

Arterial	**Venous**
ATHEROMA	IMMOBILITY
SMOKING	TRAUMA/SURGERY
HYPERTENSION	MALIGNANCY
MYELOPROLIFERATIVE DISORDERS	ORAL CONTRACEPTIVES
	OBESITY

THE LYMPHOID SYSTEM

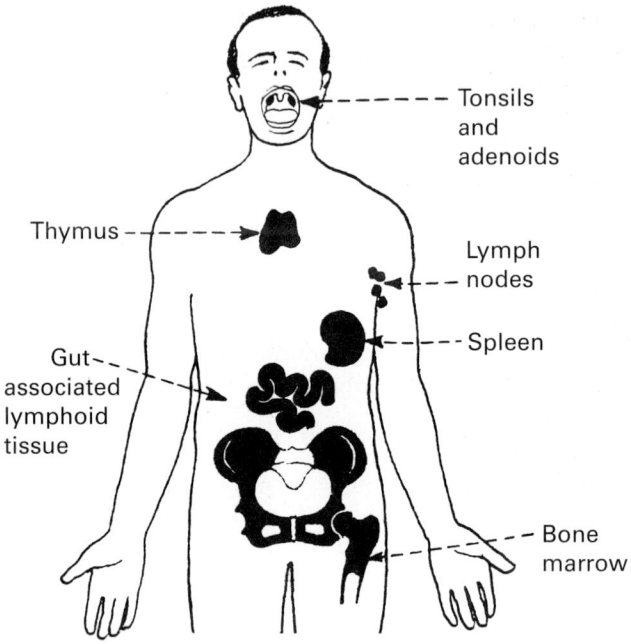

The lymphoid organs are principally involved in:

(a) Production and maturation of lymphocytes — thymus (T cells) and bone marrow (B cells).

(b) Antigen presentation and the immune response.

(c) 'Filtration' and phagocytosis of micro-organisms and particulate material.

LYMPH NODES

The basic structure reflects the main functions.

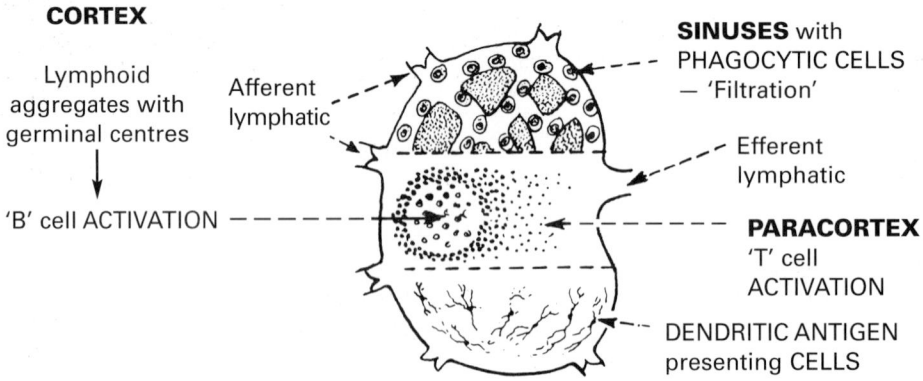

LYMPHADENOPATHY

Lymph node enlargement may be **localised** or **generalised.** It may be due to:
(a) reactive hyperplasia e.g. — infection by bacteria or viruses,
— particulate material,
— immune stimulation e.g. Rheumatoid arthritis,
— draining degradation products from a cancer.
(b) due to neoplasia e.g. — secondary deposits of carcinoma,
— primary lymphoid tumours.

REACTIVE HYPERPLASIA

The changes include three basic and several subsidiary:

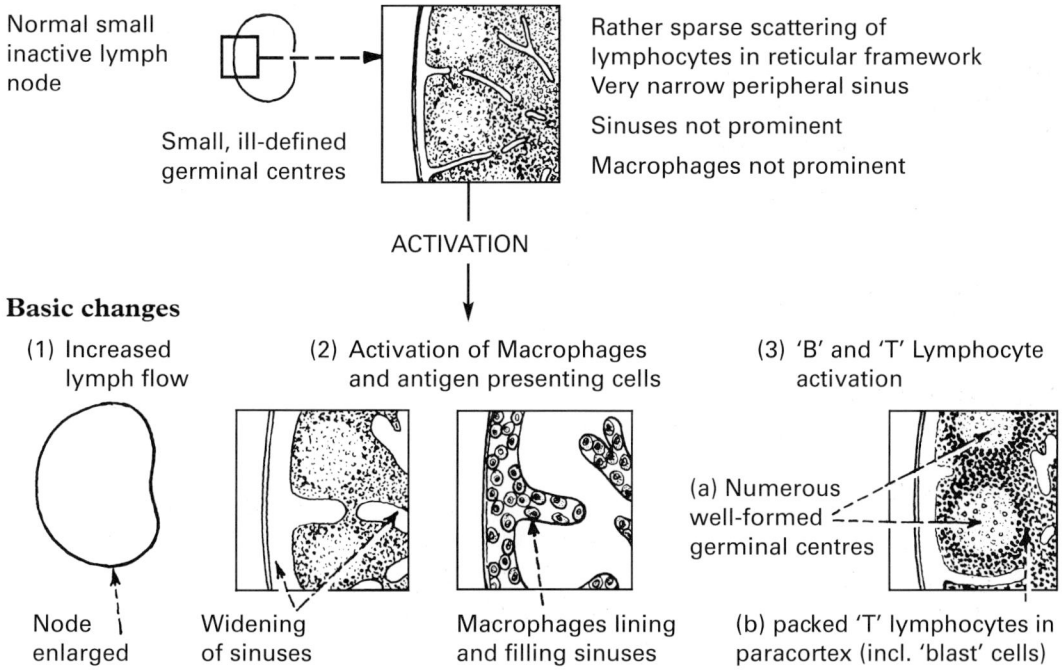

Subsidiary changes

1. Infiltration by neutrophils (in acute inflammation)
2. Increased blood flow (prominent venules)
3. Increased plasma cells
4. Increased eosinophils

} → Chronic inflammation

The qualitative and quantitative variations and combinations of these changes are very numerous; in most reactive states the appearances are non-specific. In only a few instances do particular patterns of response reflect a specific stimulus.

LYMPHADENOPATHY – INFECTIONS

ACUTE BACTERIAL LYMPHADENITIS

This is seen draining an infected area.

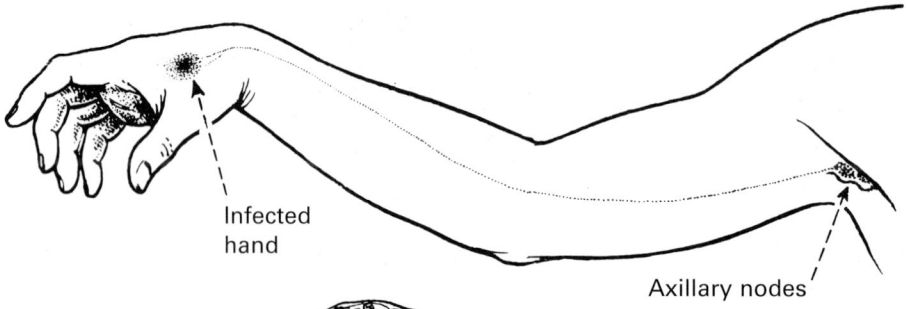

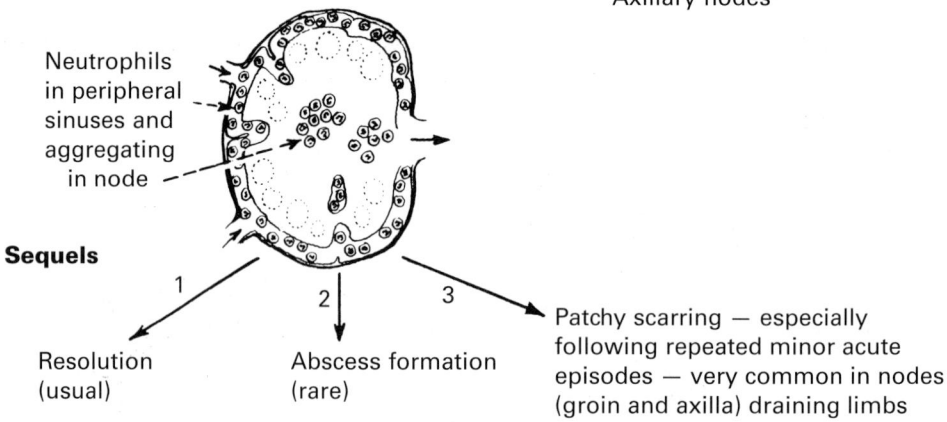

In **LYMPHOGRANULOMA VENEREUM (LGV)**, the enlarged lymph nodes show a striking histological appearance.

LGV is an infection by chlamydia trachomatis. The portal entry is by venereal contact and the disease runs a subacute course.

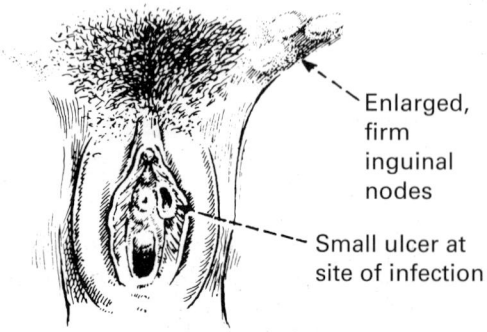

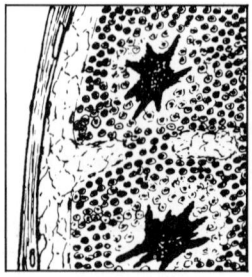

Granulomatous reaction with typical stellate abscess (neutrophils)

The diagnosis has to be confirmed by a skin test (Frei test) or a complement fixation test.

In **CAT SCRATCH FEVER**, the nodes draining the scratched area show similar histological changes. The organism Bartonella henselae is thought to be responsible.

LYMPHADENOPATHY

TUBERCULOSIS is associated with a granulomatous response, often with caseation due to delayed type sensitivity.

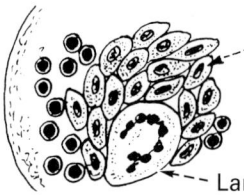

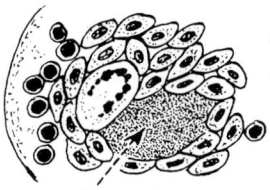

VIRAL LYMPHADENITIS — Many infections induce paracortical hyperplasia — with activation of T cells.

In **GLANDULAR FEVER** (Infectious mononucleosis), an infection by Epstein-Barr virus of young adults, the cervical lymph nodes are particularly involved.

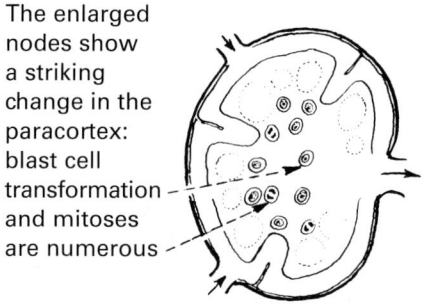

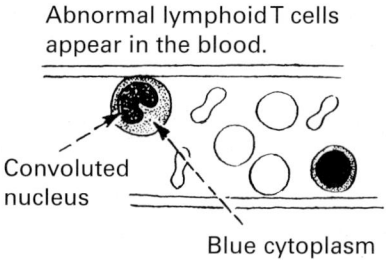

In **MEASLES**, the reactive nodes and lymphoid tissues generally contain unusual, multinucleate **giant cells** (Warthin-Finkeldey).

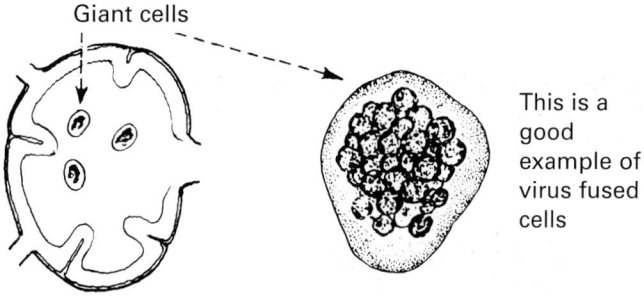

In **TOXOPLASMOSIS**, a protozoal disease (*Toxoplasma gondii*) which may cause serious damage to the fetus or neonate and present with lymph node enlargement in the adult, the histological appearances in the node may indicate the aetiology. The diagnosis is confirmed by serological tests.

In addition to the usual reactive changes

↓

A scattering of small epithelioid granulomas

↓

Numerous smaller monocytoid 'B' cells in the sinuses

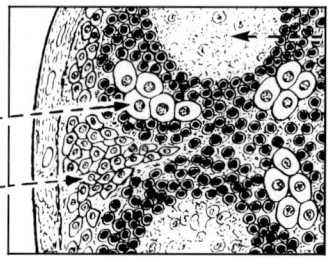

LYMPHADENOPATHY – NON-INFECTIVE CAUSES

FOREIGN MATERIAL

Lymph nodes to which foreign particulate material drains often show marked enlargement due to accumulation of macrophages which have ingested the foreign material.

For example: — carbon and silica in hilar lymph nodes
— silicon e.g. in axiliary lymph nodes in patients with prosthetic joints.

CHRONIC SKIN DISEASE (so-called Dermatopathic lymphadenopathy) e.g. psoriasis, eczema and mycosis fungoides (p. 452).

The following may be seen lying free and in macrophages:
- Fat
- Melanin – from damaged skin
- Haemosiderin – from minor bleeding in skin

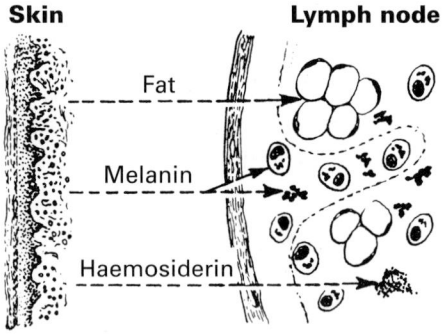

SARCOIDOSIS

In this disease of unknown aetiology (possibly infective?) non-caseating granulomas are seen.

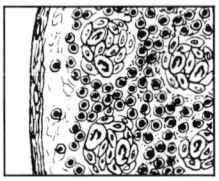

The appearances clearly resemble tuberculosis, but the follicles remain discrete and there is no caseation.

Sarcoid type granulomas are also seen in the lymph nodes of patients with other granulomatous diseases e.g. Crohn's disease and in lymph nodes draining tumours.

SPLEEN

The anatomy of the spleen reflects both its basic function, which is filtration of the blood, and sequential functions of phagocytosis and the immune response. Normal average weight — 150 g.

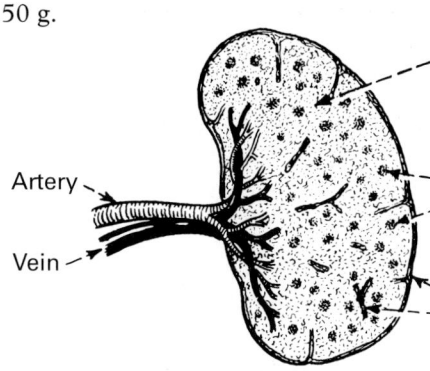

Microscopic appearance

Lymphoid aggregate — mediates IMMUNE RESPONSE.

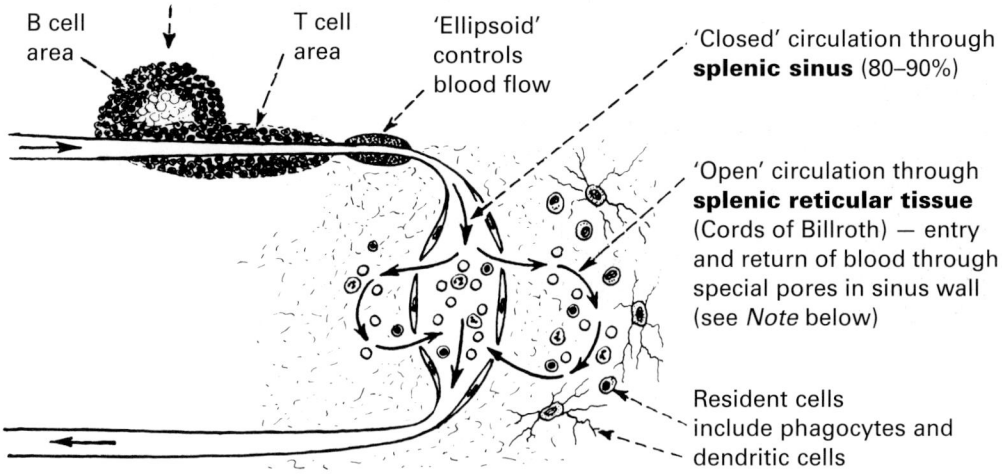

The red pulp is the site of filtration and phagocytosis of the following:

1. Effete cells and cell debris — especially blood cells but also cell debris derived from the body generally
2. Microbes and their toxins
3. Abnormal or excess material derived from metabolic processes.

Note: The special pores allowing re-entry of RBCs to the circulation have a 2μ aperture: abnormal RBCs (e.g. spherocytes) cannot pass through and are trapped.

SPLENOMEGALY

Enlargement of the spleen is an important and common clinical sign. Increase in the red pulp due to increased numbers of phagocytes and/or increased numbers of blood cells is the major component; in chronic infections particularly, hyperplasia of the lymphoid tissue contributes.

An aetiological classification under 5 broad headings is convenient.

Enlargement associated with:
1. INFECTIONS
2. CIRCULATORY DISTURBANCES
3. STORAGE DISEASES and DEGENERATIONS
4. NEOPLASIA — primary and secondary
5. DISORDERS OF THE BLOOD.

1. INFECTIONS

In acute systemic bacterial infections the spleen shows slight to moderate enlargement (200–400 g).

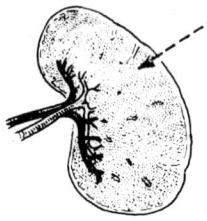

Cut surface uniform pink or red — white pulp obscured due to:
CONGESTION
↑ PHAGOCYTES
↑ NEUTROPHILS

↓

After death the enzymes rapidly digest splenic tissues

'SEPTIC' spleen at autopsy

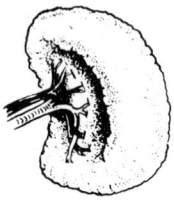

Soft with wrinkled capsule

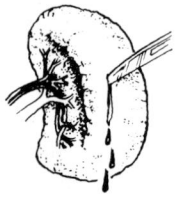

Red fluid flows from cut surface

Sequels

(a) Resolution as infection resolves.
(b) Occasionally spreads through capsule (perisplenitis) to adjacent tissues, with or without abscess formation.
(c) Only extremely rarely does abscess formation occur within the spleen.

In non-pyogenic and chronic infections, there may be moderate enlargement.

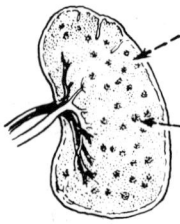

Firm

Cut surface shows lymphoid aggregates

Red pulp contains increased PHAGOCYTES often PLASMA CELLS

Examples: Subacute infective endocarditis
Tuberculosis
Typhoid fever
Infectious mononucleosis
Brucellosis
Malaria } protozoal
Kala-azar } diseases
— often massive enlargement

SPLENOMEGALY

2. CIRCULATORY DISTURBANCES

Congestive splenomegaly occurs in two main conditions:

(1) **Congestive cardiac failure**

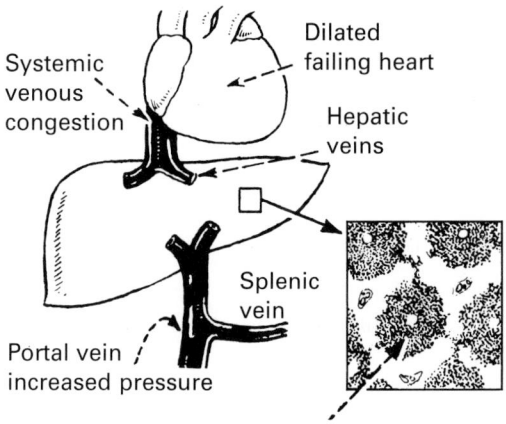

Centrilobular congestion is reflected through the liver to the portal vein

(2) **Hepatic cirrhosis**

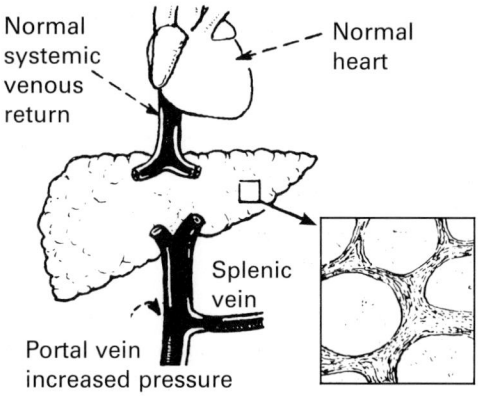

Obstruction to portal venous flow due to fibrosis in liver

SPLENIC ENLARGEMENT

Moderate — rarely exceeds 500g

Consistency — firm to hard; so-called 'cricket ball' spleen

Cut surface purple; white pulp just visible

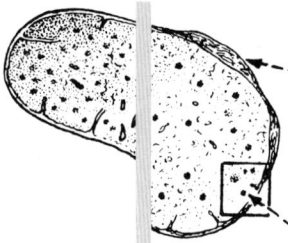

May be severe, e.g. 1000+ g
May be focal capsular thickening

Consistency — firm to hard
Cut surface — pink to purple depending on amount of fibrous tissue

Small lymphoid aggregate

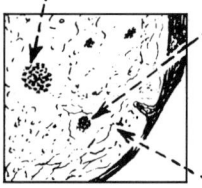

May be flecked with small brown spots (Gandy-Gamna nodules) due to organisation of old haemorrhages

Permanently dilated sinuses

The type of splenomegaly associated with portal venous hypertension may have serious haematological effects (see Hypersplenism).

SPLENOMEGALY

3. STORAGE DISEASES AND DEGENERATIONS

The diseases associated with this type of enlargement are rare.

Examples are:

Amyloidosis (see pp.21–24)

Lipid storage diseases, (see p.20) including Gaucher's disease, Niemann Pick disease and Tay-Sachs disease.

Some disorders of glycogen storage.

4. NEOPLASIA

(a) PRIMARY — the spleen is rarely the seat of primary tumour growth.

(b) SECONDARY — the spleen is rarely affected by secondary tumour, e.g. carcinoma and sarcoma, but it is commonly affected during the systematised spread of **lymphomas** and **leukaemias.**

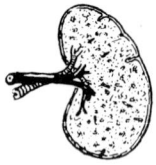

Normal spleen 150 g

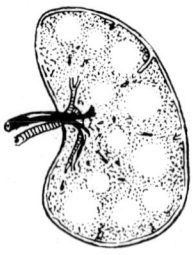

Moderate enlargement 500 g

Nodules of white lymphoma tissue e.g Hodgkin's disease

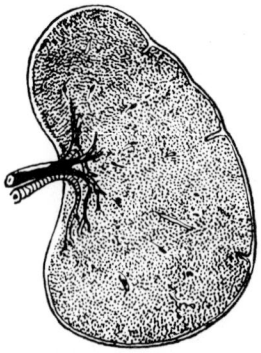

Massive enlargement 1500 g

Uniform, beefy, cut surface in chronic leukaemia

Splenic enlargement may be a feature of histiocytosis-X (Langerhans cell histiocytosis).

SPLENOMEGALY

5. DISORDERS OF THE BLOOD

Splenic enlargement is associated with blood disorders in two main circumstances:

1. Splenic enlargement causing blood disorders

ENLARGED SPLEEN from any cause, but particularly in cases of **portal hypertension** → Increased capacity for sequestration of blood cells → Reduction in circulating blood cells, i.e. *anaemia, leucopenia, thrombocytopenia,* separately or together, i.e. **pancytopenia** → Marrow hyperplasia

This syndrome is called **hypersplenism** (splenic anaemia)

2. Blood disorder causing splenic enlargement

(a) Production of abnormal blood cells, e.g. in haemolytic anaemias: idiopathic thrombocytopenia (antibody coated platelets) → Increased demand on sequestration function of spleen → Increase in spleen size

(b) In leukaemias and lymphomas → Infiltration of spleen by neoplastic cells / Increased sequestration of abnormal cells → Increase in spleen size

(c) In chronic marrow failure due to fibrosis or secondary tumour infiltration → Resumption by spleen of fetal blood forming role → Increase in spleen size — may be massive (500–2,000 g)

Note: When a blood disorder initiates splenic enlargement the disability may be compounded by a superimposed hypersplenism, e.g.

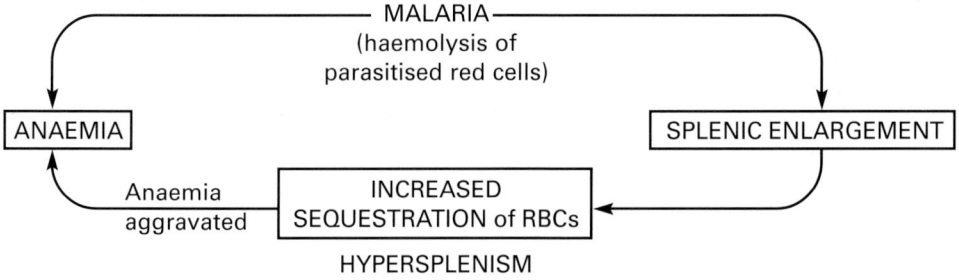

DISEASES OF THE SPLEEN – MISCELLANEOUS

HYPOSPLENISM

Hyposplenism is not usually a cause of major disability. It occurs following splenectomy and in cases of splenic atrophy.

The effects are considered under two main headings:

1. **On the cells of the blood**

Loss of splenic sequestration function
↓
Deficiency in disposal of abnormal cells

Red cell series:
(a) increased acanthocytes
(b) increased Howell-Jolly bodies
(c) increased number of iron-containing cells

Neutrophils: may be leucocytosis

Platelets: may be thrombocythaemia

Seen especially after splenectomy — usually not permanent

2. **On resistance to infection**

Loss of filtration of bacteria from blood → Occasional cases of **septicaemia** — especially caused by *streptococcus pneumoniae* — young children are particularly susceptible

CIRCULATORY AND VASCULAR CHANGES

(a) *Infarction*

(i) Embolism causing infarction is not uncommon but usually clinically unimportant.

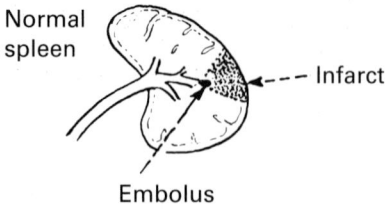

(ii) Enlarged spleens are particularly susceptible to infarction without embolism.

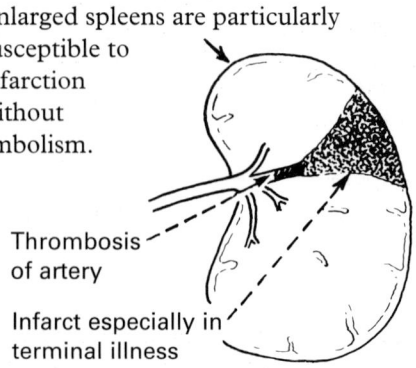

(b) *Hyalinisation of splenic arterioles*

This is an almost invariable concomitant of ageing and is not related to systemic arteriosclerosis or hypertension.

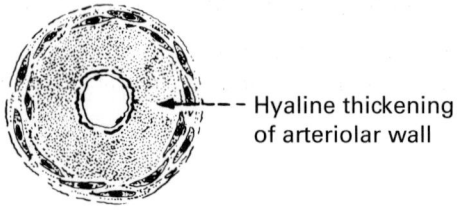

THYMUS

This 'primary' lymphoid organ is concerned with the development and processing to maturation of the long-lived T lymphocytes which are then distributed to the lymphoid tissues and to the circulating pool of T lymphocytes.

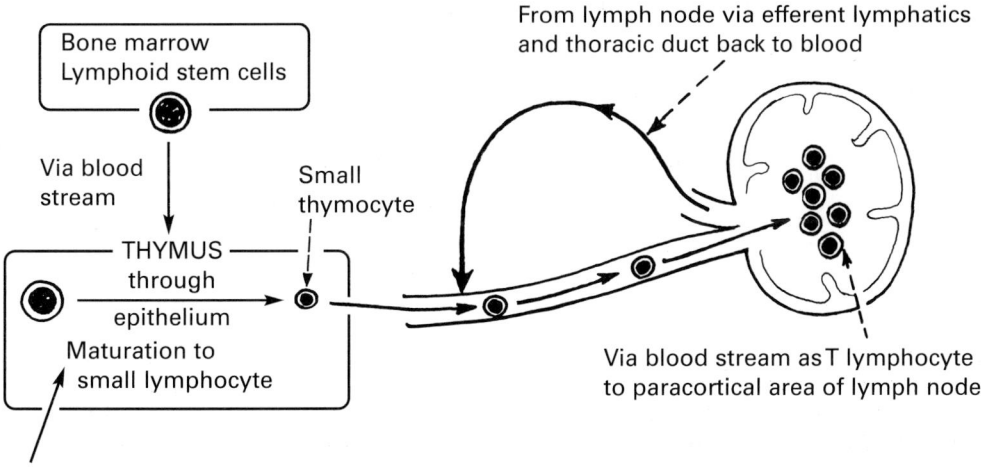

Mechanism — stimulation by hormones formed locally by thymic epithelial cells.

This activity is maximal in the fetal and childhood stages. Involution is rapid after puberty.

Childhood

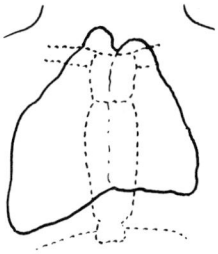

Large cellular organ overlying pericardium (av. wt. 25 g)

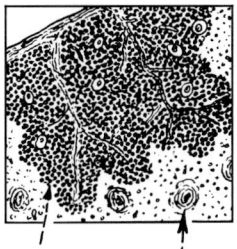

Lymphocytes

Epithelial cells (Hassall's corpuscles)

Adult

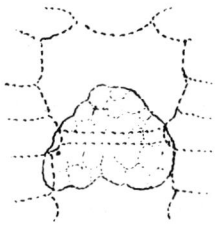

Relatively small, ill-defined — in upper anterior mediastinum (av. wt. 15 g) (3 g corrected for fat)

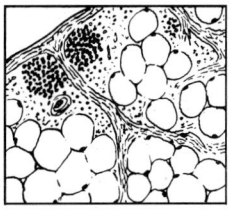

Small foci of lymphocytes and occasional Hassall's corpuscles in large tracts of fatty tissue.

Congenital thymic aplasia or hypoplasia

The resulting T cell deficiency is associated with disordered cell-mediated immune response.

Note: Thymectomy in adult life has little pathological significance since the T lymphocytes produced in childhood are long enough lived to obviate serious immune deficiency.

THYMUS

Thymic hyperplasia

Assessment by weight alone is unsatisfactory due to the variability of the fat content in adult life. A weight over 35 g probably represents hyperplasia, but the appearance of lymphoid follicles with germinal centres is a more reliable indication of hyperplasia.

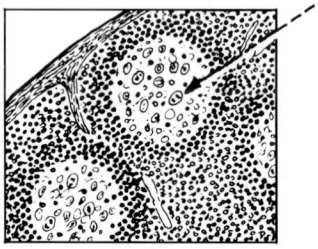

Associated conditions:
- Auto-immune disorders,
- e.g. Systemic lupus erythematosus
  - Addison's disease
  - Thyrotoxicosis
  - Pancytopenia
  - and *NB* MYASTHENIA GRAVIS

Thymic tumours

Thymomas are rare tumours: they are essentially low-grade carcinomas with an admixture of lymphoid cells: they rarely metastasise. They may have an auto-immune component similar to thymic hyperplasia.

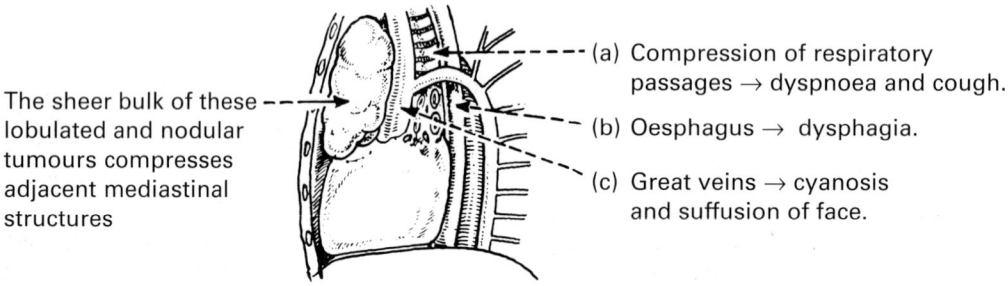

Other primary tumours arising in the thymus are;
(1) T cell lymphoblastic lymphomas (adolescent males).
(2) Hodgkin's disease.
(3) Germ cell tumours (e.g. teratoma).
(4) Carcinoids.

The thymus in Myasthenia Gravis (MG)

MG is a disease of voluntary muscles in which weakness is the main feature. The association with the thymus is striking in that 80% of all cases of MG have either thymic hyperplasia or thymoma.

Follicular hyperplasia (80%) — seen especially in young females.
Thymoma (20%) — seen especially in middle aged males.
The results of thymectomy in MG patients are very unpredictable.

The detailed pathological changes in MG and the mechanisms by which the thymus is linked with the disease are described on pages 110, 609.

NEOPLASTIC LYMPHADENOPATHY

Lymph node enlargement may be due to

(a) Invasion by SECONDARY TUMOURS — especially CARCINOMAS —
or (b) Primary lymphoid tumours — LYMPHOMAS.

SECONDARY TUMOUR invasion
Carcinoma of the breast is taken as an example.

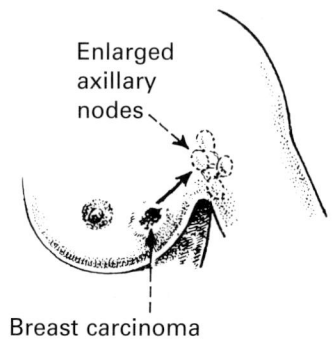

Note:

(i) The nodal enlargement is not necessarily due to secondary tumour.

Reactive hyperplasia is also common in nodes draining tumours especially if there is ulceration. The distinction between these 2 causes of node enlargement can only be made with certainty by **histological examination.**

(ii) The invasion of a group of nodes occurs in a step-wise fashion: a single node (the SENTINEL node) is invaded initially and spread to adjacent nodes follows.

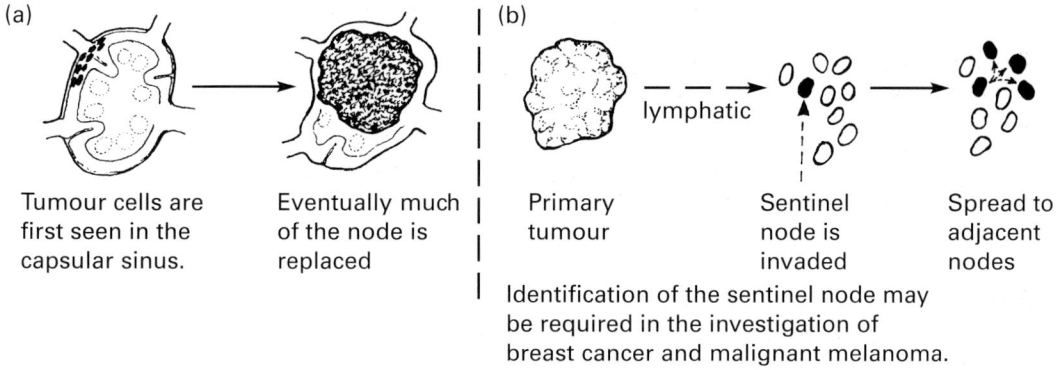

Identification of the sentinel node may be required in the investigation of breast cancer and malignant melanoma.

LYMPHOMAS

Lymphomas are malignant tumours derived from lymphoid cells. They may arise within lymph nodes or at other sites (extra-nodal lymphomas).

Classically, they are divided into 2 main groups.

(a) Hodgkin's disease 20–25%
- almost always of lymph node origin.
- characterised by the presence of Reed-Sternberg cells.

(b) Non-Hodgkin's disease 75–80%
- three-quarters arise in lymph nodes

In recent years, modern immunocytochemical, molecular biology and cytogenetic techniques have been applied to the study of lymphomas. The traditional division between Hodgkin's and non-Hodgkin's lymphoma has been challenged but remains of major clinical importance.

NON-HODGKIN'S LYMPHOMAS

These solid tumours mainly affect middle aged to elderly patients.

They may arise

(a) Within lymph nodes or (b) in extra-nodal sites.

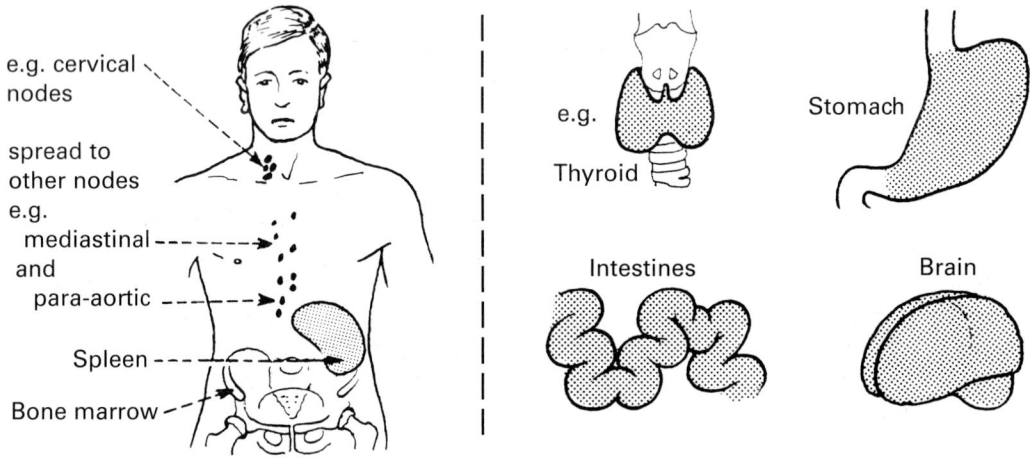

Eventually a generalised spread with involvement of liver, lungs and heart may occur.

DEGREE OF MALIGNANCY

The natural history tends to separate lymphomas into two main groups which have links with the morphological appearances.

1. *Low grade malignancy* associated with well differentiated relatively inactive cell types,
— progress of years.

2. *High grade malignancy* associated with primitive actively proliferating cells,
— progress over weeks or months.
Tend to respond well to chemotherapy.

PATHOLOGICAL COMPLICATIONS

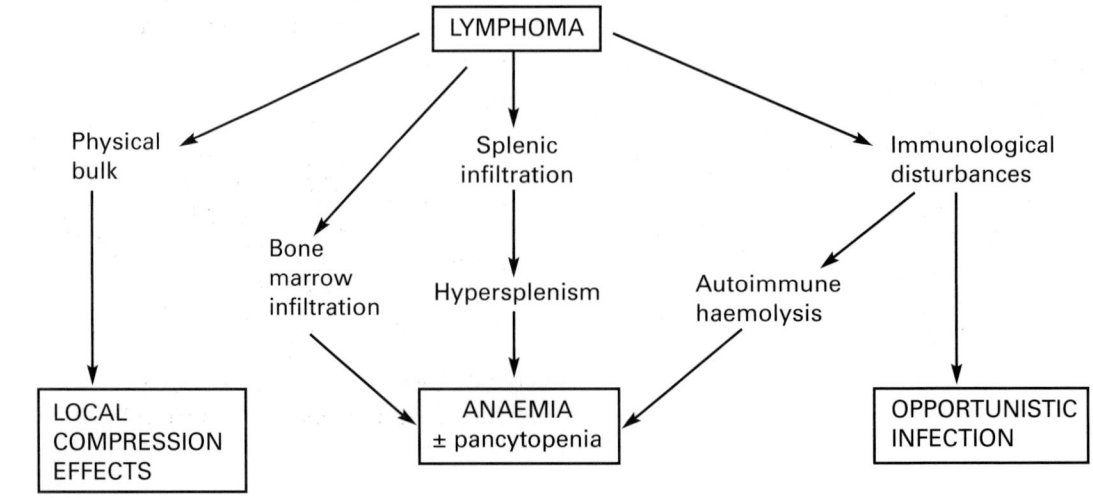

NON-HODGKIN'S LYMPHOMAS

Classification

This is a confusing area. Traditional classifications relied on morphology alone. Many clinicians now use the REAL (Revised European American Lymphoma) classification which includes immunohistochemistry and genetic data. A simplified version follows:

NON-HODGKIN's LYMPHOMAS

B CELL (> 90%)

- Small lymphocytic lymphoma (equivalent to B CLL, p. 459).
- Immunocytoma (lymphoplasmacytic) lymphoma.
- Mantle cell lymphoma.
- Follicle centre lymphoma.
- Burkitt's lymphoma.
- Large B cell lymphoma.
- MALT lymphomas (Mucosa Associated Lymphoid Tissue).
- Myeloma/Plasmacytoma.

T CELL (< 10%)

- Peripheral T cell lymphoma.
- Adult T cell leukaemia.
- Angioimmunoblastic lymphoma.
- Anaplastic large cell lymphomas (some do not express T cell markers).
- Intestinal T cell lymphoma.
- Mycosis fungoides (skin).
- Angiocentric lymphoma.

According to this classification each type is considered separately for treatment purposes.

The classification relies on cell surface markers which distinguish the B and T cells and their subsets. B and T cell monoclondality can be detected by gene rearrangements.

Subtyping of lymphoma

IMMUNOHISTOCHEMISTRY

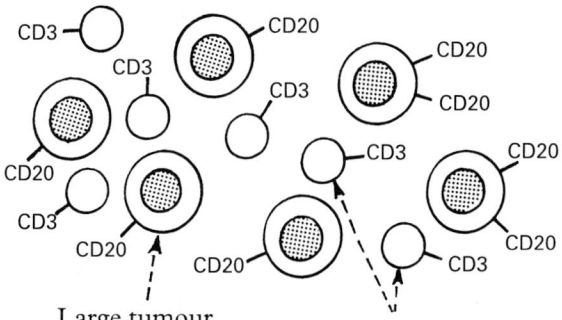

Large tumour cells of B cell type express B cell markers e.g. CD20

Frequently small reactive T cells are seen — they express CD3

MOLECULAR GENETIC ANALYSIS

In B cell differentiation different immunoglobulin genes are found by gene rearrangements, while in T cell differentiation a similar process occurs with T cell antigen receptors (p. 93).

In a polyclonal (reactive) population many different genes are found.

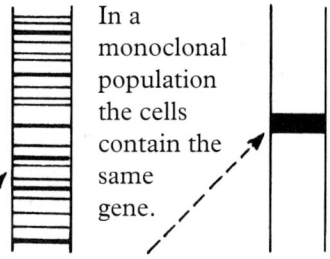

On DNA gel, many different bands.

In a monoclonal population the cells contain the same gene.

One strong monoclonal band.

NON-HODGKIN'S LYMPHOMAS

FOLLICLE CENTRE LYMPHOMA

This is one of the commonest forms — a 'B' cell lymphoma.

The neoplastic follicles are the malignant equivalent of normal germinal centres.

The tumour cells express the anti-apoptosis gene bc1–2 which immortalises them. There is often a translocation t (14;18) which joins the bc1–2 gene to the immunoglobulin heavy chain gene.

The lymphoma is slowly progressive but often eventually fatal. Occasionally it transforms into a diffuse large 'B' cell lymphoma.

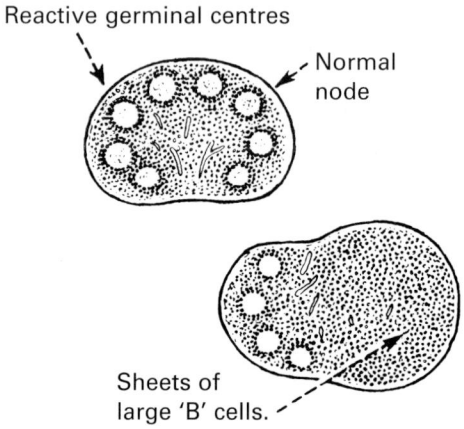

BURKITT'S LYMPHOMA

This is a high grade lymphoma found mainly in Equatorial Africa, New Guinea and other malaria endemic areas. Similar tumours are seen in AIDS patients. The relationship with Epstein Barr virus has already been discussed (p. 81) — as has the translocation t (8;14) which activates the c-myc oncogene (p. 152).

The histological appearance is typical and striking.

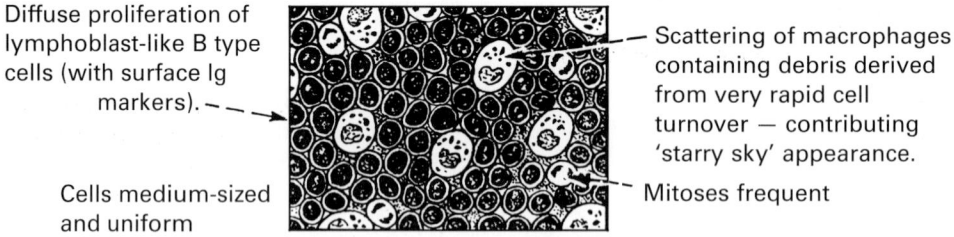

Endemic (African type) Burkitt's lymphoma typically presents with lesions in the jaw, or in the abdomen, e.g. ovary, liver, gastrointestinal tract. The less common cases in the West typically involve lymph node, marrow and gut.

The disease may respond dramatically to aggressive treatment.

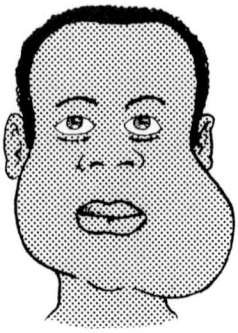

NON-HODGKIN'S LYMPHOMAS

The LYMPHOPLASMACYTOID LYMPHOMAS

These low grade tumours, arising particularly in lymph nodes, but sometimes in the alimentary tract, synthesise and may secrete monoclonal immunoglobin (Ig) into the plasma.

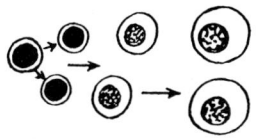

Monoclonal proliferation of cell line showing differentiation to various stages

Synthesis and secretion of whole molecules of Ig — always monoclonal, usually IgM, very rarely others.

Extremely rarely only parts of the molecule are produced resulting in 'heavy chain disease' e.g. alpha chain disease.

Pathological effects may result from the presence of these products

WALDENSTRÖM'S MACROGLOBULINAEMIA is the classic example. It affects the lymph nodes, marrow and spleen in the late middle aged and elderly, with a preponderance of males. In addition to the usual pathological complications of low-grade lymphomas, the production of IgM in large quantity produces special complications.

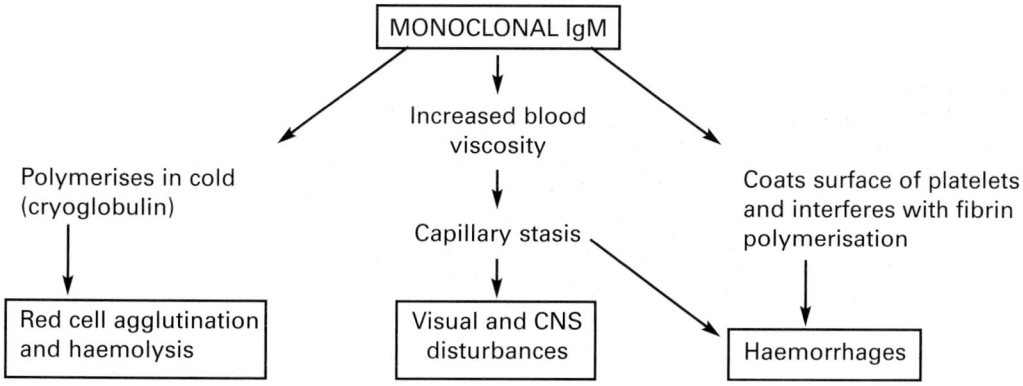

PLASMA CELL TUMOURS

SOLITARY PLASMACYTOMA

A very small number of plasma cell tumours present as solitary growths, e.g. in a long bone, the nasopharynx, a lymph node, alimentary tract. It is likely that these slow-growing tumours have been present for long periods before they present clinically. In some cases, dissemination particularly to the bone marrow ensues.

MULTIPLE MYELOMA (MYELOMATOSIS)

The great majority of plasma cell tumours present as widespread deposits in the bone marrow. Classically the lesions are seen as punched out defects in the bones — the skull showing this appearance particularly well. These focal proliferations of plasma cells usually occur against a background of more diffuse infiltration throughout the marrow.

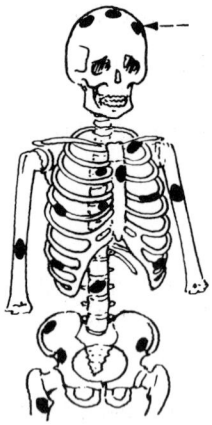

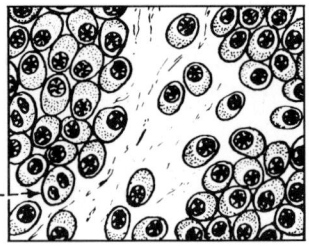

The disease has an incidence similar to Hodgkin's disease, with an age peak in the 5th and 6th decades.
After initial presentation, the progress is usually fairly rapid, leading to death in 2 to 4 years without treatment.

Pathological effects are considered under two main headings:

1. **Tumour growth and its effects**

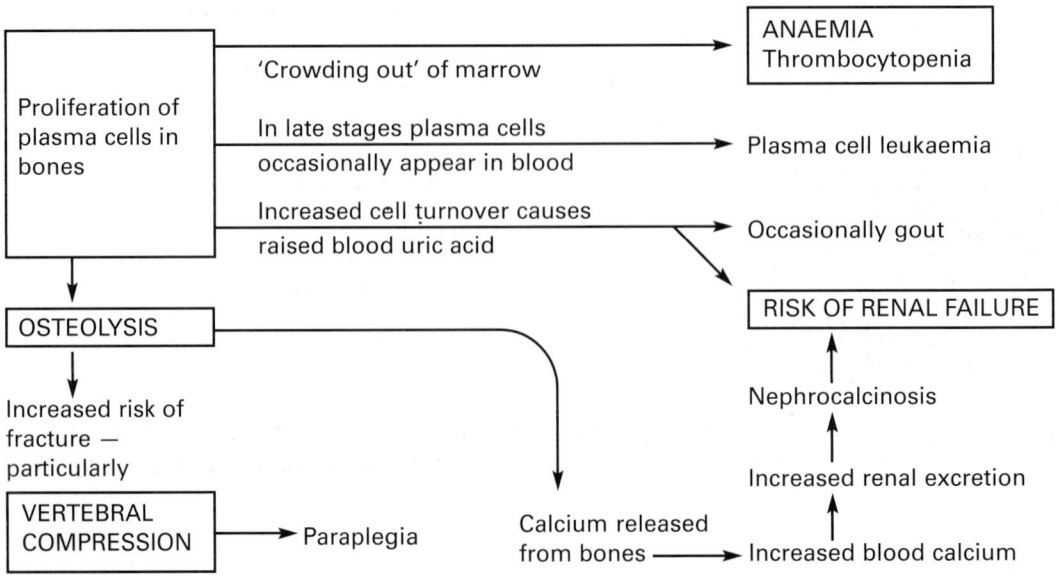

PLASMA CELL TUMOURS

Pathological effects (continued)

2. Synthesis of immunoglobulin and its effects

Myelomatosis, being a monoclonal tumour, will produce a single Ig, but the type of Ig varies from case to case, unlike Waldenström's macroglobulinaemia where the immunoglobulin is always IgM. The common heavy chains are G (60%) and A (20%). Light chains of K type are encountered more frequently than λ reflecting the normal K:λ ratio, i.e. 65:35. Thus myeloma of IgGK is the most frequent.

The presence of a single type of Ig is reflected in the electrophoretic pattern

The other normal immunoglobulins are always decreased.

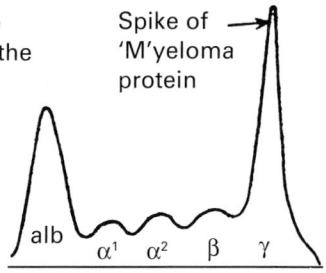

In most cases high levels of 'M' protein cause:
1. High ESR
2. Marked rouleaux formation
3. Depending on type of Ig — increased blood viscosity.

Note: 'M' stands for myeloma and it does not signify IgM.

Release of light chains

In many myelomas, some of the Ig molecules are incompletely formed, and unattached light chains are released with important effects. Because of their low molecular weight the light chains:

(1) Pass through the glomerular filtrate,
(a) appearing *in the urine* as Bence-Jones protein (precipitates during heating — redissolves between 90°–100°C).
(b) During passage through the tubules the protein precipitates as casts and also damages the epithelial cells.

↓

Myeloma kidney

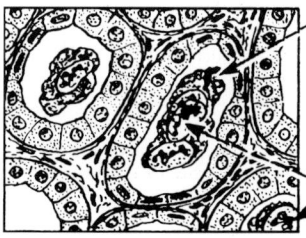

Note giant cells

(2) Pass through capillaries

Light chains

↓

These are incorporated in AMYLOID.

↓

Damage to many organs

↓

Including kidneys

Infections, often of opportunistic type, and particularly pneumonias are common because the immune response is deficient since the high levels of 'M' protein are non-functioning.

NON-HODGKIN'S LYMPHOMA – T cell

MYCOSIS FUNGOIDES

This is a primary T cell (CD4) lymphoma of the skin occurring usually in middle aged men. It presents as a scaly, red macule progressing to skin plaques and then nodules.

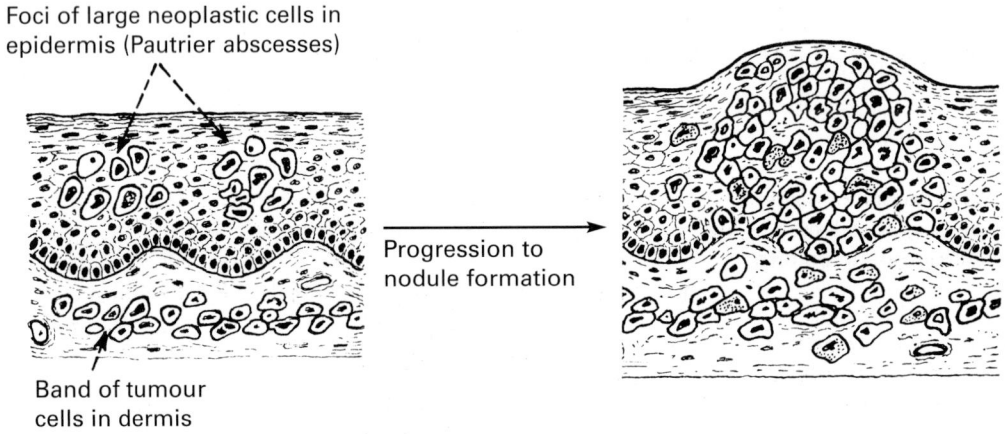

After many years the lymphoma may become generalised or exfoliate into the blood (Sézary syndrome).

ANAPLASTIC LARGE CELL LYMPHOMA

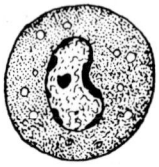

The large malignant T cells (usually expressing surface marker CD30) often spread within the sinuses of the node and, in the past, were mistaken for secondary carcinoma cells.

Some of the large tumour cells mimic the cells in Hodgkin's disease.

Although three-quarters of cases are of T cell type, the remainder are 'null' cell type, i.e. they express neither T nor B cell markers, causing further diagnostic difficulties.

The tumour shows 2 age peaks.

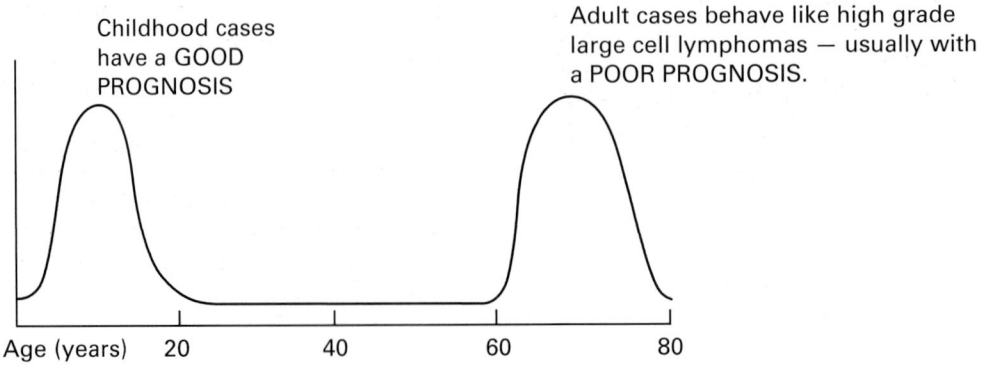

HODGKIN'S DISEASE

Incidence
This disease accounts for 20% of lymphomas. It may occur at any age but there are 2 peaks of incidence. The overall average incidence is 30 cases/ million population but there are wide geographical variations.

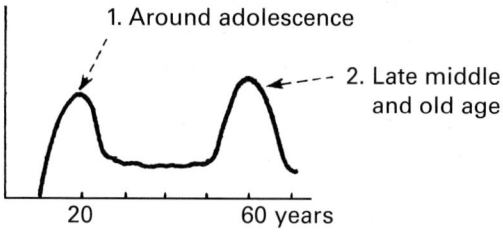

Presentation
Most patients present with painless enlargement of one or more lymph node groups — cervical, axillary, mediastinal. One quarter complain of systemic 'B' symptoms (see Staging) — fever, night sweats, weight loss, itch. The risk of infections is increased by immunosuppression.

Spread and Staging
The disease spreads from one group to the next directly connected by lymphatics.

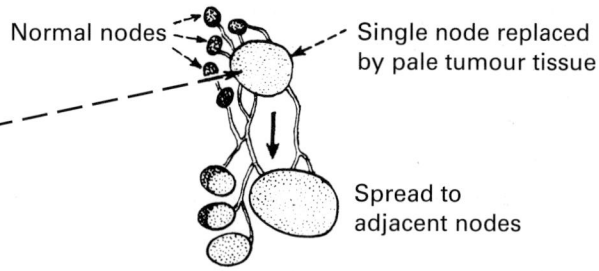

Disease beginning in lymph node

Spreading to
1. Other lymphoid tissue
   (a) Nodes in central axis
   (b) Spleen
2. Other organs
   (a) Marrow
   (b) Liver
   (c) Miscellaneous, e.g. alimentary tract

Staging (Ann Arbor system)

Stage I	Disease involving single node or group of nodes
Stage II	Disease in more than one site — all lesions either below or above the diaphragm
Stage III	Disease on both sides of diaphragm
Stage IV	Widespread involvement of extralymphoid sites ± lymph node involvement

The suffix (E) to the numeral indicates Extranodal disease, (A) denotes absence of systemic symptoms, (B) presence of these (see above).

HODGKIN'S DISEASE

The diagnosis of Hodgkin's disease and the presence or absence of spread can only be made with certainty by microscopic examination of tissues.

The disease presents a considerable variety of histological patterns, but the one constant feature is the presence of Reed-Sternberg (RS) cells, the nature of which remains uncertain.

Typical RS cell

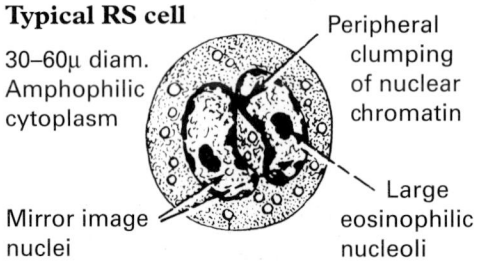

The further histological classification of Hodgkin's disease depends on the recognition of histological patterns.

The RYE classification

1. *Lymphocyte predominant (10%)*

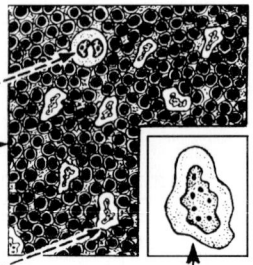

2. *Nodular sclerosing (30–60%)*

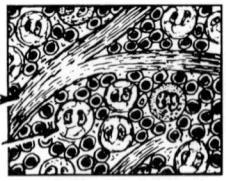

3. *Mixed cellularity (20–30%)*

Plasma cells and eosinophils present in addition to RS cells and lymphocytes

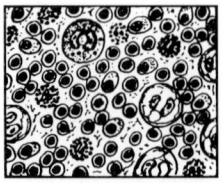

4. *Lymphocyte depleted (<2%)*

Very numerous RS and mononuclear Hodgkin's cells — few lymphocytes ± diffuse fibrosis

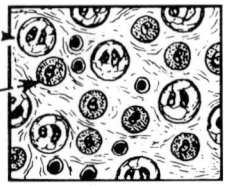

Cells closely related to the RS cell

1. The lacunar cell

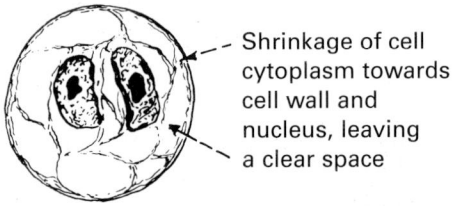

2. Mononuclear Hodgkin's cell

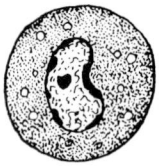

Nuclear characteristic similar to RS cell but smaller

These cells are not specifically diagnostic of Hodgkin's disease.

Lymphocyte predominant and nodular sclerosing types have a relatively good prognosis. Lymphocyte depletion indicates serious disease.

Note: Lymphocyte predominant HD may progress to a B cell lymphoma (large cell type): this and marker studies suggest that it is an unusual type of B cell lymphoma.

LEUKAEMIAS

Leukaemias are primary malignant tumours of haemopoietic cells.

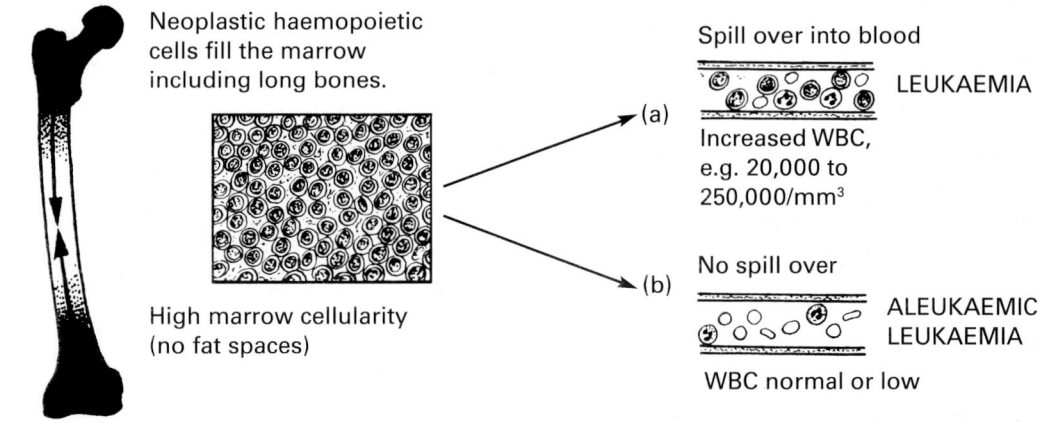

Clinical Effects

The neoplastic cells replace the normal bone marrow

1. Deficiency of red cells ⟶ anaemia.
2. Deficiency of platelets ⟶ thrombocytopenia ⟶ bleeding.
3. Deficiency of white cells ⟶ infection.
4. Increased cell turnover ⟶ ↑DNA breakdown ⟶ ↑uric acid ⟶ gout.

Spread of leukaemia

Leukaemic cells circulate in blood and/or lymph and can therefore spread anywhere in the body. Nodular deposits are, however, uncommon.

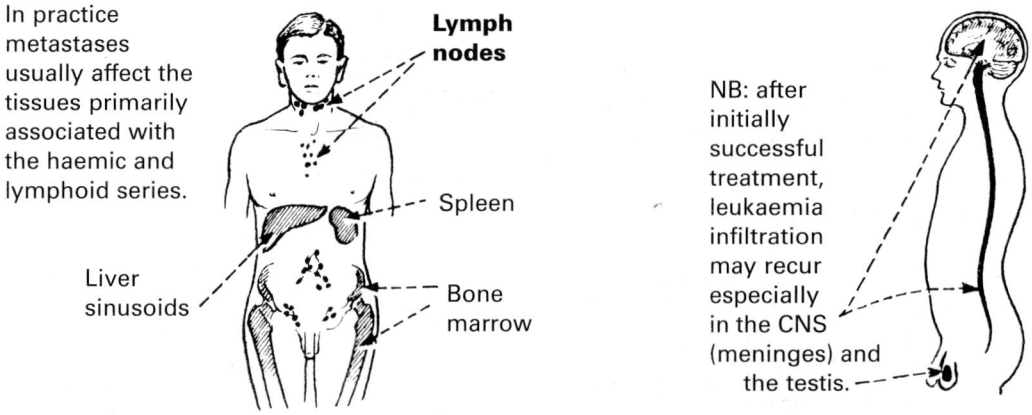

LEUKAEMIAS

Classification

Leukaemias are classified according to the rate of progression and the lineage of the tumour cells. The 4 main forms are:

	MYELOID (granulocyte: monocyte series)	LYMPHOID (B and T lymphocyte series)
ACUTE LEUKAEMIA — Rapid progression — Numerous primitive 'blast' cells.	(i) ACUTE MYELOBLASTIC LEUKAEMIA	(iii) ACUTE LYMPHOBLASTIC LEUKAEMIA
CHRONIC LEUKAEMIA — Slow progression — Cells almost mature.	(ii) CHRONIC MYELOID LEUKAEMIA	(iv) CHRONIC LYMPHOCYTIC LEUKAEMIA

Rare leukaemias affect red cells, megakaryocytes and plasma cells.

Aetiology

In most cases, the cause is unknown. Risk factors include:

1. Radiation e.g. post Hiroshima, Chernobyl, therapeutic X-ray.
2. Chemicals e.g. chemotherapy, benzene.
3. Genetic e.g. Down's syndrome.
4. Virus e.g. Human T-cell Leukaemia Virus-1.

CELL KINETICS

Even in acute leukaemias, increased cell longevity beyond the normal (due to failure of response to mechanisms controlling ageing and destruction) is as important as proliferative rates in increasing the marrow cell population.

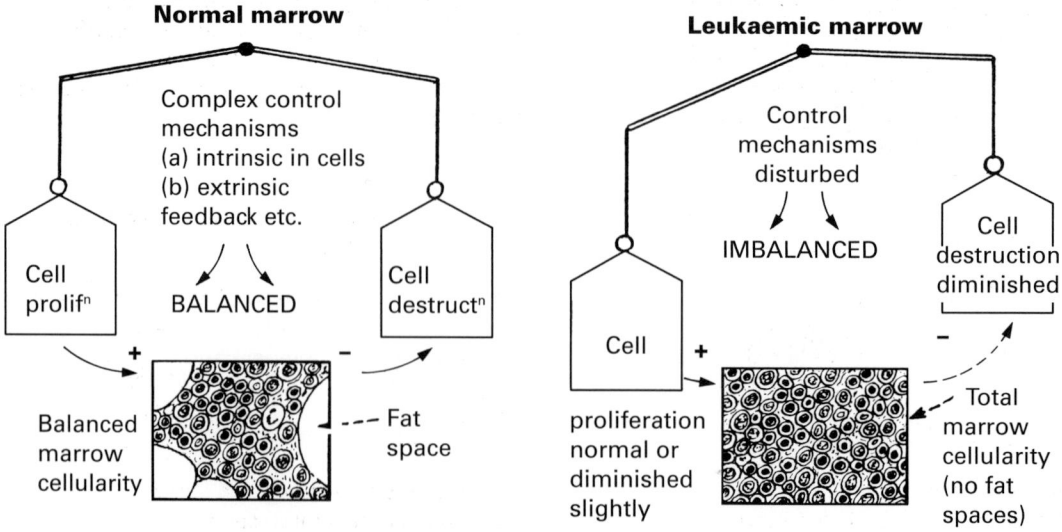

ACUTE MYELOBLASTIC LEUKAEMIA

This is the commonest acute leukaemia of adults — 80% of patients are over 60 years old. Young adults and children may also be affected.

It may arise de novo or in association with chronic myeloid leukaemia, myeloproliferative disorders, myelodysplasia. The onset and progression to marrow failure is rapid, clinically presenting as anaemia, haemorrhage or serious infection.

Classification

The French-American-British (FAB) classification describes 8 different subtypes depending on the degree of differentiation of the cells involved.

TYPE	DIFFERENTIATION	DESCRIPTION OF CELLS
M_0	Undifferentiated	Cells so poorly differentiated that their myeloid nature is not apparent.
M_1	Undifferentiated myeloid	Very primitive myeloid cells.
M_2	Myeloid with granulocytic differentiation	Myeloblasts with granules.
M_3	Promyelocytic	Further myeloid differentiation.
M_4	Myelomonocytic	Both granulocytic and monocytic differentiation.
M_5	Monocytic	Large primitive monocytes.
M_6	Erythroleukaemia	Many red cell precursors.
M_7	Megakaryoblastic	Primitive megakaryocytes.

PATHOLOGY

The marrow

Over-run by blast cells

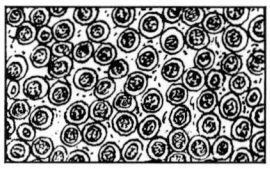

The blood

Decreased platelet count — **thrombocytopenia.**

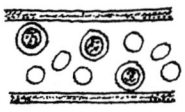

2/3 cases: WBC 20,000—50,000 blast cells
1/3 cases: **aleukaemic**

Other organs may be involved: Splenomegaly, hepatomegaly and lymph node enlargement.

More specific pathological clinical complications are seen in 2 subtypes.

M_3 — Promyelocytic

Primitive cell with primary myeloid granules

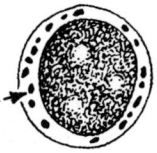

A typical chromosomal translocation t(15:17) is found.

Patients often develop disseminated intravascular coagulation.

M_4 — Myelomonocytic and M_5 — Monocytic.

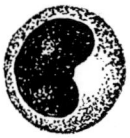

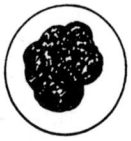

Infiltration of the gums and central nervous sytem is often seen.

CHRONIC MYELOID LEUKAEMIA (CML)

This form of leukaemia arises from malignant transformation of a primitive stem cell — but with the production of differentiated cells — particularly neutrophils.

This is a disease of middle age. There are 3 phases:

1. **Chronic phase** — a period of slow evolution — 2–6 years is typical.
2. **Accelerated phase** — an increase in immature cells.
3. **Blast phase** — transformation to an acute leukaemia — myeloblastic or, very rarely, lymphoblastic.

Rarely patients develop myelofibrosis with marrow failure.

Marrow

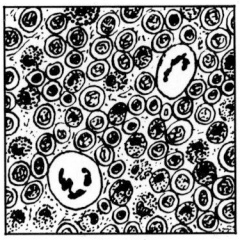

Total cellularity: cells of granulocyte series – late forms numerous (including eosinophil and basophil types). Often increase in megakaryocytes; may be increased fibrosis. Increased pressure in bones may cause clinical tenderness and pain.

Blood

(a) WBC: 75,000–250,000/mm^3
Differential WBC
Blasts } <5%
Promyelocytes }

Majority of cells are late myelocytes and mature granulocytes

(b) ANAEMIA

(c) THROMBOCYTOPENIA (sometimes thrombocytosis)

Splenomegaly

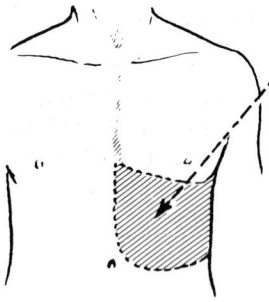

Firm, may be massive, e.g. 3 kg

May be infarction

↓

Clinically painful

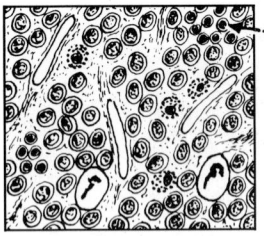

Lymphoid follicles inconspicuous

Red pulp with cells of granulocyte series ± megakaryocytes ± red cell precursors

Philadelphia (Ph) chromosome

In over 95% of cases of CML there is a specific cytogenetic change with the formation of the 'Ph chromosome'.

The change involves a translocation of the c-abl gene (an oncogene) from chromosome 9 to chromosome 22 where hybridisation with the bcr gene occurs.

CHRONIC LYMPHOCYTIC LEUKAEMIA

This is a common form of leukaemia (25% of all cases) and particularly affects middle aged and elderly patients. It is a monoclonal proliferation of small lymphocytes and is best regarded as the leukaemic form of lymphocytic lymphoma.

Most cases are of B cell type — less than 5% are of T cell lineage.

There is typically lymph node enlargement and splenomegaly.

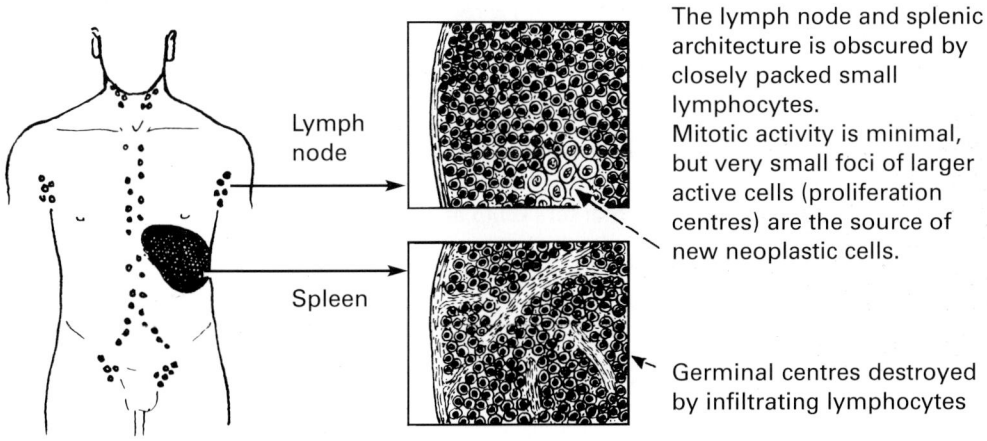

In some cases the lymphoid enlargement precedes the leukaemic phase.

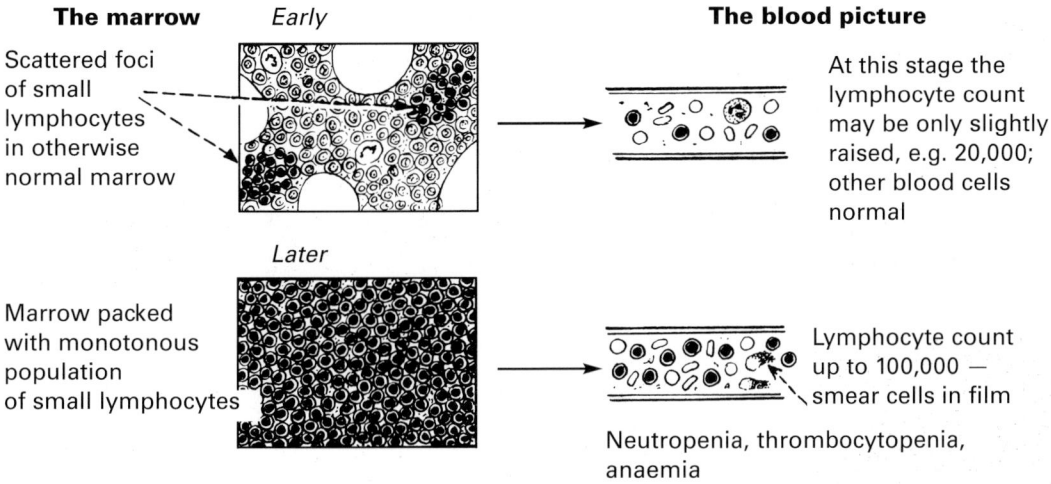

In addition to anaemia these patients often suffer recurrent infections due to defective immunity.

In a minority of cases (approximately 5%) transformation to a high grade 'B' cell lymphoma results (Richter syndrome).

ACUTE LYMPHOBLASTIC LEUKAEMIA (ALL)

This term describes a group of leukaemias of lymphocytic precursors. ALL is the commonest form of childhood leukaemia but is also seen in adults.
Using immunological markers there are 5 main types:

1. **Common ALL** — distinguished by expression of CD10, the Common ALL Antigen (CALLA)

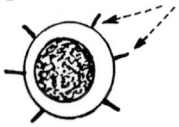

2. **Null ALL** — no markers — a very primitive cell type, commoner in adults.
3. **Pre B-ALL** and **early B-ALL** — primitive B cells
4. **B-ALL** — showing full B cell differentiation
5. **T-ALL** — expression of T cell markers CD3 and CD7.

CD19, CD22.

In addition, distinctive cytogenetic abnormalities — translocations — are of prognostic importance.

ALL in Childhood
This is usually of Common ALL type

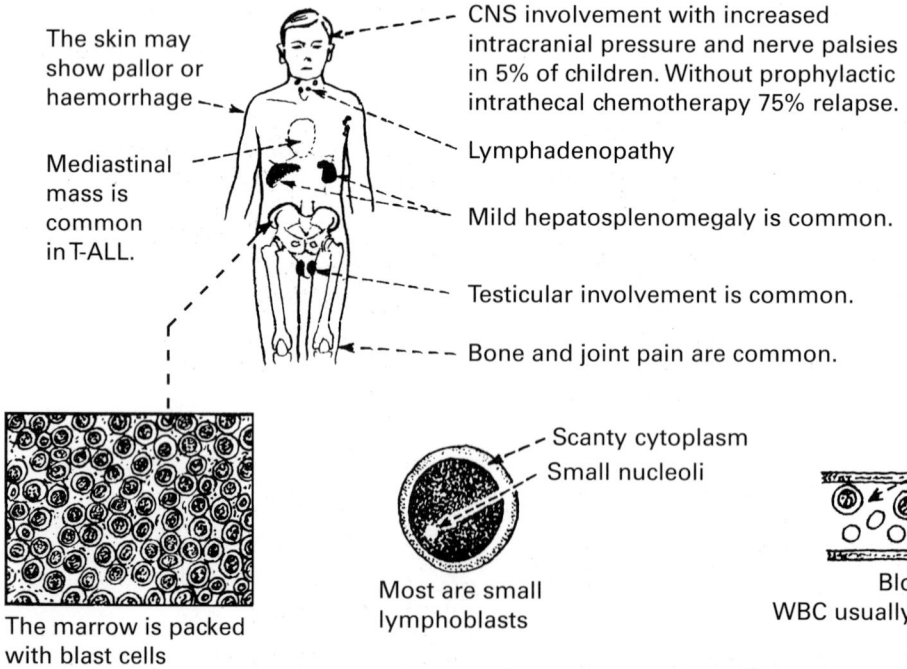

Childhood ALL is now potentially curable — 70% survive 5 years.

ALL in Adults
This is often of Null type. Adults have a much worse prognosis and often require bone marrow transplantation as well as chemotherapy.

MYELOPROLIFERATIVE DISORDERS

In this group of diseases, neoplastic transformation of a haemopoietic precursor cell may lead to excess production of erythrocyte, leucocyte or white cell precursors. In many cases more than one element is affected. This can be summarised as follows:

Abnormal marrow proliferation

- Erythroid precursors → ↑RBC → Polycythaemia rubra vera
- Myeloid precursors → ↑WBC → Chronic myeloid leukaemia
- Megakaryocytes → ↑Platelets → Essential thrombocytosis
- Megakaryocytes → ↑Production of platelet derived growth factor → Excessive marrow fibroblastic proliferation → Myelofibrosis
- ↑Platelets → ↑Production of platelet derived growth factor

In these conditions excess marrow proliferation may be seen in liver, spleen and other organs — EXTRAMEDULLARY HAEMOPOIESIS (EHM).

MYELOFIBROSIS

In this rare affection of the elderly, the haemopoietic cellular proliferation is overshadowed by progressive FIBROSIS of the marrow; SPLENOMEGALY (often of massive proportions) due to EXTRAMEDULLARY HAEMOPOIESIS (myeloid metaplasia) is a usual concomitant.

Marrow: ordinary marrow puncture usually results in a 'dry tap', therefore trephine or cutting needle biopsy is required

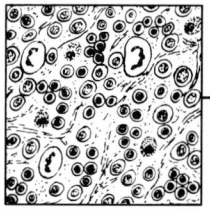

Total cellularity — all types of cell — very early reticulin increase.

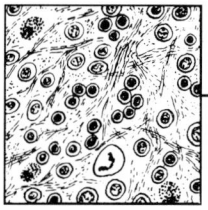

Reticulin++ — early fibrosis — cellularity decreasing.

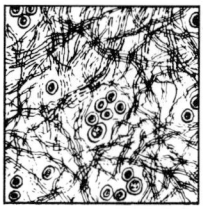

Established fibrosis — only small foci of haemopoietic cells remaining.

At this stage bone changes may be seen on X-ray — OSTEOSCLEROSIS.

Blood findings

RBC	WBC	Platelets
low	may be increased	may be increased

as marrow cells are replaced

↓

Progress to PANCYTOPENIA (this is exaggerated by enlarged spleen)

Film — *Leucoerythroblastic blood picture*

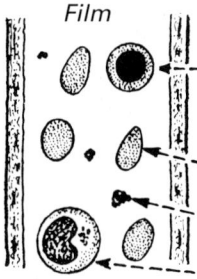

- Nucleated reds
- Poikilocytosis
- 'Tear drop' cells
- Abnormally large platelets
- Myelocytes

2. MYELODYSPLASTIC SYNDROMES (MDS)

These are primary disorders of stem cells associated with several different chromosomal abnormalities. They lead to ineffective haemopoiesis of varying types, with the appearance in the peripheral blood of abnormal cells. A significant number progress to LEUKAEMIA.

CHAPTER 12

GENITOURINARY SYSTEM

Kidney — Structure and Function ... 464
Glomerulus — Structure and Function ... 465
Glomerular Diseases ... 466
Acute Diffuse Proliferative Glomerulonephritis. ... 467
Rapidly Progressive Glomerulonephritis ... 468
Focal Glomerulonephritis ... 469
Membranous Glomerulonephritis ... 470
Mesangiocapillary (Membranoproliferative) Glomerulonephritis. ... 471
Chronic Glomerulonephritis ... 472
Glomerulonephritis — Disease Mechanisms ... 473
Glomerular Disease in Systemic Disorders ... 474
The Kidney and Hypertension ... 475, 476
Chronic Renal Failure ... 477, 478
Infections of the Kidney ... 479
Acute Pyelonephritis ... 480
Chronic Pyelonephritis ... 481, 482
Tuberculosis of the Kidney ... 483
Intercurrent Renal Conditions .. 484, 485
Renal Tubules — Structure and Function ... 486
Acute Tubular Necrosis ... 487, 488
Tubulo-Interstitial Diseases ... 489
Tubular Lesions of Metabolic Origin ... 490
Haemolytic Uraemic Syndrome ... 491
Pathological Complications of End-Stage Therapies ... 492
Congenital Disorders ... 493
Congenital Cystic Disease ... 494
Renal Calculi ... 495, 496
Tumours of the Kidney ... 497, 498
Diseases of Urinary Tract ... 499
Urinary Tract Infection ... 500
Tumours of the Urinary Tract ... 501
Female Genital Tract — Anatomy and Physiology. ... 502
Cyclical Endometrial Changes ... 503
Diseases of the Endometrium ... 504, 505
Endometrial Hyperplasia ... 506
Endometrial Carcinoma ... 507, 508
Diseases of the Myometrium ... 509
Diseases of Cervix ... 510
Cervical Intraepithelial Neoplasia (CIN) ... 511
Carcinoma of Cervix ... 512, 513
Diseases of Vagina and Vulva ... 514, 515
Diseases of Fallopian Tube ... 516
Diseases of Ovaries ... 517, 518
Common Epithelial Ovarian Tumours ... 519
Carcinoma of Ovary ... 520
Tumours of Ovary — Miscellaneous ... 521–523
Ectopic Pregnancy ... 524
Trophoblast Diseases ... 525
Benign Diseases of the Breast ... 526, 527
Benign Breast Tumours and In Situ Carcinoma ... 528
Carcinoma of the Breast ... 529–531
Diseases of Male Genitalia ... 532–540
Infertility ... 541

KIDNEY – STRUCTURE and FUNCTION

The kidney has several functions:

1. Eliminating waste products.
2. Controlling electrolyte and fluid balance.
3. Contributing to acid-base balance.

} By filtering plasma and modifying the filtrate to produce urine.

It produces several hormones:

(i) *Renin*, which influences vascular tone and blood pressure.
(ii) *Erythropoietin*, which increases red blood cell production.
(iii) *1, 25 dihydroxy Vitamin D* — The active form is produced by 1α hydroxylation in the kidney. It promotes calcium absorption from the gut and is required for normal bone mineralisation.

Tests of renal function:

1. **Blood analysis**

Many substances will show altered values in renal failure, but the following are always elevated and are commonly used in estimating the progress of the disease.

(i) Urea — normal range 2.5–7.0mmol/1. (20–40 mg/100 ml)
(ii) Creatinine — 50 –100 mmol/1. (0.6–1.2 mg/100 ml)

2. **Urine examination**

(a) Tests for the presence of protein, red cells, haemoglobin and neutrophils in the urine. Estimation of specific gravity and measurement of urinary output.
(b) Urinary casts. These are composed of foreign elements of various types which are moulded into cylindrical form by passage along tubules and are seen in microscopy.

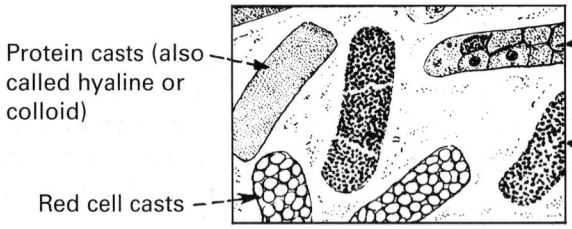

In jaundice, casts of bile-stained debris may be found and other solids may be seen floating freely.

3. **Clearance Tests** (typically creatinine clearance) give an indication of glomerular filtration rate: this is not absolute since some creatinine is secreted by renal tubules. The following formula is used to calculate the volume of blood cleared:

$$\text{Clearance} = \frac{UV}{P} \text{ where}$$

U = urinary concentration,
V = volume of urine per minute,
P = plasma concentration.

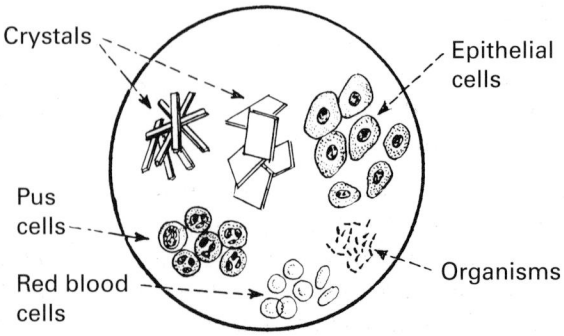

GLOMERULAR STRUCTURE AND FUNCTION

The glomerulus consists of an invagination of a capillary network, derived from the afferent arteriole, into Bowman's capsule — the beginning of the proximal tubule.

The glomerulus is an efficient filter with a large surface area — controlled by the structure of the glomerular capillaries.

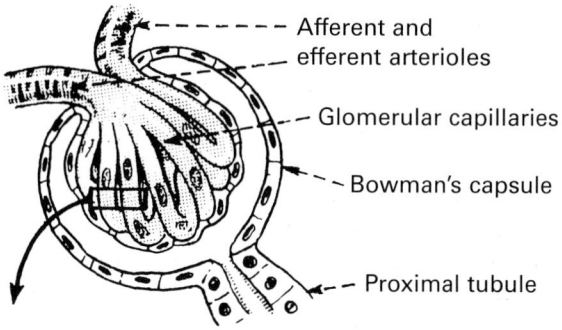

Ultrastructure

The barrier separating blood from the lumen of the nephron consists of 3 layers:

1. Endothelium (fenestrated)
2. Basement membrane
3. Epithelium

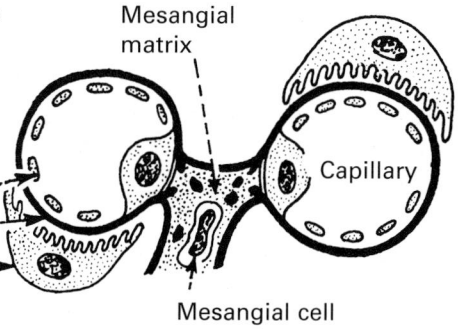

Mesangial cells are of two types:
1. Contractile smooth muscle cells which control blood flow, and
2. Phagocytic (macrophage) cells — normally few in number — which ingest proteins and immune complexes (p. 102).

These layers form a complicated sieve controlling glomerular permeability. Wide pores in the endothelium allow all components to reach the basement membrane.

The basement membrane has a strong anionic (negative) charge which repels major plasma proteins (also anionic). It has a central dense layer (lamina densa).

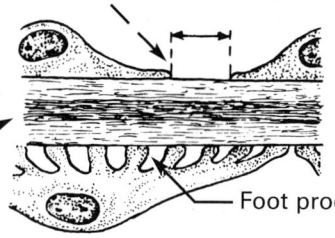

The epithelial cells are attached to the basement membrane by foot processes, separated by gaps 30–60 nm in diameter covered by a fine 'slit diaphragm'.

Filtration

The glomerular filtrate is virtually protein free plasma. Its rate of production is dependent upon:

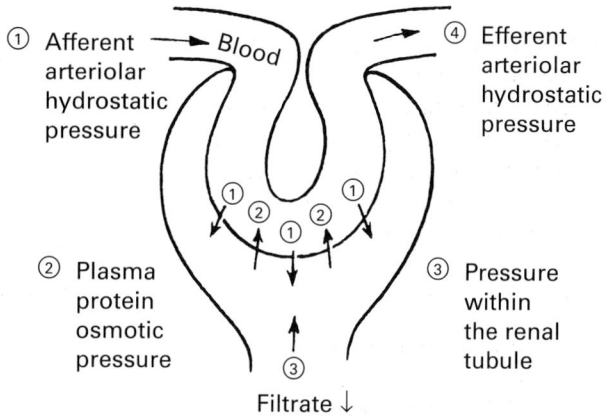

Variation in any of these factors affects the output of urine. Diminished urinary output results from a reduction in renal blood flow as in shock, from an increase in osmotic pressure as in haemoconcentration, or from obstruction to the outflow of urine.

GLOMERULAR DISEASES

Glomerular damage

The usual consequences of this are threefold:

1. Reduction in urinary output.
2. Proteinuria.
3. Haematuria.

The mechanism underlying these changes is probably as follows:

Swelling of endothelium
↓
Diminished blood flow
↓
Reduction in urine

Inflammation altering permeability of layers
↓
Proteinuria

Focal loss of epithelium and endothelium
↓
Haematuria

These lead to 3 main clinical syndromes.

1. The NEPHRITIC SYNDROME — characterised by moderate proteinuria, haematuria, oedema, oliguria and often renal impairment. Hypertension is common.
2. THE NEPHROTIC SYNDROME
   Heavy proteinuria ⟶ Hypoalbuminaemia ⟶ Oedema
3. RENAL FAILURE — usually chronic in type.

The main causes are:

(a) IMMUNE DAMAGE ⟶ GLOMERULONEPHRITIS
(b) DIABETES MELLITUS
(c) AMYLOIDOSIS
(d) MULTIPLE MYELOMA

The cause is best determined by renal biopsy.

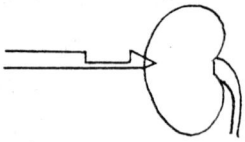

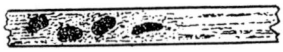

The core of tissue obtained is examined by:

1. **Light microscopy**

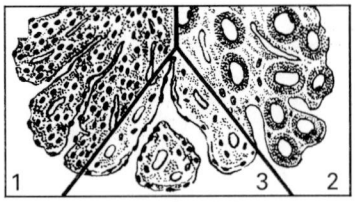

Shows 1. Increase in cells,
2. Details of basement membrane and
3. Mesangial matrix.

2. **Immunofluorescence**

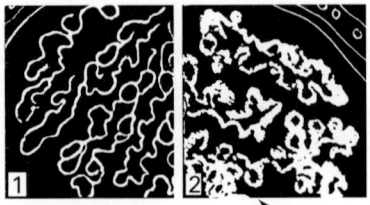

Immune complexes can be detected.
1. Linear
2. Granular

3. **Electron microscopy**

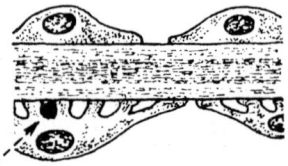

Detailed cellular and membrane damage can be seen.

The main forms of glomerular disease are described in the following pages.

ACUTE DIFFUSE PROLIFERATIVE GLOMERULONEPHRITIS

This disease classically follows 2–3 weeks after an infection — usually pharyngitis due to Group A haemolytic streptococci. It is commonest in children and young adults who develop the NEPHRITIC SYNDROME: oliguria, proteinuria, haematuria (urine is smoky and dark), moderate hypertension and facial (periorbital) oedema. This disease is now uncommon in fully developed countries.

The lesion is essentially acute inflammation of the glomerulus — all are affected.

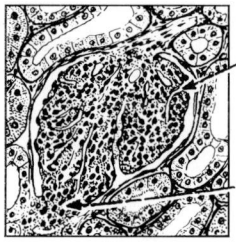

Glomerulus large, fills capsular space: solid and cellular

Projects into tubule

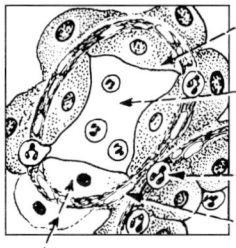

Endothelial cells swollen and more numerous

Capillary lumen narrowed

Neutrophils sometimes present

Oedema, basement membrane swollen

Necrosis of individual endothelial and epithelial cells occurs

Immune complexes are identified by:

1. **Electron microscopy**

Electron-dense granular deposits constantly seen in subepithelial position

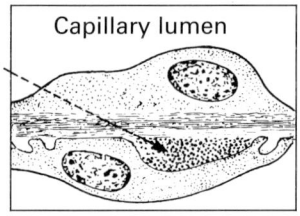

and 2. **Immunofluorescence** — demonstrates granular deposition of IgG and C3 (complement component 3)

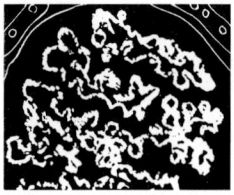

The clinical findings can be correlated with pathology as follows:

Glomerular capillary obstruction → Reduced blood flow → Stimulation of juxtaglomerular apparatus → Rise in blood pressure

Reduced blood flow → Diminished filtration → Oliguria → Raised blood urea

Reduced blood flow → Tubular epithelial damage → Fluid retention → Oedema

Damaged glomerular endothelium → Focal increase in permeability → Unselective proteinuria

Damaged glomerular endothelium → Escape of red cells → Haematuria

Unselective proteinuria, Haematuria → Casts → Epithelial, Protein, Red cell

Prognosis — The disease usually resolves in 1–2 weeks, particularly in children, but in adults complications may occur.

(1) Mild proteinuria persisting for a month or two → RECOVERY

(2) Rapidly progressive glomerulonephritis (rare) → Poor prognosis

(3) Cardiac failure or uraemia → DEATH in acute phase **(very rare)**

(4) Persisting proteinuria and haematuria → CHRONIC NEPHRITIS → DEATH years later

RAPIDLY PROGRESSIVE GLOMERULONEPHRITIS (RPGN)

As the name suggests, this disease progresses to end-stage renal failure in weeks or months. The histological hallmark is **crescent formation** in >50% of glomeruli.

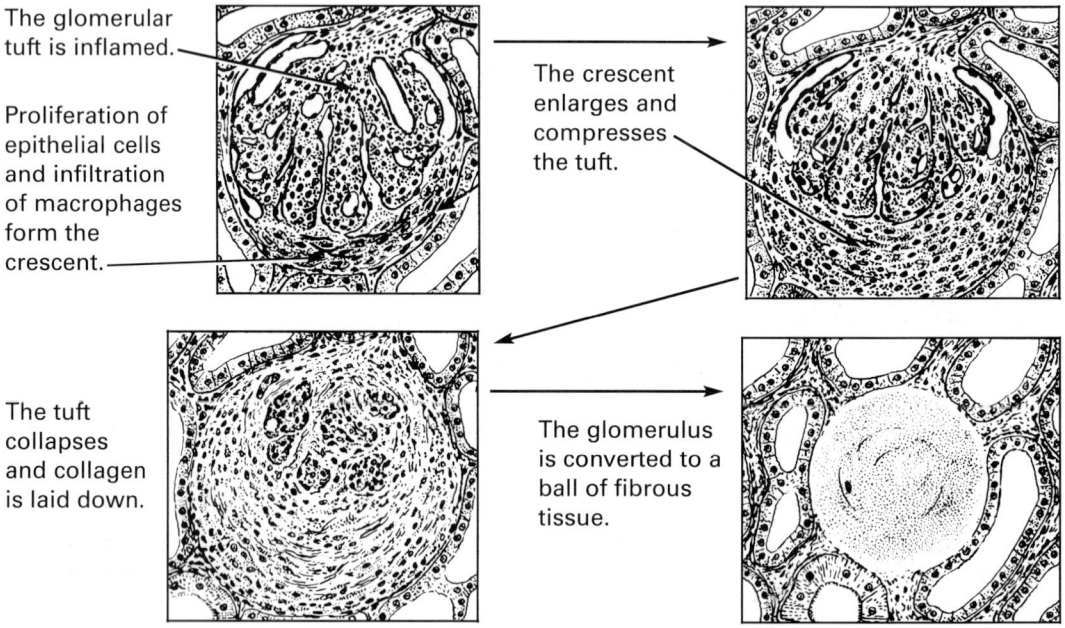

RPGN may complicate most types of glomerulonephritis. It occurs in several circumstances:

1. **Goodpasture's syndrome**
   In this serious disorder there is both renal and pulmonary damage. Immunofluorescence shows the essential cause — an antibody to glomerular basement membrane (anti-GBM) which also damages pulmonary alveolar membranes.

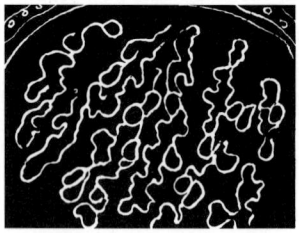
Linear deposits of IgG, IgM and C3 in the capillary basement membranes

Anti-GBM antibody → Renal damage (RPGN) / Lung damage (haemorrhage) } Renal and/or Pulmonary failure

Note: In some cases the lungs are not affected.

RPGN may complicate:

2. **Vasculitis** — e.g. Wegener's granulomatosis, microscopic polyarteritis nodosa.
3. **Systemic Lupus Erythematosus.**
4. **Acute diffuse proliferative glomerulonephritis,** especially in adults.

Prognosis — Without treatment, most patients die within 6 months.
Immunosuppressive drugs (e.g. prednisolone, cyclophosphamide) and plasma exchange (to remove anti-GBM antibodies) improve the prognosis but many patients require dialysis or transplantation. Hypertension is a further serious complication.

FOCAL GLOMERULONEPHRITIS

In this form of glomerulonephritis the changes do not affect all glomeruli. Almost all or only a small number may be affected. In addition, within an affected glomerulus the damage is focal and usually affects only one or two lobules of the glomerulus.

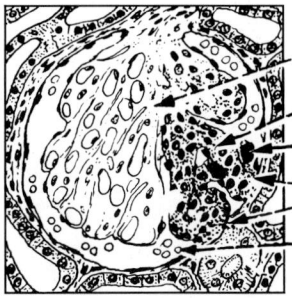

The commonest form is **IgA nephropathy** (Berger's disease) — a disease typically of young males. There is proteinuria and recurrent episodes of mild haematuria often follow sore throats. The IgA blood level is raised and the glomerular damage is due to IgA immune complexes retained within the glomerulus.

Mechanism

IgA immune complexes in blood → Glomeruli → **Focal** deposition → Activation of complement (C3) → **Focal damage**

Immunofluorescence

Shows deposits of IgA and C3 within the mesangium: the capillary loops are not usually affected.

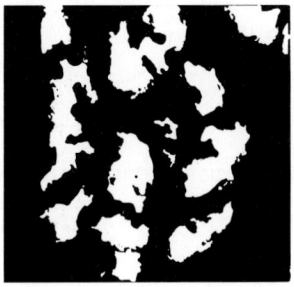

Note: The focal deposition is dependent on the molecular size of the complex and failure of mesangial clearance.

Prognosis

In childhood, this is usually good although proteinuria, haematuria and hypertension may persist.

In adults, there is often slow progression to renal failure over 10–20 years but sometimes over 3–5 years.

Focal glomerulonephritis is also seen in Henoch-Schönlein purpura, polyarteritis nodosa, systemic lupus erythematosus and other disorders.

MEMBRANOUS GLOMERULONEPHRITIS

This accounts for around 30% of cases of the nephrotic syndrome in adults; some patients present with asymptomatic proteinuria.

Aetiology

1. Around 70% of cases are IDIOPATHIC.
2. Drugs e.g. penicillamine and gold — in treatment of rheumatoid arthritis.
3. Tumours e.g. carcinoma of lung, lymphomas.
4. Infections e.g. malaria.

Pathology — There is generalised thickening of capillary basement membrane.

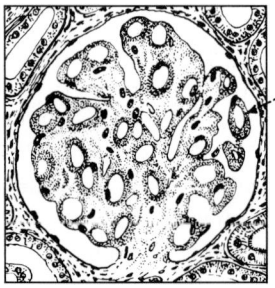

Tuft enlarges

Diffuse hyaline thickening of capillary

Glomeruli not hypercellular

Specific silver staining of the basement membrane shows a typical pattern.

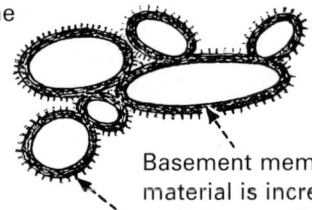

Basement membrane material is increased and shows spikes

Immunofluorescence reveals deposition of IgG and IgM in the capillary walls.

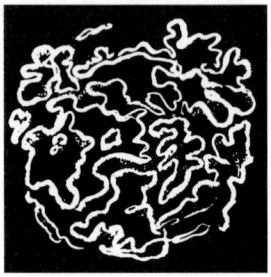

Electron microscope findings explain this appearance.

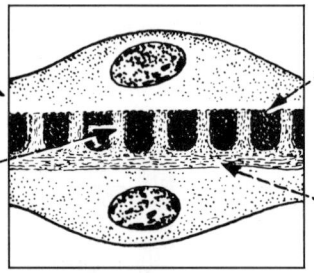

Loss of foot processes

Basement membrane material between deposit ≡ spikes

Subepithelial deposits

Single layer of basement membrane

In the later stages there is a massive increase in basement membrane material.

Silver staining shows

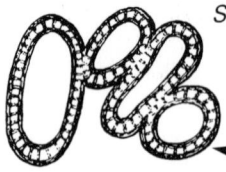

Basement membrane shows a double contouring with joining spikes (rail track)

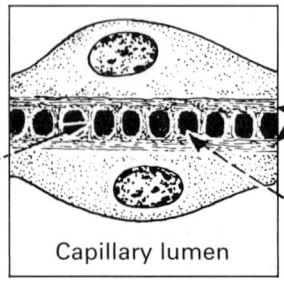

Electron microscope shows

Two layers of basement membrane

Deposits

Capillary lumen

Tubular changes — In the early stages, protein droplets and lipid globules appear in the tubular epithelium. Lipid is also found in the interstitial tissue. Foamy macrophages and giant cells form granulomas in association with cholesterol deposits. If the disease progresses, narrowing of the glomerular capillaries causes ischaemic atrophy of the tubules and interstitial fibrosis.

Prognosis — In about 25% of patients the disease remits spontaneously, while 25% continue to have proteinuria. In 50% chronic renal failure eventually supervenes.

MESANGIOCAPILLARY (MEMBRANOPROLIFERATIVE) GLOMERULONEPHRITIS

In this form of glomerulonephritis there is an increase both in **cells** and **mesangial matrix** within glomeruli.

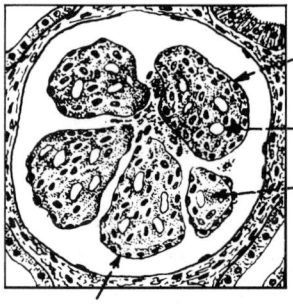

Tufts are lobulated and hypercellular

Capillaries narrow

Increase of mesangium between capillaries; sometimes areas of hyalinosis

Epithelial cells swollen; occasionally crescents form

Silver staining of basement membrane

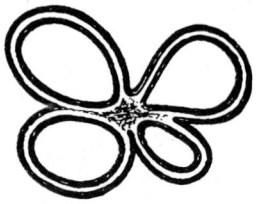

Duplication of basement membrane as in membranous glomerulonephritis, but without spikes.

These changes are due to **'mesangial interposition'**

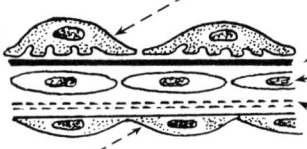

Epithelial layer

Basement membrane

Mesangial cells growing between endothelial layer and basement membrane

A **new layer** of basement membrane is laid down

Endothelial layer

Using electron microscopy and immunofluorescence, 2 types are identified.

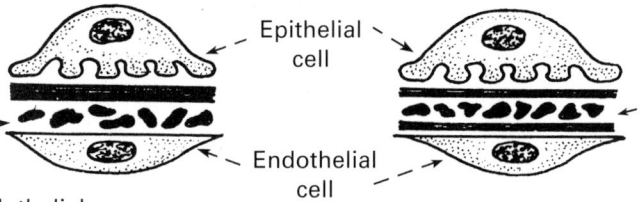

Type 1

Type 2

Epithelial cell

Endothelial cell

Electron dense material within basement membrane **'Dense deposit disease'** consisting of C3 but no immunoglobulin.

Subendothelial deposits of C3 and IgG

Aetiology

Complement activation is a feature of both forms. In Type 1 this is due to immune complexes by the classical pathway (p. 99). In Type 2 there is activation by the alternative pathway by an autoantibody which stabilises C3 converting enzyme. Serum C3 is low in both forms.

Clinical features

Children and young adults usually affected, display **nephrotic syndrome** or simple proteinuria or the nephritic syndrome.

Progression to renal failure (with hypertension) is common.

CHRONIC GLOMERULONEPHRITIS (GN)

This is the end stage of many forms of glomerulonephritis.

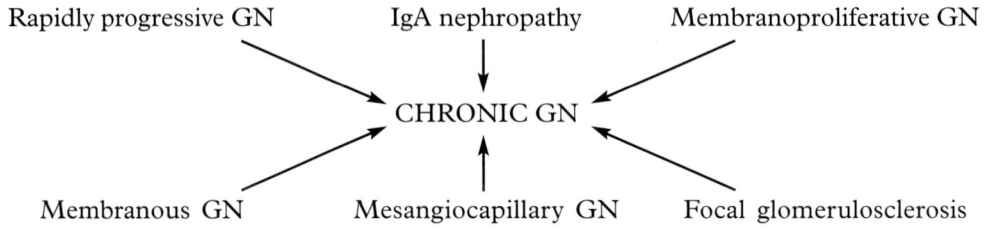

Pathology The kidneys are both small — Granular contracted kidney.

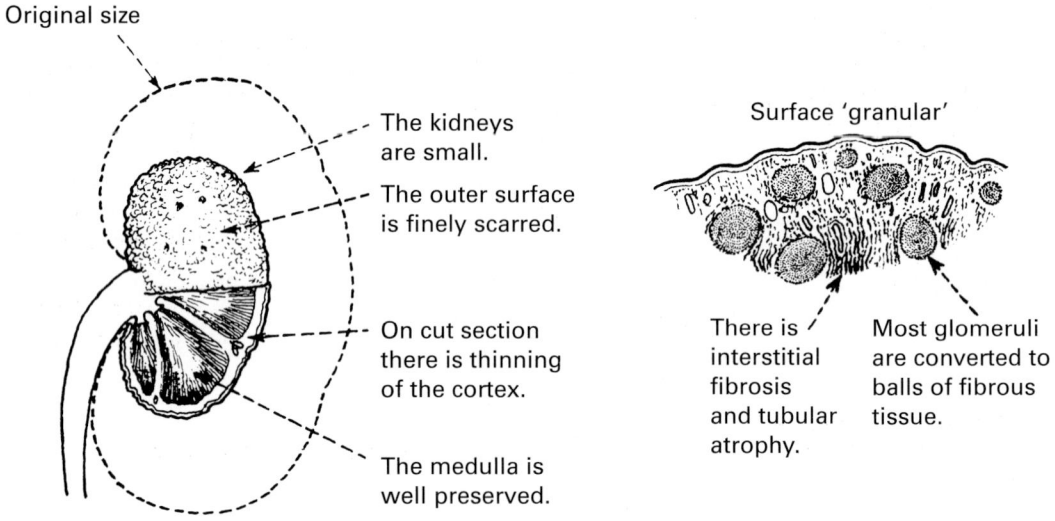

In chronic glomerulonephritis a vicious cycle is set up.

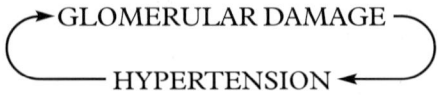

Patients may first present with chronic renal failure, or this may develop after years of glomerulonephritis.

GLOMERULONEPHRITIS (GN) – DISEASE MECHANISMS

The mechanism in most forms of GN is:

Immune complex formation → Activation of **complement** → **Cell damage** / **Neutrophil** activation → Glomerular injury

The glomerulus is central to immune complex deposition and formation due to its **fenestrated endothelium** and **high intraluminal pressure**.

Immune complexes can occur in glomeruli as follows:

1. Deposition of circulating complex.
2. In situ formation of complexes
   (a) Deposited antigens. (b) Glomerular antigens.

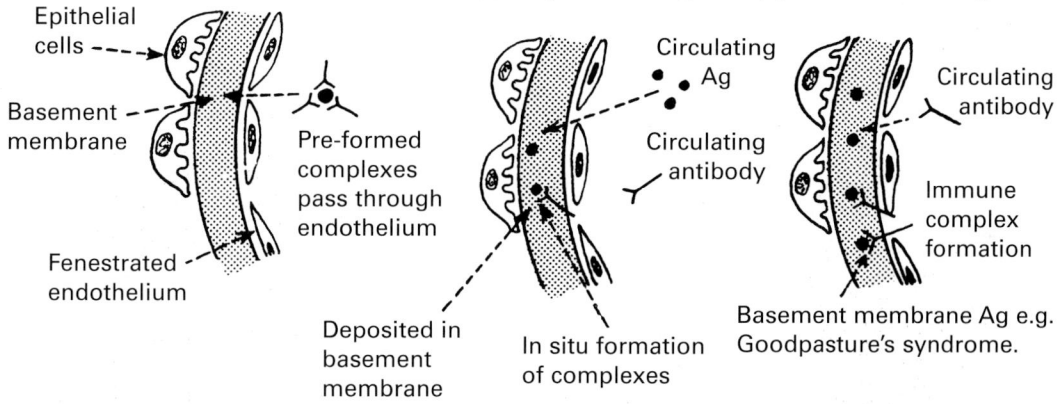

Localisation of complexes

This depends on the size of the complexes and their ability to penetrate the basement membrane.

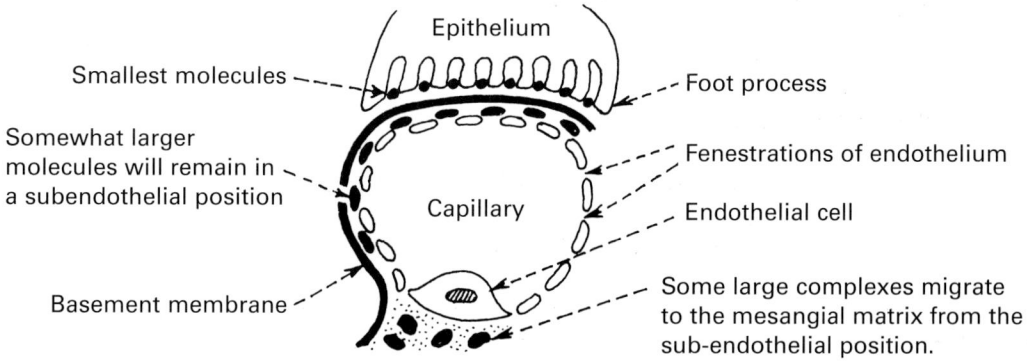

Other factors modifying the pathological changes are:
(i) Amount of antigen and its persistence, (ii) Intensity of the immune reaction and rate of antibody production, (iii) Type of antibody (especially IgA), (iv) Availability of complement.

Note: In addition to its damaging consequences, complement activation does **solubilise complexes** allowing their disposal. Thus complement deficiency may predispose to immune complex disease e.g. in systemic lupus erythematosus (SLE).

GLOMERULAR DISEASE IN SYSTEMIC DISORDERS

SYSTEMIC LUPUS ERYTHEMATOSUS (SLE)

At least 50% of patients with SLE have clinical evidence of renal involvement, and almost all will have abnormalities on renal biopsy.

The main consequences are (1) Proteinuria ⟶ nephrotic syndrome.
(2) Microscopic haematuria.
(3) Hypertension.
(4) Progression to renal failure.

The renal changes form a spectrum.

Minimal abnormalities		Diffuse proliferative glomerulonephritis
MILD	Focal glomerulonephritis ⟶	**SEVERE**

On immunofluorescence, IgG, C3 are almost always present and IgA, IgM, Clq and C4 are often also seen.

AMYLOIDOSIS

The general features of amyloidosis have already been described. Amyloid is deposited around the capillary basement membranes of the glomeruli and in the renal vessels and interstitium.

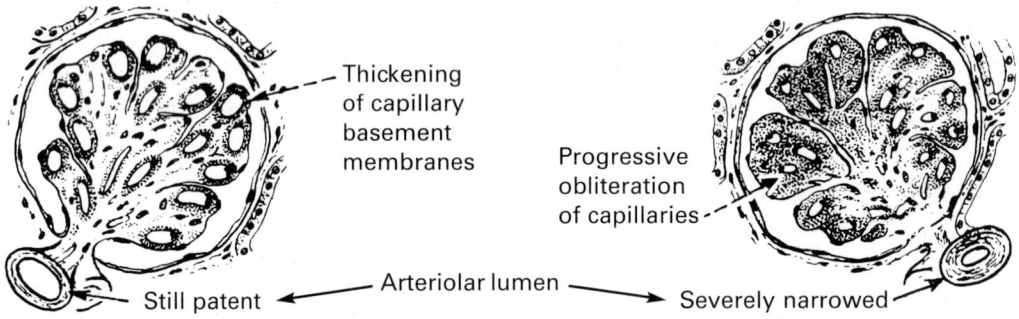

Gross proteinuria leading to a nephrotic syndrome is common. Interstitial fibrosis results from tubular degeneration and ischaemia due to glomerular and arteriolar lesions. Chronic renal failure results. Renal vein thrombosis can occur in amyloidosis causing acute renal failure.

Parasitic glomerulopathies

The kidney and particularly the glomeruli are damaged in many parasitic infections in the tropics. **Malaria** and **schistosomiasis** are especially important.

Mechanism

Parasitic antigen + antibody (IgM in early stages; then IgG, IgE)
(Immune complex)
↓
glomerulus ⟶ membranous GN ⟶ progression to chronic GN.

Clinically

Progression from mild proteinuria ⟶ nephrotic syndrome / ⟶ nephritic syndrome } ⟶ renal failure

THE KIDNEY and HYPERTENSION

There are two aspects to the relationship of the kidney and high blood pressure.

(a) Many renal diseases lead to hypertension (p. 199).

(b) Hypertension leads to renal damage.

A vicious circle can be set up:

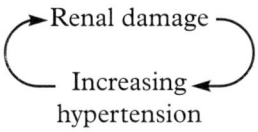

Activation of the Renin-Angiotensin system is important.

The renal consequences of benign and malignant hypertension differ, but in each vascular changes are important.

BENIGN HYPERTENSION

Afferent arterioles

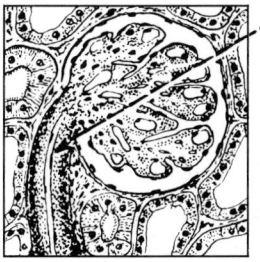

Intimal thickening due to plasmatic vasculosis

Hyaline material (fibrin) is deposited in subendothelial layer, reducing the lumen.

Interlobular arteries

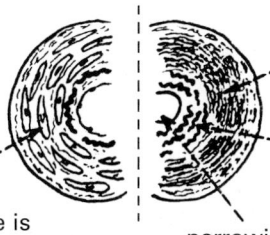

The early change is medial hypertrophy

Later: fibrosis of media,

fibro-elastic thickening of intima,

narrowing of lumen.

These arteriolar changes lead to glomerular ischaemia.

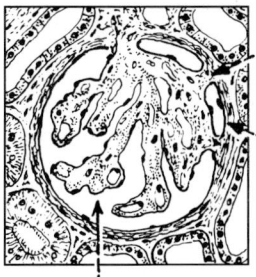

Adhesions develop

Increasing fibrosis of capsule

Capillaries collapse and disappear

Late

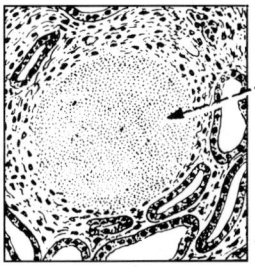

Glomerulus completely sclerosed

The tubules atrophy and there is interstitial fibrosis.

These changes are patchy in distribution so that renal failure rarely occurs.

THE KIDNEY and HYPERTENSION

BENIGN HYPERTENSION (continued)

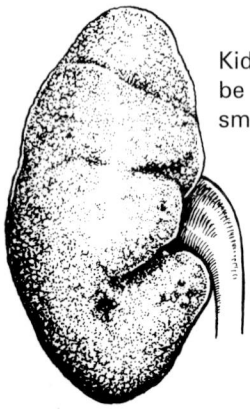

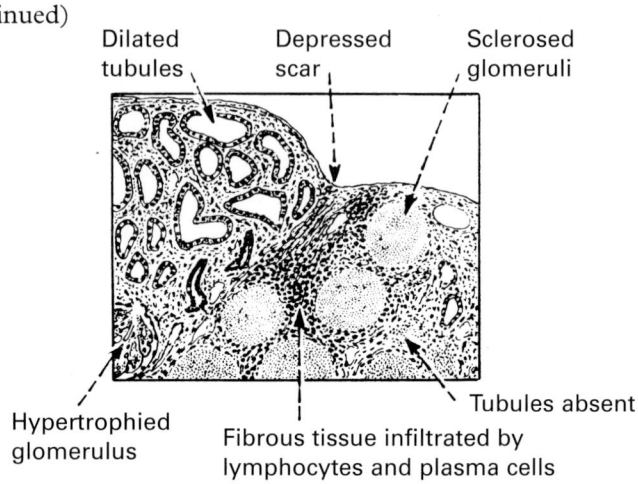

It is now thought that small emboli from atheroma of the aorta are responsible for much of the scarring in benign hypertension.

MALIGNANT HYPERTENSION

In this form of hypertension, the blood pressure rises very rapidly and damages renal arteries, arterioles and glomeruli. Renal failure is common unless the disease is treated.

Afferent arterioles: the hallmark is **fibrinoid necrosis.**

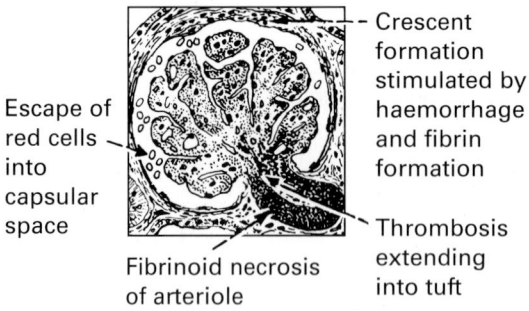

Fibrinoid necrosis heals with the production of an 'onion-skin' lesion.

Interlobular arteries

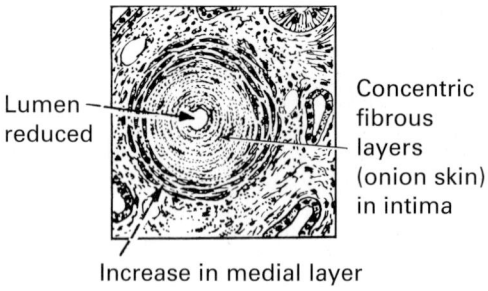

These changes account for the gross appearance.

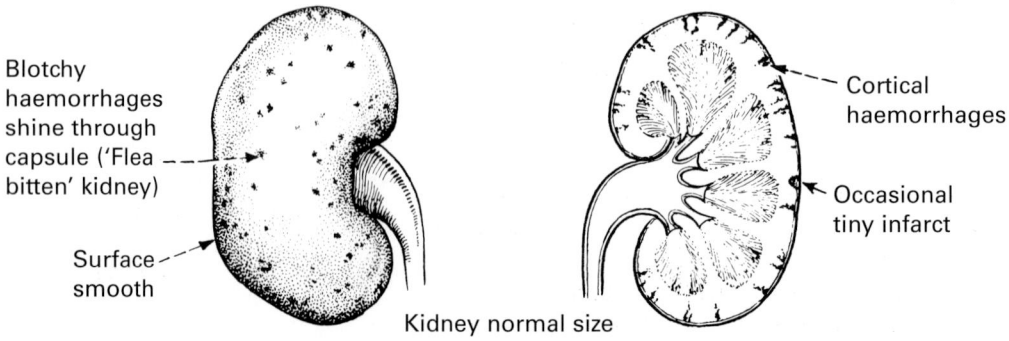

CHRONIC RENAL FAILURE

Progressive renal damage in many kidney diseases eventually leads to chronic renal failure. The major causes include:

(a) Chronic glomerulonephritis.
(b) Chronic pyelonephritis and interstitial nephritis.
(c) Diabetic nephropathy.
(d) Obstructive uropathy.
(e) Polycystic kidneys.

In many cases the underlying cause cannot be determined.
The severity of renal failure is monitored by the serum urea, creatinine and by the glomerular filtration rate (GFR).

GFR (normal approximately 100 ml/min)

50 —
Mild renal failure — usually asymptomatic, hypertension may develop.
30 —
Moderate — anaemia, fatigue and hypertension.
10 —
Severe — marked fluid retention, anorexia, vomiting.
5 —
End stage — pulmonary oedema, coma, death
0 —

The rate of decline depends on the underlying cause

Compensatory mechanisms:
As nephrons are lost, the surviving nephrons show (1) COMPENSATORY HYPERTROPHY and are (2) CONTINUALLY ACTIVE with no 'down time'. (In the normal kidney, the nephrons do not all function simultaneously.)

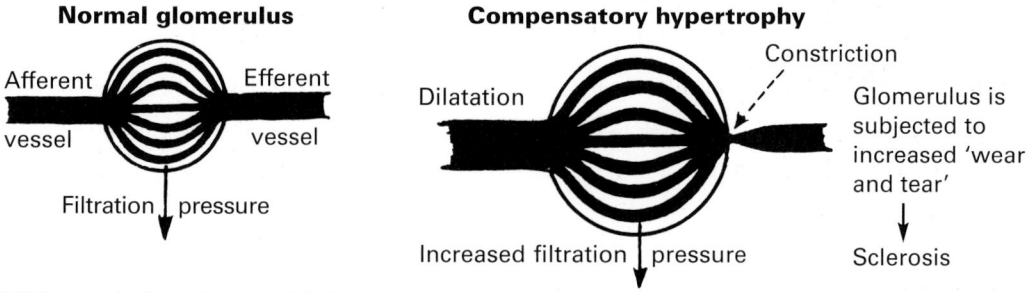

Effects of chronic renal failure:
1. **WATER and ELECTROLYTE BALANCE**

Loss of tubular resorptive power

↓ Glomerular filtration rate
↓
Retention of Na^+ → Retention of water
↓
Hypertension

↓ Excretion of K^+
↓
Hyperkalaemia
↓
Cardiac arrhythmias

Urine concentration is lost — with production of urine of fixed specific gravity — 1010.

CHRONIC RENAL FAILURE

Effects of Chronic Renal Failure (continued)

2. **DISTURBANCE OF ACID BASE BALANCE**

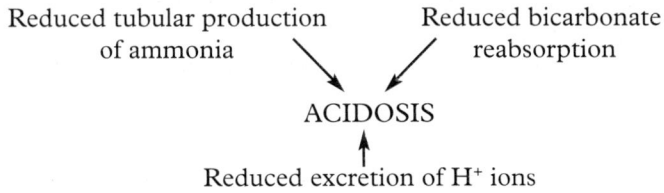

3. **URAEMIA**
   The kidney also fails to excrete nitrogenous waste products, which accumulate. Although urea concentrations rise and are used to monitor renal function, retention of urea is not in itself harmful.
   In uraemia, patients are lethargic. Anorexia, nausea and vomiting are common, with confusion, convulsions and death.

4. **HORMONAL ABNORMALITIES**
   Three main hormones are involved: Erythropoietin, parathormone and vitamin D.

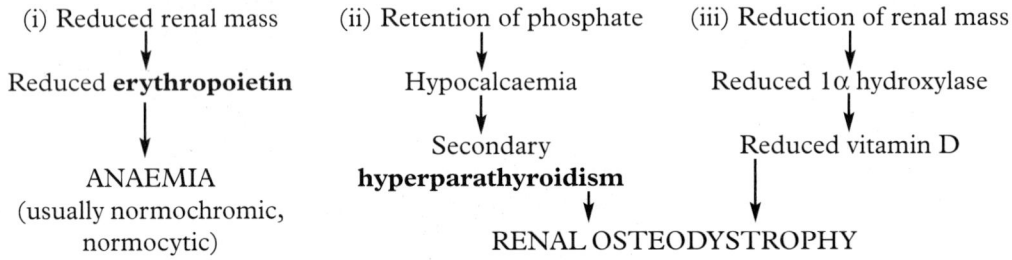

5. **HYPERTENSION** — This is almost inevitable and several consequences are possible.

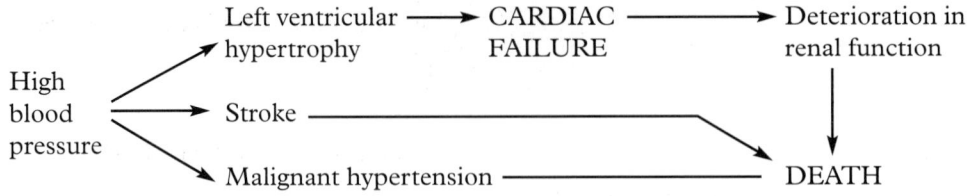

6. **Fibrinous exudates, e.g. fibrinous pericarditis, 'uraemic pneumonitis' with pleural exudate, uraemic colitis.**

7. **Haemorrhagic ulcers** of the gastro-intestinal tract.

8. **Depression of immunological reaction.** Infections are common and will in turn affect renal function. Claims are made that the lack of reaction is beneficial in that there may be less likelihood of a renal transplant rejection.

INFECTIONS OF THE KIDNEY

The kidney can become infected through 2 main routes.

(1) **Ascending infection** usually associated with **lower urinary tract infection** (obstruction and/or vesico-ureteric reflux are often present). This is by far the commoner route and gives rise to PYELONEPHRITIS.
(2) Blood borne (haematogenous) infection by pyogenic organisms (e.g. from septicaemia) or in tuberculosis.

ACUTE PYELONEPHRITIS

This is an acute ascending pyogenic infection and the patient exhibits the usual general features of pyrexia, nausea, vomiting, headaches, rigors, etc., plus localising signs, e.g. frequency, dysuria, loin pain and sometimes haematuria.

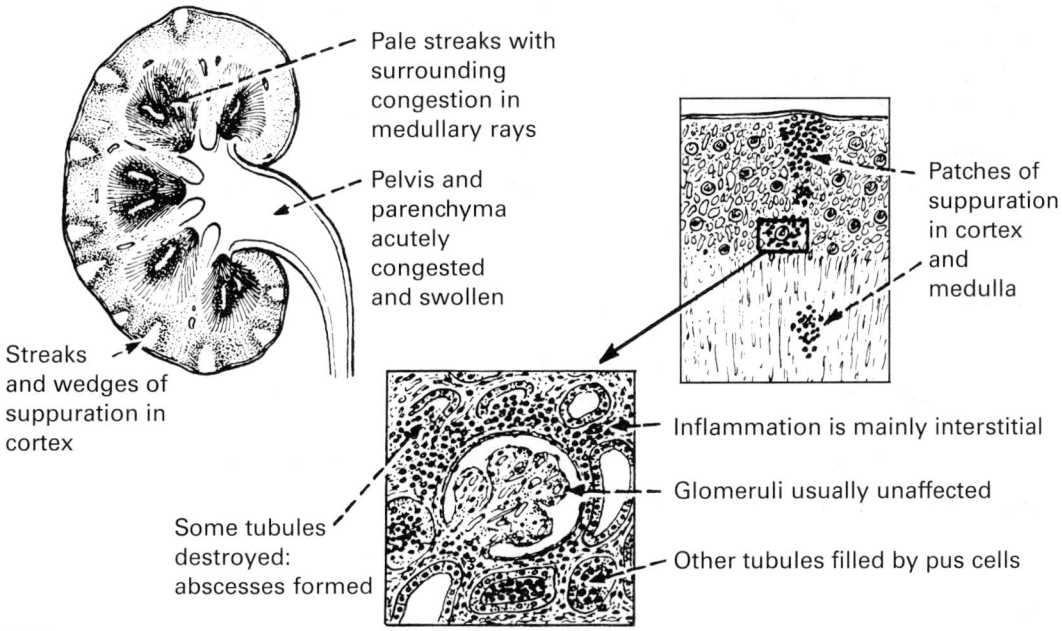

Urine

1. **Microscopy**

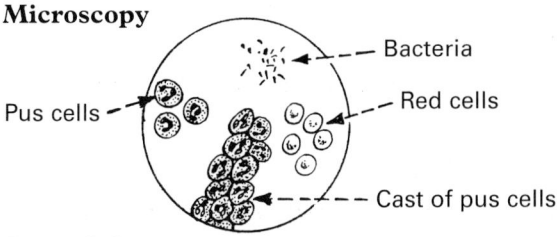

2. **Chemical** — protein, blood

3. **Bacteriology**

Large numbers of bacteria are found in the urine, several hundred thousand per ml in the acute phase.

The commonest infecting organism is *Escherichia coli*, but other faecal bacteria may also be found, e.g. pseudomonas, *Streptococcus faecalis.*

ACUTE PYELONEPHRITIS

Causes

In women, cystitis is common, particularly in the sexually active. Ascending infection is often provoked by vesico-ureteric reflux during micturition. Pregnancy or tumour of the uterus or ovaries may be causes of obstruction.

In men, urinary tract obstruction is usually found, typically due to prostatic enlargement. A number of causes of obstruction are seen in both sexes e.g. calculi or tumours in renal pelvis, tumours pressing on ureter, calculi in ureters and tumours of bladder.

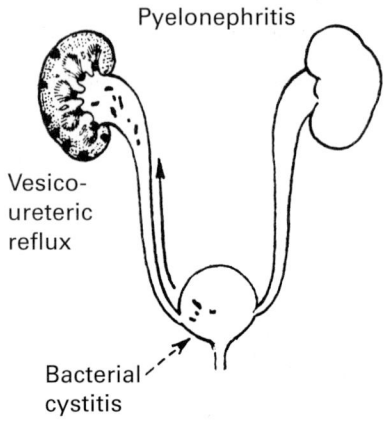

Influence of urinary tract obstruction

Obstruction of the urinary tract acts in 3 ways to promote infection:

1. The urine tends to stagnate and encourage growth of bacteria.
2. A tendency to vesicoureteric reflux during micturition develops especially when cystitis occurs.
3. Catheterisation is commonly carried out in these cases and can introduce infection. In this case the infection is likely to be mixed.

Progress The possibilities are as follows:

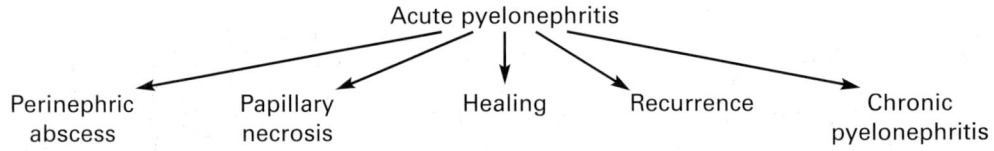

Perinephric abscess and papillary necrosis are now rare due to specific antibiotic therapy.

Papillary necrosis (maximal at the kidney poles) is most apt to occur in cases associated with urinary obstruction, diabetes, analgesic nephropathy (e.g. aspirin and phenacetin), sickle cell anaemia and severe hypotension.

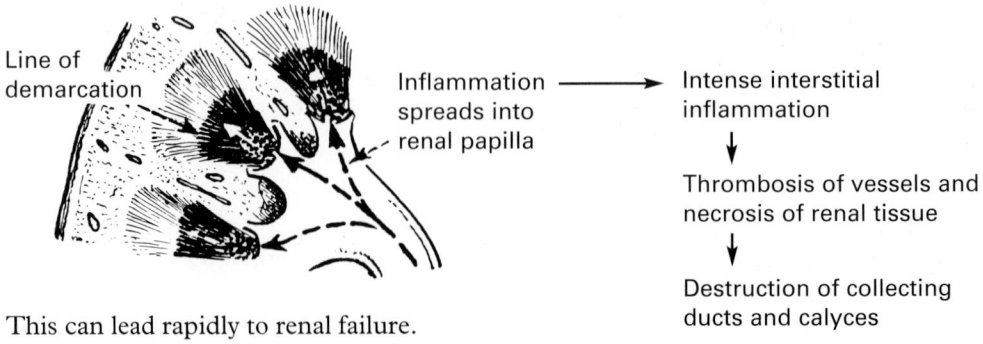

This can lead rapidly to renal failure.

CHRONIC PYELONEPHRITIS

Chronic pyelonephritis is essentially the result of repeated attacks of inflammation and healing. The process can be visualised as follows:

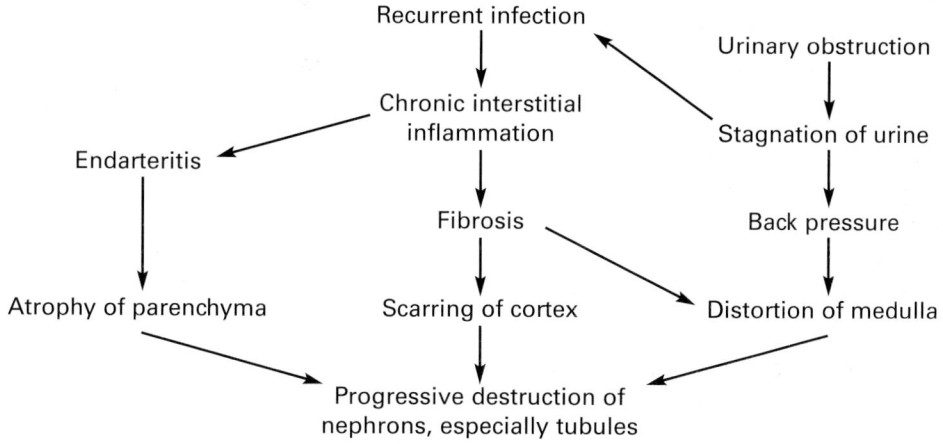

Kidney structure and function may be further prejudiced by the onset of hypertension. In cases with urinary obstruction, the external size of the kidney may remain normal or even be increased. Those with no underlying abnormality, commoner in the female, show progressive contraction of the kidney which becomes greyish white. The majority of cases are of this type.

Obstructive type

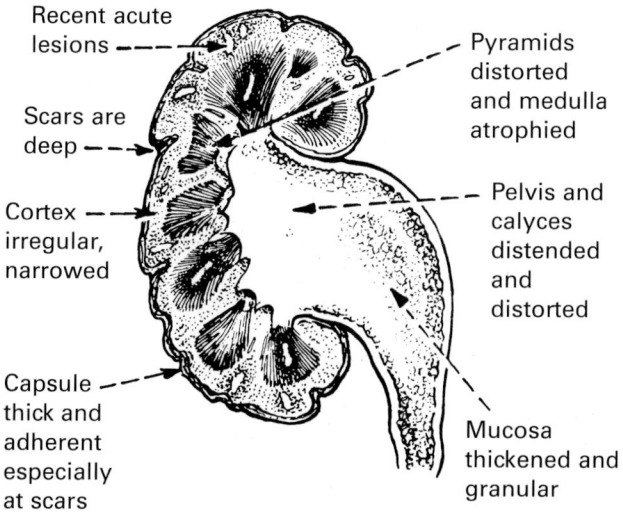

Non-obstructive type

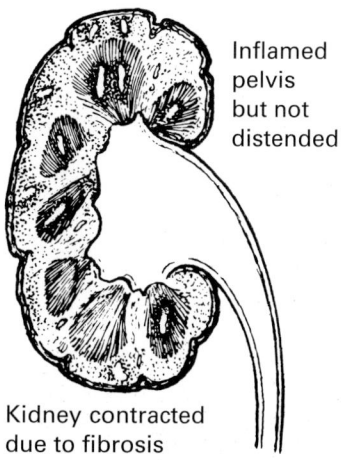

Depending on the cause, only one or both kidneys may be affected to variable degrees (c.f. chronic glomerulonephritis).

CHRONIC PYELONEPHRITIS

Microscopically, 3 types of lesion are seen in most cases:

1. Extensive interstitial fibrosis, inflammation and parenchymal loss.

2. Occasionally acute suppurative lesions due to recent infection.

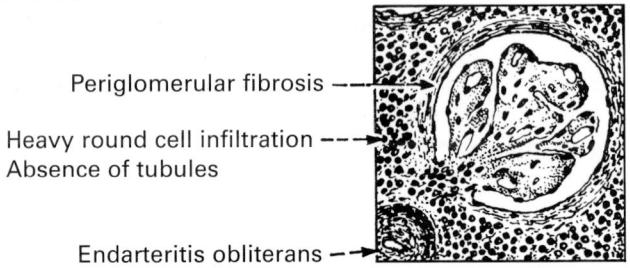

3. Foci of dilated tubules in the cortex. This is due to destruction of the collecting tubules so that they end blindly. Upper tubules dilate, develop colloid casts and come to resemble thyroid tissue. The patchy inflammation results in fibrosis and atrophy irregularly distributed throughout the cortex and medulla.

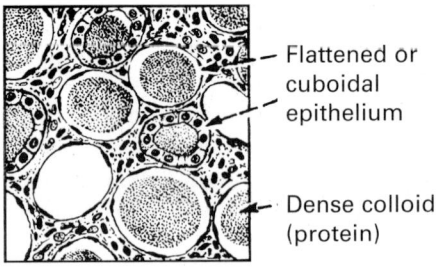

Clinical effects

These are due to destruction of tubules and distortion of the anatomy of the renal medulla.

1. There is a progressive loss of the renal concentrating power.

2. The sodium pump effect of the counter-current mechanism is upset (see p.486); base is lost thus causing acidosis. In children this can interfere with calcium metabolism.

Renal failure with uraemia develops, although the patient may still be passing relatively large quantitites of dilute urine. Chronic pyelonephritis is probably the commonest cause of fatal uraemia. Where unilateral obstruction is the cause only one kidney is affected and uraemia is not a feature.

3. Hypertension is common. Ninety per cent of patients are hypertensive when renal failure occurs. Equally striking, malignant hypertension develops in at least 15% of cases of severe chronic pyelonephritis. Where the inflammation is confined to one kidney, its removal relieves the hypertension in some cases.

TUBERCULOSIS of the KIDNEY

This is now uncommon in many Western countries, due to BCG vaccination for tuberculosis and the effect of specific treatment. It is due to **blood spread of infection** from another site, e.g. the lungs. Alternatively, but much less commonly, there may be an ascending infection from some other part of the genitourinary system, e.g. epididymis.
As usual, the tuberculous process develops slowly and lesions in the lungs which are the source of infection may have healed and disappeared by the time kidney damage is clinically apparent. The disease is commonly unilateral.

Stages

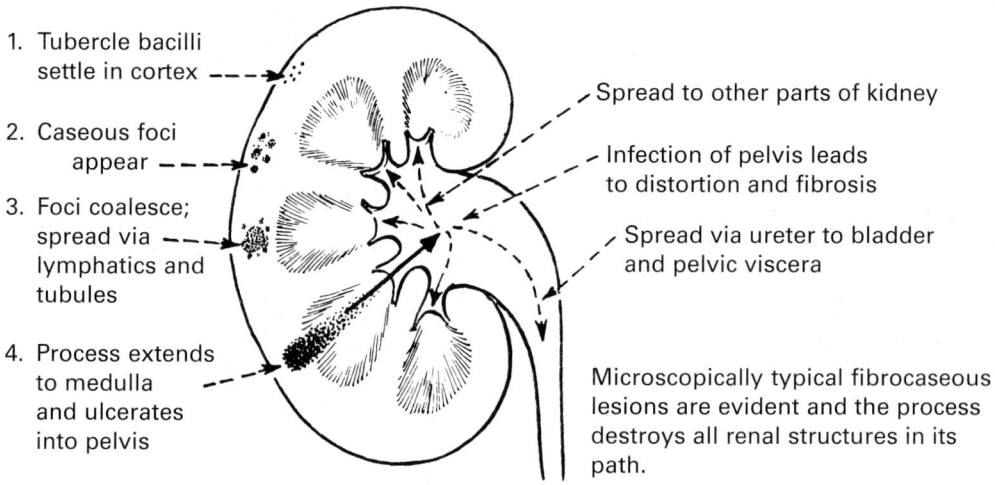

Clinical features
There may be no localising features, the patient merely showing the general features of tuberculous infection — fever, night sweats and loss of weight. Lumbar discomfort or pain, dysuria and haematuria can develop. Secondary pyogenic infection is common leading to pyuria. Tubercle bacilli can usually be demonstrated in the urine either on direct microscopic examination or by culture. If, however, the ureter is blocked by caseous material, the urine, now coming solely from the uninfected kidney, may be sterile.

The danger is that infection may spread to the unaffected kidney and lead to renal failure.

INTERCURRENT RENAL CONDITIONS

DIABETES

Renal complications are common in diabetes. Up to 30% of diabetics develop proteinuria, usually after many years. In most cases the kidneys show typical changes.

The renal lesion is essentially a special form of the 'small vessel disease' seen systemically in insulin dependent diabetes e.g. diabetic retinopathy.

Diabetic glomerulosclerosis This takes one of two forms:

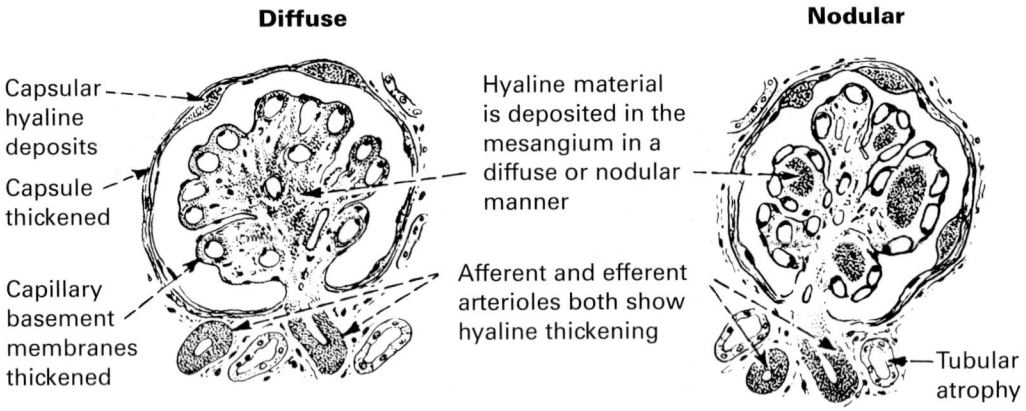

Deposited material is PAS-positive and resembles amyloid. The nodular form is often termed the Kimmelstiel-Wilson lesion. Progressive closure of capillaries can occur together with fibrous obliteration of the capsular space and the whole glomerulus. The changes in the afferent arterioles are an important factor in this process. Secondary tubular atrophy follows.

Clinical effects

Proteinuria may lead to the nephrotic syndrome. Hypertension leads to further renal damage: control of blood pressure, and of diabetes itself, is important to delay the onset of renal failure.

Pyelonephritis

This is common in diabetes and may be complicated by papillary necrosis.

Atheroma

This disease is common in the renal arteries and their branches in diabetes. It increases the renal ischaemia.

INTERCURRENT RENAL CONDITIONS

RENAL FUNCTION AND PREGNANCY

Four conditions affecting renal function may arise in pregnancy.

1. **Acute pyelonephritis** is relatively common, possibly due to (a) the effects of uterine pressure on the ureters and (b) relaxation of smooth muscle allowing ureteric dilatation and reflux.

2. **Pre-eclampsia and eclampsia.** This is a syndrome characterised by hypertension, increasing unselective proteinuria and oedema. The essential kidney lesion is glomerular; tubular changes are secondary.

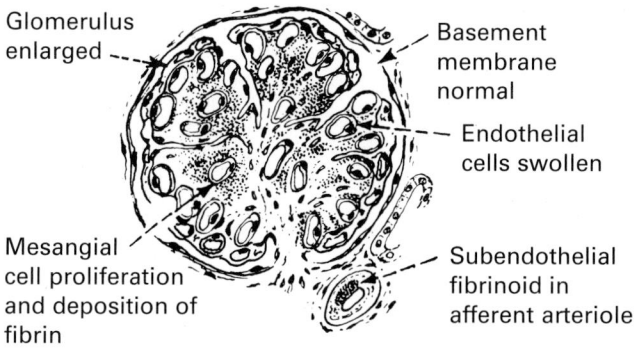

EM examination shows mesangial deposits of fibrin, fibrinogen, IgM and complement.

The lesion appears to resolve rapidly after parturition. So far as kidney function is concerned, the danger of eclampsia lies in the occasional development of acute renal failure from '3' and '4' below.

In addition there is often severe liver damage and cerebral injury indicated first by convulsions.

3. **Acute tubular necrosis.** This is associated with complications of pregnancy causing SHOCK e.g. septic abortion, retroplacental haemorrhage and postpartum haemorrhage.

4. In more severe cases **bilateral cortical necrosis** may occur especially if disseminated intravascular coagulation (DIC) is superadded.

RENAL TUBULE – STRUCTURE AND FUNCTION

The renal tubules modify the glomerular filtrate. Initially isotonic and neutral, it becomes hypertonic and quite strongly acid. Within 24 hours, 180 litres of filtrate are reduced to 1.5 litres of urine. The main functions of this process are:

(a) to get rid of waste products, particularly those of protein metabolism.
(b) to aid in maintaining the normal acid-base balance.
(c) to conserve fluid, electrolytes and other essential substances.

Three mechanisms are involved:

1. Active absorption of substances from the filtrate by the tubular epithelium.
2. Passive interchange between the filtrate and the interstitial tissues to maintain osmotic equilibrium.
3. Secretion by the tubular epithelium.

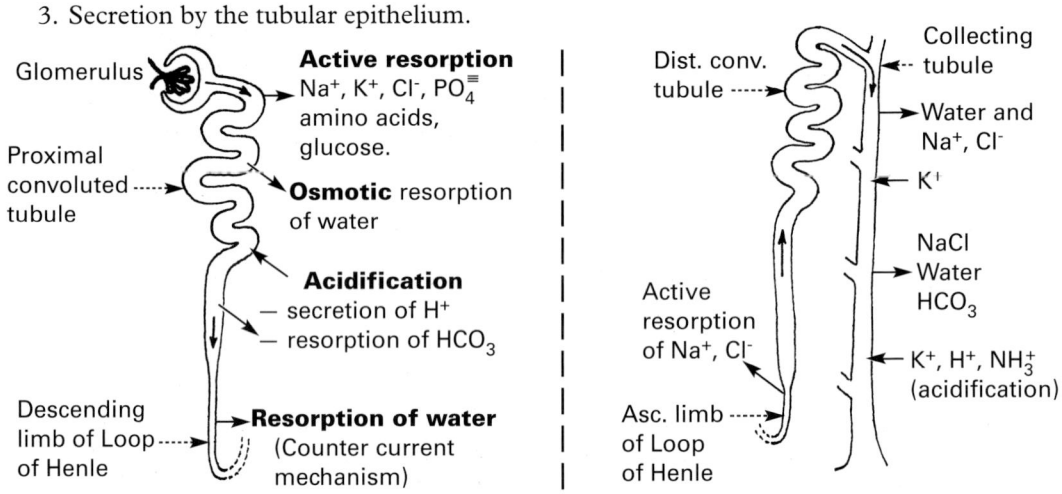

Note: 1. Active reabsorption requires energy, and there is a limit to the capacity of the process — maximal tubular capacity (Tm). When this is exceeded, the particular substance involved will appear in the urine. Glucose is an example. In diabetes, the amount of glucose in the filtrate far exceeds the absorptive capacity, and glycosuria results.

2. **Urinary acidification**
H ions, excreted by distal tubule, take part in 3 reactions:

$$\left.\begin{array}{l} 1.\ H + HCO_3 = H_2CO_3 \\ 2.\ H + NH_3Cl = NH_4Cl \\ 3.\ H + HPO_4 + Na = NaH_2PO_4 \end{array}\right\} \text{Urinary excretory products}$$

Effects of tubular damage

Damage to the tubules results in gross biochemical changes.

1. Loss of mechanisms controlling balance of electrolytes, water and urea.
2. Upset in acid-base balance.
3. Loss of substances in urine normally completely or almost completely reabsorbed — glucose, potassium, amino acids.

Glomerular lesions and pathological changes in the renal pelvis also upset tubular function by interfering with blood supply.

ACUTE TUBULAR NECROSIS

This arises in 2 circumstances:

1. During a state of shock, e.g. due to haemorrhage, burns, trauma, acute intestinal obstruction, incompatible transfusion and abdominal operations.
2. Following administration of toxic substances, e.g. carbon tetrachloride, ethylene glycol, compounds of mercury, uranium, chromic acid and various drugs e.g. antibiotics.

The gross appearance of the kidneys is the same in both groups, although the type and distribution of the lesions are different.

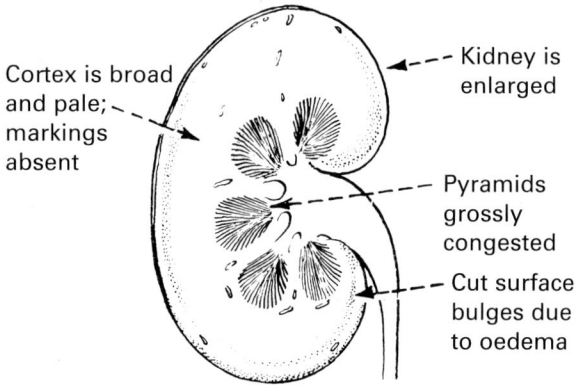

Shock cases

The lesions are the result of ischaemia, and this determines the part of the kidney affected and the portion of the tubule damaged.

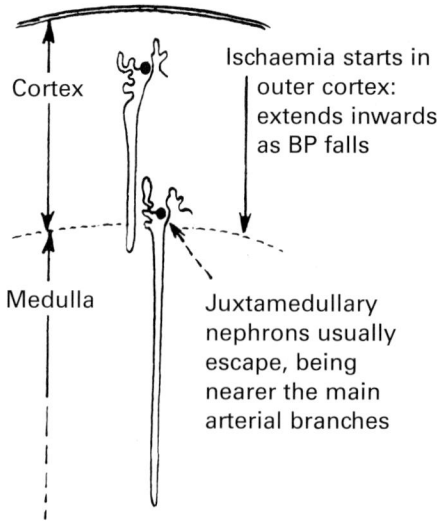

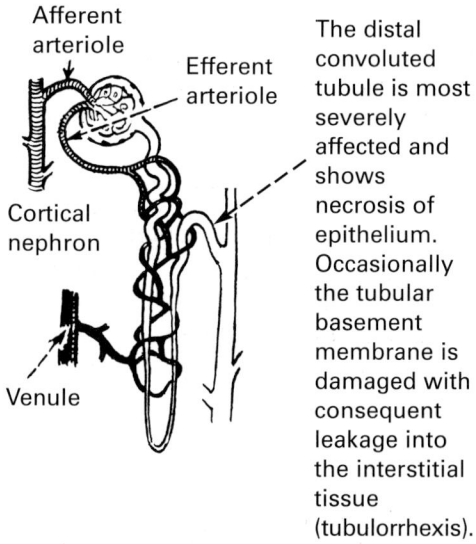

Casts are found in the distal tubules, protein, haemoglobin or myoglobin according to the cause.

TUBULAR LESIONS OF METABOLIC ORIGIN

This type of lesion is brought about by a metabolic defect which may arise outside the kidney (primary) or be the result of renal dysfunction (secondary).

The basic pathological mechanism is very similar in many of the conditions:

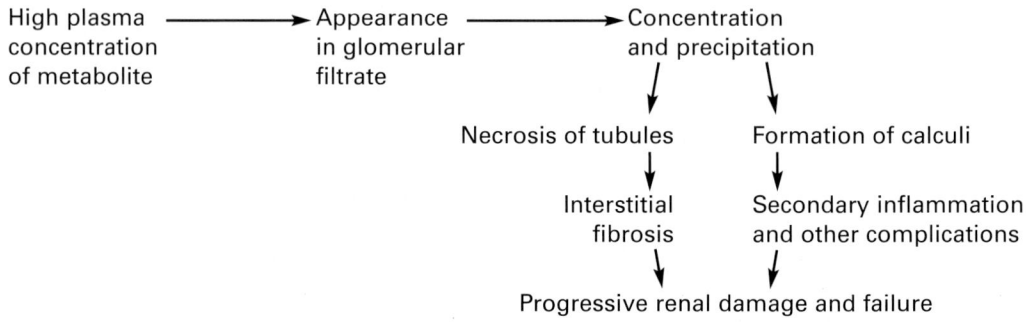

The following are some examples:

(a) **Hypercalcaemic nephritis**

Calcium is deposited in tubular epithelial cells with subsequent fibrosis and calcification—**nephrocalcinosis.**

The usual causes of hypercalcaemia are malignant tumours, primary hyperparathyroidism, hypervitaminosis D and sarcoidosis.

(b) **Urate nephropathy** occurs particularly in **gout.**

Increased primary secretion of uric acid leads to uric acid crystal formation in the acid environment of the distal tubule.

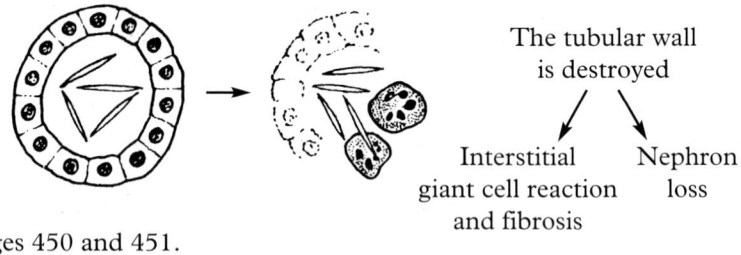

(c) **Myeloma kidney**

This is dealt with on pages 450 and 451.

RENAL TUBULAR ACIDOSIS

The tubules, either due to an inherited defect or to damage secondary to other renal diseases, are unable to produce an acid urine.

There are 2 main forms:

1. In Type I the defect is in the distal tubule.
2. In Type II the function of the proximal tubule is abnormal and there are usually other abnormalities in addition to acidosis e.g. in the Fanconi syndrome there is aminoaciduria, glycosuria and hypophosphataemia.

HAEMOLYTIC URAEMIC SYNDROME

This is a rare complication of many apparently dissimilar conditions. The mechanism appears to be as follows:

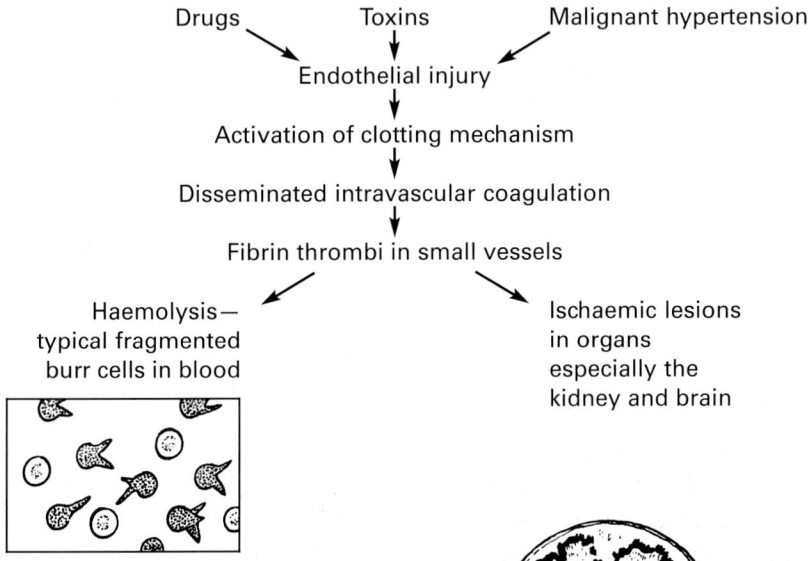

The renal lesions are similar to those seen in malignant hypertension. There is fibrinoid necrosis of the afferent arterioles and capillaries of the glomeruli, and resulting areas of tubular necrosis. In the most extreme cases, bilateral cortical necrosis of the kidneys may occur. The underlying pathology is sometimes termed thrombotic microangiopathy. Clinical manifestations are varied. Renal failure, haemolytic anaemia, hypertension, and sometimes purpura with thrombocytopenia are the main features, but lesions in other organs and the symptoms of the initiating disease produce a complicated picture.

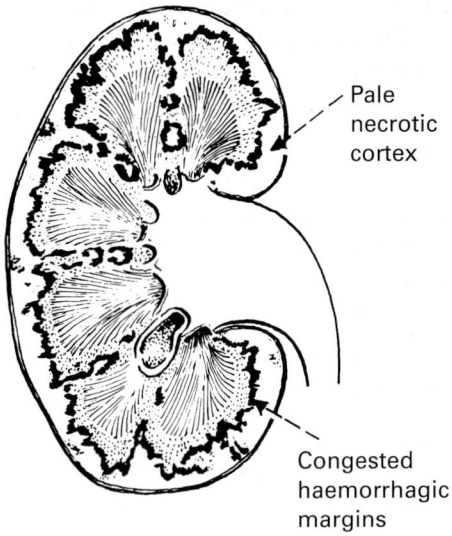

Aetiology

Activation of the clotting system can occur in many differing circumstances:

1. In children there is a close association with alimentary infections: particularly by *E.coli* 0157 which produces a verocytotoxin.
2. Shock conditions, e.g. following abruptio placentae in pregnancy, endotoxic shock.
3. Malignant hypertension. This can be a sequel to the syndrome and equally can predispose the patient to it.
4. Drugs e.g. contraceptive pill, immunosuppressive drugs.

PATHOLOGICAL COMPLICATIONS OF END-STAGE THERAPIES

The prognosis of end-stage renal failure has been greatly improved by (1) Dialysis and (2) Renal Transplantation. The following possible pathological complications are important:

Dialysis

(a) ***Haemodialysis***

(i) ***Local*** — infection and thrombosis at site of vessel access.

(ii) ***Systemic*** — aluminium toxicity: historically, severe dementia or severe osteomalacia was caused by using water containing excess aluminium. Aluminium and other impurities are now removed.

In some cases of long-standing dialysis, small amounts of absorbed aluminium may be associated with mild mental deterioration.

Amyloidosis affecting synovial tissues (e.g. carpal tunnel syndrome: joint stiffness) due to raised circulating β_2 microglobulin.

(b) ***Continuous Ambulatory Peritoneal Dialysis (CAPD)*** — peritonitis: especially due to Staphylococci, Gram -ve organisms and fungi.

Renal Transplantation

Rejection is the main complication. The mechanism is described on page 112.
Depending on the time after transplantation, rejection is classified as
(1) HYPERACUTE — within minutes/hours:
(2) ACUTE — within a few weeks:
(3) CHRONIC — after months/years.

Hyperacute rejection

Pre-existing humoral antibodies against donor MHC or ABO incompatibility → Type 2 or Type 3 Hypersensitivity reaction → Platelet and neutrophil aggregation → Thrombosis and haemorrhage

Acute rejection → Type 2 and cell mediated reaction (Type 4) → Vascular and cellular rejection → Oedema and necrosis

Chronic rejection → continuation of above → Lobular arteries gradually occluded, glomerular damage → Ischaemia

Other complications

1. Cyclosporin toxicity
2. Opportunistic infections
3. Increased incidence of tumours, particularly LYMPHOMAS

Associated with therapeutic immuno-suppression.

Note: Many lymphoproliferative disorders are due to Epstein Barr virus infection and some respond to reduction in immuno-suppressive therapy.

4. Recurrence of original renal disease e.g. IgA nephritis in transplanted kidney.

Note: Similar complications occur in other transplant situations.

CONGENITAL DISORDERS

Malpositions and malformations of the kidney are relatively common and the variations are numerous. Some of the commoner are:

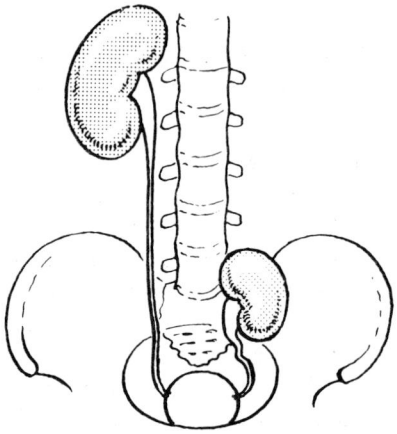

1. **Ectopic kidney (pelvic kidney)**
   One or both kidneys fail to reach the normal adult position. The condition causes difficulty:
   (a) During parturition
   (b) In differential diagnosis of pelvic neoplasms and infections
   (c) When the renal artery originates at the normal level and the long vessel creates problems in arterial supply.

2. **Fusion of kidneys**

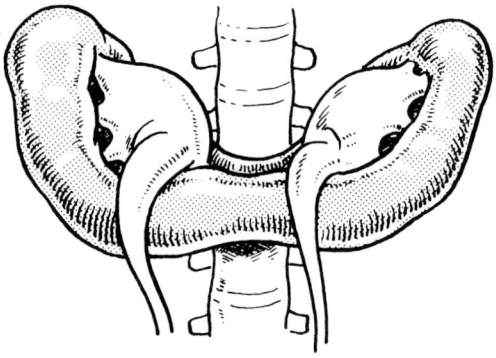

This is usually partial, producing the so-called 'horse-shoe' kidney. The ureters may be partially obstructed leading to hydronephrosis, infection and calculus formation. Frequently the kidneys are also ectopic, adding another hazard.

3. **Single kidney**
   This may be a form of fusion and there may be two ureters. In other cases, there is absence (agenesis) of one kidney, usually the left. There is no interference with renal function unless, of course, the single kidney becomes diseased.

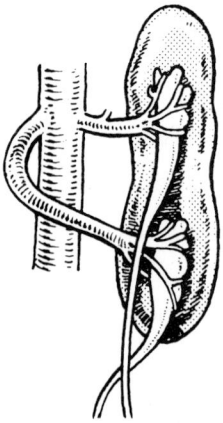

4. **Bilateral agenesis (Potter's syndrome)**
   This is incompatible with life. The affected infants have a distinctive appearance, with low set ears, receding chin, parrot beak nose and wide set eyes.

CONGENITAL CYSTIC DISEASE

This occurs in two main forms:

1. **Adult polycystic disease**
   This is relatively common, and varying degrees of the change may be seen from single cysts up to the classical type where the kidneys are converted into a mass of cysts.
   It is an inherited autosomal dominant trait due to a gene (PDK-1 gene) on chromosome 16 in 85% of cases.

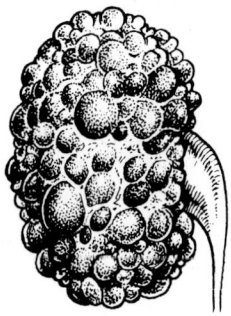

Kidney greatly enlarged: (often exceeds 1 kg)

Cysts vary in size (largest 5 or 6 cm)

Many are brownish (fluid serous or mucoid)

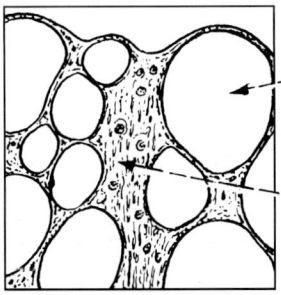

The defect is in the branching of some of the collecting tubules, causing a mixture of normal and abnormal nephrons. Cystic change develops after birth and is progressive, resulting in atrophy of normal nephrons by pressure. The cystic change may not be primarily due to obstruction, but opinion varies.

Intrahepatic cysts are often present but rarely numerous. Death from cerebral haemorrhage is more frequent than expected, partly due to the hypertension secondary to the kidney disorder and in some cases to aneurysms of cerebral arteries.

Clinical Findings

(a) Usually discovered during 3rd and 4th decades, rarely in childhood.
(b) Atrophy of the normal nephrons leads to chronic renal failure, uraemia and hypertension. Progress varies with the number of normal nephrons.

2. **Infantile polycystic disease (Polycystic kidney of the newborn)**
   This is a rare condition.

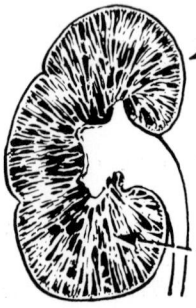

Fetal lobulation preserved

Cystic change extends from medulla to cortex

Uniform spongy appearance

The nephrons are said to be normal in number and formation. Cystic dilatation is situated in the terminal branches of the collecting tubules. The disease, if severe, is incompatible with life, and death occurs shortly after birth. It is due to an autosomal recessive trait. Small liver cysts and multiplication of the intrahepatic bile channels are often present.

RENAL CALCULI

Three basic types of renal calculi are recognised.

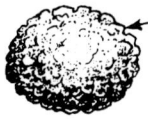

Surface is rough; colour brown, probably due to old blood pigment

(1) **Calcium oxalate**

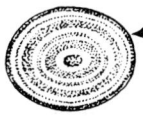

Smooth light brown colour

(2) **Uric acid and urates**

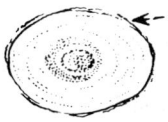

Flaking surface, greyish white

(3) **Triple phosphates** (magnesium, ammonium and calcium)

Commonly the stones are mixed.

1. Urate stones frequently have a rough covering of oxalate.
2. Both oxalate and urate stones tend to develop a covering of phosphates.

Sites of formation. Two suggestions have been made.

1. Precipitates form in the collecting tubules and pass into the renal pelvis where they enlarge.
2. Deposits are formed in the lymphatics of the renal papillae and are extruded into the renal pelvis (this is a less likely explanation).

Mode of formation. This is complex, but the the following is one modern theory:

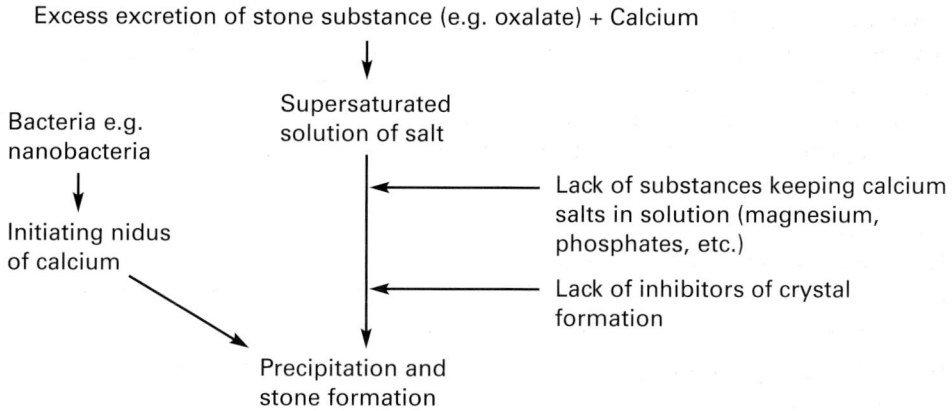

Predisposing factors

1. **Urinary pH.** Urate and oxalate stones form in an acid urine; phosphate stones in alkaline urine.
2. **Dehydration** — causing increased urinary concentration.
3. **Stasis.** Obstruction to urine flow encourages salt precipitation.
4. **Renal disease.** The pH of the urine is frequently disturbed, and the composition of the urine is always altered.
   (a) Renal infection is one of the most important factors. In many cases of renal sepsis, the urine becomes alkaline, favouring phosphate precipitation. Ischaemia causing degeneration and necrosis induces calcification in many chronic renal diseases, and this may lead to stone formation.
   (b) Renal tumours encourage stone formation. Areas of tumour necrosis may calcify, and tumours tend to cause urinary stasis.

RENAL CALCULI

Predisposing factors (continued)

5. **Metabolic factors.** These can operate by altering the pH of the urine and especially by increasing the output of substances e.g.
   (a) Hypercalcuria and hyperphosphaturia. These may be caused by:
   Hyperparathyroidism, primary or secondary to renal failure
   Vitamin D overdosage
   Diet, e.g. excessive milk and alkalis over years in peptic ulcer cases
   Immobilisation leading to loss of calcium from bones.
   (b) Oxaluria. Due to:
   Congenital metabolic defect
   Poisoning by ethylene glycol.
   (c) Urate excess
   (d) Rare stones, e.g. custine, xanthine, are related to inborn metabolic defects.

Effects and complications
These are related to passage of the stone and develop in two situations.

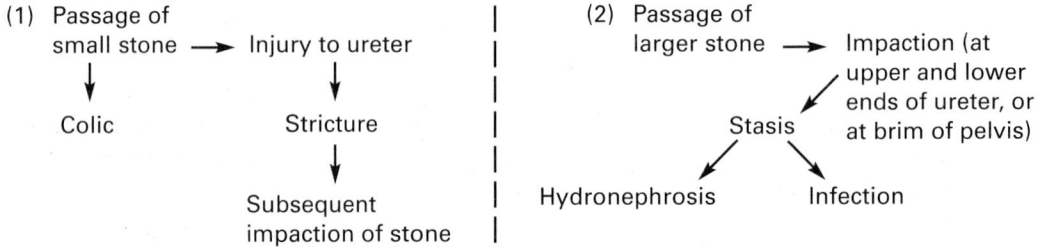

With the development of stasis and infection, further stone formation is encourgaged. This can lead to some peculiar results, e.g.:

Staghorn calculus
This large single stone is associated with suppuration and ulceration of the pelvis and calyces. It is composed mainly of phosphates.
Stones and infection in the pelvis can lead to squamous metaplasia of the epithelium. In a few instances this may develop into squamous carcinoma.

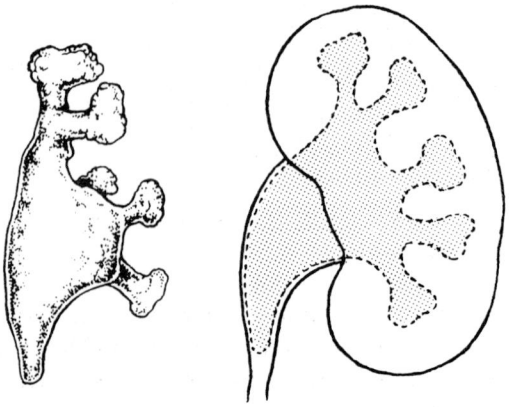

BLADDER CALCULI

These may have passed down the ureter. In the bladder they can increase greatly in size. Cystitis is common and the enlargement is due to deposit of phosphates. Stones may actually form in the bladder when there is urethral obstruction and chronic cystitis.

TUMOURS OF THE KIDNEY

MALIGNANT TUMOURS

Three are of importance: renal cell carcinoma, transitional cell carcinoma and nephroblastoma.

Renal cell carcinoma (hypernephroma)

This is the commonest primary malignant renal tumour. It usually has a typical appearance.

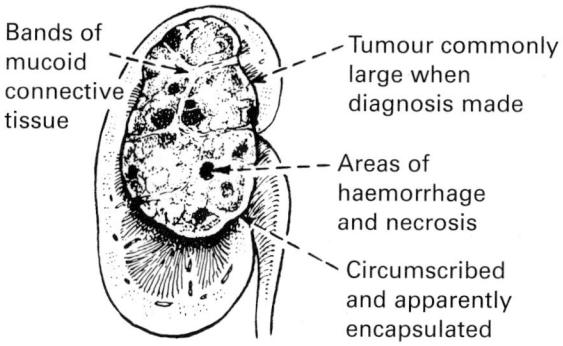

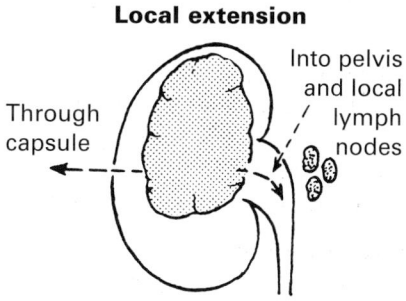

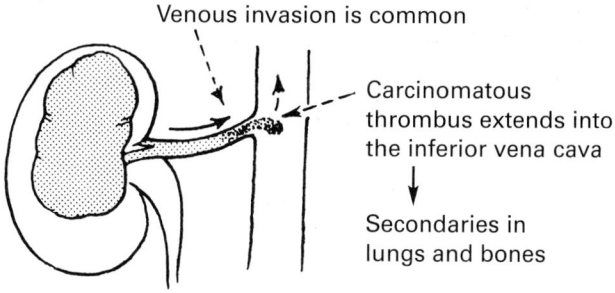

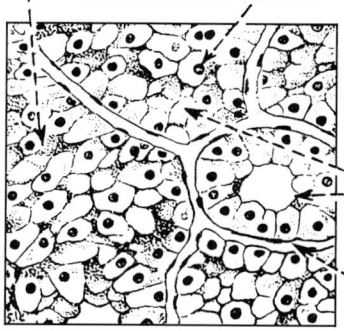

Aetiology: Renal cell carcinoma is associated with:

(a) Cigarette smoking,
(b) Obesity,
(c) Cystic change in patients on haemodialysis,
(d) Genetic predisposition e.g. the von Hippel-Lindau syndrome (renal cysts, cerebellar haemangioblastoma) — associated with a gene on chromosome 3.

Systemic effects

Rarely, patients with renal carcinoma show:

(i) Hypercalcaemia — parathyroid related hormone peptide production (PTHrP).
(ii) Hypertension — increased renin production by tumour or in adjacent kidney.
(iii) Polycythaemia — increased erythropoietin.

TUMOURS OF THE KIDNEY

Malignant (continued)

Transitional cell carcinoma
This tumour arises from the epithelium of the renal pelvis and is similar to the commoner transitional cell carcinoma of the bladder, with which it shares aetiological factors.

Patients usually present with haematuria.

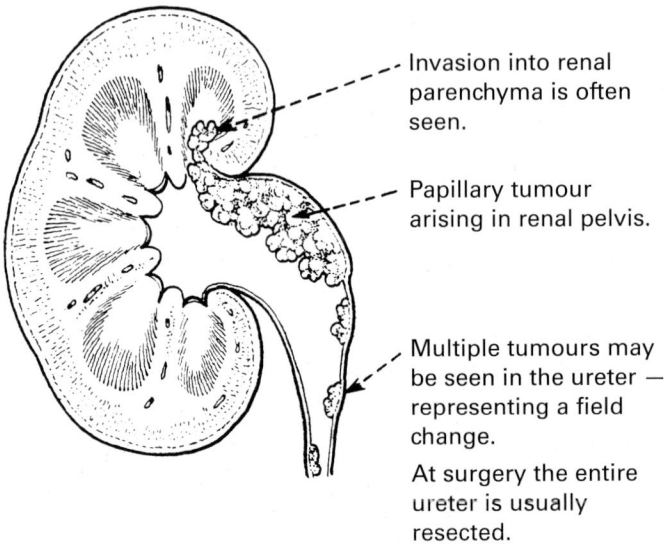

Nephroblastoma (Wilm's tumour)
This is one of the commonest malignant tumours of childhood. It is an embryonic type of tumour derived from kidney rudiments, and forms a large well-circumscribed growth which rapidly invades blood vessels, giving rise to pulmonary secondaries. With modern therapy 90% long-term survival rates are achieved.

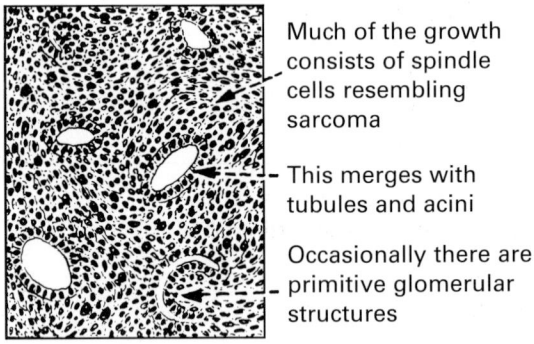

There may be masses of striped muscle.

Mutation of a gene (WT-1) on chromosome 11 appears to be responsible for the development of this tumour.

BENIGN TUMOURS

1. **Fibroma.** This is the commonest simple tumour arising from interstitial cells. It is found incidentally at autopsy in the medulla as a tiny round white nodule, usually less than 1 cm in diameter.
2. **Adenoma.** This is a small nodular proliferation of tubular type epithelium. Histologically they are similar to renal cell carcinomas. It is arbitrarily stated that a tumour smaller than 2 cm in diameter is benign: larger than 3 cm may behave as a metastasising carcinoma.

DISEASES OF URINARY TRACT

The urinary tract is essentially a collecting and discharge system. There are 4 main pathological processes affecting its function: (1) obstruction, (2) infection, (3) calculus formation and (4) neoplastic disease.

Congenital anomalies, which are relatively rare, produce their effects by one or other of these processes.

Obstruction

Acute obstruction, if complete, causes rapid cessation of urine production. If both kidneys are involved, renal failure quickly follows. Chronic obstruction is more common and leads to anatomical changes, with sequels.

Hydronephrosis

This is a dilatation of the renal pelvis and calyces, due to chronic incomplete or intermittent obstruction.

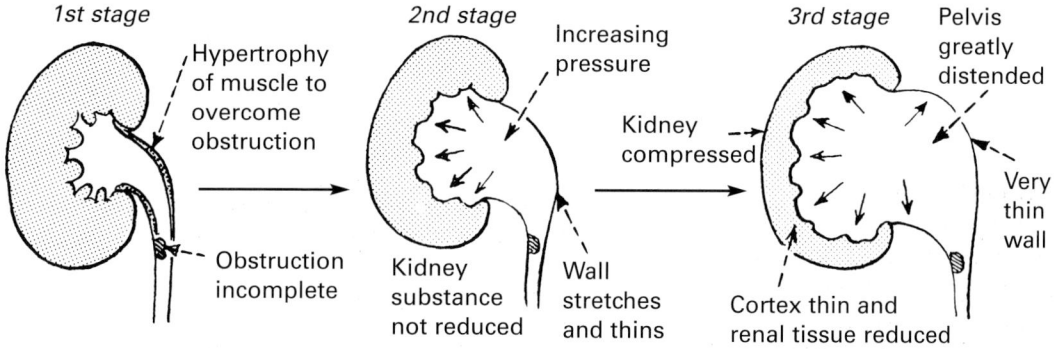

Microscopically, there is tubular atrophy and glomerular scarring. Superimposed infection is common and aggravates the renal damage.

Aetiology

The condition may affect one or both kidneys. This is related to the site of obstruction.

Unilateral obstruction:
above the bladder

Common sites:

1. Pelvi-ureteric junction.
2. At pelvic brim.
3. At entrance to bladder.

Causes:

1. Calculus.
2. Tumour growth.
3. Inflammatory stricture.
4. Congenital abnormality.

Gross hydronephrosis is more commonly unilateral.

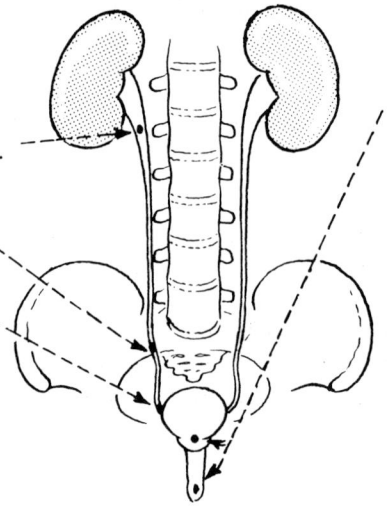

Bilateral obstruction:
in or around bladder or urethra. The ureters are also affected and become dilated and tortuous.

Causes:

1. Prostatic enlargement.
2. Tumour of bladder.
3. Urethral stricture.
4. Pelvic neoplasm.
5: Retroperitoneal fibrosis.

URINARY TRACT INFECTION

Pyelonephritis has already been considered. Inflammation of the ureters is due to extension upwards from an infection of the bladder and urethra.

Acute cystitis

The bladder shows the usual signs of inflammation. Small haemorrhages are common in the oedematous mucosa. The following points are important:

1. It is common in females, especially frequent in pregnancy: and also associated with sexual intercourse.
2. In males it is usually secondary to obstruction, e.g. due to enlarged prostate or a urethral stricture.
3. Obstruction encourages infection, enhances its effects and prolongs the inflammatory process.
4. In non-obstructive cases, infection is usually due to *E. coli*. Mixed infections, proteus and staphylococcus, are common in obstructive cases.
5. Vesicoureteric reflux is very important allowing retrograde spread of infection to the kidneys. It occurs as a congenital defect in children but also may be secondary to cystitis.

Chronic cystitis

This is the result of repeated attacks of acute cystitis, but it is usually associated with obstruction of the urethra causing stasis of urine.

Mixed infection including *B* proteus is common and, together with urea-splitting organisms forming ammonia, result in an alkaline urine. Phosphates precipitate and can form crumbling whitish calculi.

Tuberculous cystitis

This is always secondary to a tuberculous infection elsewhere, usually in the kidney. Less commonly, the epididymis is the source of infection. Small tubercles form in the submucous layer, usually at the bladder base. These ulcerate and secondary infection is common.

Urethritis

Acute inflammation of the urethra is commonly due to the gonococcus, but another form is now more common in Western countries: so-called non-specific urethritis is often due to chlamydia infection.

In Reiter's syndrome, in addition to urethritis, there is arthritis and conjunctivitis.

TUMOURS OF THE URINARY TRACT

Transitional cell carcinomas occur in the bladder, ureters and renal pelvis. They arise from the stratified transitional epithelium lining the tract and are all considered to be CARCINOMAS but show a wide spectrum of malignant potential. They are graded I to III as follows, according to the World Health Organisation (WHO) classification.

GRADE I — These are **Papillary Tumours.** Tumours at the benign end of the spectrum have a uniform, well-differentiated epithelial covering showing no mitotic activity. They have a slender stalk and delicate branching fronds. With this structure, and their fine vascular connective tissue, haemorrhage is common.

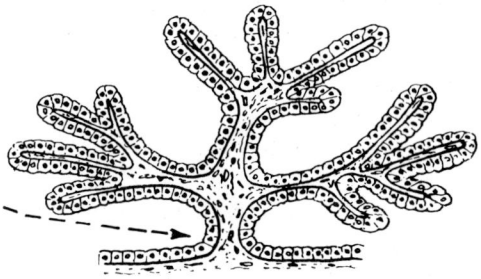

GRADE II — These also are **Papillary.** The stalk of the tumour is broader and the epithelial cells show mitoses and variability. Early stromal invasion may be present.

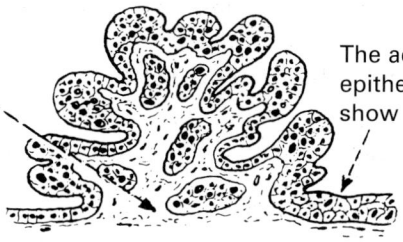

GRADE III are **Solid Sessile Tumours:** They are distinguished by the degree of cellular anaplasia, mitotic activity and aggressive growth. Infection with ulceration and necrosis is common: local penetration into the bladder muscle and lymphatic invasion are usual.

Squamous carcinoma and adenocarcinoma are rare tumours. Rhabdomyosarcoma may occur in the bladder in children.

Aetiology

Bladder tumours are an industrial hazard:

(a) in aniline dye manufacture due to beta-naphthylamine
(b) in the rubber industry
(c) in manufacturing processes involving benzene.

SMOKING and CHRONIC ANALGESIC ABUSE are important associations. In the MIDDLE EAST chronic infestation by ***Schistosoma haematobium*** is an important association, particularly of squamous carcinoma.

Mechanism

KIDNEY → UROTHELIUM → FIELD CHANGES → **CARCINOMA**

KIDNEY: Excretion of carcinogen (i) direct elimination or (ii) metabolite concentration in urine

UROTHELIUM: chronic exposure particularly in bladder

Note: (i) Urothelial tumours are often multiple and recurrence is common: long term surveillance is important.
(ii) Progression from a low grade to higher grades is frequent.

FEMALE GENITAL TRACT – ANATOMY AND PHYSIOLOGY

The ovaries, fallopian tubes, uterus, vagina and vulva form an integrated system which is unique in that full function is limited to a period of roughly 40 years from puberty to menopause. A two-tier system of hormonal control operates. Secretion of steroids by the ovary prepares the uterus for pregnancy, and the ovarian secretion is controlled by the anterior pituitary and hypothalamus.

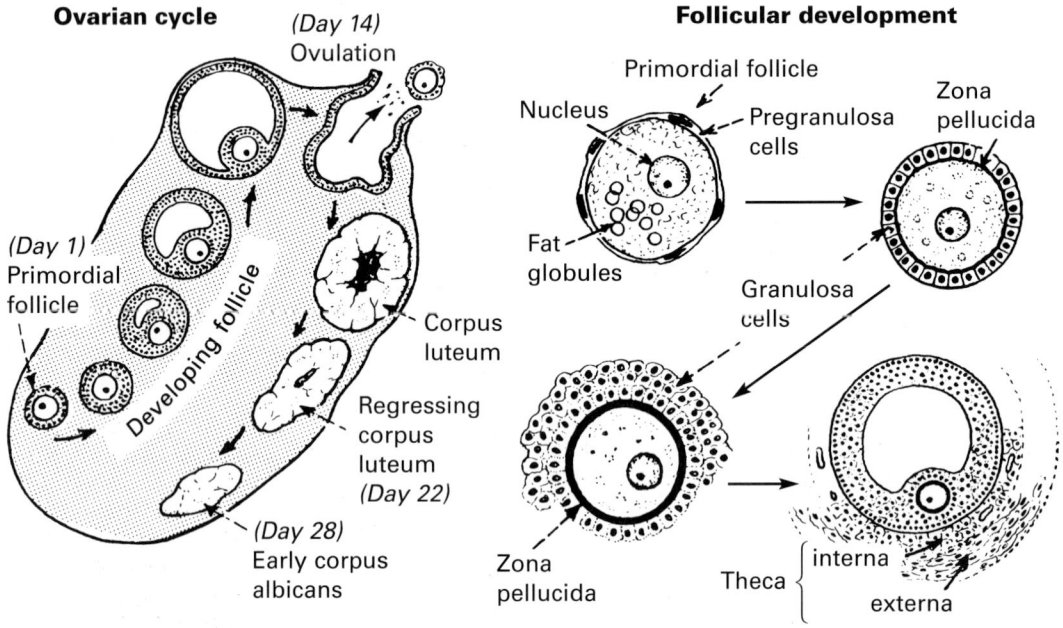

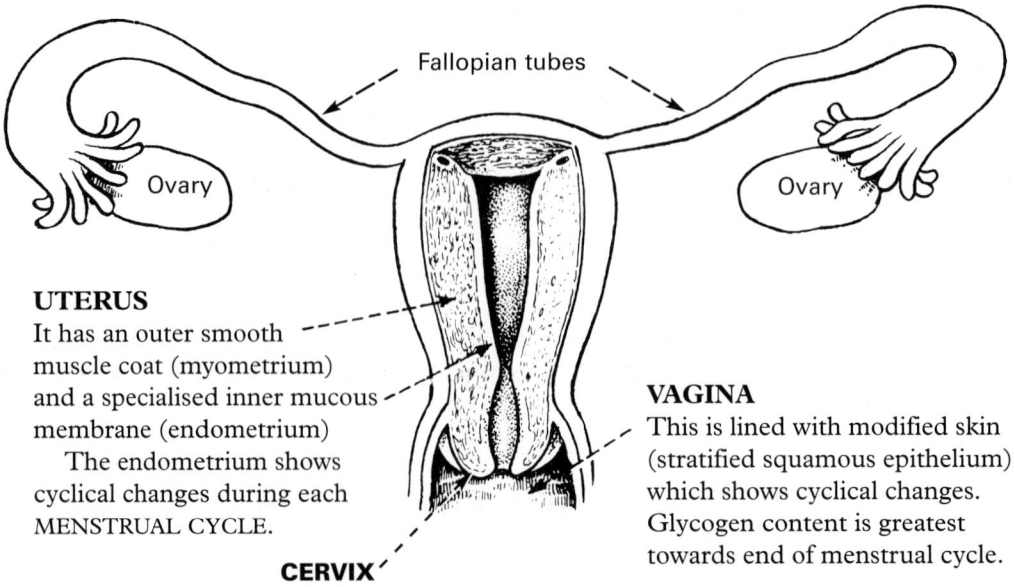

CYCLICAL ENDOMETRIAL CHANGES

Menstruation

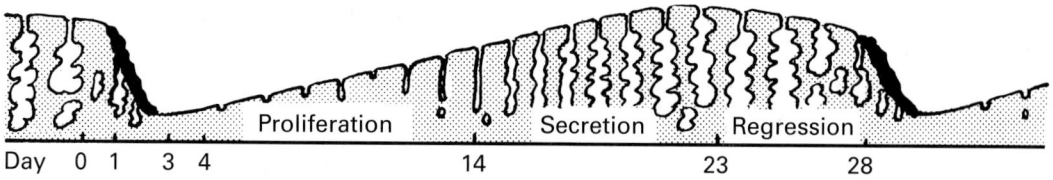

ASSOCIATED OVARIAN STEROID SECRETION

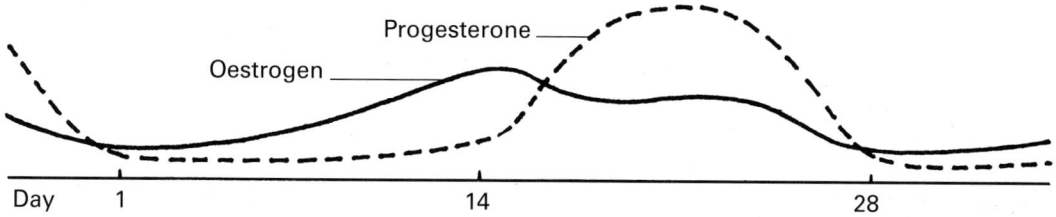

Proliferative phase
This is induced by oestrogen produced by developing ovarian follicles, stimulated by FSH from the pituitary.

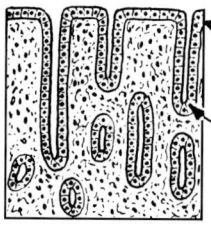

Secretory phase
Progesterone produced by the corpus luteum stimulates secretion by the glands. Oestrogen is also produced. The stromal cells enlarge (pseudo-decidual change), oedema is present and vascularity greatly increased.

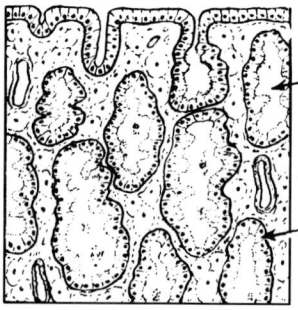

Premenstrual regressive phase
Endometrial growth ceases 5–6 days before menstruation. Prior to menstruation, it shrinks due to decreased blood flow and discharge of secretion. This increases the tortuosity of glands and blood vessels.

DISEASES OF THE ENDOMETRIUM

Endometritis is now an unusual condition.

Acute infection is almost confined to infection associated with parturition and abortion — often related to retention of products of conception. Historically, criminal abortion in non-sterile conditions led to severe infection. Gonococcal infection does not commonly extend beyond the cervix but can lead to acute endometritis. Chlamydia may cause acute or chronic endometritis.

Chronic endometritis

This is a rare lesion as a primary condition. It can follow an acute endometritis which may be mild. The uterine changes occur in 2 phases:

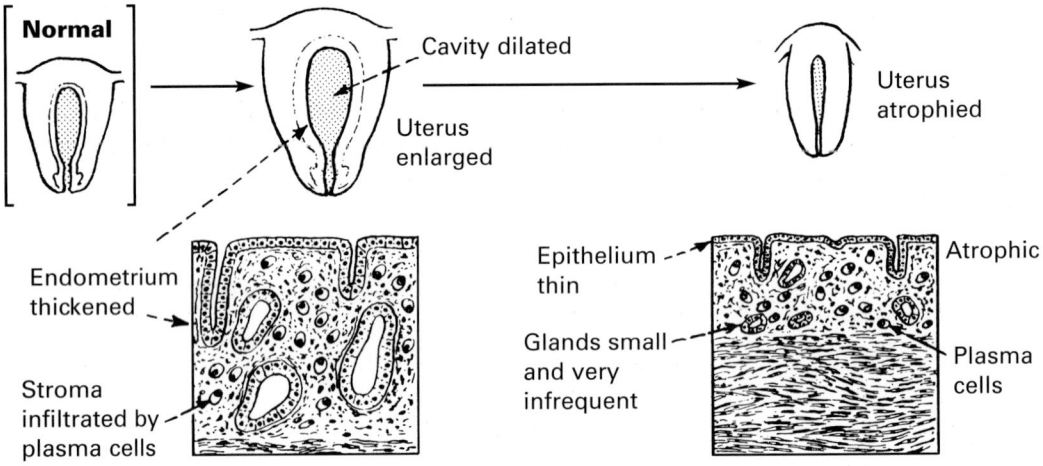

The normal cyclical changes may fail to take place.

Tuberculous endometritis

This is now uncommon in the British Isles. It is the result of infection spreading from the fallopian tubes. If the patient is still menstruating, the tubercles are shed each month: diagnostic curettage should be done as late in the cycle as possible to allow new tubercles to develop. In some cases, menstruation ceases and caseation occurs.

Intrauterine anti-fertility devices

A mild chronic inflammation may be associated with the use of these devices. There may be focal atrophy with mild plasma cell infiltration. Irregular bleeding may result.

Oral contraceptives

These are commonly a combination of an oestrogen with a progestogen. They tend to induce atrophy of the endometrium, the glands becoming small, inactive and infrequent. The stroma appears relatively abundant. On stopping the 'pill', amenorrhoea, sometimes intractable, may follow. Mild hypertension occasionally develops while taking oral contraceptives.

DISEASES OF THE ENDOMETRIUM

ENDOMETRIOSIS

This consists of deposits of endometrium outside of the uterine cavity.

In most cases, the disease is confined to the pelvis and the genital tract.

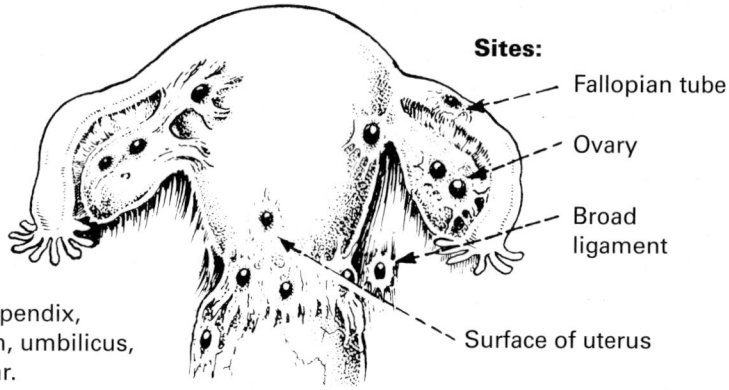

Other sites: Caecum and appendix, bladder, rectum, umbilicus, laparotomy scar.

These deposits react to the stimulus of ovarian steroids and show cyclical changes. The result is haemorrhage into the local tissues at the time of menstruation. Adhesions develop, often leading to infertility. Malignant change to endometrioid adenocarcinoma occurs uncommonly.

Aetiology

In some instances deposits are formed in laparotomy scars after uterine operations, but in most cases there has been no surgical interference. Three theories have been proposed.

1. Retrograde spill of menstrual debris.
2. Metaplasia of tissues into Müllerian duct elements.
3. Lymphatic and blood borne emboli of endometrial tissue.

ADENOMYOSIS

This is a condition of ectopic endometrial deposits in the myometrium. There is an accompanying overgrowth of muscle and connective tissue. Two macroscopic forms occur:

1. **Diffuse**
   Deposits are confined to inner part of myometrium.
   Foci of endometrium often brownish in colour

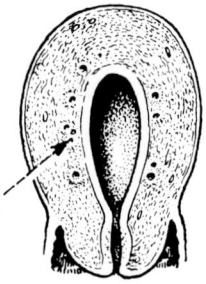

2. **Localised**
   Resembling fibroid but with brownish foci

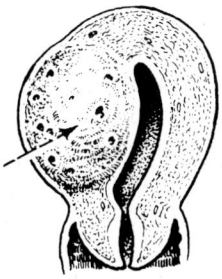

The endometrial deposits communicate with the uterine cavity, but despite this they often contain altered blood in the glands which become cystic. The diffuse type is commoner. Adenomyosis is *not* related to endometriosis.

ENDOMETRIAL HYPERPLASIA

Endometrial hyperplasia occurs in 3 forms: Simple hyperplasia, complex hyperplasia and atypical hyperplasia. Of these, atypical hyperplasia is most important as it is associated with an increased risk of malignancy.

SIMPLE HYPERPLASIA

This tends to occur in the peri-menopausal period. It is due to excess oestrogen stimulation — particularly associated with **anovulatory** cycles, but rarely with oestrogen therapy or oestrogen-secreting tumours.

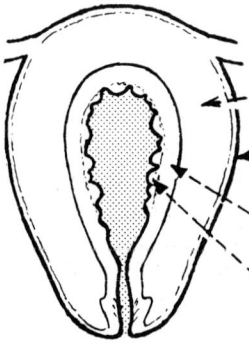

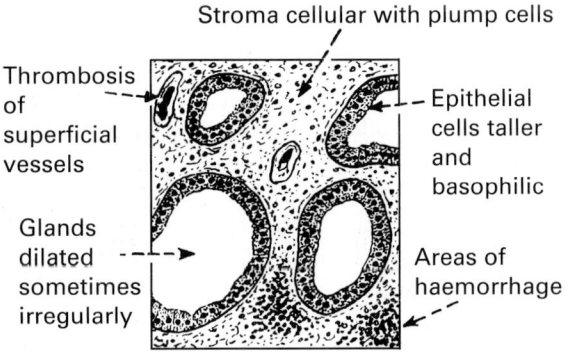

Clinically, there is irregular, frequent and heavy bleeding.

COMPLEX HYPERPLASIA

In this form, hyperplasia is often focal and glands but not stroma are affected. Thus the glands appear crowded, but show **no** atypia. There is no increased risk of malignancy.

ATYPICAL HYPERPLASIA

In this condition the hyperplasia is focal and cytological atypia with mitotic figures is common.

Intervening endometrium may show simple hyperplasia. The importance of atypical hyperplasia is its relationship to the development of adenocarcinoma i.e. it is considered to be pre-cancerous, with a risk of around 20%.

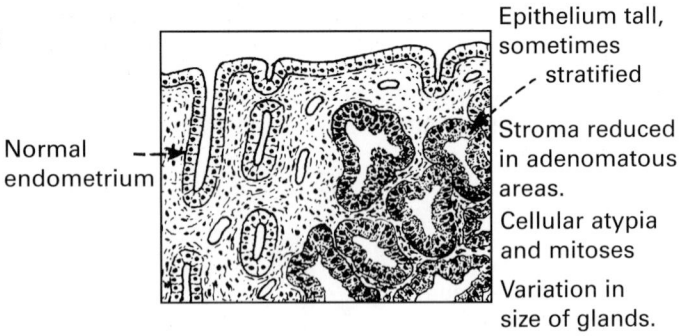

ENDOMETRIAL POLYP

This is a localised proliferation of endometrial glands which becomes pedunculated.

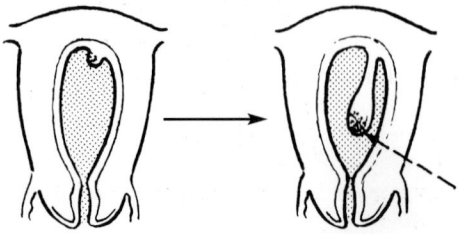

Sometimes polyps are associated with general endometrial hyperplasia. Progressive elongation of the pedicle jeopardises the blood supply. Compression by the uterine muscle results in venous congestion at the tip leading to bleeding and necrosis.

ENDOMETRIAL CARCINOMA

This common gynaecological cancer particularly affects postmenopausal patients, who typically present with vaginal bleeding.

CARCINOMA
This growth may form a *localised* plaque or polyp.

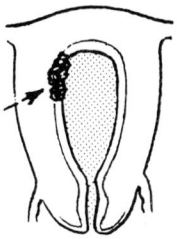

In some cases, however, it appears as a *diffuse* change involving much of the endometrium. It grows initially within the endometrial layer, bulging into the uterine cavity. Surface necrosis occurs at an early date.

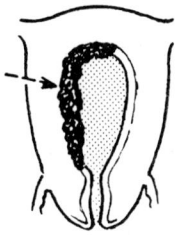

Most growths are well-differentiated adenocarcinomas

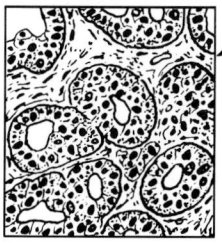

but anaplastic growths are not uncommon

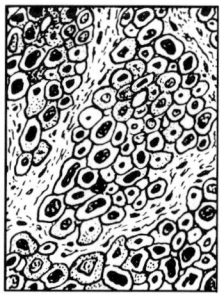

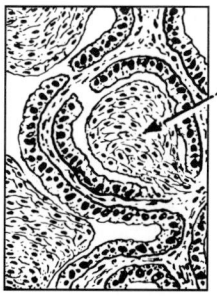

Areas of squamous metaplasia are relatively common (adeno-acanthoma); they have no prognostic implication

In some cases with a particularly poor prognosis malignant squamous epithelium is admixed with the adenocarcinoma — so-called ADENOSQUAMOUS carcinoma.
The endometrium possesses no lymphatics and invasion of the myometrium takes place slowly.

Local extension: this may take place in several directions.

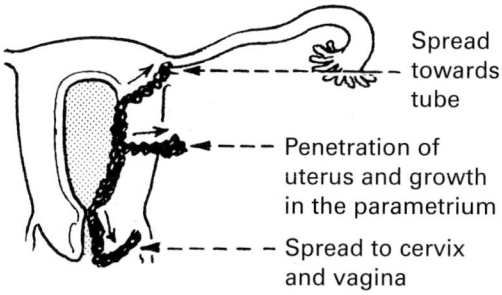

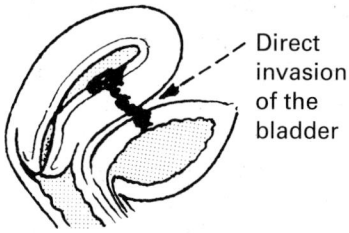

Metastases

1. **Via lymphatics**

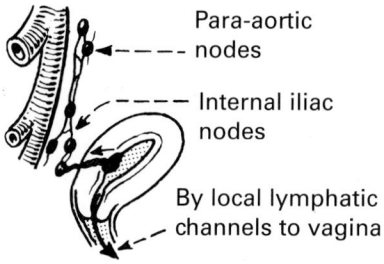

2. **Via blood vessels**
Secondary deposits in the vagina and ovaries may be due to this mode of spread

3. **Via fallopian tube**

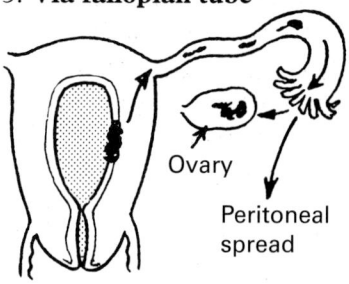

4. **Distant metastases.** At a late date, secondaries may appear in the liver, lungs and bones. These may be the result of lymphatic or blood spread.

ENDOMETRIAL CARCINOMA

Prognosis

Post-menopausal bleeding may give early warning of the disease. Lack of lymphatics in the endometrium limits extension for some time. The most important prognostic factor is the **stage** of the tumour, usually expressed in the FIGO (International Federation of Gynaecology and Obstetrics) system. The histological grade and subtype are also important. Overall a 60% 5 year survival is seen.

Aetiology

Endometrial carcinoma is uncommon before the 5th decade. The most important factor is prolonged OESTROGENIC stimulation due to:

(a) endogenous overproduction e.g. in cases of oestrogen-secreting ovarian tumours.
(b) exogenous oestrogen therapy.
(c) in OBESITY: increased conversion of androstenedione (from adrenals) to oestrone,
(d) ATYPICAL HYPERPLASIA is an important precancerous stage.

Other endometrial malignancies:

ENDOMETRIAL STROMAL SARCOMAS

These rare tumours may be of low grade or high grade.

Low grade tumours — infiltrate extensively through the lymphatics of the myometrium. The cells are cytologically bland and mitoses are few. About one fifth of patients eventually die from the disease.

High grade stromal sarcomas — are highly malignant spindle celled tumours, with poor prognosis. It may be difficult to separate these from uterine leiomyosarcomas.

MIXED MESODERMAL TUMOURS

These uncommon tumours can differentiate both into endometrial carcinoma and stromal sarcoma. They often present as soft fleshy masses protruding from the cervix into the vagina.

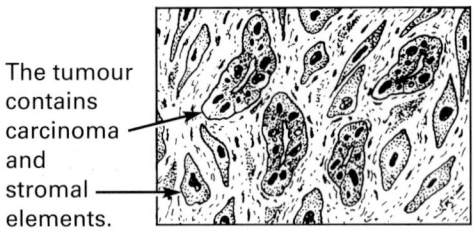

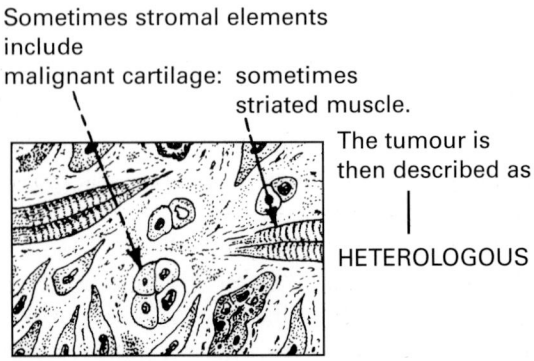

DISEASES OF THE MYOMETRIUM

MYOMETRIUM

The myometrium is never a primary site of inflammation, acute or chronic. It is involved secondary to lesions in the endometrium or peritoneum. Tumours however are quite common.

LEIOMYOMA (Myoma, fibromyoma, fibroid)

This is a circumscribed growth derived from uterine muscle.

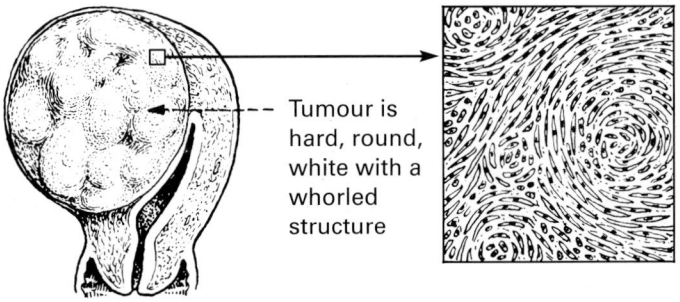

They vary in size from tiny (mm) growths to several cm in diameter and are frequently multiple. Apparent encapsulation is due to compression by adjacent muscle.

Fibroids may be found in any part of the uterus.

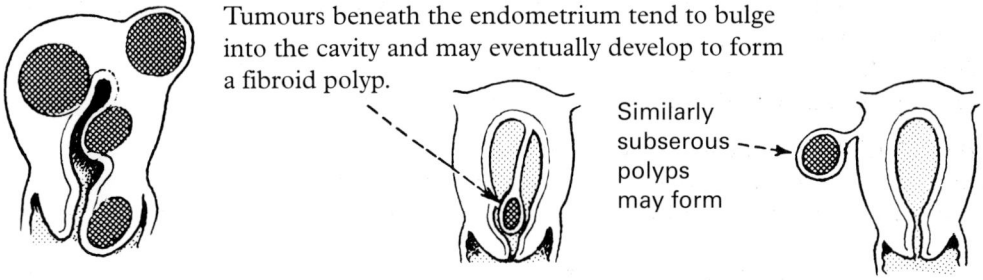

Complications

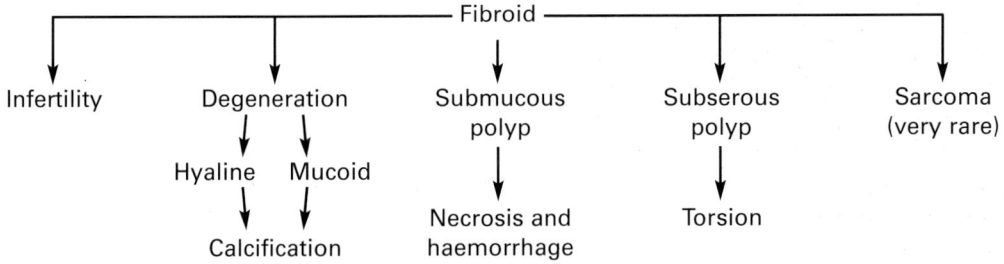

Leiomyoma is one of the commonest tumours, occurring in 15–20% of women over the age of 35. Growth ceases at the menopause.

LEIOMYOSARCOMA

This is a rare tumour which may arise from a preceding leiomyoma, but usually does not. Some tumours are highly malignant but in others with few mitotic figures it is difficult to predict the outcome — these are known as Smooth Muscle Tumours of Unknown Malignant Potential (STUMP).

DISEASES OF CERVIX

The cervix constitutes the lower one third of the uterine body.

It is in two parts: endocervical and vaginal or ectocervical. The dividing line is quite sharp and is determined by the character of the lining epithelium.

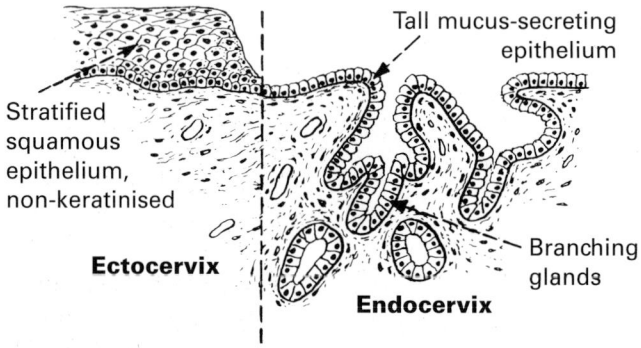

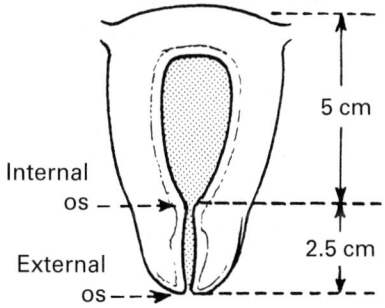

The remainder of the cervical wall consists of circular smooth muscle lying in abundant fibroelastic tissue.

At the internal os, the structure gradually merges with that of the uterus proper, the branching glands giving place to the simple tubules of the endometrium, and the proportion of muscle increases greatly.

CERVICITIS

Inflammation of the cervix may be acute or chronic. Acute cervicitis may be due to gonorrhoea or follow cervical laceration at childbirth.

Chronic cervicitis is commoner. Candida, trichomonas (p. 514) and Chlamydia may be responsible. The last is associated with reactive lymphoid follicles (follicular cervicitis).

Viral infections of the cervix include Herpes Simplex Virus (Type II) and human papilloma viruses (HPV). The latter can cause simple viral warts or be associated with cervical intraepithelial dysplasia and neoplasia (CIN) and invasive carcinoma (p. 512).

CERVICAL POLYP

This is a local proliferation of endocervical mucosa which becomes pedunculated and may protrude through the cervix.

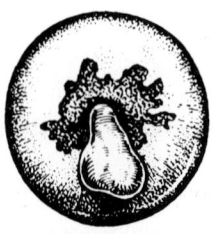

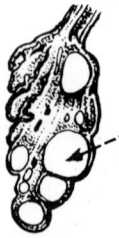

Cystic glands are common due to obstruction by chronic inflammation

CERVICAL INTRAEPITHELIAL NEOPLASIA (CIN)

The transformation zone

From puberty onwards and particularly in pregnancy the squamo-columnar junction presents on the vaginal surface of the external os. This is the area where **squamous metaplasia** occurs. It is important because cervical squamous carcinoma and its precursor **cervical intraepithelial neoplasia** (CIN) begin there. Within this metaplastic epithelium, **dysplastic** changes may develop. They are graded as CIN I, II and III. Later, in some cases, invasive squamous carcinoma develops.

CIN I = Mild dysplasia.

Upper $^{2}/_{3}$: Stratified.

Basal $^{1}/_{3}$: High nucleo-cytoplasmic ratio; pleomorphic nuclei

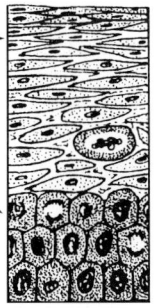

CIN II = Moderate dysp.

Superficial stratification

Cellular abnormalities extending up into middle one third

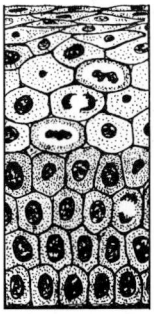

CIN III = Severe dysp. and Carcinoma in situ.

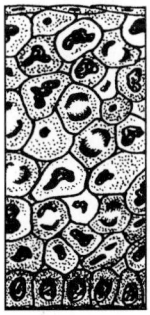

May be 1 or 2 layers of stratified epithelium on surface.

Remainder: Immature; large nuclei; mitoses.

Koilocytes (cells with a wrinkled pyknotic nucleus and perinuclear cytoplasmic clearing) are often seen in the suprabasal layers indicating HPV infection.

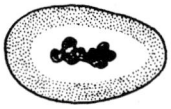

CYTOLOGY and CIN

The cervical screening programme aims to detect CIN and thus prevent the development of invasive carcinoma. Smears from the squamo-columnar junction obtained by a wooden spatula are stained by Papanicolaou's method. The cells can be examined for dysplasia — so-called dyskaryosis. Inflammatory changes e.g. due to candida infection may be seen.

Normal smear

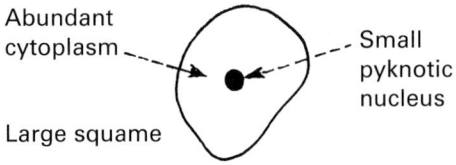

Dyskaryosis

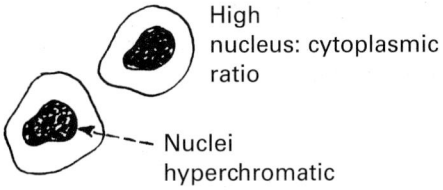

The cytology is a SCREENING TEST. Patients with abnormalities are referred for colposcopy where abnormal epithelium turns white on exposure to acetic acid (acetowhite). Punch biopsy to assess dysplasia is often followed by laser ablation. New techniques to identify proliferating and malignant cells are being rapidly developed.

CARCINOMA OF CERVIX

CARCINOMA

This is the most common malignant tumour of the female genital tract, even where there is a vigorous campaign for early diagnosis and eradication of carcinoma in situ. The growth is a squamous carcinoma in 70% of cases, a squamous carcinoma with an adenocarcinoma component (adeno-squamous carcinoma) in 20% and a pure adenocarcinoma in 10%. Most squamous carcinomas arise at the squamo-columnar junction: a minority (20%) and most adenocarcinomas arise within the endocervical canal.

The cervix becomes very indurated; necrosis and ulceration commonly follow quickly.

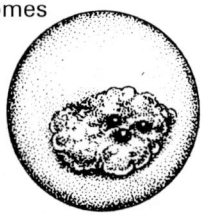

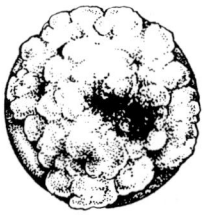

Later, a large fungating mass is produced. Sloughing may leave an excavated crater.

Microinvasive carcinoma is the earliest stage of invasive cancer — where spread is less than 5 mm in depth. This is associated with an excellent prognosis.

Spread

Until a very late stage, the disease is confined to the pelvic cavity. The patient commonly dies before distant metastases appear.

Local spread takes place in several directions:

1. **Downward extension.**

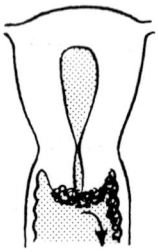

The ureters come very close to the cervix in their travel to the bladder, and are apt to be involved in extension of the growth to the parametrium. The ureters may be obstructed by pressure or invasion. Renal infection and failure follow.

2. **Lateral extension.** The anatomy of this region is important.

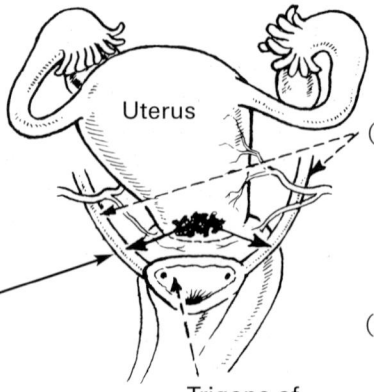

(a) The growth encircles the external os. In some cases it causes obstruction of the cervical canal and pyometra may develop.

(b) Extension to the vagina takes place in direct continuity.

CARCINOMA OF CERVIX

Spread of carcinoma (continued)

3. **Anterior and posterior extension**

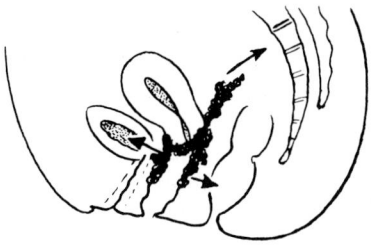

Direct invasion of the bladder or rectum results in fistulous communications. Spread along the uterosacral ligaments involves the sacral nerves, causing intractable pain.

4. **Lymphatic spread**
This occurs early and involves the chains of lymph nodes in the pelvis.

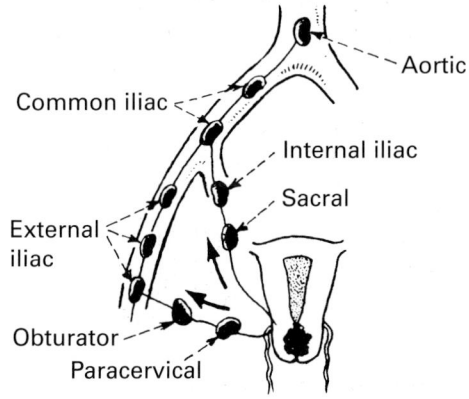

Prognosis
With modern treatment there is an 80% 5-year cure rate when the disease is diagnosed early i.e. confined to the cervix: it falls significantly if spread to the pelvis has occurred.

Previously death was commonly due to a combination of renal failure and sepsis: fatal haemorrhage from eroded vessels also occurred. With better local control death is usually due to metastases.

Aetiology
1. ***Epidemiological facts***
   (a) The disease is rare in virgins (in a community of nuns, no cases were seen) and the incidence is highest in prostitutes. The disease is rare in strictly orthodox Jewish women and significantly increased in less strict Jewish communities.
   (b) Historically the disease was seen most commonly in the 4th and 5th decades. Nowadays, in Western Societies, dysplasia and carcinoma are seen in younger women (3rd decade) and the prevalence has greatly increased. These changes are statistically related to sexual promiscuity and early age of first coitus.
   (c) The use of barrier methods of contraception is associated with a decreased incidence.

2. ***Virus Infection***
   In the great majority of cases HUMAN PAPILLOMA VIRUS (HPV) is associated with cervical carcinoma and is the postulated carcinogenic agent with male to female transmission.

Associations

HPV types 6, 11, 31 and others	CIN I and condylomata
HPV types 16 or 18	CIN III and invasive carcinoma

3. Of other possible co-factors or mutagens ***Tobacco*** heads the list.
4. It seems likely that in many cases initiation of the progression to cancer begins at an early age before the cervical muco-squamous junction has stabilised.

DISEASES OF VAGINA AND VULVA

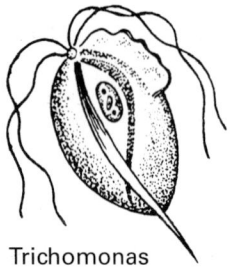

Trichomonas vaginalis

Vaginal discharge is a common complaint especially in parous women. In many cases it is related to chronic cervicitis. There are however a number of inflammatory conditions which arise primarily in the vagina.

Gonococcal infection may produce an acute inflammation with purulent discharge but it is often asymptomatic.

Purulent discharge is also associated with infection by a protozoon, Trichomonas vaginalis. The discharge tends to be frothy. It is commonly transmitted during sexual intercourse. The male can also be infected.

Candida albicans infection is common in pregnancy and in patients undergoing antibiotic or immunosuppressive therapy.

PRIMARY TUMOURS of the VAGINA are rare. Squamous carcinoma occurs in the upper vagina of women and may lead to fistula formation between the vagina and the bladder or rectum. Vaginal intraepithelial neoplasia (VAIN) may be associated with CIN and VIN.

Historically, clear cell carcinoma was sometimes found in adolescent girls. It has been traced to the effect on the fetus of administration of diethylstilboestrol to the patient's mother during early pregnancy. It arises in a background of vaginal adenosis — a proliferation of glands within the vaginal wall.

VULVAL INFLAMMATION is common in post-menopausal women. It is related to atrophy of the skin, which has very thin epithelial covering at this phase of life and is easily abraded. Inflammation at other periods of life frequently involves Bartholin's gland.

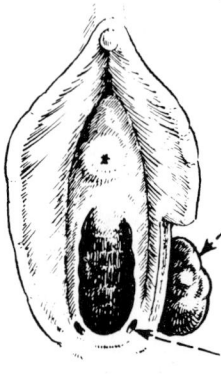

The duct which opens into the vagina in front of the hymen is apt to become blocked. If the inflammation subsides a simple cyst of the duct arises but an abscess may form.

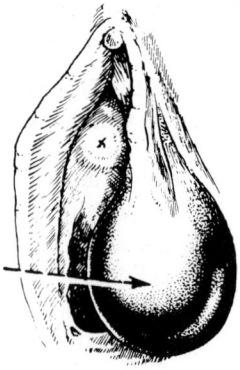

Two conditions which mainly occur in the tropics and are seen only very occasionally in temperate countries are:

1. **Lymphogranuloma venereum.** This is a chlamydial infection which starts as an ulcer on the vulva or in the vagina. It heals in a short time, only to be followed by a chronic suppurative reaction in the inguinal and sometimes pelvic lymph nodes. This leads to extensive scarring and sometimes fistulous openings in the pelvic viscera.
2. **Granuloma inguinale.** This begins as a papule on the vulva, perineum or vagina. It ulcerates and can spread widely, causing extensive destruction of tissue. Histologically, it is a granuloma and the infecting organism (Calymmatobacterium granulomatosis) can be seen in macrophages.

DISEASES OF VAGINA AND VULVA

LEUKOPLAKIA AND PREMALIGNANCY

Leukoplakia is a descriptive term meaning white patches. These are common on the vulval and perineal regions in almost any chronic inflammatory skin condition due to the local moist conditions, e.g. chronic dermatitis (lichen simplex), fungal infection and lichen sclerosis.

There is however one type of lesion appearing as white patches in this region which shows epithelial dysplasia and is premalignant.

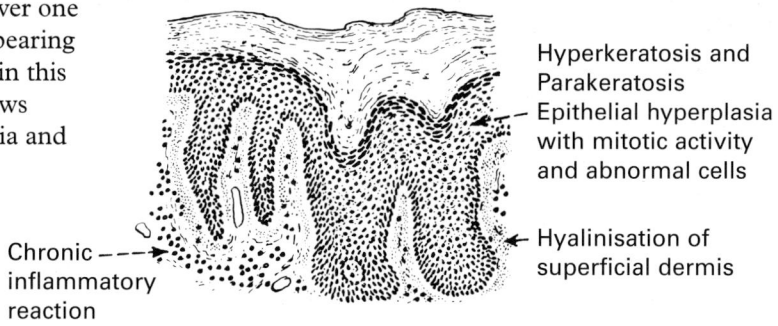

The degree of dysplasia varies, amounting to carcinoma in situ in some cases.

These changes are now numerically graded VIN I, II and III, i.e. Vulvar Intraepithelial Neoplasia (analogous to CIN).

TUMOURS OF THE VULVA

Simple tumours are common. CONDYLOMATA ACUMINATA are papillary proliferations due to infection by Human Papilloma Virus (HPV) types 6 or 11. Koilocytosis (see p. 511) in the superficial keratinocytes is the histological marker.

Sweat gland tumours (hidradenomas) may also occur.

Carcinoma of vulva

This is a rare condition found usually in women in the 6th and 7th decades of life.

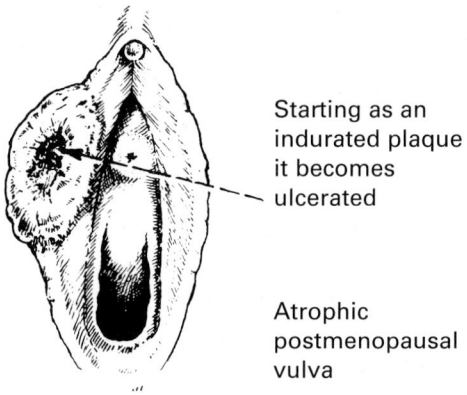

The inguinal glands on both sides are invaded at an early date. The growth is usually a squamous carcinoma.

DISEASES OF FALLOPIAN TUBE

Acute Salpingitis

The inflammation is the result of ascending infection from the endometrium: some cases follow abortion and puerperal infection. In addition to the infecting organisms causing acute endometritis (see p. 504) members of the Chlamydia and Mycoplasma species are now known to cause acute salpingitis.

The inflammation is usually bilateral and primarily involves the tubal plicae which are congested and oedematous: there is a purulent exudate.

If resolution of the acute inflammation does not occur (antibiotic therapy is important) chronic salpingitis and its possible complications are established. The term 'pelvic inflammatory disease' is used.

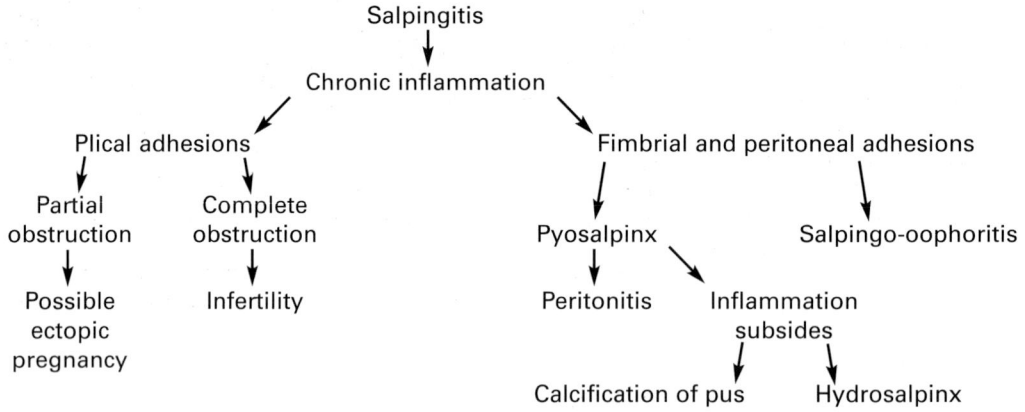

Tuberculous salpingitis

Tuberculous infection of the female genital tract, for some unexplained reason, almost always starts in the fallopian tube. It is usually due to blood spread from some other site: only very occasionally it is secondary to tuberculous peritonitis.

The complications are these expected of a chronic salpingitis with the added element of caseation.

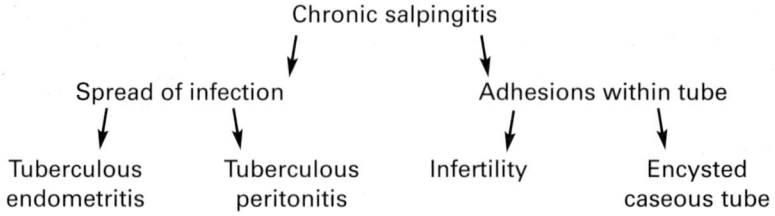

Tumours of the fallopian tube

Benign tumours such as fibroma and myoma occasionally occur. Small cysts of congenital origin are common around the fimbrial ends of the tubes.

Carcinoma, usually a papillary adenocarcinoma, is extremely rare. There may be a profuse watery secretion which appears as a vaginal discharge.

DISEASES OF OVARIES

Oophoritis

Inflammation of the ovaries is always secondary to disease of the fallopian tubes or peritoneum. In the case of the tube, the inflamed fimbrial end becomes adherent to the ovary and direct spread of infection occurs. Tubo-ovarian inflammation is also associated with the presence of an intra-uterine contraceptive device (see p. 504). Important local complications may follow.

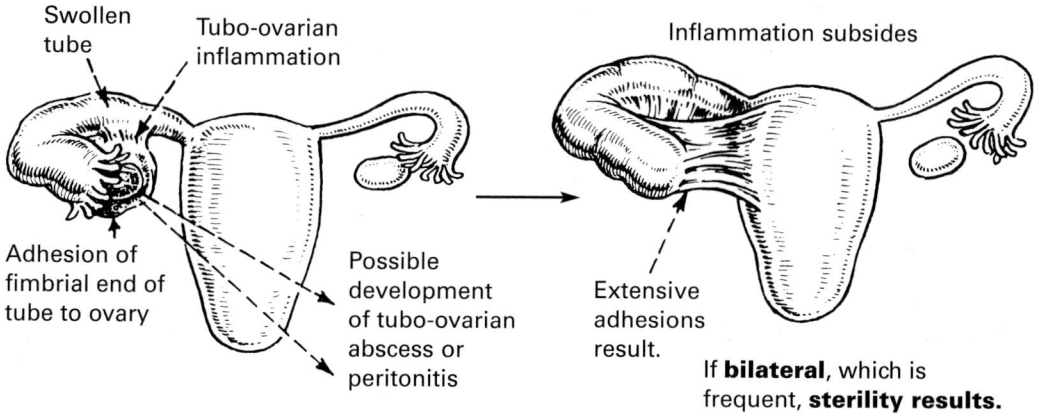

The ovary may be similarly involved in tuberculous salpingitis, and caseating lesions can occur.

Ovarian changes of functional origin

The control mechanisms of ovarian function frequently develop faults resulting in abnormalities of structure:

Follicular cysts

These may be single or multiple. The maximum diameter of a normal Graafian follicle is 1.5–2 cm. Single follicular cysts may be several centimetres in diameter. Amenorrhoea is common in such instances. Multiple follicular cysts, usually small, are associated with endometrial hyperplasia.

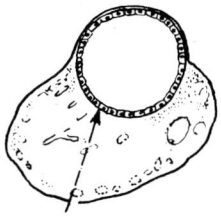

Theca lutein cysts

These are cysts from which the granulosa cells have disappeared, leaving cysts surrounded by luteinised thecal tissue. Bilateral, multiple small cysts of this nature occur in polycystic ovarian disease and are associated with obesity, hirsutism and oligomenorrhoea (Stein-Leventhal syndrome).

DISEASES OF OVARIES

A multiplicity of types of ovarian tumours exists. Various classifications have been suggested; none is completely satisfactory. The following is a simple working classification:

1. Epithelial tumours (derived from surface epithelium).
2. Sex cord/stromal tumours.
3. Germ cell tumours.
4. Secondary (metastatic) tumours.

COMMON EPITHELIAL TUMOURS

These comprise 60% of all ovarian tumours and 90% of malignant tumours and are found in adult life, very rarely in children.

Histogenesis: The ovarian surface epithelium and the various mature Müllerian structures have a common origin in EMBRYONAL COELOMIC epithelium. The ovarian surface epithelial stem cells retain the ability to differentiate along different pathways: this explains the histological appearance of these tumours.

EMBRYONAL COELOMIC EPITHELIUM → MATURE OVARIAN SURFACE EPITHELIUM

	Mature Müllerian tissues	*analogous TUMOURS*
e.g.	1. Tubal epithelium →	SEROUS
	2. Endocervical epithelium →	MUCINOUS
	3. Endometrial epithelium →	ENDOMETRIOID
	4. Transitional epithelium →	BRENNER

The histological features relate to a spectrum of behaviour:

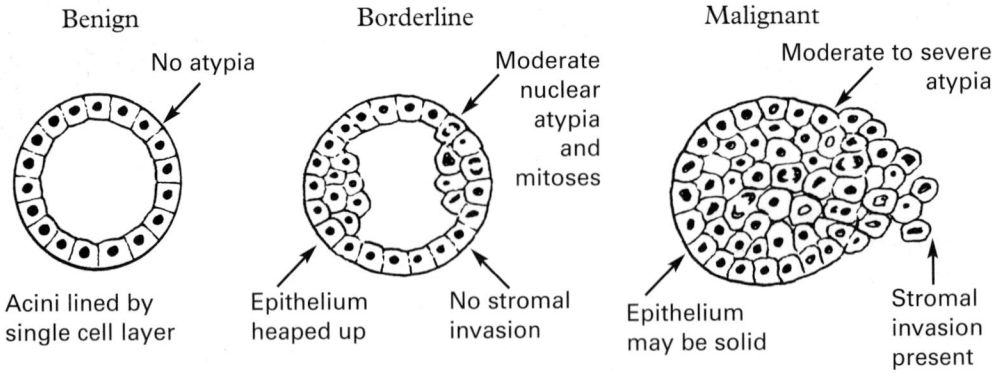

Prognosis:	Excellent (100%)	Usually good (90% at 5 years)	Poor (10–20% at 5 years)

COMMON EPITHELIAL OVARIAN TUMOURS

Serous cystadenoma

Twenty-five per cent of all ovarian tumours are of this variety. In a third of cases they are bilateral, but they almost never reach the large size of the mucinous growths.

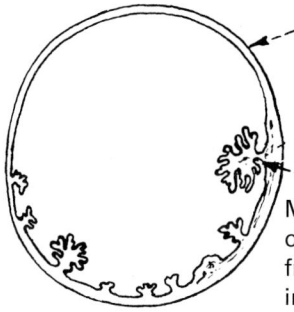

Smooth surface

(Unilocular or multilocular)

Intracystic papilla. May be few and sessile or pedunculated with fronds often complex in structure

Some tumours have small loculi with papillary formations making them appear solid.

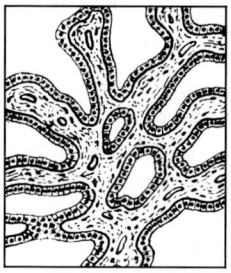

Epithelium cuboidal with central nuclei. Fluid is watery.

Psammoma bodies with concentric layers of calcification are commonly seen.

Complications

1. Torsion may occur
2. Malignant transformation is common and 30% of malignant tumours are bilateral.

Mucinous cystadenoma

This accounts for 20% of all ovarian tumours. It can reach a very large size and is typically multilocular. 25% are bilateral.

Slightly nodular due to loculi

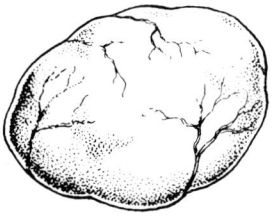

Smooth peritoneal covering

The cut surface shows the multilocular mosaic pattern

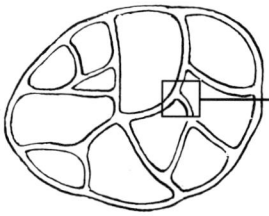

The tumour is usually unilateral

Mucin secretion

Nuclei basal

Tall columnar epithelium (septa from the capsule support cyst)

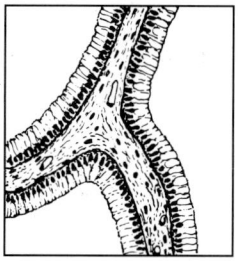

Complications

1. **Torsion of the pedicle.** This is not uncommon with a large ovarian tumour of any type.
2. **Rupture.** This may lead to seeding of the mucin-secreting epithelium on the peritoneum. It continues to secrete, leading to the condition 'pseudomyxoma peritonei', with a peritoneal cavity filled with mucin.

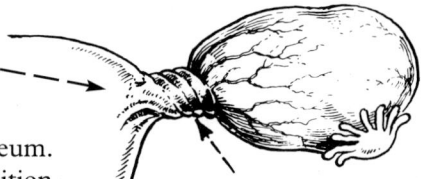

Congestion, often infarction due to interruption of blood flow

3. **Malignant transformation** including borderline tumours. Cells are large, with large irregular nuclei. Mitoses are common; slight secretion present (see over).

Brenner tumours

These are essentially benign and show islands of transitional epithelium in a fibrous stroma.

CARCINOMA OF OVARY

Mucinous cystadenocarcinoma

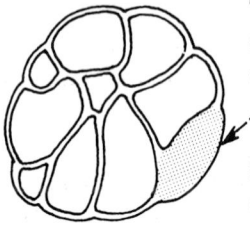

This accounts for 20% of all cases of primary carcinoma of the ovary. It almost always arises as a malignant transformation of a benign cystadenoma.

Areas of solid growth appear in the cyst wall.

Frequently in the malignant areas, florid papillary structures are formed and where the change is widespread it may be difficult to differentiate it from the malignant form of papillary cystadenoma.

Papillary (serous) cystadenocarcinoma

This is the commonest malignant tumour of the ovary — responsible for 40% of the total. Usually it takes the form of exuberant papillomatous growths extending over the surface and obliterating the ovarian structure. It is often bilateral.

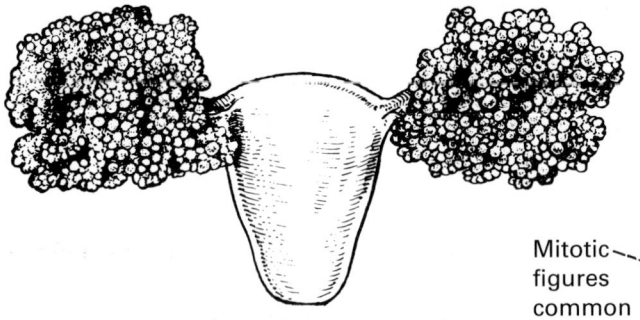

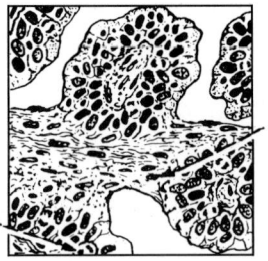

Endometrioid carcinoma

In a considerable number of cases, ovarian carcinoma has a solid or semi-solid appearance and as such starts off as a growth smaller than either of the cystic tumours.

Microscopically, they are frequently anaplastic, but sometimes they show differentiation towards an endometrial pattern and are termed 'endometrioid'. There is no 'benign' equivalent, but some cases arise in endometriosis.

Progress in ovarian carcinoma

Spread of ovarian cancer in the early stages is by direct extension to the pelvic peritoneum. The papillary serous cancer seeds widely in the peritoneal cavity and only later are lymphatics invaded and metastases appear.

The mucinous variety rarely spreads by lymphatics.

The overall 5-year survival rate for ovarian cancer is only 30% and death often takes place within 2–3 years due to cachexia and interference with intestinal and renal function.

Aetiology

Most cases are sporadic. Nulliparous women with a late menopause have an increased risk. There is a family tendency — especially in women with mutation of the BRCA-1 gene.

Tumour marker

CA125 is a glycoprotein: serum levels are raised in about 50% of patients with ovarian carcinoma.

TUMOURS OF OVARIES – MISCELLANEOUS

SEX CORD and STROMAL TUMOURS

These may be divided into two broad groups:

1. Those tending to produce excess oestrogen: granulosa cell tumours and thecomas.
2. Those producing androgens and virilisation: Sertoli-Leydig cell tumours, hilus cell tumours and lipid cell tumours.

Granulosa cell tumour

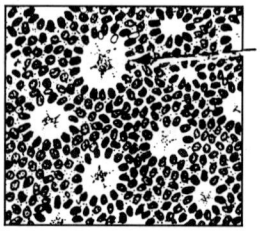

Rosettes of cells with nuclei radially arranged are common (Call-Exner bodies)

This is composed of cells resembling the granulosa cells lining Graafian follicles. They vary in size from a few mm to large cystic structures. Commonly, the smaller varieties are found deep in the ovarian substance.

This tumour may be found at any age: 5% occur in children; 50% in the child-bearing years; 40% postmenopausally.

All granulosa cell tumours are potentially malignant — they may recur, sometimes many years after removal.

Measurement of serum **inhibin** (a glycoprotein produced by granulosa cells) is useful in following progress.

Thecoma

This is a growth consisting of spindle cells. They are found mainly during the 3rd, 4th and 5th decades of life. They are benign and rarely recur.

Function of these tumours varies widely. Oestrogenic manifestations consist of:

1. Precocious puberty in children.
2. Hyperplasia of endometrium. This may be atypical and carcinoma is said to develop occasionally.
3. Enlargement of breasts.

Fibromas are histologically similar but do not produce hormones. They may be associated with pleural effusion (Meig's syndrome).

Sertoli-Leydig cell tumours (androblastoma, arrhenoblastoma)

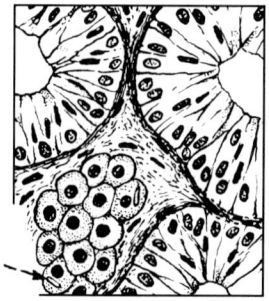

Tubules lined by SERTOLI cells, sometimes pyramidal with clear cytoplasm.

LEYDIG cells occasionally with Reinke crystalloids in their cytoplasm

This typifies the virilising tumour group. It is a rare tumour. The degree of virilisation varies. Usually a small yellow tumour within the ovarian substance, it has a characteristic microscopic structure.

Some of these tumours are malignant and consist of poorly differentiated spindle cells with occasional tubule formations.

The androgens, if secreted, result in:

1. Atrophy of breasts and external genitalia
2. Deepening of voice, temporal recession of hair
3. Growth of facial and body hair
4. Enlargement of clitoris.

BENIGN BREAST TUMOURS AND IN SITU CARCINOMA

Duct papilloma

This tumour may develop in any part of the duct system of the breast, but is most common in the lacteal sinuses at the nipple. Two forms exist:

1. **Solitary papilloma.** These are almost always near the nipple.

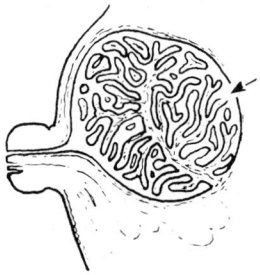

Complex branching pedunculated tumour filling lacteal sinus

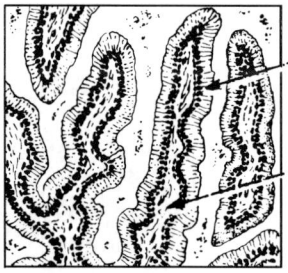

Columnar epithelium with underlying myoepithelium

Connective tissue core

Prominent myoepithelium gives a double layer of cells covering the fronds.

2. Multiple papillomata

These may be distributed throughout the duct system. In this form, multicentric carcinoma occasionally develops.

In both forms, there may be discharge from the nipple which may be haemorrhagic. Examination of the discharge will reveal the tumour epithelial cells which are benign. Other benign breast tumours are rare.

Intra-duct carcinoma

This is a carcinoma in situ of the ducts. It may be visible as greyish-white material filling the dilated ducts, and central necrotic debris may be squeezed out of the ducts (comedocarcinoma).

Solid or cribriform cylinders of cells show the usual features of malignancy — variation in size and shape of both cell and nucleus, relatively greater size of nuclei, mitotic figures, etc. The condition has to be differentiated from atypical ductal hyperplasia.

Solid proliferation of pleomorphic cancer cells

Necrotic debris

No myoepithelium

Thinning of duct wall

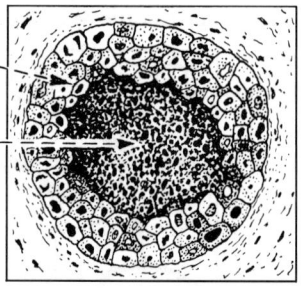

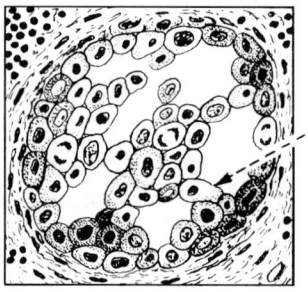

Cribriform pattern with rigid 'Roman bridges'

This form has a higher risk of invasive malignancy.

Lobular carcinoma in situ. This lesion is usually multifocal and bilateral. The breast acini of affected lobules are distended by fairly uniform carcinoma cells which grow into the duct system or break through basement membrane to become infiltrative carcinoma, either of lobular or ductal type.

CARCINOMA OF THE BREAST

This is the commonest form of malignancy in the female. It may be found in any part of the breast but most frequently it is in the upper outer quadrant.

INFILTRATING DUCTAL CARCINOMA

This, the commonest form, presents as a firm to hard lump. The following illustrations show a large carcinoma with significant local spread. It is emphasised that modern screening methods aim to detect the disease at a much earlier stage.

Gross appearance

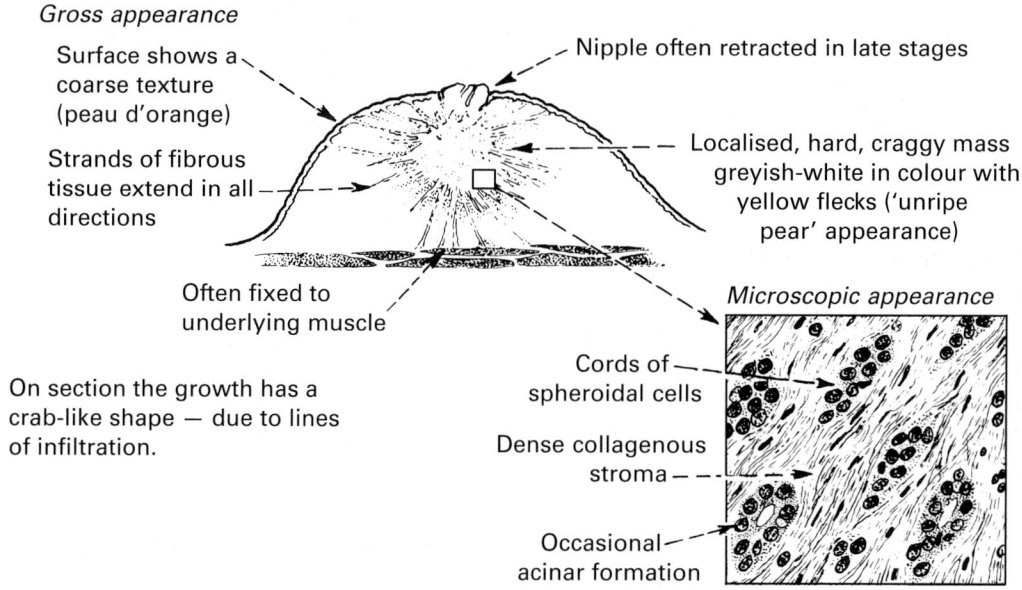

On section the growth has a crab-like shape — due to lines of infiltration.

INFILTRATING LOBULAR CARCINOMA

Ten per cent of breast cancers are of this type. Based on distribution of the 'in situ' precursor, this tumour may be multicentric within the breast and there is a 30% chance of a similar tumour arising in the contralateral breast. Microscopically the tumour infiltrates the tissues as single files of malignant cells.

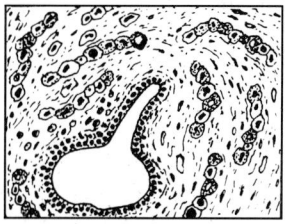

Infiltrating lobular carcinoma

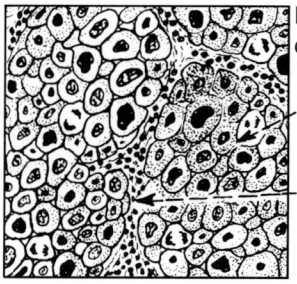

More rare forms of breast cancer are TUBULAR CARCINOMA — showing well differentiated cells often with intra-tubular calcification: MEDULLARY CARCINOMA — a highly cellular tumour with a florid lymphocytic infiltrate, and MUCOID CARCINOMA where the malignant cells lie in pools of mucin.

CARCINOMA OF THE BREAST

Local Spread: Breast cancers are usually slow growing: tumour size is proportional to duration. In late stages local infiltration causes skin ulceration and there may be direct penetration of the chest wall. In addition, intra-epithelial spread occurs. The classical example is **PAGET'S DISEASE OF THE NIPPLE** — which may complicate intra-duct carcinoma. (Occasionally an infiltrating component is absent.)

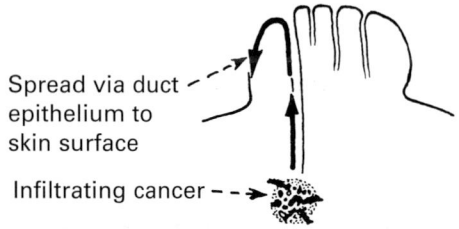

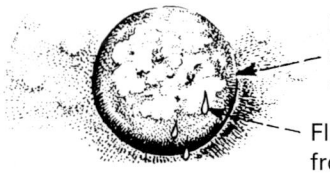

Microscopic examination reveals:

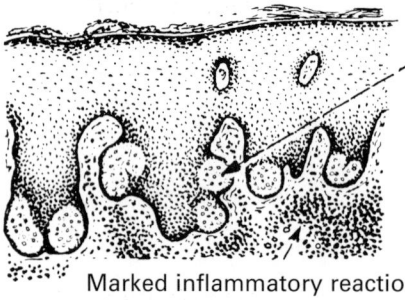

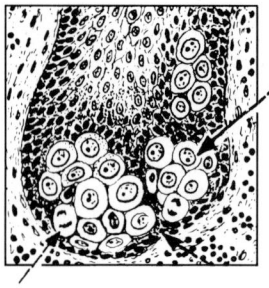

Metastatic Spread: This is by lymphatic and blood streams.

Early
(When the tumour is still small)

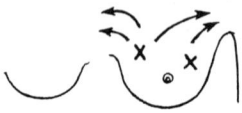

via LYMPHATICS

1. To axillary nodes from all sites of breast.
2. Through internal mammary lymphatics to thorax (esp. in cancers sited medially).

via BLOOD STREAM

? to bone marrow where cells can lie dormant for long periods.

Late

Local spread via skin lymphatics causing:

(a) Widespread lesion — skin becomes stiff and board-like: 'cancer-en-cuirasse'.

(b) Blockage of dermal lymphatics: oedema of skin except at anchorage points, giving a fine mamillated appearance: 'peau d'orange' (see p. 245).

Secondaries appear in many viscera, particularly liver, lung and BONE (spinal column).

CARCINOMA OF THE BREAST

Prognosis
Crude mortality rates are 40% at 5 years: 60% at 10 years and 75% at 25 years.
Important factors which influence these crude rates are: 1. Number of involved lymph nodes. 2. Size —lesions under 1 cm rarely metastasise. 3. Grade (graded 1,2,3). 4. Oestrogen receptor status — positive tumours have an improved response to anti-oestrogens e.g. tamoxifen.

Aetiology
Breast cancer is uncommon below the age of 30 years. The risk increases with age, the maximal incidence being in the later decades.
The important risk factors are:

1. ***Genetic:***
   There is a strong familial association. Mutation of genes, BRCA1 on chromosome 17 and BRCA2 on chromosome 11, are responsible for many cases of breast cancer in young women with a positive family history. Deletion of tumour suppressor genes has been identified (mutation of suppressor gene p53 is common) — Li Fraumeni syndrome.

2. ***Sex hormone associations:***
   (a) Commoner in nulliparous women.
   (b) Early menarche and late menopause increase risk — ? prolonged cyclical exposure to sex hormones.
   (c) Breast feeding reduces risk.

Screening for Breast cancer
The aim of screening is to detect either pre-malignant conditions or cancer at an early stage and is very important where there is a family history of cancer. Mammography is capable of detecting intra-duct carcinoma and pre-cancerous lesions. Focal calcification is an important indicator but is not diagnostic of malignancy because it also occurs in benign lesions. Whatever method of screening is used the diagnosis must be established on morphological evidence using fine needle aspiration, needle biopsy and, sometimes, open biopsy.

Other rare tumours of the breast include PHYLLODES TUMOUR — large and usually benign, affecting elderly women: occasionally sarcoma of the stroma is present. Soft tissue sarcomas and primary lymphoma are exceedingly rare.

THE MALE BREAST
The breast is seldom the seat of disease in males. Abnormal enlargement — gynaecomastia — may occur in a temporary form at puberty or as a permanent feature in intersex states, e.g. Klinefelter's syndrome (XXY). Oestrogen metabolic upsets (e.g. in liver disease) or excess intake (e.g. treatment of prostatic cancer) are other causes. All tumours are rare.

DISEASES OF MALE GENITALIA

The male genital tract consists of a number of structures connected by ducts opening into one another. These interconnections are important in the spread of infection.

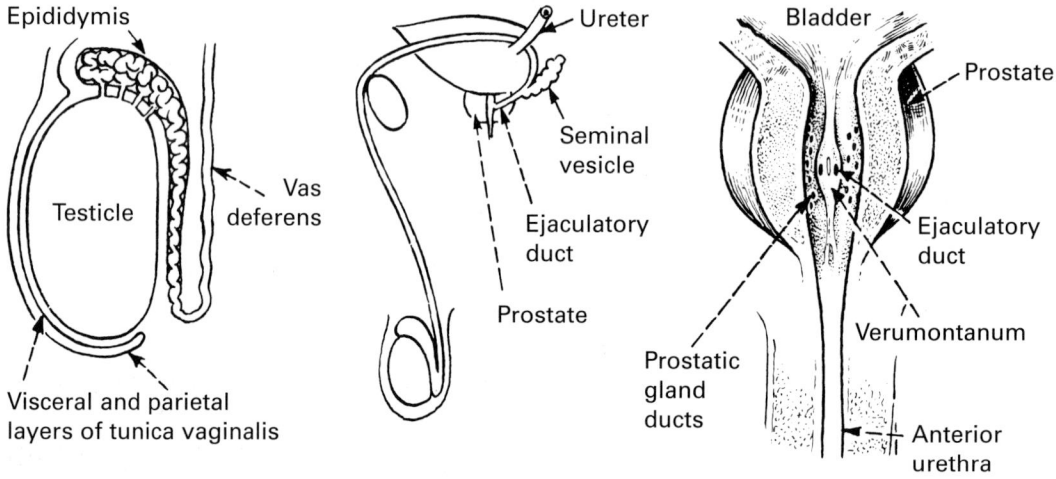

Inflammation of the genital tract may start in the posterior urethra and spread to other structures.

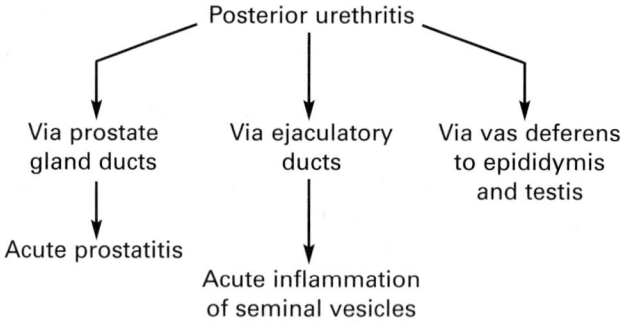

The condition in these instances is secondary to urinary infection associated with urethral obstruction caused by an enlarged prostate or urethral stricture. This is indicated by the fact that in 80% of cases of prostatitis, the infecting bacterium is *E.coli*. In the remaining 20%, various organisms may be isolated — staphylococci, streptococci, pseudomonas and proteus. Frequent catheterisation is an aetiological factor.

Anterior urethritis is almost always a sexually transmitted disease. Gonococci, trichomonas, mycoplasma and chlamydia are the usual agents. In the case of gonorrhoea, infection may spread back to the posterior urethra and thence to other structures.

DISEASES OF MALE GENITALIA

GONORRHOEA

This has been relatively uncommon in Western countries in recent years but is now becoming somewhat more prevalent due to the emergence of drug resistant strains of *Neisseria gonorrhoeae*.

Gonorrhoeal infection is important because of the complications which may arise:

1. Chronic urethritis ⟶ urethral stricture
2. Prostatitis, acute and chronic
3. Occasionally epididymitis and orchitis
4. Blood spread leading to arthritis, endocarditis, etc
5. Infection of sexual partner ⟶ endometritis and sterility
   ⟶ gonorrhoeal ophthalmitis of newborn.

PROSTATITIS

The prostate consists of five ill-defined lobes:

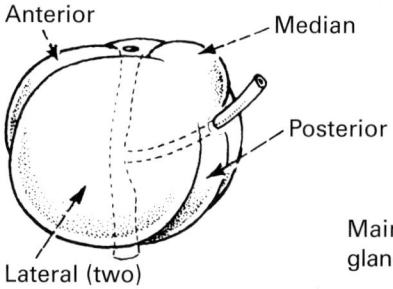

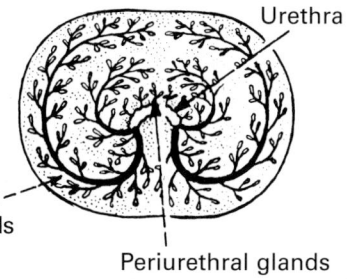

Its internal structure is a series of branching glands in a fibromuscular stroma.

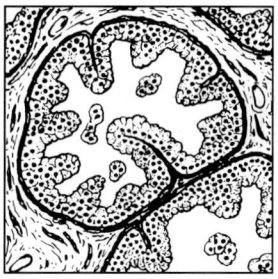

Inflammation of the prostate always involves the posterior urethra and seminal vesicles. The usual congestion, exudation and neutrophil infiltration take place and may proceed to abscess formation. These abscesses are usually small, but if they coalesce and extend they may rupture in several directions. *E. coli* is most commonly responsible.

CHRONIC PROSTATITIS may follow an acute episode but it is often of insidious onset. Subsequent fibrosis may cause urethral obstruction. *Neisseria gonorrhoeae* or Chlamydia may be responsible.

Abscesses may also form in the seminal vesicles.

DISEASES OF MALE GENITALIA

EPIDIDYMITIS AND ORCHITIS

Acute inflammations due to bacteria are less common in these organs, but spread via the vas deferens does occasionally take place and may result in destructive suppuration.

In 20% of adult cases of mumps, the epididymis and testis become acutely inflamed. The condition is usually unilateral, but if bilateral there is a distinct danger of subsequent infertility.

Acute inflammation of the testis may be confused with **torsion.** Torsion generally occurs within the tunica vaginalis and leads to obstruction of the testicular vessels. Infarction results, with destruction of the tissue. Recurrent minor degrees of torsion can cause atrophy. Since the torsion may be bilateral, prophylactic surgery may reduce the risk of a second event.

Chronic inflammations are important, although rare, in this region.

Chronic granulomatous orchitis

This is a condition of unknown origin. The testis is infiltrated by macrophages, plasma cells and lymphocytes. Atrophy of the germinal epithelium occurs and the testis becomes fibrotic.

TUBERCULOSIS

In this disease, the epididymis is usually the first part of the genital tract to be affected.

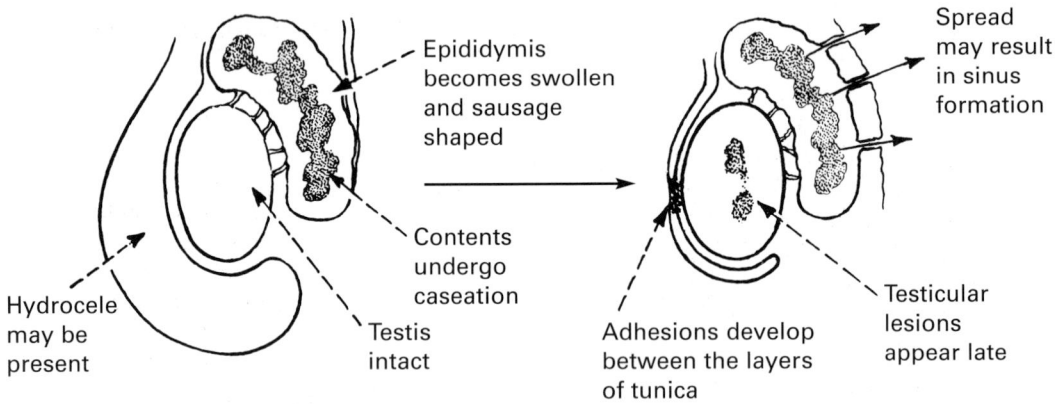

Infection is almost always haematogenous from some other focus in the body. Subsequently the process may spread along the vas deferens to the seminal vesicles, prostate and bladder. In rare cases the infection is in the opposite direction — kidney → bladder → prostate → vas → epididymis.

DISEASES OF MALE GENITALIA

SYPHILIS

Apart from the primary sore which appears on the penis, the only other genital site of syphilitic lesions is the testis. These are common in the tertiary stage, their incidence being only second to those in the aorta at this phase. Two types of lesion are found:

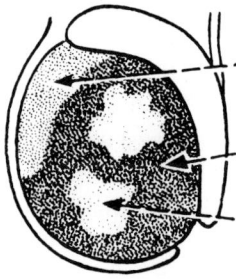

1. **Gumma**
2. **Granulomatous lesion** leading to scar formation with destruction of seminiferous tubules.

The primary lesion of lymphogranuloma venereum (see p. 514) appears on the penis and, as in the female, it spreads and causes chronic suppuration in the inguinal lymph nodes. But late complications are less drastic in their effects.

BENIGN PROSTATIC HYPERPLASIA

Different forms may be seen. The central area of the gland is most affected: the changes present as a firm nodularity and may affect all prostatic lobes.

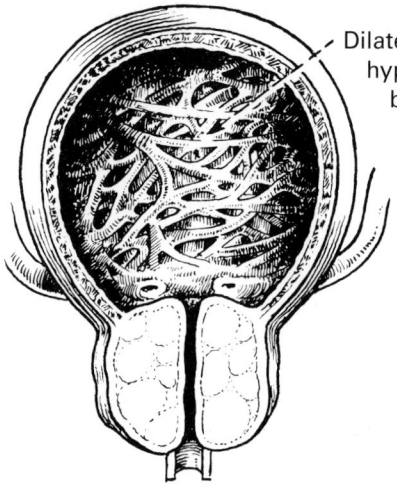

Nodularity of lateral lobes with compression of urthera.

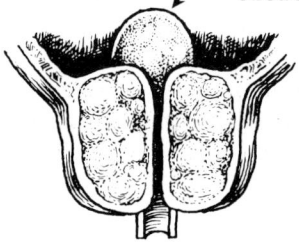

DISEASES OF MALE GENITALIA

Benign prostatic hyperplasia (continued)

In practice, the appearances are very variable and can include two or more of the forms illustrated on the previous page.
There is a hyperplasia of both the glandular tissue and fibromuscular stroma, the relative proportions varying greatly. Section of the prostate reveals:

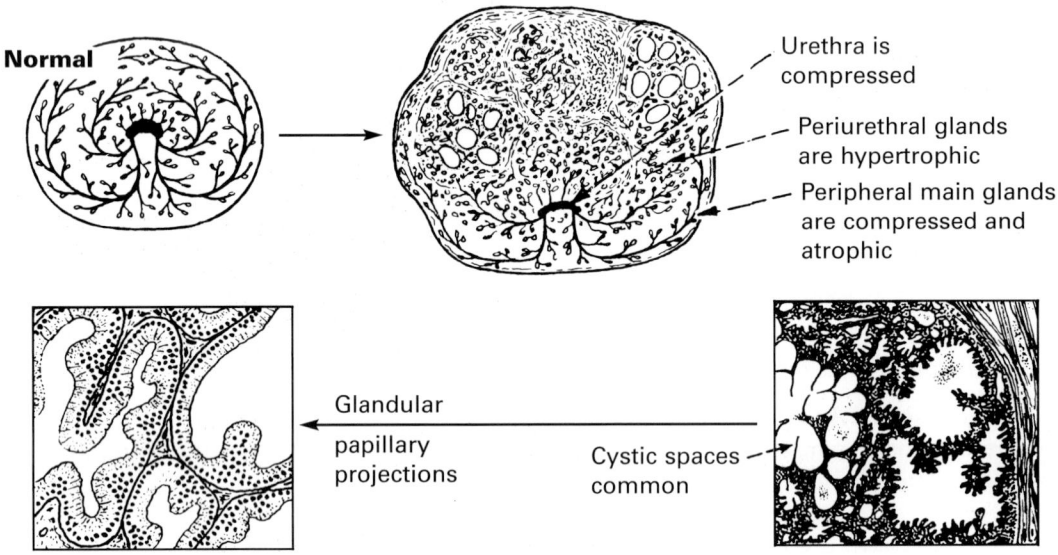

The atrophic compressed peripheral tissue forms a false capsule from which the hypertrophied mass can be shelled out.

Aetiology

This is obscure. It is a disease of the elderly and there is often asymptomatic prostatic enlargement in old age. The periurethral glands are said to predominate at this period and hyperplasia may be an exaggeration of this process. It has also been claimed that the central glands are sensitive to oestrogen and hence the hyperplasia may be related to the normal drop in androgens in old age, leaving the action of oestrogen, normally present, unopposed. On the other hand, it has been noted that prostatic enlargement is never seen after castration and does not occur in patients suffering from hepatic cirrhosis (oestrogens are not inactivated).

Complications

1. Chronic retention of urine.
2. Attacks of acute retention are common, usually due to oedema and congestion of the prostatic urethra.
3. Cystitis and pyelonephritis.
4. Hydronephrosis.
5. Bladder stone.
6. Bladder diverticulum.

DISEASES OF MALE GENITALIA

CARCINOMA OF THE PROSTATE

This is a common cancer and is the fifth most common cause of male death.

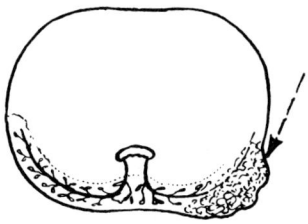

It takes origin from the subcapsular region, i.e. where the main glands are found. Often the prostate also shows benign hyperplasia, but this is coincidental and not causally related. It is almost always an adenocarcinoma.

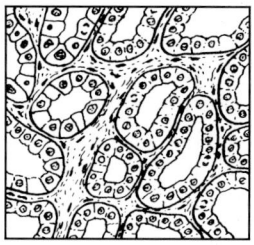

Closely set small irregular acini lined by a single layer of epithelium

Histological grading:

The GLEASON system (Grades 2 through 10) indicates the degree of differentiation from (2) very well differentiated to (10) aggressive anaplastic tumours.

Spread

1. Direct spread occurs throughout the prostate and outwards to the pelviprostatic tissue.
2. Lymphatic spread is the main mode of extension. There is a rich lymphatic plexus and the perineural lymphatics are particularly affected. The pelvic nodes are invaded and subsequently the abdominal chain.
3. Bone metastases tend to be common, especially in the vertebrae. This is due to retrograde spread from the prostatic venous plexus to the vertebral veins. These secondaries are often characterised by the formation of new dense bone around them (osteosclerosis).

Biochemical tests

1. Prostatic specific antigen (PSA) measured in the blood using an immuno-histochemical technique is a useful diagnostic marker.
2. These tumours produce prostatic acid phosphatase and, when metastases are present, an increased level may be found in the blood. When bones are invaded, blood alkaline phosphatase may also rise due to osteoblastic activity.

Latent carcinoma

Small subcapsular foci with the histological features of very well differentiated carcinoma may be found in a prostate showing benign hyperplasia. They are discovered incidentally at autopsy in cases dying from causes unconnected with prostate disease. The incidence increases with age and reaches 90% at age 80. Although invasion of local peri-neural spaces may be seen there is never any metastatic growth.

Prostatic intraepithelial neoplasia (PIN), analogous to CIN (p. 511), has been recognised as a pre-invasive stage of the disease.

DISEASES OF MALE GENITALIA

TUMOURS of the PENIS

Papillomatous proliferations (condylomata acuminata), sometimes sessile but often florid, usually arise in the coronal sulcus or glans. They are due to sexually transmitted infection by Human Papilloma Virus (HPV) Types 6 and 11, and are analogous to similar lesions in the female genitalia

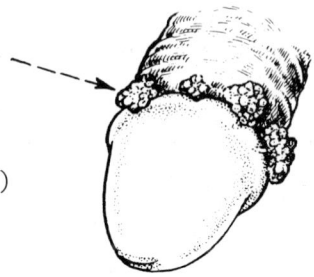

Peyronie's disease is a cellular fibromatosis related to Dupuytren's contracture.

Precancerous lesions

So-called leukoplakia and Bowen's disease are occasionally found on the penis. Another condition involving epithelial hyperplasia is Queyrat's erythroplasia. The histological appearances vary in these lesions, but all show epithelial dysplasia and usually amount to carcinoma-in-situ.

Carcinoma of the Penis

Accounts for less than 2% of all male malignancy. The site of growth is usually in the preputial area, often in the coronal sulcus, but it extends to involve the glans penis. Two forms of growth occur:

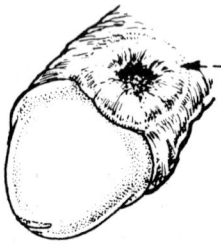

Ulcer with sloughing base and hard rolled edges; usually it is adherent to the underlying tissues

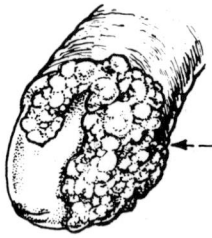

Soft cauliflower growth

The growth spreads by the lymphatics to the regional nodes. Distant metastases occur late. The prognosis is reasonably good, the 5-year survival rate being greater than 50%.

Aetiology

1. Early circumcision virtually confers immunity against carcinoma; the risk is greatly increased in the presence of poor penile hygiene.
2. Human Papilloma Virus (HPV) Types 16 and 18 are the initiating carcinogens. Inspissated smegma trapped behind the foreskin may be an important promoter (cofactor).

CANCER of the SCROTUM

This is a lesion which is rarely seen nowadays. Previously it was an occupational disease due to exposure to carcinogenic agents, e.g. soot, industrial oils, arsenic, etc.

DISEASES OF MALE GENITALIA

GERM CELL TUMOURS of the TESTIS

These tumours are by no means uncommon and the incidence is rising steeply in Western countries. They are the commonest form of malignancy in young men. Tumours are more common in cases of undescended testicles.

The 2 main tumour types are SEMINOMA and TERATOMA.

Seminoma This corresponds to the dysgerminoma in the female. It is rare before puberty and has its peak incidence in adults in their 30's. It accounts for 50% of all testicular tumours.

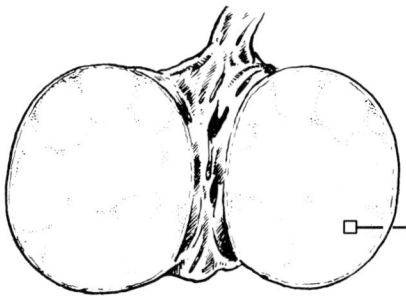

The testis is uniformly enlarged; the surface is smooth. On section it has a faint lobular appearance and is often described as the 'potato' tumour because of its white solid appearance.

Spread is principally via the lymphatics along the spermatic cord.

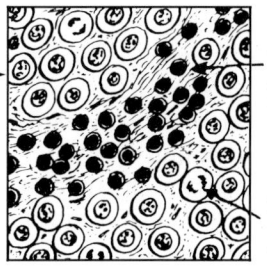

Fine stroma infiltrated by lymphocytes

Large germ cells sometimes in mitosis

The growth is extremely radiosensitive and chemosensitive. Orchidectomy and adjuvant therapy give a >95% cure rate. In older men 'spermatocytic seminoma' is a rare variant but has an excellent prognosis.

Malignant teratoma (non-seminomatous germ cell tumour)

This type represents 35% of malignant testicular growths. It takes origin from totipotent germ cells capable of differentiating into derivatives of ectoderm, endoderm and mesoderm. It is customary to classify them according to the degree and type of differentiation exhibited. The lack of differentiation indicates the malignancy of the tumour.

The tumours form a spectrum of well differentiated to anaplastic highly malignant growths and are classified in various ways. The following is often used:

MALIGNANT TERATOMA (MT)

- SOMATIC DIFFERENTIATION
  - MTD — D=well differentiated; WHO equivalent =mature teratoma
  - MTI — I=intermed.diff.; WHO=immature teratoma or teratocarcinoma
- EXTRA-EMBRYONIC DIFFERENTIATION
  - Yolk sac
  - MTT — Choriocarcinoma; T=trophoblast
- NO DIFFERENTIATION
  - MTU — U=undifferentiated; WHO=embryonal carcinoma

→ INCREASING MALIGNANCY →

DISEASES OF MALE GENITALIA

Malignant Teratoma (continued)
These tumours, unlike seminoma, are usually irregular in shape and show focal haemorrhage and necrosis: in the better differentiated tumours small cysts are common.

1. **MTD** — In this tumour organoid differentiation is easily recognisable (e.g. formation of intestinal glands, squamous epithelium, cartilage etc.): it is unlike its ovarian counter-part in important respects, however (a) it is very rare and (b) although apparently histologically benign, metastases may occur.
2. **MTI** — In addition to mature organised tissue this tumour contains varying amounts of clearly malignant tissue (e.g. adenocarcinoma)

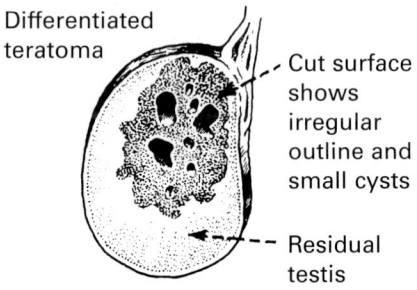

3. **MTU** — These tumours are almost completely anaplastic showing only focal areas of poor attempts at differentiation.
4. **Yolk sac and Trophoblastic elements** occur commonly in malignant teratomas: pure forms are rare. α-fetoprotein (from yolk sac elements) and chorionic gonadotrophins (from trophoblastic elements) are used in diagnosis and monitoring progress.
5. **Combined Germ-Cell Tumours** — Between 10 and 15% of germ-cell tumours consist of a mixture of seminomatous and teratomatous elements.

Spread
Lymphatic spread to paraortic lymph nodes is the usual mode of spread: vascular invasion with lung metastases also occurs.

Prognosis
Modern therapy has greatly improved the overall prognosis.

Intratubular germ cell neoplasia
There is an 'in situ' form of germ cell tumour, often found in association with the malignant tumours described above and thought to represent a precursor form.

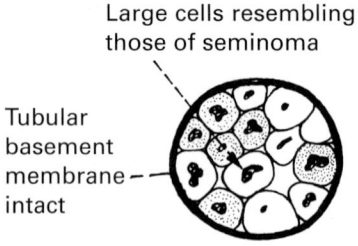

MISCELLANEOUS TUMOURS
The following tumours are rare: Sertoli tumours,
Leydig cell tumours,
Lymphoma.
It should be remembered that leukaemia often involves the testes (p.455).

INFERTILITY

There are numerous causes which affect females or males. The causes are classified as follows:

1. **Pregonadal** — usually endocrine disorders of pituitary or adrenal origin.

Anterior pituitary

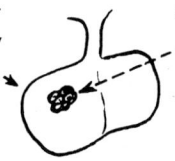

Small pituitary adenoma producing **Prolactin**

Adrenal cortical adenoma or genetic abnormality —

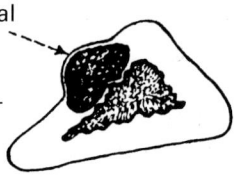

— excess androgen secretion causes virilisation in females.

2. **Gonadal** — failure of production of gametes.

	Male	Female
(i) *Chromosomal defects*	**Klinefelter's syndrome** XXY	**Turner's syndrome** XO
(ii) *Germ cell aplasia*	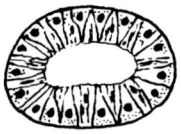 Tubules lined only by Sertoli cells: — spermatocyte arrest, — often maldescent.	Gonadal dysgenesis — ovaries represented by small slender functionless tissue — **'Streak gonads'** Polycystic ovary syndrome (Stein Leventhal syndrome) 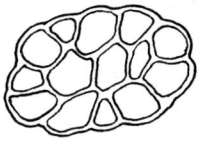 Ovarian tissue replaced by multiple cysts.

(iii) *Iatrogenic causes:* **Irradiation, chemotherapy,** hormones e.g. the 'pill' and oestrogens in treatment of prostatic carcinoma.

3. **Postgonadal** — obstruction of passage of gametes.

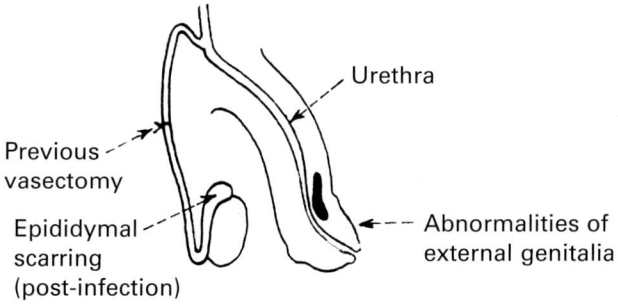

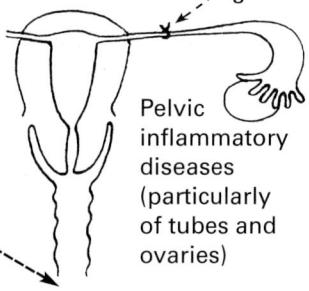

Note: In some cases of infertility no cause can be detected.

CHAPTER 13

NERVOUS SYSTEM

Nervous System — Anatomy and Physiology 544, 545
Neuronal Damage 546
Glial Reactions 547
Demyelination 548
Increased Intracranial Pressure 549, 550
Cerebral Oedema 551
Increased Intracranial Pressure 552
Circulatory Disturbances 553
Cerebral Infarction 554, 555
Brain Damage due to Cardiac Arrest 555
Cerebral Infarction 556
Cerebral Haemorrhage 557
Subarachnoid Haemorrhage 558
Hypertension 559
Head Injury 560–563
Ageing and Dementia 564
Alzheimer's Disease 565
Dementia 566
Infections 567
Bacterial Infection 568, 569
Tuberculous Meningitis 570
Virus Infections 571–575
Prion Diseases 576
Miscellaneous Infections and Infestations 577, 578
Demyelinating Diseases 579, 580
Parkinson's Disease 581
Miscellaneous Disorders 582, 583
Diseases of Spinal Cord 584, 585
Disorders of Motor Pathways 586
Motor Neurone Disease 587
Mixed Motor and Sensory Disorders 588
The Peripheral Nerves 589
The Neuropathies 590, 591
Hydrocephalus 592–594
Developmental Abnormalities 595
Tumours of the Nervous System 596
Secondary Brain Tumours 597
Primary Brain Tumours 598
Tumours of the Nervous System 599–601
Tumours of Peripheral Nerves 601, 602
Epilepsy 603
Cerebrospinal Fluid 604

NERVOUS SYSTEM – ANATOMY AND PHYSIOLOGY

Considerations of anatomy and physiology have important applications to diseases of the central nervous system (CNS), particularly their effects and spread.
The anatomy of the various coverings is important.

The skull and vertebrae form a rigid compartment protecting the delicate CNS tissues.

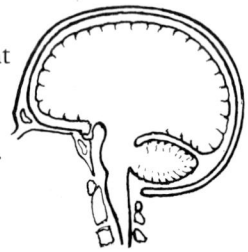

This rigidity has serious disadvantages when pressure inside the skull increases, e.g. an expanding lesion soon takes up the small reserves of space available and the delicate brain tissues are progressively compressed, with very serious results.

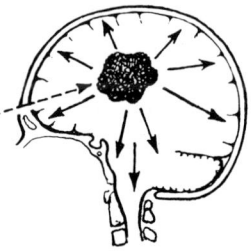

Meninges and cerebrospinal fluid (CSF)

The CSF circulating freely in the subarachnoid space over the whole CNS surface and in the ventricular system acts as a protective water bath.

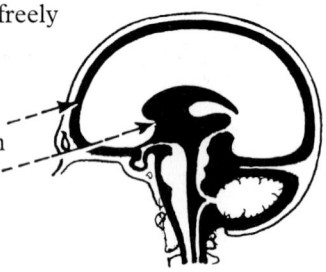

Diseases (particularly infections) at this site are usually *widespread* over the whole brain and cord surfaces, e.g. meningitis. Impediment to the flow of CSF causes serious effects — hydrocephalus.

The detailed arrangement of the meninges is important.
The thick **dura**, closely applied to the skull, acts as the periosteum — its rigid reflections (falx cerebri and tentorium cerebelli) complicate the effects of increased intracranial pressure.

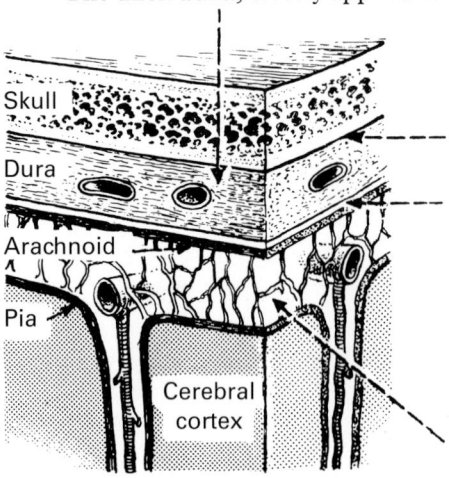

Extradural lesions tend to be localised; they have to strip the dura from the bone.
Subdural lesions remain local but can spread more widely since the arachnoid and dura are loosely attached.
The **arachnoid**, a delicate membrane, is loosely attached to the dura and sends trabeculae across the subarachnoid space which contains the cerebral blood vessels and the CSF.
Disease in the **subarachnoid** space can spread widely over the whole surface of the brain and spinal cord but is prevented from penetrating into the brain tissue by the **pia**.

NERVOUS SYSTEM – ANATOMY AND PHYSIOLOGY

The **pia** is invaginated into the brain substance along with the small penetrating vessels.

The dura, arachnoid and pia act as barriers which selectively separate the CSF and the blood from the CNS tissues.

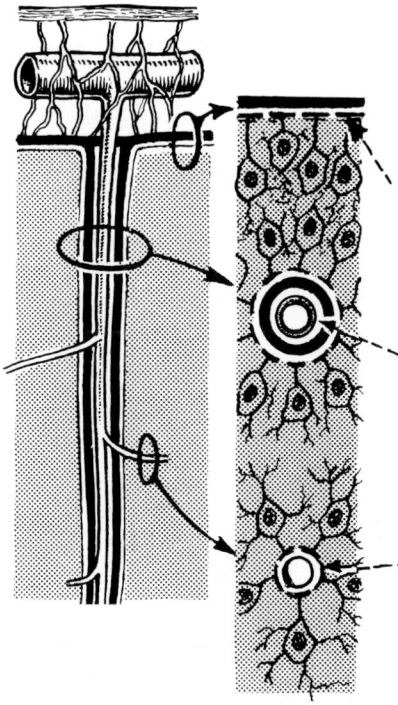

The pia's barrier function is reinforced by the membrane formed by the foot processes of astrocytes:

1. on the brain surface
2. around the penetrating vessels. The potential space between the vessel wall and the pia is called the Virchow Robin space.
3. at capillary level the pia is not present, but the foot processes along with the capillary endothelium and basement membrane form a specialised and selective 'blood-brain barrier'.

It is important to understand that, although the CSF is very similar in composition to the extracellular fluid of the brain, changes in the CSF only very indirectly reflect changes in the CNS in disease.

Thus the pia and the membrane formed by the foot processes of the astrocytes separate types of tissue derived from two embryological layers.

Pia

(1) **Neuroectodermal**
i.e. CNS tissue consisting of
Neurones
Neuroglia — Ependyma, Astrocytes, Oligodendroglia

(2) **Mesodermal**
i.e. Blood vessels, meninges (fibrous tissues)

and

MICROGLIA (most are resident round blood vessels) ← MACROPHAGES

During embryological development these enter the CNS tissues proper and become microglia

These SPECIALISED tissues are subject to INJURY and DEGENERATIVE processes.

These tissues behave similarly to mesodermal tissues elsewhere in the body, e.g. INFLAMMATORY RESPONSE.

NEURONAL DAMAGE

NEURONES are sensitive to damage by a wide variety of agents including anoxia, hypoglycaemia, virus infections and intracellular metabolic disturbances (e.g. associated with vitamin B deficiencies).

There are two main types, depending on the rapidity of the changes.

1. *Rapid NECROSIS* — associated with acute failure of function.

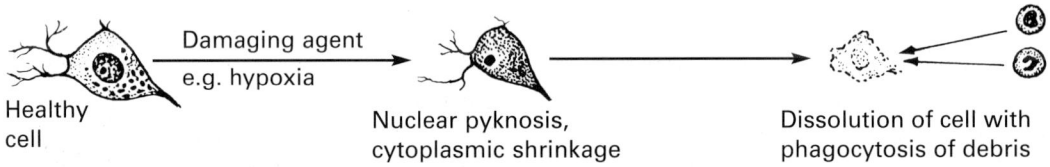

2. *Slow ATROPHIC CHANGES* — associated with gradual loss of function.

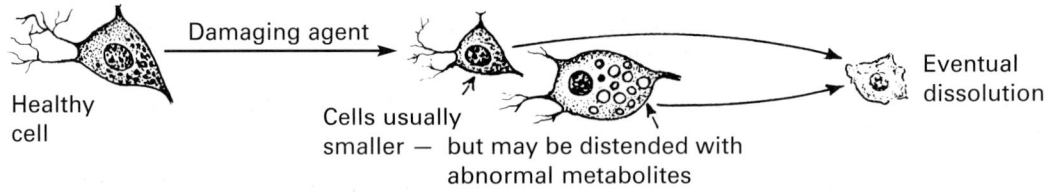

The process of ageing involves cumulative atrophy and disappearance of neurones; in some individuals the process is speeded up resulting in ***presenile dementia***.

NB There is *no* regeneration of destroyed neurones.

A large group of disorders of cerebral function seen in psychiatric practice have (as yet) no morphological evidence of nerve cell damage. They are caused by disturbances of poorly understood biochemical control mechanisms within the brain.

In addition to the PRIMARY degenerations described above, neurones are subject to SECONDARY degeneration in certain circumstances.

1. ***Retrograde degeneration*** — when the main axon is damaged there is degeneration of the neurone as well as the classical distal degeneration of the axon.

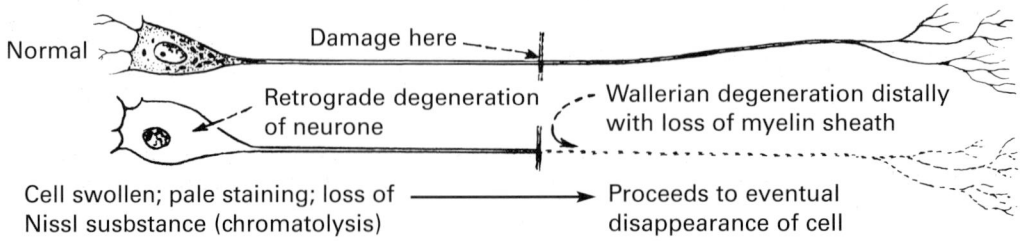

2. ***Trans-synaptic degeneration*** — in closely integrated neurone systems, neurone loss may be followed by degeneration of associated neurones across synapses.

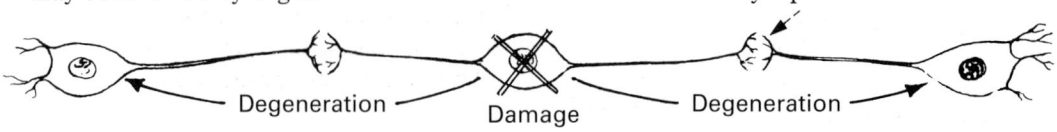

GLIAL REACTIONS

The glial cells react vigorously in many diseases of the CNS.

1. The **NEUROGLIAL** cells have supportive and nutritive functions.

(a) The **astrocytes** with their numerous fibrillary processes give structural support. They are less susceptible to damage than neurones.

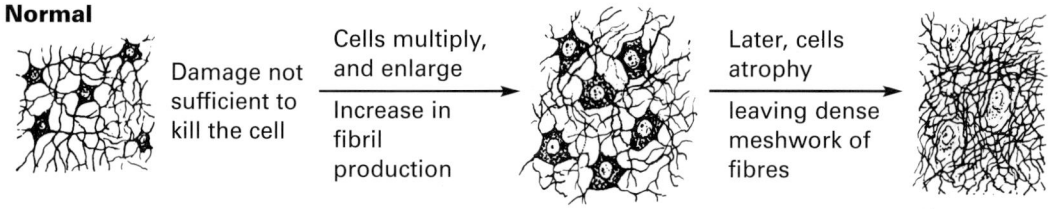

This process is called GLIOSIS. It is a feature of many diseases and is analogous to scar tissue. These cells and fibres contain Glial Fibrillary Acidic Protein (GFAP), recognition of which, using antibodies, is useful in histological sections.

Note: Collagenous scar tissue is only formed in the CNS when mesodermal structures such as large blood vessels are damaged.

(b) The **oligodendrocytes** — small cells with short processes — have a nutritive function in respect of neurones and especially myelin. This reaction is best seen when neurones are damaged.

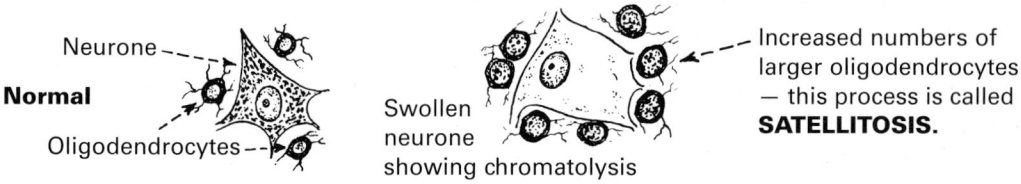

2. The **MICROGLIAL** cells are members of the mononuclear-phagocytic system. Reaction is best seen when there is necrosis of tissues.

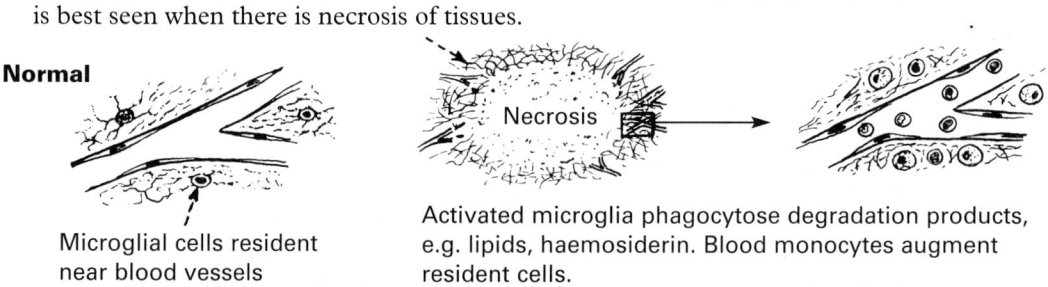

Microglial cells are well seen in and around infarcts; the activated cells which have ingested lipids are strikingly different from the small inactive microglia.

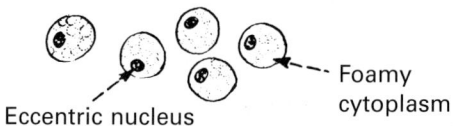

These cells have been given a variety of names: e.g. 'gitter' cells, or lipophages (lipid phagocytes).

DEMYELINATION

Loss of the myelin sheath may occur in two main circumstances:

1. **Primary** specific destruction of myelin.
   Demyelination precedes any axon damage. It is usually not related to specific nerve tracts.
   The mechanism is not clear; it may be autoimmune reaction or virus infection, or both.
   This type, although rare, occurs in an important group of diseases — the DEMYELINATING DISEASES (p.579).

2. **Secondary** loss following nerve cell and axon destruction. This type usually affects nerve tracts in an anatomically predictable way.
   The mechanism is similar to that described in peripheral nerves (Wallerian degeneration, p. 56).
   This type occurs in many disease processes, e.g. the nerve tract degeneration following regional infarction (p. 585).

The pathological sequels which are influenced by time factors are similar in both types.

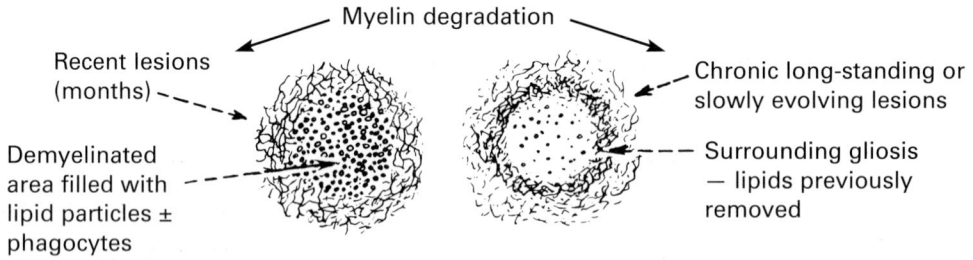

Demonstration of demyelination

Because routine histological stains are unsuitable, special methods are required. The following example, showing descending degeneration (and demyelination) of the corticospinal tract in the cord following infarction of the internal capsule in the brain, illustrates the two main methods.

1. *'POSITIVE'* method used in **recent** (months) lesions. The lipid particles are stained, e.g. Marchi's method or Sudan black stain.

2. *'NEGATIVE'* method — used in lesions of **any duration**. Absence of staining using stains for normal myelin, e.g. Weigert-Pal or Loyez methods.

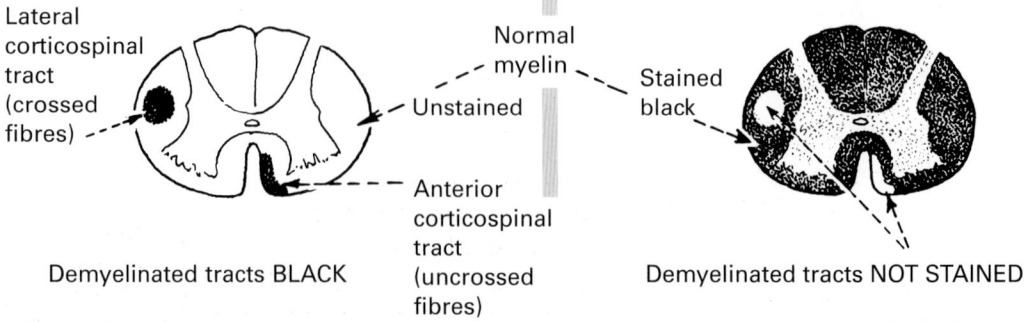

INCREASED INTRACRANIAL PRESSURE

INCREASED INTRACRANIAL PRESSURE (ICP) occurs in two main circumstances:
1. Due to the presence of an EXPANDING LESION
2. Due to obstruction of the free flow of the CSF — this causes hydrocephalus and is dealt with on page 592.

INTRACRANIAL EXPANDING LESIONS

These lesions may occur within the brain substance or in the meninges. Important examples are:

INTRACEREBRAL		MENINGEAL	
Haemorrhages and haematomas	→ Traumatic or → Spontaneous	Haemorrhages and haematomas (a) Extradural (b) Subdural (c) Subarachnoid	→ Usually traumatic
Infarction			
Tumours	→ Primary cerebral → or secondary	Very occasionally meningioma.	

The situation is often aggravated by cerebral OEDEMA.
The severity of the effects is modified by two important factors:
(1) the size of the lesion and (2) the rapidity of expansion.
There are three stages in the progress of increased intracranial pressure ICP.

(1) The stage of **Compensation**

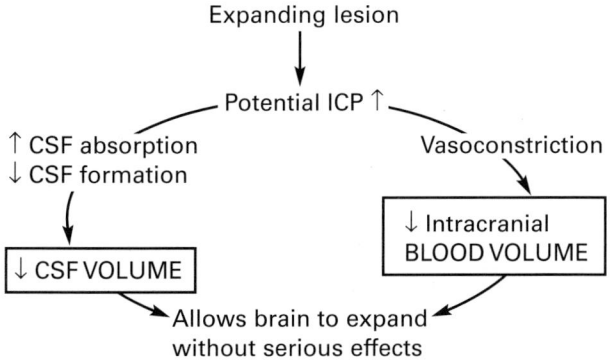

(2) The stage of **Decompensation**

At this stage there are herniations and distortions of the brain with their associated complications. The systemic blood pressure is raised and the pulse slows ('Cushing' effect).

(3) A vicious circle is established leading to the stage of **vasomotor paralysis.**

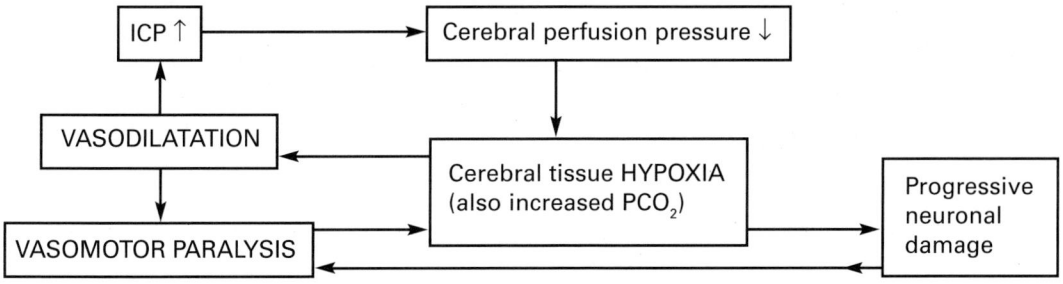

INCREASED INTRACRANIAL PRESSURE

Effects

DISTORTIONS and DISLOCATIONS of the brain substance

These are to some extent dependent on the site of the initiating lesion; the effects of a unilateral expanding lesion are illustrated.

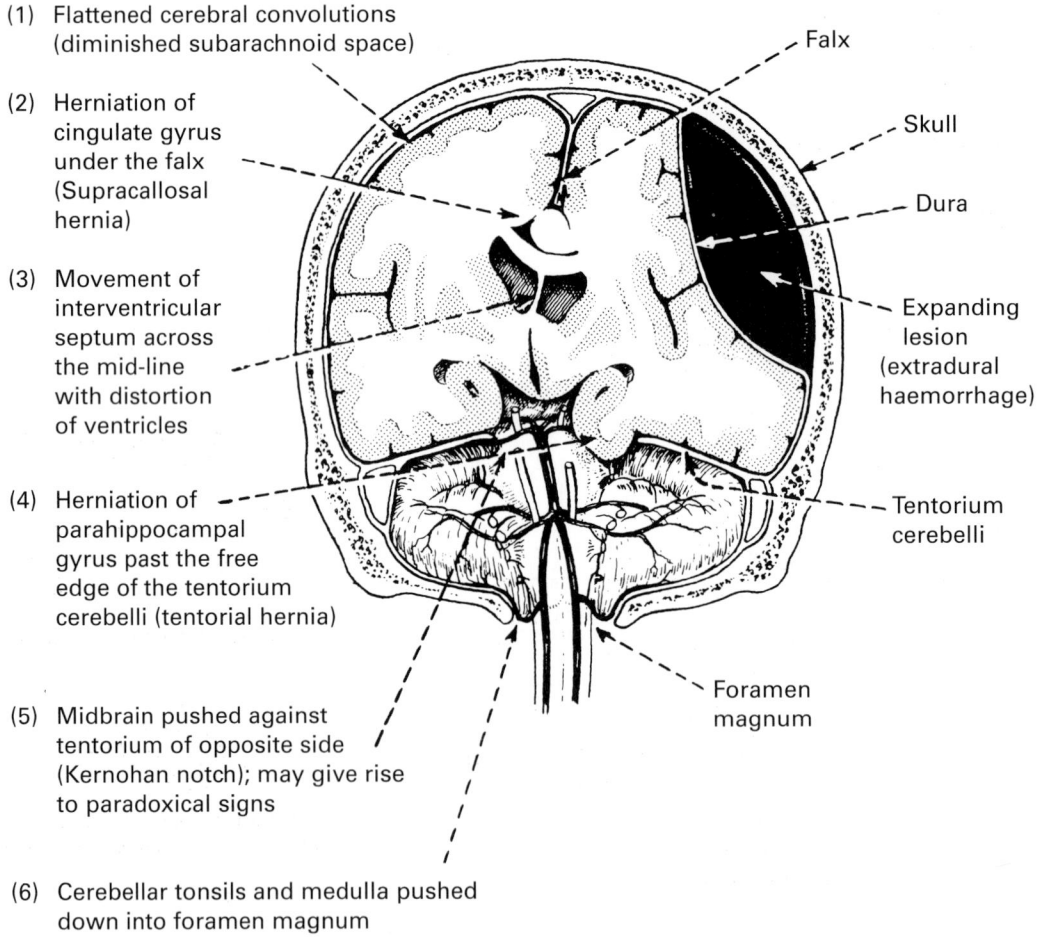

NB The sudden removal of even small amounts of CSF by **LUMBAR PUNCTURE** may precipitate medullary 'coning' with fatal results due to damage to the 'vital centres'.

CEREBRAL OEDEMA

Swelling of the brain, of which oedema is the major component, is an important complication of many brain diseases because the enlargement either initiates or aggravates increased intracranial pressure.

The process may be localised or generalised depending on the type of initiating disorder.

Localised conditions
Examples:
- Infarcts, and local ischaemia
- Haematomas (due to vessel rupture and injury)
- Tumours

Generalised conditions
Examples: Intoxications
- Metabolic disturbances, e.g. hypoglycaemia
- Generalised hypoxia
- Severe head trauma
- Malignant hypertension

The pathological mechanism is as follows:

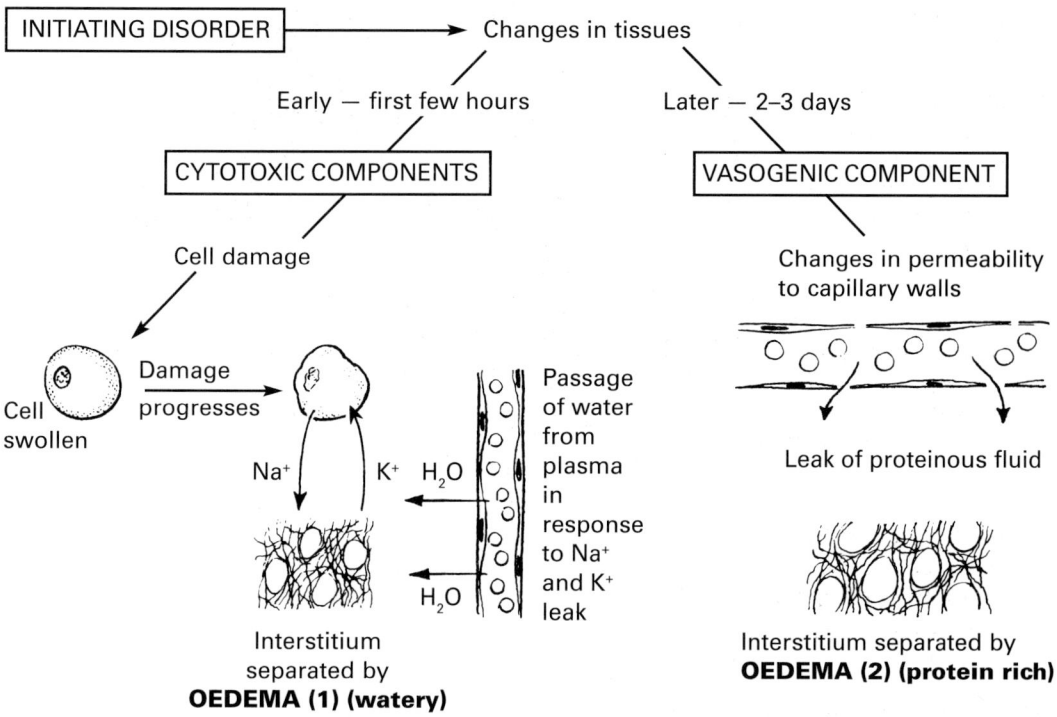

Notes

(a) Components (1) and (2) overlap.
(b) The oedema fluid tends to spread in the white matter.
(c) The severity of oedema formation is very variable and unpredictable clinically.
(d) In clinical practice, therapy has two aspects:
  1. Treatment of the initiating disorder by any appropriate means.
  2. Minimising the formation of oedema by the use of
     (i) osmotic agents, e.g. urea or mannitol
     (ii) steroids (the mechanism is not known).

INCREASED INTRACRANIAL PRESSURE

SECONDARY COMPLICATIONS

1. **Vascular damage**
   (a) Compression of the central retinal vein causes PAPILLOEDEMA, an important clinical sign of raised ICP. *Note:* Axonal flow in the optic nerve is reduced, contributing to swelling of the optic disc.

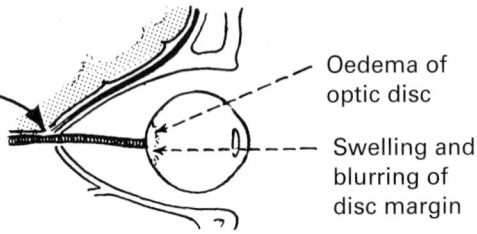

   (b) Stretching and compression of blood vessels may cause haemorrhage and infarction quite remote from the initiating lesion — secondary midbrain and calcarine infarction and haemorrhage are common.

2. **Intracranial nerve damage**
   Oculomotor (III) and abducens (VI) nerves are particularly prone to damage, giving rise to paralysis of ocular movements in varying combinations.
   The VIth nerve is specially vulnerable due to its long subarachnoid course. It is often the nerve on the side opposite the lesion which is stretched giving rise to paradoxical signs.

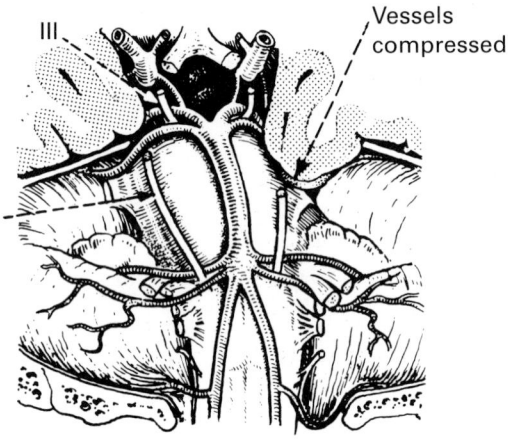

3. **Obstruction of flow of CSF**

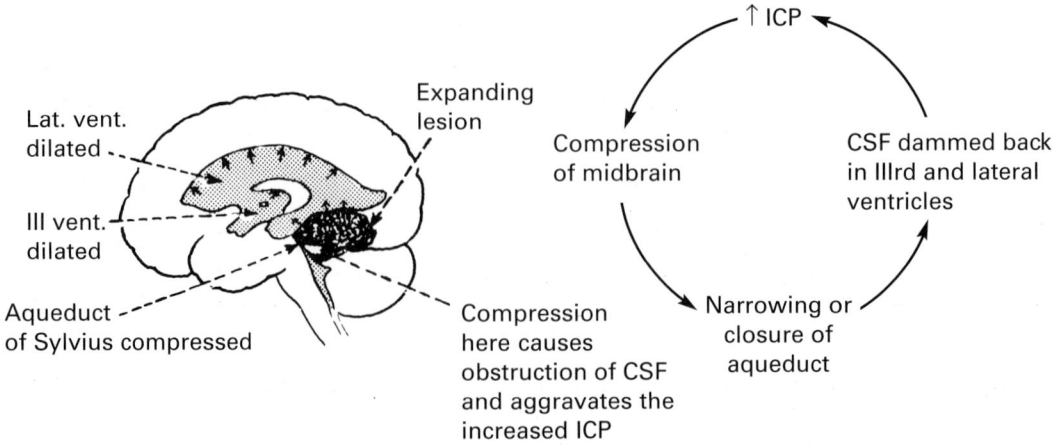

4. **Changes in the skull bones**
   Long continued ICP causes bone erosion and thinning visible on X-ray.
   (a) Erosion of posterior clinoid processes of sphenoid bone.
   (b) In children, before the skull is fully ossified, the inner table is thinned at the sites of convolutional pressure giving a striking X-ray appearance.

CIRCULATORY DISTURBANCES

(1) Hypoxia and ischaemia and (2) intracranial haemorrhage are the important and common mechanisms causing brain damage.

ACUTE HYPOXIC DISORDERS

Blood supply: 20% of cardiac output is delivered via carotid and vertebral arteries

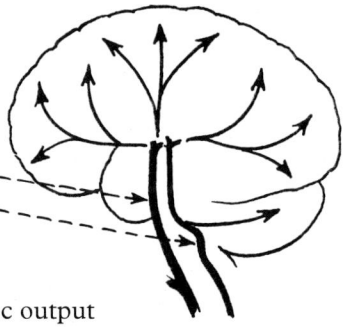

When the cardiac output falls, an autoregulatory vascular control mechanism protects the cerebral blood supply — the arterial BP must be kept above 50 mmHg.

Neuronal aerobic metabolism of glucose

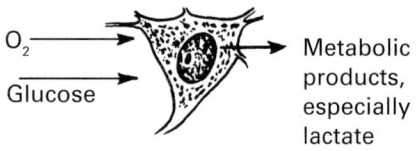

There are no reserves of O_2 or glucose in the brain, therefore a constant delivery via arterial blood is necessary.

Neurones are very susceptible to hypoxia (and hypoglycaemia); with complete O_2 deprivation neuronal **necrosis** occurs in 5–7 minutes (at normal temperatures).

The following flow diagram illustrates the factors which influence availability of O_2 and the conditions giving rise to hypoxia.

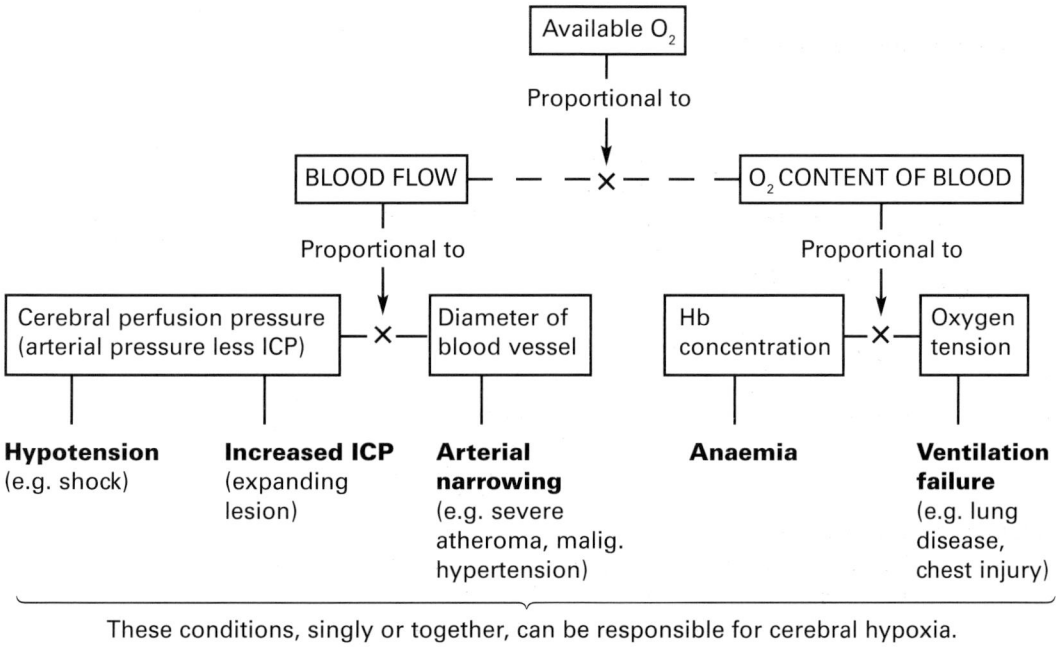

CEREBRAL INFARCTION

This condition, the commoner of the two main types of stroke (the other is spontaneous intracerebral haemorrhage), is caused by failure of the supply of oxygen (and glucose) to maintain the viability of the tissues in the territory of a cerebral arterial branch. This is not always due to simple local arterial occlusion, and very often a component of central circulatory deficiency is contributory. The lesion is essentially necrosis of all the tissues in the affected territory.

Mechanism

Precipitating condition → Perfusion failure → INFARCTION (ischaemic necrosis)

LOCAL ARTERIAL DISEASE (particularly ATHEROMA) and its complications, are the most common.

1. **Arterial occlusions**

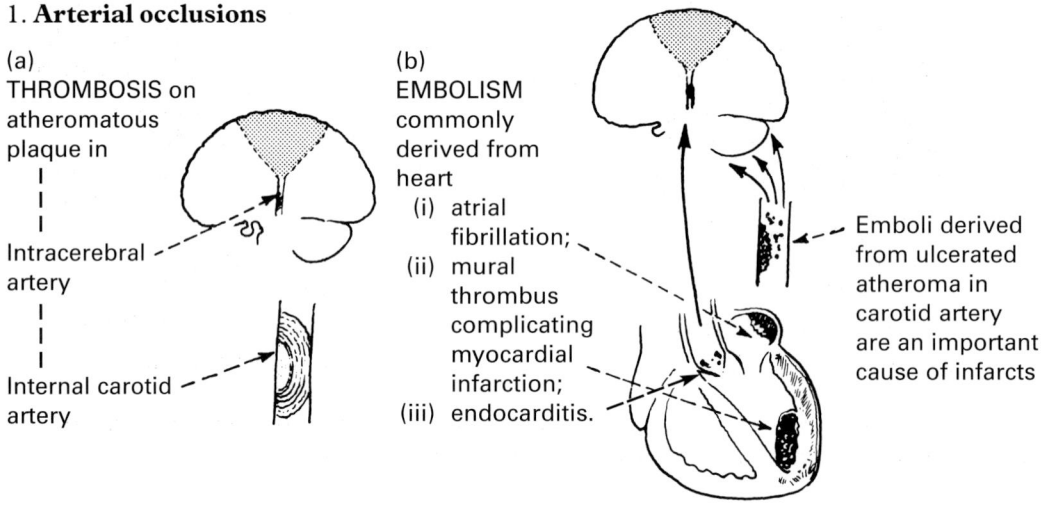

2. **Arterial stenosis**

ATHEROMA — the widespread loss of arterial lumen potentiates cerebral perfusion deficiency in two ways: (1) by distributing the normal arterial flow and (2) by prejudicing anastomotic communications.

Atheromatous stenosis alone is not usually a cause of infarction, but when central circulatory deficiency is added, infarction is common, e.g. this may vary from the slight fall in BP during sleep to the severe hypotension of shock or myocardial infarction.

Other rarer causes of arterial stenosis are dissecting aneurysm and arteritis. Arterial spasm is a rare cause.

CEREBRAL INFARCTION

SITES

While infarcts may occur anywhere in the brain, depending on the vagaries of the precipitating arterial lesions, certain sites are more commonly affected.

1. In cases of local arterial occlusion, **internal structures supplied by 'end' arterial branches** are particularly vulnerable. The cortex is often protected in variable degree by anastomoses of other cerebral arteries. This is illustrated in the territory of the middle cerebral artery.

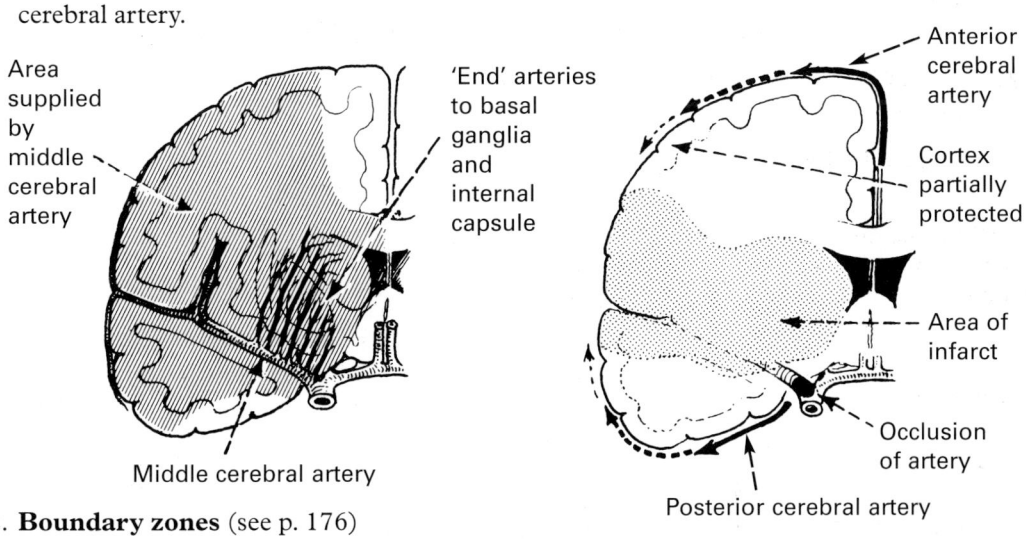

2. **Boundary zones** (see p. 176)

   The cortex in particular is damaged in boundary zone infarction. In these cases, central circulatory deficiency is an important component, e.g. hypotension.

BRAIN DAMAGE DUE TO CARDIAC ARREST

This is characterised by widely distributed selective neuronal necrosis — the neurones are more susceptible to hypoxia than the supporting cells.

Affected areas — total cortical necrosis
or
most sensitive zones — hippocampus
— layers III, V, VI of cortex
— within sulci
— Purkinje cells of cerebellum.

Note: (a) These changes do not become apparent unless the patient survives at least 12 hours after the arrest.
(b) Similar types of neuronal damage can be seen in severe acute hypoglycaemia, carbon monoxide or barbiturate poisoning.

CEREBRAL INFARCTION

The diagram below illustrates the evolution of an infarct, e.g. in the territory of the middle cerebral artery. Up to 24 hours there is virtually no visible change.

18-24 hr	After 24 hours	After a few days	After weeks/months
Gross appearances			
Very difficult to see	Less difficult to see Slight swelling Blurring of white/grey junction	Line of demarcation seen Necrotic tissue. Soft to touch; usually pale but may be congested if blood has permeated in (haemorrhagic infarct)	Demolition + scarring Cyst with pale or yellowish fluid Shrinkage of scarred area: compensatory dilatation of ventricle
Microscopic appearances			
Early neuronal damage	Early neuronal damage ↓ Necrosis of neurones	Organisation of infarct begins Macrophages appear; capillary sprouting; oedema diminishing	Organisation well established; neurones disappear; numerous macrophages; gliosis
Clinical associations			
	FUNCTIONAL LOSS		

Effects are maximal in the early stages when oedema and circulatory disturbance in the adjacent tissues augment the functional loss caused by infarct. Larger infarcts may be associated with loss of consciousness.

The prognostic assessment of final functional loss cannot be made until the changes have subsided and any possible functional compensations have been established. This takes many weeks. Complete clinical recovery may follow small infarcts.

CEREBRAL HAEMORRHAGE

Spontaneous intracranial bleeding is the second main type of stroke. In the great majority of cases there is localised arterial disease aggravated by hypertension. A small number are associated with cerebral tumours, systemic bleeding diathesis or arteriovenous malformations.

In most hypertensives over middle age, **microaneurysms** are found in the very small cerebral arteries. It is believed that rupture of one of these aneurysms is the immediate cause of intracerebral haemorrhage.

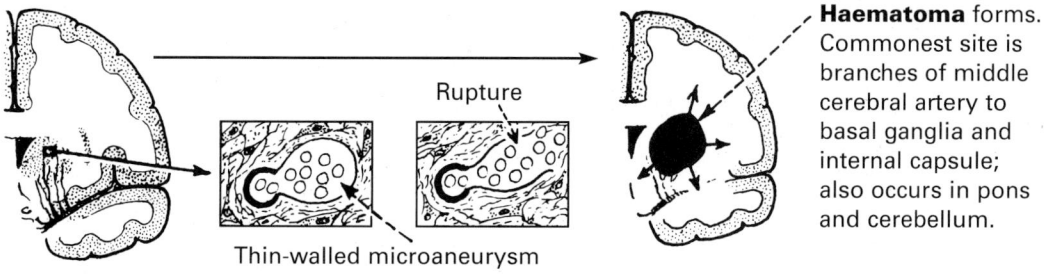

Progress
The onset is usually sudden with headache and, because of the high blood pressure, progress is rapid and the haemorrhage large.

↓

Associated raised ICP effects

↓

Death in many cases

When the bleeding is limited, there is survival with varying residual paralysis.

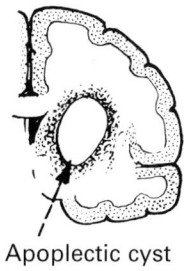

Final outcome
Cystic space containing yellow-brown fluid walled off by gliosis.

NB Intracerebral bleeding may track irregularly and often reaches the subarachnoid space and ventricles.

SUBARACHNOID HAEMORRHAGE

This is commonly but not exclusively the result of rupture of a 'berry' aneurysm at or near the circle of Willis. The basic abnormality is a congenital weakness of the elastic tissues in the arterial wall; only rarely is an aneurysm present at birth, and while subarachnoid haemorrhage does occur in young people, the incidence increases with age. Hypertension is an important contributing factor.

Sites

Often multiple, near arterial junctions.

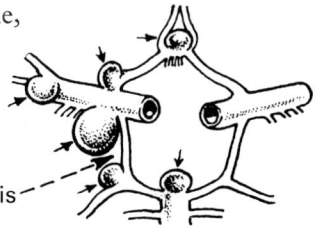

Circle of Willis

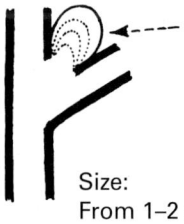

Thin walled aneurysm developing at site of deficiency in arterial wall

Size:
From 1–2 mm up to 1–2 cm

Not all aneurysms rupture; they are found incidentally at autopsy.
Massive haemorrhage may be preceded by one or more small leaks — marked by headache and no functional loss.

Progress

Haemorrhage spreading throughout subarachnoid space — generalised ICP increased; blood-stained CSF.

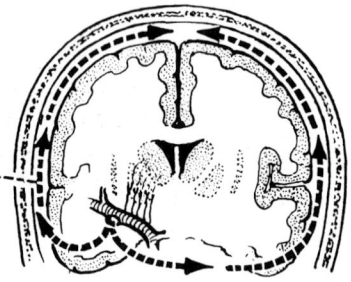

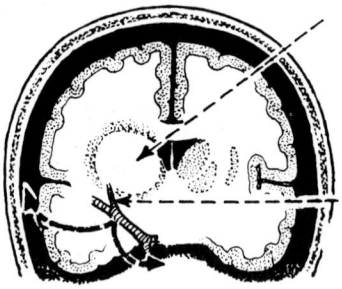

Local infarction may be a complication

Irritant effect of haemorrhage causes local arterial spasm

NB The aneurysm may rupture directly into the brain and mimic an intracerebral haemorrhage.

CSF findings

1–24 hours — blood stained; blood content constant in sequential samples (distinguishes blood derived from a traumatic tap)
— centrifuge supernatant — may be pink due to haemolysis.

24 hours onwards — supernatant shows xanthochromia (yellow colour due to presence of blood degradation products).

Other causes of cerebral haemorrhage of either type are vascular malformations and coagulation disorders.

HYPERTENSION

The incidence of strokes in hypertensive subjects is very significantly increased.

1. **Intracranial haemorrhage**

Mechanism

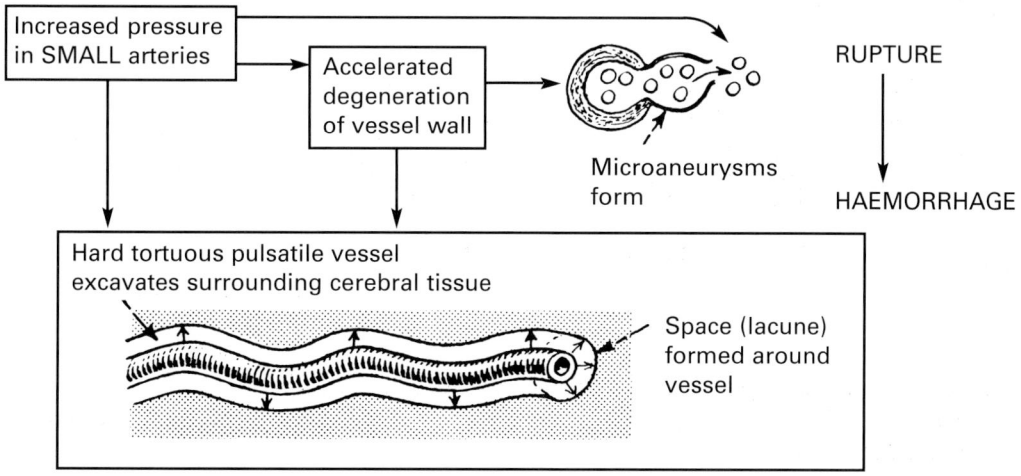

2. **Cerebral infarction** — risk increased indirectly.

Mechanism

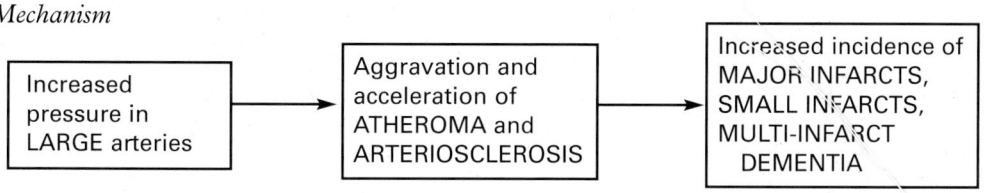

In MALIGNANT HYPERTENSION, an additional dimension, HYPERTENSIVE ENCEPHALOPHATHY, is added.

Mechanism

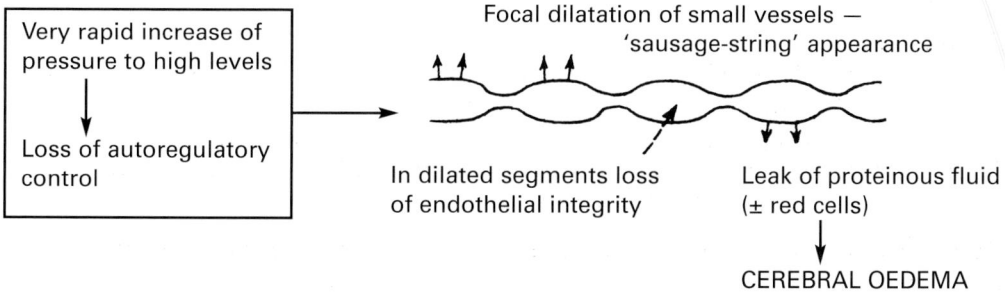

Clinically, signs of cerebral 'irritation' including convulsions progress through stupor to coma. Papilloedema, evidence of increased intracranial pressure, is always present.

HEAD INJURY

Head injuries of varying severity are common nowadays, particularly as a consequence of road traffic accidents. Immediate damage is caused by two main mechanisms which overcome the protection of the vulnerable cerebral tissues provided by the skull and the CSF 'water cushion'.

1. **Direct blows to the head** (e.g. **missile head injury**)

   usually cause injury to the soft tissues of the scalp and often fracture of the skull with contusion or laceration of the underlying brain.

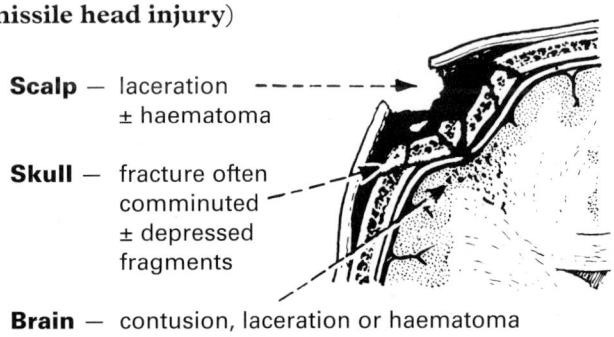

2. **Non-missile head injury**

   Since the head is usually freely moveable on the neck, the sudden application of forces derived from **acceleration**, **deceleration** and, particularly, **rotation** of the head often causes serious brain injury.

   (a) **Skull fractures**

   (i) *Skull damage*

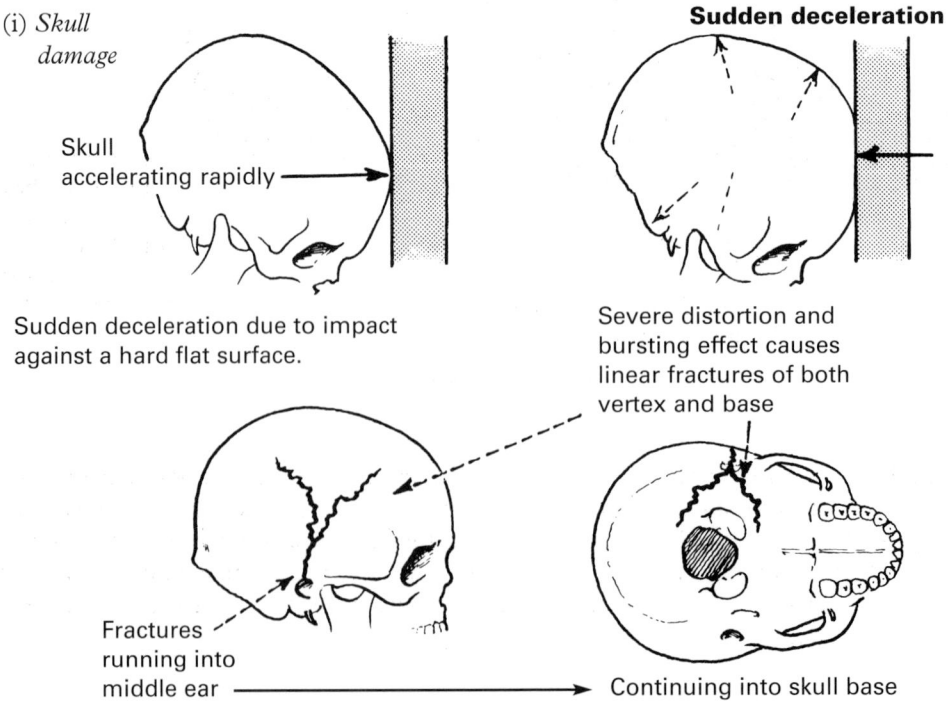

HEAD INJURY

Acceleration/deceleration injury

(ii) *Brain damage*

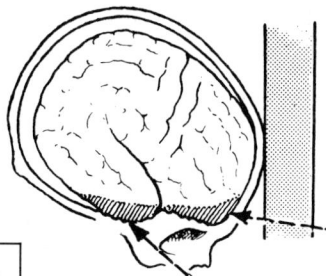

The brain continues to move forward and is contused by the rough surface of the middle fossa and orbital plate

Frontal contusion

Temporal contusion

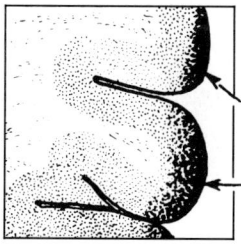

The damage is characteristically on the surface of gyri, the sulci being spared

(b) **Rotation**

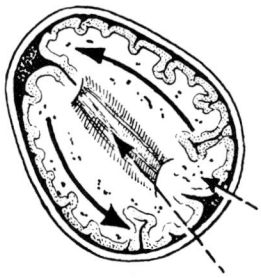

Rotary movement of cerebral emispheres causes:

(i) variable diffuse damage to the cerebral tissues; presents as minute haemorrhages

(ii) shearing injury to the corpus callosum:

axonal bulbs from where axons have been sheared.

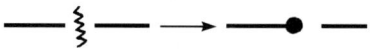

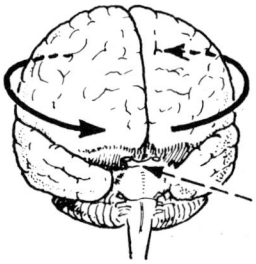

Sudden torsion of the midbrain (± vascular damage) may be fatal, but decerebrate survival sometimes occurs

Note:

It will be appreciated that more serious cerebral damage is the result of interaction of complex physical forces and anatomical features. An understanding of these mechanisms explains why serious cerebral injury is not uncommon in the absence of damage to the scalp or fracture of the skull, and also why brain damage may be remote from the site of impact: so-called 'contre-coup' injury is sustained when the brain tissue opposite the site of impact is contused.

HEAD INJURY

DELAYED COMPLICATIONS

In addition to damage sustained immediately at the time of impact, certain serious complications may supervene over the next hours or few days.

1. **Haemorrhages**

(a) **Extradural haematoma**

This type of haemorrhage classically occurs as a complication of linear fracture of the skull vault when the middle meningeal artery is torn.

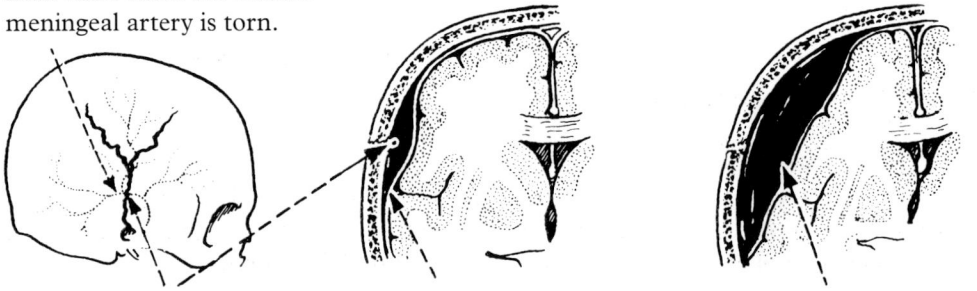

The classical clinical association is a direct blow to the head from which recovery is rapid. After a lucid interval of varying duration up to several hours, signs of increased intracranial pressure supervene. This chain of events is explained by the time taken for the haemorrhage to accumulate by stripping the dura from the skull.

(b) **Subdural haematoma.** This may occur at any site and is often extensive because of the loose attachment of the dura and arachnoid membranes. It is usually due to rupture of small bridging veins.

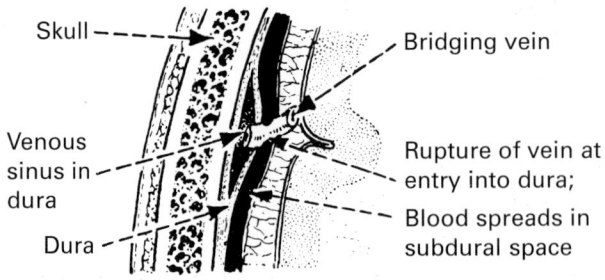

These acute subdural haematomas are often associated with subarachnoid haemorrhage and cerebral contusions.

(c) **Intracerebral haematomas** occur in association with the cortical contusions particularly in the temporal and frontal lobes, but also at random deep within the hemispheres due to shearing at the time of impact. Large haematomas are uncommon.

HEAD INJURY

Delayed complications (continued)

2. **Cerebral oedema** is an important complication.
   ↓
   Increased intracranial pressure → Cerebral hypoxia.

3. **External leakage of CSF** (and blood) from the ear and nose may complicate fractures of the skull base. This complication may be of long duration and is always a potential entry for infection.

4. **Local infection** may complicate compound fractures and proceed to meningitis.

LATE COMPLICATIONS

1. **Scarring and Epilepsy**

   During the healing process, resorption of necrotic tissues and blood degradation products is gradually effected, leaving pigmented scars. These may act as trigger foci for epilepsy, particularly if the meninges are adherent to the underlying brain.

2. **Chronic subdural haematoma**

   A thick layer of fluid and partially clotted blood gradually accumulates between the dura and arachnoid membranes which show considerable reactive thickening.

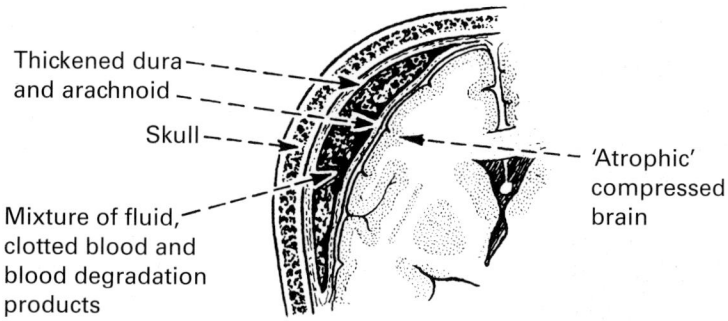

The precise cause is not known; most cases occur in alcoholics or in elderly people already suffering from cerebral atrophy, and it is possible that the small bridging veins are unduly stretched and become more susceptible to damage.

The clinical signs are usually insidious in onset and progressive, and in many cases there is a history of either no or only very trivial injury.

AGEING and DEMENTIA

Normal Brain Ageing

With normal ageing the brain becomes atrophic, but the morphological changes described below are not necessarily accompanied by loss of intellect.

Changes in old age

Gross as seen naked-eye at autopsy

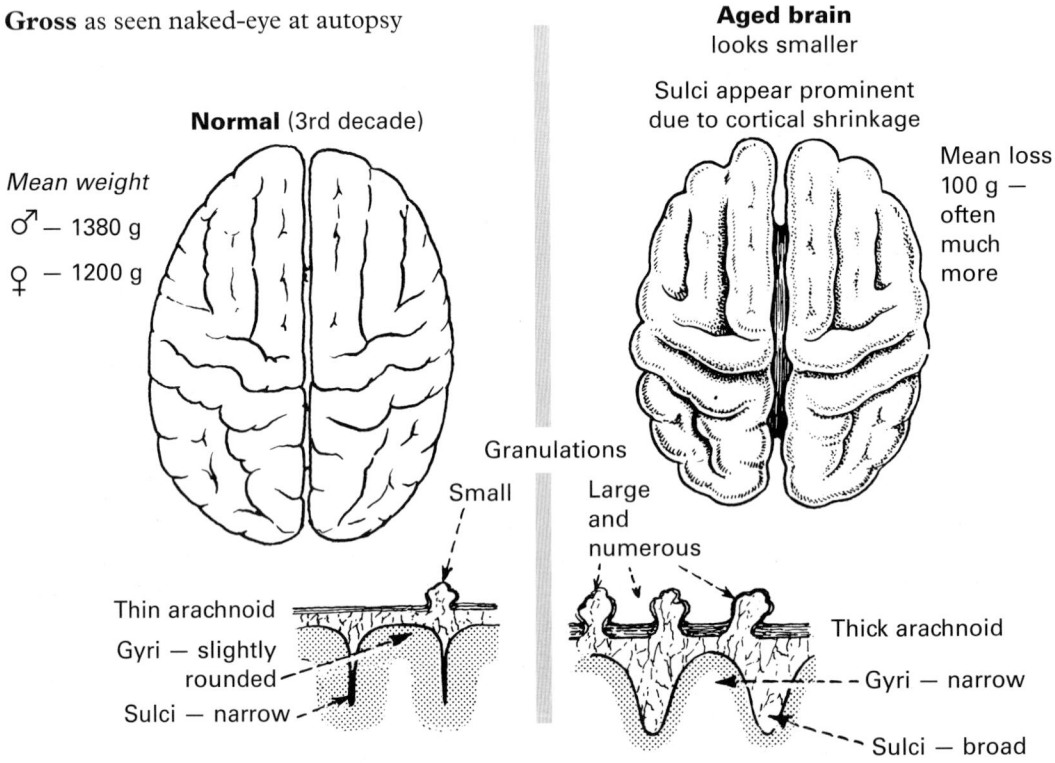

There is compensatory enlargement of the lateral ventricles.

Dementia

Dementia is defined as 'an acquired progressive global impairment of intellect, memory and personality, without impairment of consciousness'. Around 5% of the population over 65 years are affected and the proportion rises to over 20% of these over 80 years.

There are numerous causes among which are:

1. Alzheimer's disease } These are the two main causes and often co-exist.
2. Multi-infarct dementia
3. Dementia associated with AIDS — the commonest cause in younger adults worldwide.
4. Pick's disease } These are rare hereditary forms.
5. Huntington's disease
6. Creutzfeld-Jacob disease. This rare dementia is topical because a recently described variant appears to be linked to bovine spongiform encephalopathy (B.S.E.) (p. 576).

ALZHEIMER'S DISEASE

This disease accounts for around 60% of cases of dementia. While typically a disease of the elderly, especially females, it is also seen in patients under 60 years, in whom there is often a family history. Almost all patients with Down's syndrome who survive to 50 years develop Alzheimer's (suggesting that chromosome 21 is important).

Pathology

The changes of Alzheimer's resemble those of normal ageing, but are greatly exaggerated in the temporal and parietal lobes and in the hippocampus.

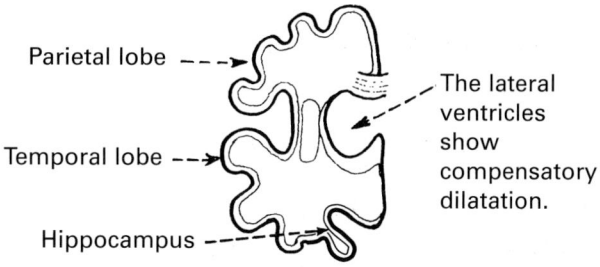

The histological hallmarks are:

1. Extracellular senile plaques.

(Silver stain)

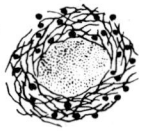

Tangled aggregates of distended neurites presenting as black dots and rods with a centre core of amyloid

2. Intracellular neurofibrillary tangles.

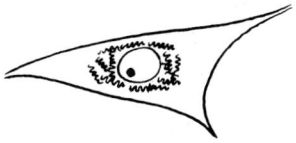

Helical strands of neuroprotein form around the nuclei of neurones.

3. Amyloid angiopathy.

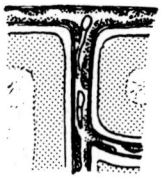

Deposited in meninges and blood vessel walls

Aetiology

This remains unclear, but there are both genetic and acquired factors.

Genetic factors — several genes are involved

1. Amyloid precursor protein (chromosome 21) — early onset Alzheimer's.
2. Presenilin 1 and 2 (chromosome 14 and 1) — proteins involved in binding amyloid precursor proteins.
3. Apolipoprotein E — the e4 allele is associated with late onset disease — it may determine the age of onset.
4. α-2 macroglobulin — may be involved in clearance of amyloid proteins.

Acquired factors

1. Toxic substances e.g. aluminium.
2. Reduced nerve growth factors and diminished repair.
3. Impairment of calcium dependent K^+ channels in neurones.
4. Repeated head injury.
5. Free radical injury.
6. Coexistent vascular disease.

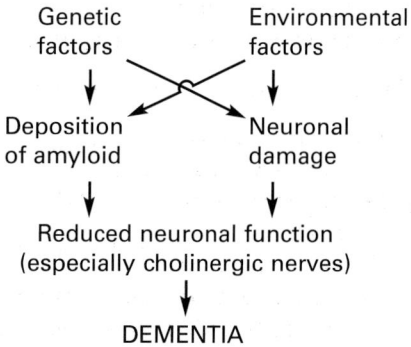

DEMENTIA

MULTI-INFARCT DEMENTIA

This form of dementia is associated with vascular disease — with infarcts often in the middle cerebral arterial distribution. The volume of brain loss appears to be important.

Loss of >100ml of brain correlates with dementia.

Hypertension is an important underlying factor.

LEWI BODY DEMENTIA

This recently recognised disorder accounts for 5-10% of dementia especially in younger patients. There is widespread neuronal loss in the cerebral cortex. In the surviving neurones the histological marker is the LEWI BODY containing UBIQUITIN and similar to those seen in the substantia nigra in Parkinson's disease.

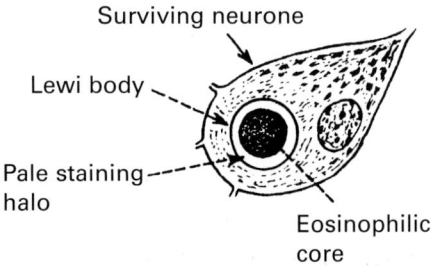

PICK'S DISEASE

This uncommon form of dementia has a strong familial (autosomal dominant) component. There is typically severe atrophy of the temporal and frontal lobes. The histological marker in the surviving neurones is the Pick body.

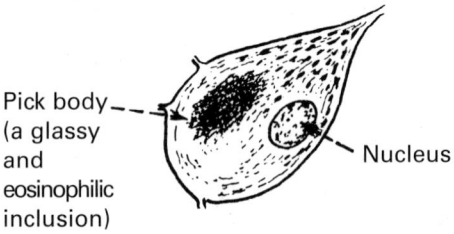

HUNTINGTON'S DISEASE

This is an uncommon autosomal dominant condition beginning in the 3rd or 4th decade and characterised by psychiatric disorders, progressive dementia and in some patients bizarre writhing movements (chorea).

Pathology

There is atrophy of the brain particularly marked in the caudate nucleus.
The responsible gene (IT 15) lies on chromosome 4 and encodes a protein known as Huntingtin.
Genetic screening is now available

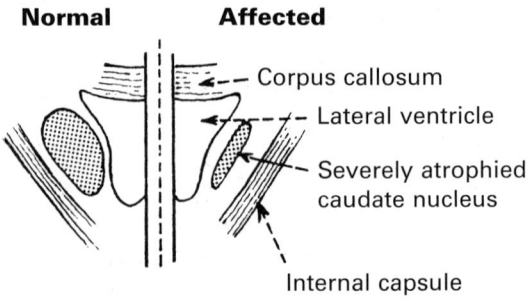

PUNCH DRUNK SYNDROME

Professional boxers may develop dementia due to neuronal damage caused by repeated blows to the head.

INFECTIONS

Compared with the high incidence of infection generally, infection of the central nervous system is uncommon. The pathological effects may be slight and wholly recoverable as in some virus infections, or severe, leading to permanent damage or death.

Anatomically, infections fall into two main groups which tend to remain separated due to the intervention of the **pial** barrier (see p. 545).

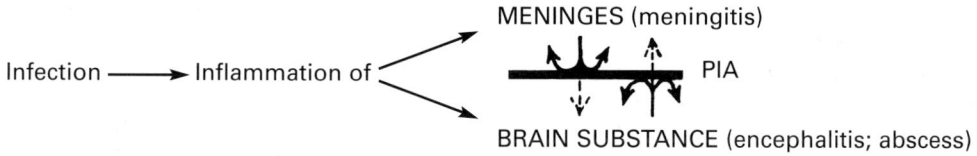

Infections will be considered in three broad aetiological groups:
(1) Bacterial, (2) Viral and (3) Miscellaneous types.

BACTERIAL INFECTIONS

1. Most commonly by the blood stream

Bacteria settling in subarachnoid space

Meningitis

(a) Pyogenic types, e.g. meningococcus, pneumococcus, haemophilus
(b) Granulomatous types, e.g. tubercle bacillus, treponema pallidum

Bacteria settling in brain substance

Brain abscess

(a) Pyogenic type — miscellaneous organisms *NB Staphylococcal pyaemia*
(b) Granulomatous type — tubercle bacillus

2. From an adjacent local infected site — these are pyogenic infections.

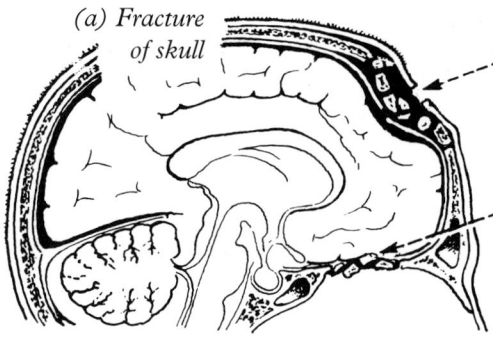

Compound depressed fracture
↓
Infection

Fracture of skull base leading into infected nasal sinus

(1) Extradural abscess
(2) Subdural abscess (empyema)
(3) Meningitis

BACTERIAL INFECTION

Bacterial infections from an adjacent local infected site (continued)

(b) *Middle ear and mastoid disease*
In untreated purulent otitis media, three serious complications may arise from spread of the inflammation.

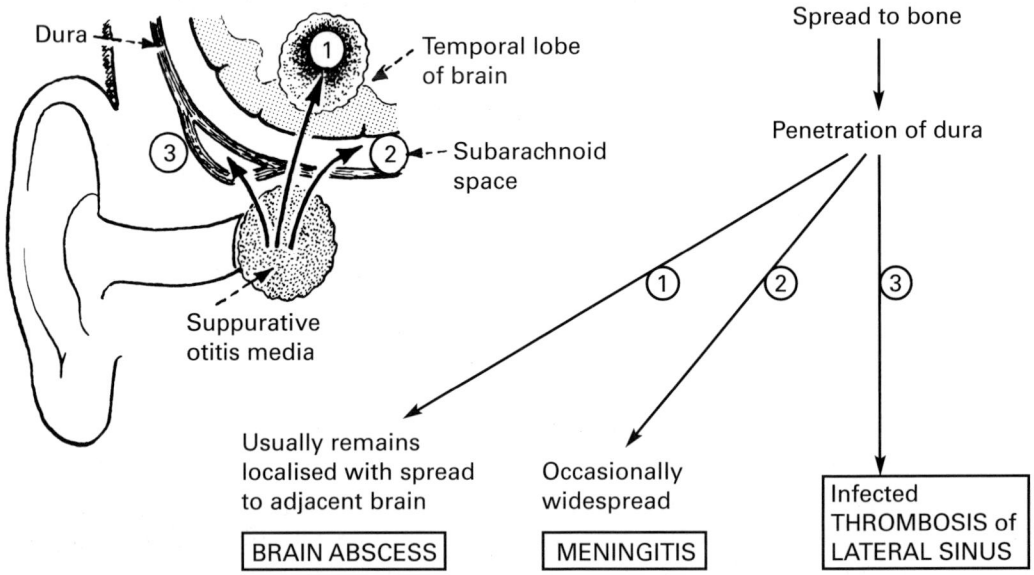

PYOGENIC MENINGITIS

The whole subarachnoid space contains purulent exudate which is maximal in sulci and around the brain base cisternae.

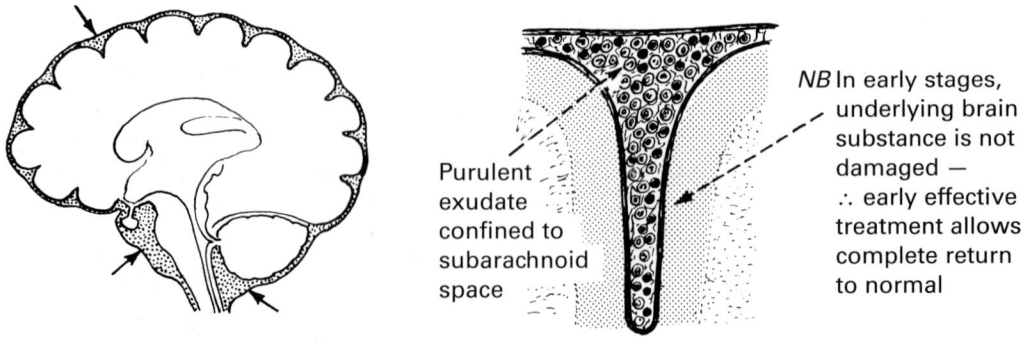

In untreated or ineffectively treated patients who survive, complications include cranial nerve damage, hydrocephalus and variable brain damage.

The CSF in the acute stage contains neutrophils and the infecting organism can usually be demonstrated.

BACTERIAL INFECTION

PYOGENIC BRAIN ABSCESS

The abscesses resulting from direct spread of adjacent infection or by blood borne infection — as seen particularly in bronchiectasis — are often well circumscribed by a pyogenic membrane.

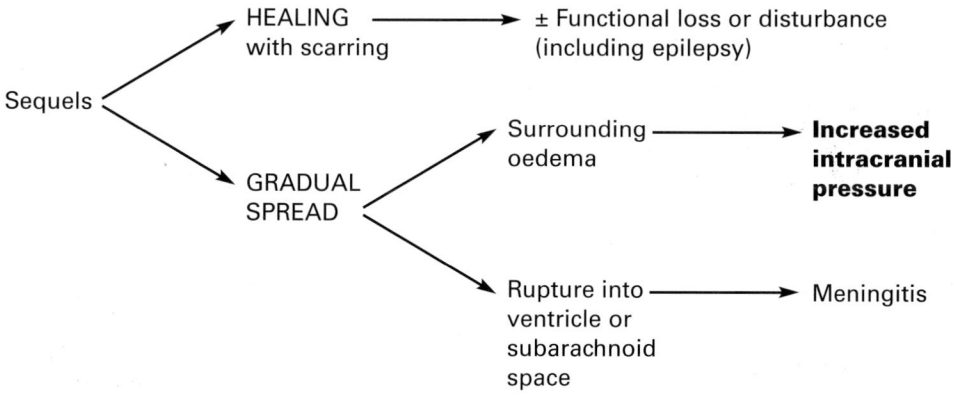

Clinical note: An abscess is often silent early in its evolution, and the infection at the site of entry may have healed before the onset of serious complications causes clinical signs.

Multiple small abscesses occur in staphylococcal pyaemia and microabscesses may complicate bacterial endocarditis. The cerebral pathology in these circumstances is only one facet of serious systemic infection.

TUBERCULOSIS

Meningitis is the result of blood borne spread, usually from a primary complex and is often the important component of generalised miliary tuberculosis (see p. 73). Although the incidence has fallen sharply in Western countries, it is emerging as a serious complication of AIDS. It remains prevalent in many parts of the world.

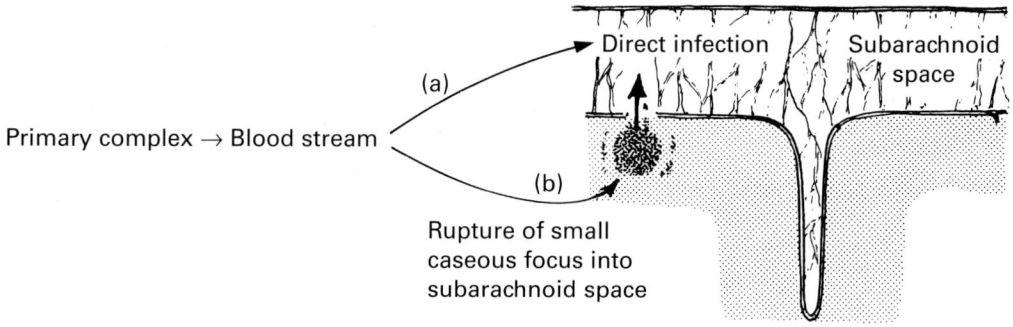

TUBERCULOUS MENINGITIS

Evolution

Before the advent of antibiotic and chemotherapy, tuberculous meningitis was invariably fatal after an illness lasting from several days to a few weeks.

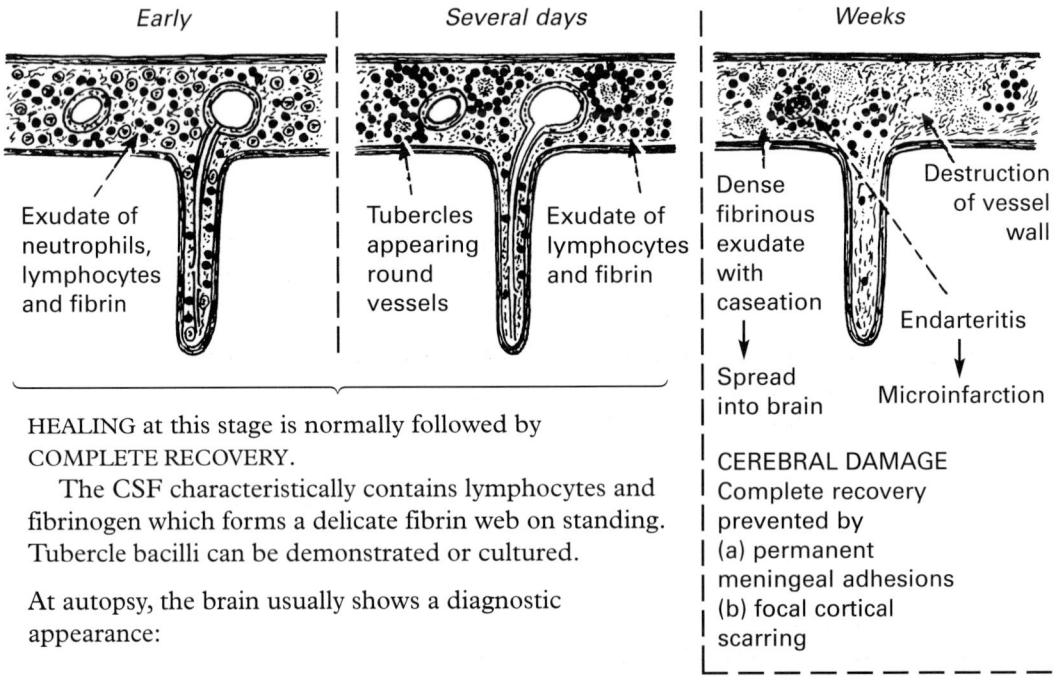

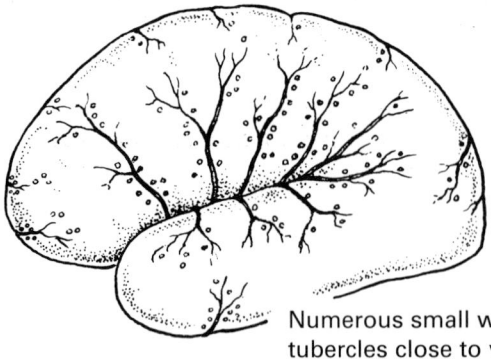

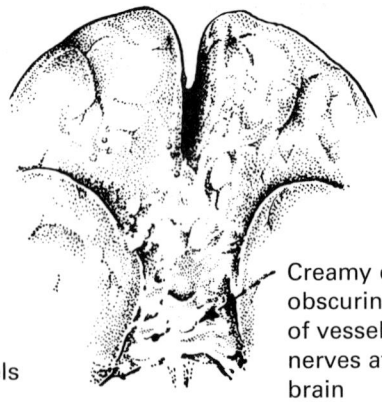

TUBERCULOMA: These localised tuberculous cerebral abscesses are now very rare.

SYPHILIS: Neurological syphilis is rare nowadays. The main pathological lesions are described on page 77.

VIRUS INFECTIONS

Compared with the incidence of virus infections in general, affection of the central nervous system is rare, even with viruses having an affinity for the CNS — **NEUROTROPIC VIRUSES**

There are 2 broad groups:-

1. **Acute**
   Cell lysis occurs towards the end of the viraemic phase of infection. This is the common type of disease. Herpes simplex, mumps, poliovirus and togaviruses are examples.

2. **Persistent**
   Viruses which usually cause damage outside the CNS behave uncharacteristically and cause continuing and active disease of the CNS over a long period (months - years). Measles, rubella and JC papovavirus are examples.

   Latent virus infection is seen in herpes zoster and possibly plays a role in the demyelinating diseases.
   Virus infection also has a possible role in oncogenesis within the CNS.

Routes of infection
Most viruses arrive at the CNS via the blood, but the factors which potentiate the establishment of disease within the CNS are poorly understood.

Primary portal of entry

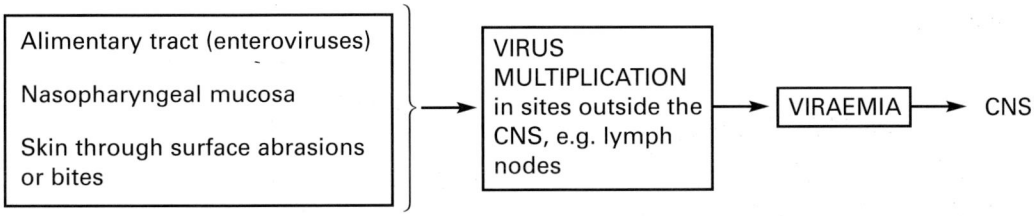

In rabies, the virus travels from the wound up the peripheral nerves to the CNS; a similar mechanism may be involved in herpes simplex encephalitis.

VIRUS INFECTIONS

BASIC PATHOLOGICAL EFFECTS

(a) **VIRAL MENINGITIS** is the commonest form of meningitis; the disease is usually mild and only the meninges are affected. Recovery is usually complete.

(b) In more severe cases, the brain substance is also damaged in varying degree — **ENCEPHALITIS** (meningoencephalitis).

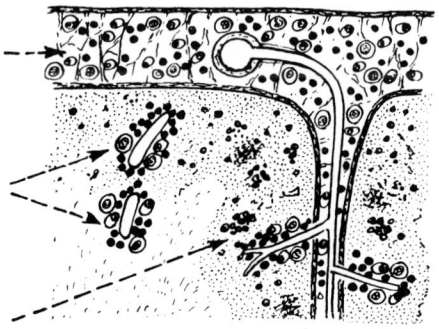

The meninges (CSF) contain increased protein, normal sugar and a mononuclear cellular infiltrate (particularly **lymphocytes**, plasma cells and large mononuclears).

In the brain the characteristic changes are:

1. PERIVASCULAR CUFFING (same infiltrate as meninges)
2. ACUTE NEURONAL DAMAGE up to complete lysis with accompanying neuronophagia and inflammatory changes. In some conditions, surviving neurones contain cytoplasmic and/or nuclear inclusions.

To these basic changes, damage to myelin and glial tissue may be added, and small focal haemorrhages may be seen. The damage is effected in two ways:

1. By the direct effects of virus on cells.
2. By a host cell mediated and humoral response to the infected cell.

Diagnosis

Examination of the CSF is helpful in establishing a diagnosis of aseptic meningitis or meningoencephalitis.

NB The findings in tuberculous meningitis are very similar except that in tuberculous meningitis the CSF **sugar is low.**

The specific virus aetiology is more difficult to establish and in severe cases brain biopsy may be required.

Clinical associations and progress

In viral meningitis, the illness is mild with fever, headache and neck stiffness the main signs. Recovery is almost always complete.

In meningoencephalitis, signs of cerebral 'irritation' and neuronal damage are seen, e.g. mental confusion, delusion, stupor, convulsions and coma, and there may be localising signs. In mild cases, recovery is complete, but in more severe cases residual paralysis and other signs indicative of permanent brain damage may follow. Death in coma with respiratory failure occurs in very severe cases.

VIRUS INFECTIONS

HERPES SIMPLEX VIRUS (HSV) ENCEPHALITIS

This is the commonest form of severe acute viral encephalitis. It occurs in 2 forms:

1. In infancy, as part of a generalised HSV infection.
2. In adults, due to reactivation of the virus in the trigeminal ganglion.
   Most cases are sporadic but immunosuppression increases the risk.

The temporal lobes are most affected. Early treatment with antiviral drugs has now greatly reduced the previous high mortality.

HERPES ZOSTER (See also p.80)

This is a disease of adults, presenting as a painful vesicular rash, usually unilateral and affecting one or a few adjacent dermatomes only. It is due to recurrence of a latent varicella (chickenpox) infection.

Mechanism

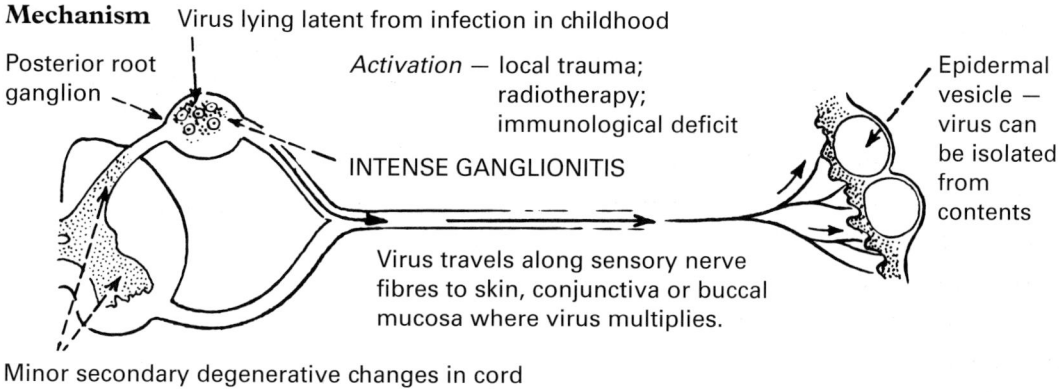

Sequels 1. An occasional sequel is intense pain with varying paraesthesia and anaesthesia long after the acute phase has healed.
2. In cases of Vth nerve herpes, serious damage to the eye may result.

RABIES

The rabies virus shows marked neurotropism and can infect most mammals. Various wild carnivores (fox, jackal, skunk, vampire bats) are the natural reservoir. Many human cases are contracted from dogs.

Mechanism

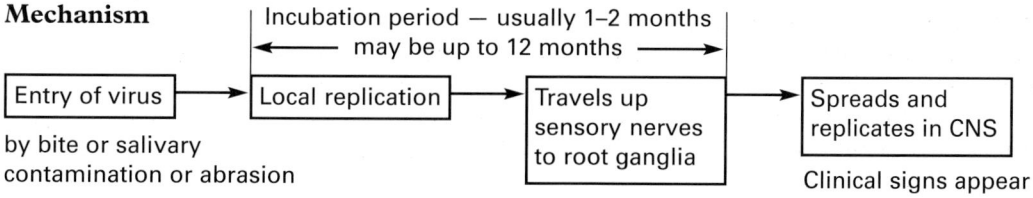

An unremitting encephalitis particularly affecting the grey matter is established. Diagnostic Negri bodies (virus inclusions) are found at autopsy in the pyramidal cells of the hippocampus and the Purkinje cells of the cerebellum.

Clinically, the encephalitis presents with extreme excitation of the sensory system. The classical hydrophobia (fear of water) is due to serious disturbance of the swallowing mechanism with muscular spasm. Without supportive therapy death occurs and is due to respiratory muscle spasm or paralysis.

VIRUS INFECTIONS

ENTEROVIRUSES

These are small RNA viruses (picornavirus group) and include POLIOVIRUSES, COXSACKIE VIRUSES and ECHOVIRUSES.

Infection is acquired by ingestion of faecally contaminated material followed by proliferation in the intestine. In only a small minority of infected cases does the virus pass the blood-brain barrier and cause disease of the CNS.

In addition to aseptic meningitis, the POLIOVIRUSES (and very occasionally Coxsackie and Echo viruses) cause the classical paralytic disease, **ANTERIOR POLIOMYELITIS**.

Pathological changes

The pathological changes are reflected in three clinical stages: (1) acute, (2) recovery and (3) permanent residual disability.

(1) **Acute** (up to 2 weeks)

Febrile illness — — — — — — — — — — — — — — Viraemia

The virus shows tropism for motor nerve cells, particularly in spinal cord

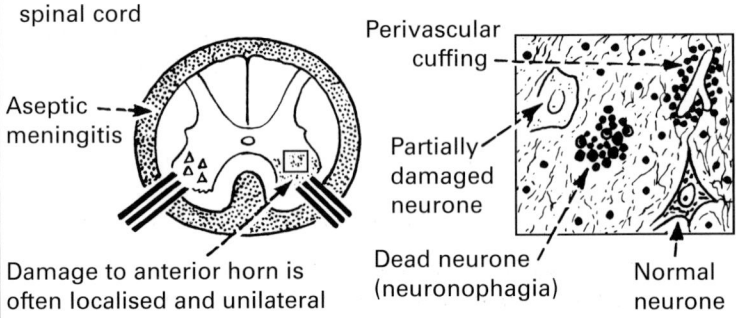

Sometimes RESPIRATORY paralysis — — — — — — — — — — — — Damage to bulbar motor nuclei

(2) **Recovery**
(Several weeks/months)
Paralyses improve — in mild cases functional recovery may be complete

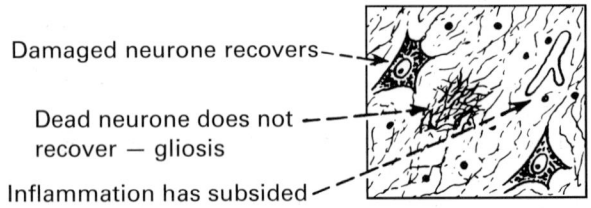

(3) **Permanent residual disability**
Wasting of muscles (neurogenic atrophy), varying deformities due to unopposed action of non-paralysed muscle

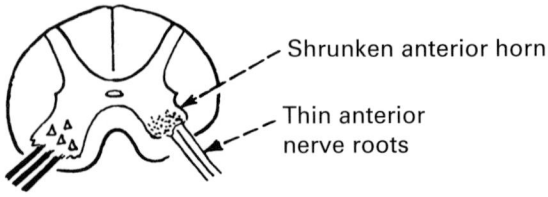

VIRUS INFECTIONS

Persistent virus infections

Subacute sclerosing panencephalitis is a very rare disorder due to persistent infection by the measles virus. It affects children and young adults and is usually fatal within 6 months. The sequence is probably as follows:

Infection by measles virus (usually under 1 year old) → USUALLY FULL RECOVERY.

↓

IN A VERY FEW INDIVIDUALS

↓

Persistent incomplete viral growth continues over approx. 10 years. — partially controlled by host defences despite high measles antibody titres.

↓

SUBACUTE ENCEPHALITIS → Numerous neurones contain nuclear inclusion bodies

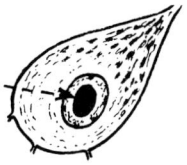

↓

DEMENTIA → DEATH

A similar disorder may follow congenital rubella infection.

Progressive Multi-focal Leukoencephalopathy

JC papovavirus, a member of the polyoma virus group, may infect the oligodendrocytes of adults who are immunosuppressed. A rapidly progressive demyelinating disease follows — with degenerative changes in the deep white matter.

HIV and the Brain

The central nervous system is commonly affected in patients with HIV infection.

(a) HIV infection of the brain. This may lead to a subacute encephalitis often with dementia.
(b) Opportunistic infections e.g. toxoplasma, fungi e.g. cryptococcus, candida and viruses e.g. cytomegalovirus.
(c) Tumours — especially cerebral lymphoma.

PRION DISEASES

This term covers a group of rare fatal brain diseases with similar histological features (SPONGIFORM change) and apparently caused by abnormalities of a cell surface protein — PRION PROTEIN (PrP) — caused by a gene on chromosome 20.

CREUTZFELDT-JACOB DISEASE (CJD) is a rare encephalopathy. The disease may be (i) **sporadic** (of unknown cause) or (ii) **acquired** through contact with infected material e.g. corneal grafts, pituitary derived hormones or (iii) **familial** due to mutation of the PrP gene.

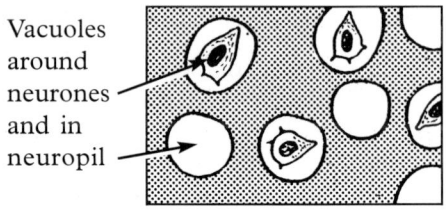

New-variant CJD is recently recognised. It occurs in younger patients, with early psychiatric symptoms and a longer clinical course. There is circumstantial evidence that ingestion of offal (particularly brain and spinal cord) from animals with **bovine spongiform encephalopathy** (**BSE**) is responsible

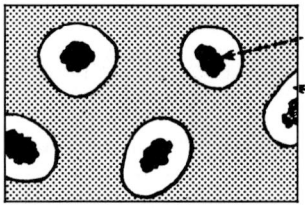

Fibrillary plaques of PrP are numerous, particularly in the occipital cortex.

Other prion diseases include KURU (historical) due to ingestion of human brain by cannibalism in New Guinea; GERSTMANN-STRAUSSLER-SCHEINKER disease; a familial dementia; BSE in cattle and SCRAPIE in sheep.

The **PRION HYPOTHESIS**

A normal cellular prion protein PrP^c is present in many cells, especially neurones. It is a glycoprotein anchored to the cell membrane. Abnormal PrPs bind to PrP^c and cause it to change its tertiary structure to an insoluble form in a β-pleated sheet (amyloid) configuration.

The diagram illustrates the ways in which normal PrP^c is converted to the abnormal form.

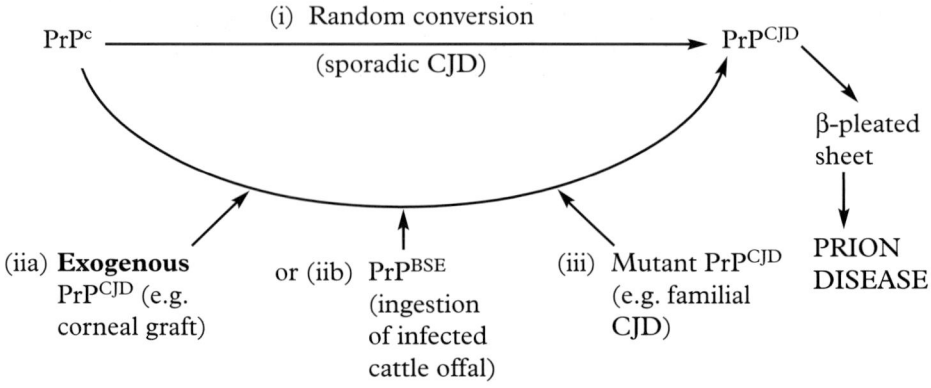

MISCELLANEOUS INFECTIONS AND INFESTATIONS

1. FUNGAL INFECTIONS

(a) **Primary infections.** In healthy adults, fungal infections are rare. Occasionally in the presence of heavy exposure to fungus, localised infection, often clinically insignificant, may occur and in very rare cases, CNS infection is a complication. In CRYPTOCOCCOSIS (*C. neoformans*), the fungus exhibits neurotropism and occasionally causes meningitis in otherwise healthy subjects.

(b) **Opportunistic infections** are becoming more common nowadays due to the use of immunosuppressive therapy and the increasing prevalence of AIDS. Various fungi including *Candida, Aspergillus nocardia* may cause serious cerebral damage.

2. PROTOZOAL INFECTIONS

(a) CEREBRAL MALARIA

Cerebral complications may occur in the severe acute malaria (falciparum type) which affects non-immune adults. Clinically, coma rapidly proceeds to death.

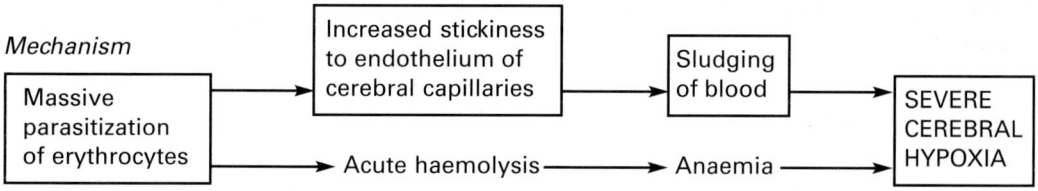

At autopsy the brain is swollen (oedema) and there may be petechial haemorrhages. Histologically, the capillaries are congested and malarial parasites and pigment easily seen.

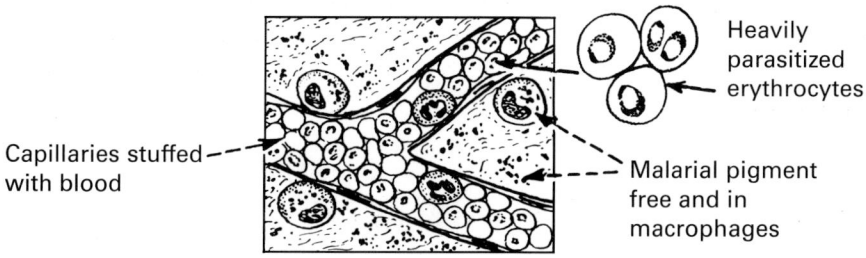

MISCELLANEOUS INFECTIONS AND INFESTATIONS

Protozoal infections (continued)

(b) **TOXOPLASMOSIS**

Although infection by T. gondii is common, serious nervous tissue damage is rare and is seen in two main circumstances. In both, it occurs as part of a systemic infection.

(i) In **congenital toxoplasmosis**, the infection is acquired by the fetus during a primary maternal infection.

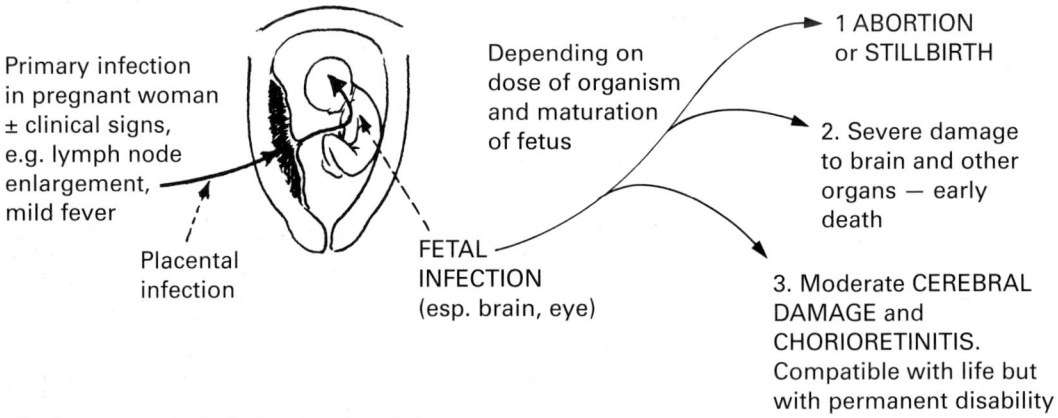

(ii) **Opportunistic infection** in adult.

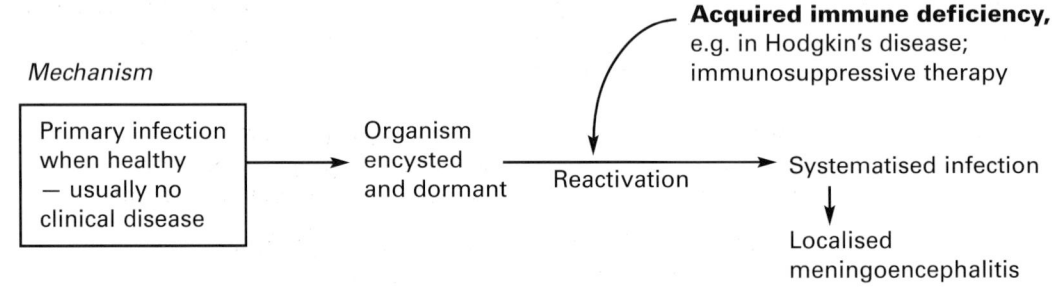

(c) **TRYPANOSOMIASIS (AFRICAN SLEEPING SICKNESS)**

T. brucei infection is transmitted to man from animal reservoirs by the Tsetse fly. The organism is neurotropic and a meningoencephalitis results. The infection is associated with excessive IgM production. The 'cuffing' infiltrate has a high component of plasma cells and also 'Mott' cells — plasma cells distended by eosinophilic globules (denatured Ig).

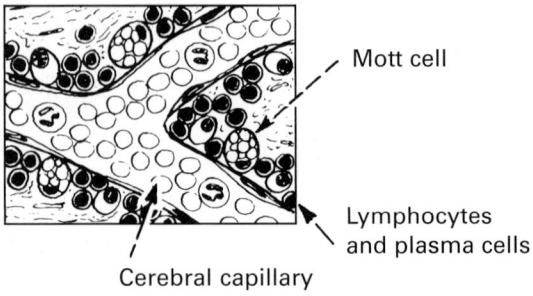

3. **METAZOAL INFESTATION**

Cysticercosis.

The larvae of *Taenia solium* may encyst in the brain and can be the cause of epilepsy.

Hydatid cyst — also occurs in the brain (see p. 366).

DEMYELINATING DISEASES

MULTIPLE SCLEROSIS (MS)

This is the commonest demyelinating disease — where the myelin sheath breaks down, leaving the axons healthy but with serious effects on their function.
Multiple sclerosis is a chronic disease of young adults.

The basic pathological change is an almost random scattering of 'plaques' of demyelination in the white matter.

The fibres of the optic nerve are often affected — retrobulbar neuritis

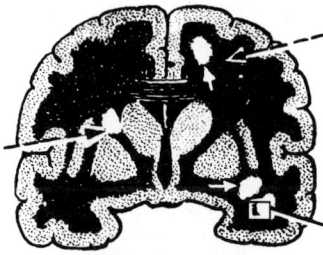

(Normal myelin stained black)

In the early stages, there may be round cell infiltrate, but in the usually seen late lesions inflammation is absent

Clinical associations
The neurological signs reflect *white matter damage* — upper motor neurone weakness and paralysis; incoordination; visual disturbances; paraesthesia. ('Grey matter' signs, e.g. aphasia, fits and muscle atrophy are rare.)

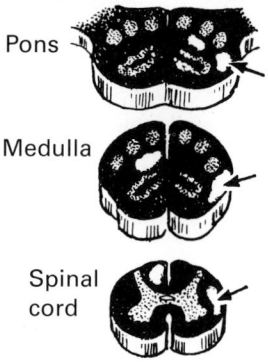

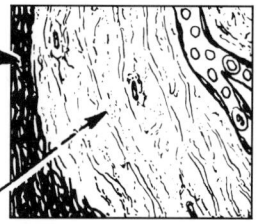

Plaque — no myelin; axons remain; glial fibres increased; few oligodendrocytes

Course of disease	*Onset*	*Progress over many years*
	Often acute; may be unnoticed.	Remission ... Relapse ... Remission → Incremental deterioration → Death

Variants are:
1. acute severe disease — rapid progress to death
2. chronic progression without remission
3. minimal signs with very long remissions.

Aetiology — This is unknown.

Geographically, the disease is common throughout temperate Europe and North America and is rare in the tropics.

A possible mechanism is:

LATENT VIRAL INFECTION
(? measles, ? EBV, ? Herpes)

GENETIC DISPOSITION
(High concordance in identical twins)

↓ ↓

Activation of CD_4^+ T cells

↓

Autoimmune attack on myelin

↓

DEMYELINATION

DEMYELINATING DISEASES

ACUTE DISSEMINATED ENCEPHALOMYELITIS

An acute encephalitis in which demyelination is a prominent and characteristic feature is a very rare sequel to many natural viral diseases and to vaccination, historically against smallpox and rabies.

Clinically, there is fever, headache, vomiting and drowsiness followed by coma. There may be clinical evidence of focal neurological damage. Pathological changes are widespread in the brain and cord and rapidly progressive.

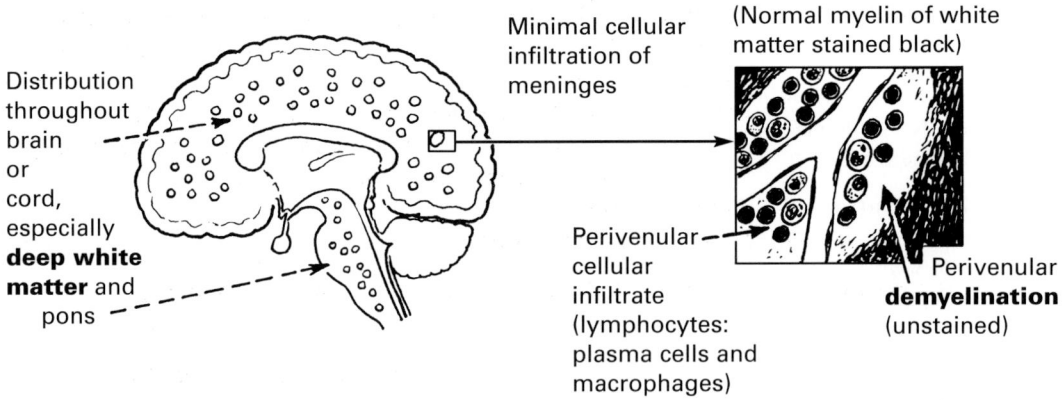

In **ACUTE HAEMORRHAGIC LEUKOENCEPHALITIS**, to these are added actual petechial haemorrhages from damaged vessels, particularly in the white matter; not all cases follow virus infection.

Mechanism. It is thought that in these disorders the damage to the myelin is not the result of direct virus attack but is an *autoimmune* reaction in which the antigen is a component of myelin and the virus in some unknown way acts as a trigger.

DISEASES due to ABNORMAL MYELIN

In this group of rare 'leukodystrophies', the molecular structure of myelin is abnormal due usually to abnormal or deficient enzyme action. Most cases are genetically determined, present in early life and progress fairly rapidly.

Abnormal metabolites which can be specifically identified accumulate in macrophages, glial cells and sometimes neurones.

e.g. 1. In **metachromatic leukodystrophy**, the accumulation of a *sulphatide* gives a metachromatic staining reaction and characteristic EM appearance.

2. In **Krabbe's disease** there are typical multinucleated histiocytes (called globoid cells) containing *cerebroside*.

In some disorders, when the loss of myelin is associated with marked gliosis, the name 'diffuse cerebral sclerosis' is applied.

PARKINSON'S DISEASE

This is a disease of the extrapyramidal system which links the higher motor centres and effector motor cells of the spinal cord. Important neurotransmitters are DOPAMINE and γ aminobutyric acid (GABA).

Aetiology — The disease occurs in 2 main circumstances:

(a) ***Idiopathic:*** occurring in people over 50 years; nowadays not infrequent in an ageing population — 1 in 200 in those over 70.

(b) ***Secondary:***
1. **Postencephalitic** (historically) i.e. as a sequel to encephalitis lethargica which occurred in epidemic form in the 1920s. Very few patients now survive.
2. **Drug induced.** The use of neuroleptic drugs may induce the syndrome temporarily (occasionally permanently), by disturbing the balance of the chemical transmitters.
3. **Arteriopathy.**
4. **Heavy metal poisoning.**

Clinically, **Parkinsonism** illustrates the classical features of extrapyramidal damage.

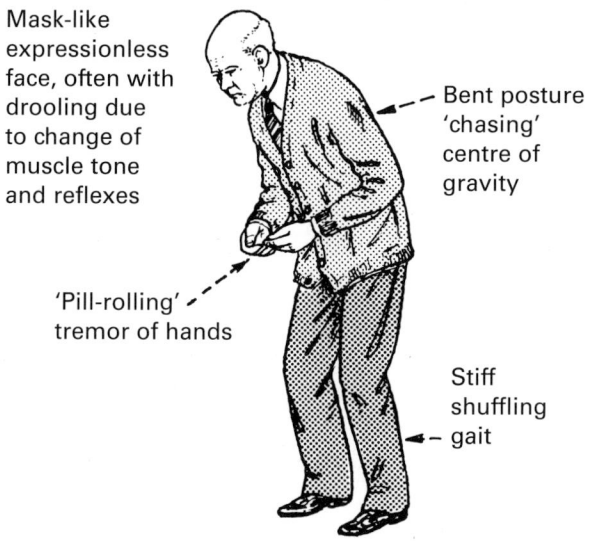

Pathological mechanism
In all cases of long-standing Parkinsonism of any type, degenerative changes are seen in the extrapyramidal nuclei. In particular, there is depigmentation of the substantia nigra.

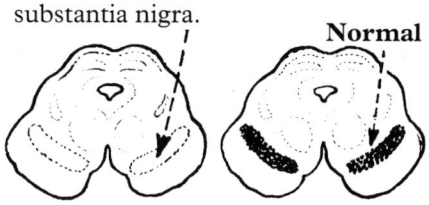

Also there is a deficiency of DOPAMINE in affected nuclei.

Histologically, there is loss of neurones, and the surviving nerve cells contain inclusions known as Lewi bodies.
Other extrapyramidal disorders include the choreas, of which there are 2 main types. Sydenham's chorea occurs in children with rheumatic fever, while chorea is a manifestation in some patients with Huntington's disease.

MISCELLANEOUS DISORDERS

NUTRITIONAL AND METABOLIC DISORDERS (ENCEPHALOPATHIES)

In the last analysis, all disorders in this group are mediated by disturbed neuronal metabolism, so that exact classification may present some difficulty. However, it is convenient to consider them in 2 broad groups.

1. NUTRITIONAL DEFICIENCY

The vitamins of the B group are important coenzymes in several intracellular oxidative pathways. Deficiency, which may arise from primary malnutrition but more commonly in association with alcohol abuse, is the cause of degenerations of the brain, spinal cord and peripheral nerves.

Wernicke's encephalopathy

Clinically, this condition presents with disturbances of consciousness, ataxia and visual disturbances, and without prompt treatment progresses to death in coma.

In Western countries, chronic alcoholism is usually present; often a particularly heavy bout of drinking precipitates the condition.

Chronic alcoholism → Poor diet → NUTRITIONAL DEFICIENCY of vit B complex, esp. THIAMIN.

Bout of heavy drinking → Vomiting → Accentuates → NUTRITIONAL DEFICIENCY of vit B complex, esp. THIAMIN.

The blood PYRUVATE level is raised.

The lesions, which are focal, consist of glial proliferations with varying neurone loss. Petechial haemorrhages may be seen.

The lesions have a characteristic anatomical distribution:

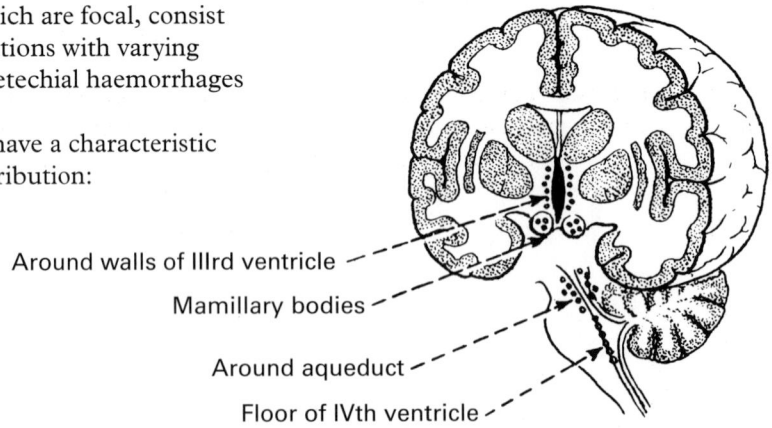

Prompt treatment with thiamin minimises the damage, but if treatment is omitted or delayed, permanent damage results. At autopsy, there is visible shrinkage of the mamillary bodies.

MISCELLANEOUS DISORDERS

2. METABOLIC DISORDERS

In the following examples, the metabolic defect causes neurological disorder, but in addition, other organs are seriously disturbed.

(a) ***Aminoacidopathies***
A wide variety of hepatic enzyme defects in the complex metabolism of amino acids have now been described. When neurological damage occurs, it is essentially non-specific and developing in the immediate postnatal period, a critical time in the development of the brain which leads to ***mental retardation.***

Phenylketonuria is an example.

The importance of this disease is that the effects can be prevented by dietary restriction of phenylalanine-containing substances, provided the treatment is begun within 60 days of birth.

Mechanism

Liver

Primary defect: ABSENCE of PHENYLALANINE HYDROXYLASE

↓

Blood

Increased PHENYLALANINE and its derivatives

→ **Kidney**

PHENYLPYRUVIC ACID in URINE — **'PHENYLKETONURIA'**

→ **Brain**

Non-specific damage: spongiosis, gliosis, demyelination — **Mental retardation**

(b) In the ***neuronal storage diseases***, which usually present during the first decade, deficiency of lysozomal enzymes leads to accumulation of intermediate metabolites in the neurones. The diagnosis of the condition often depends on the identification of the abnormal metabolite by histochemistry or EM.

Tay-Sach's disease (amaurotic familial idiocy) is an illustrative example.

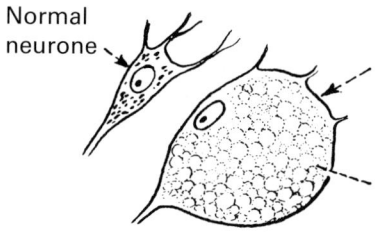

Clinically, there is progressive mental deterioration, coma or death

Note: Involvement of the retinal ganglion cells causes blindness — a *cherry red spot* at the macula is seen.

In these disorders, other organs may be mildly affected by the enzyme defect but the neurological effects are predominant.

DISEASES OF SPINAL CORD

In purely spinal lesions, basic disease processes have important anatomical and functional implications. Lack of space for expansion produces important compression effects. Examples are:

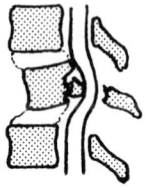

Fracture/ dislocation of vertebra

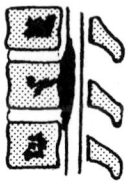

Tumour (usually secondary) in vertebrae growing into canal

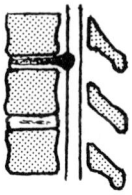

Prolapse of intervertebral disc

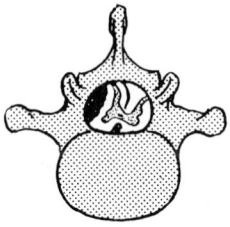

Tumour of meninges or nerve sheath

Effects

Normal

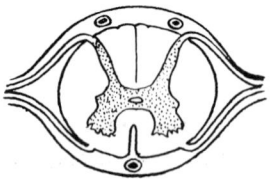

Cord, nerve roots and blood vessels loosely suspended in CSF 'water bath'

Compression

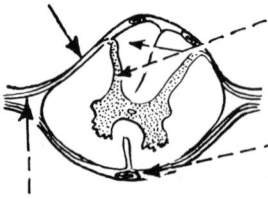

(1) *Damage to neurones and nerve tracts*
May be focal but is often transverse and complete

(2) *Vascular compression*
Impairment of circulation may be actual infarction; this is important particularly in traumatic cases

(3) *Damage to nerve roots* (radiculitis); a common complication of spondylosis

At the level of the lesion, there is loss of the sensory and motor connections which constitute the spinal reflex.

In addition, severance of the longitudinal tracts cuts off the cerebral connections to all parts below the lesion.

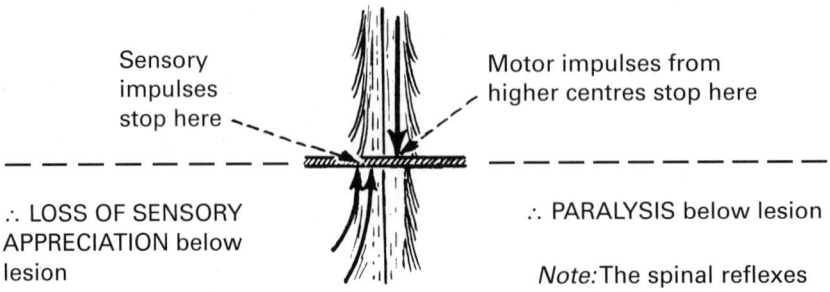

DISEASES OF SPINAL CORD

ASCENDING AND DESCENDING DEGENERATIONS

The long tract fibres which are cut off from their neurones progressively degenerate.

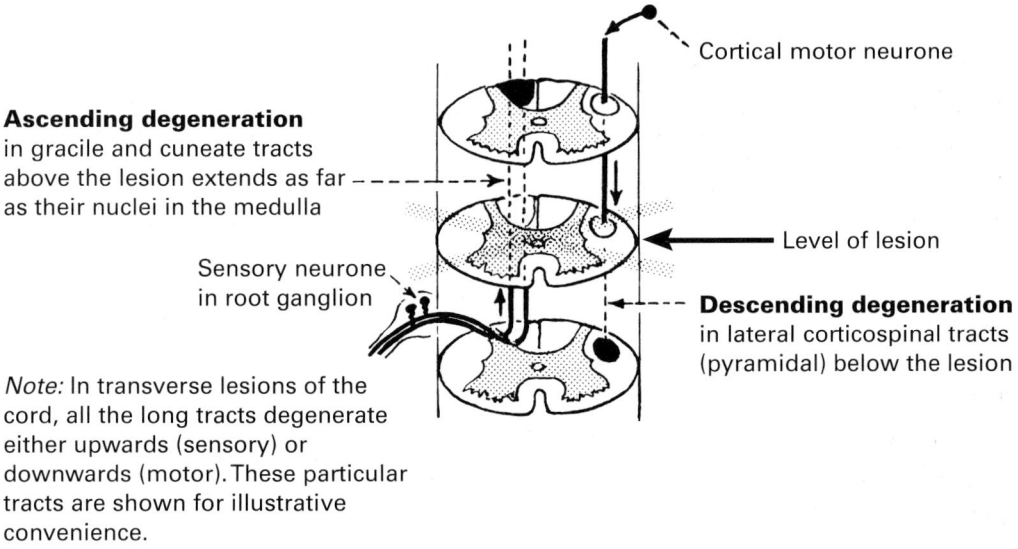

The commonest example of **descending degeneration** is seen following cerebral infarction involving the internal capsule; the degeneration extends from the lesion along the corticospinal axons to their terminations in the anterior horn.

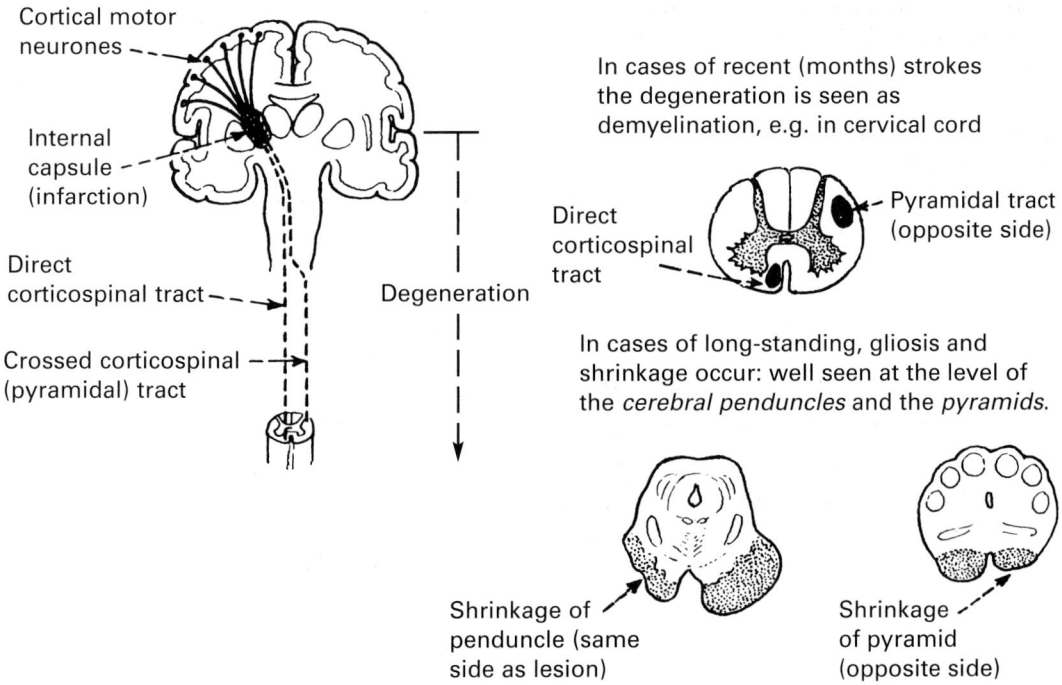

DISORDERS OF MOTOR PATHWAYS

The concept of upper and lower motor neuronal activity, based on anatomical and physiological evidence, has great clinical value in diagnosis.

The **upper motor neurones** (UMN) synapse with the **lower motor neurones** (LMN)

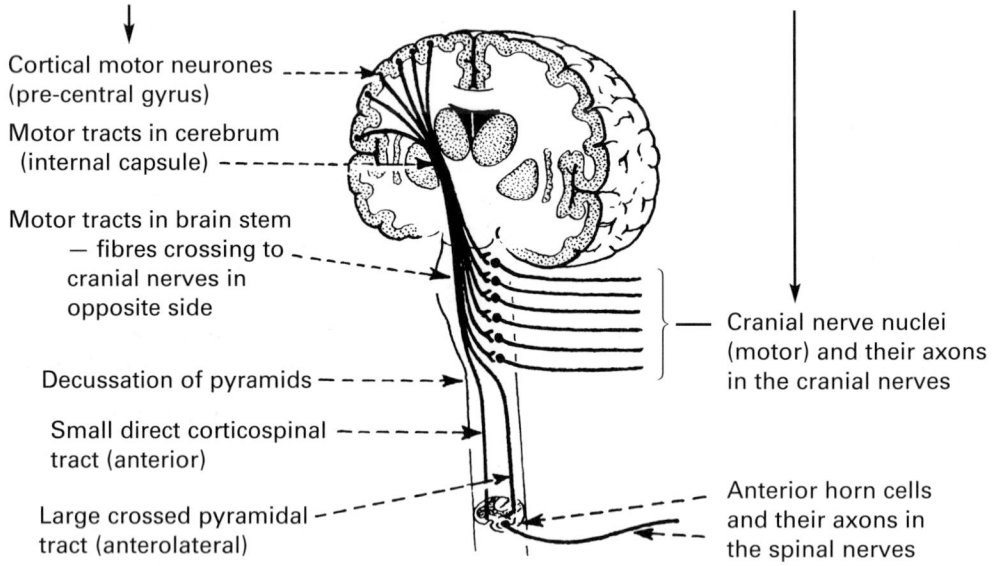

It will be appreciated that in its long course from the cerebral cortex to the anterior horn, the upper motor neurone is susceptible to damage from a variety of disease processes acting at various sites. The lower motor neurone may be damaged in the cord or in the peripheral nerve. Important illustrative examples are:

Upper motor neurone damage

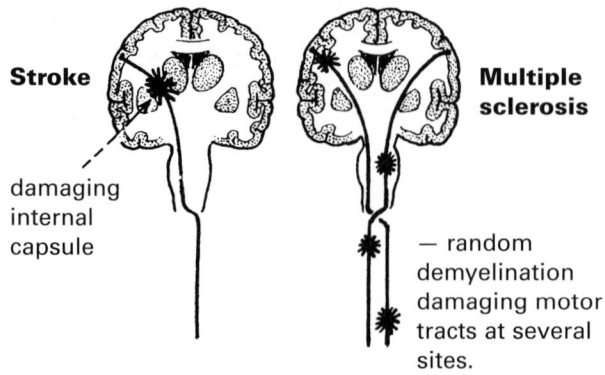

Note: Clinically, tendon jerks are increased and the plantar reflex is extensor.

Lower motor neurone damage

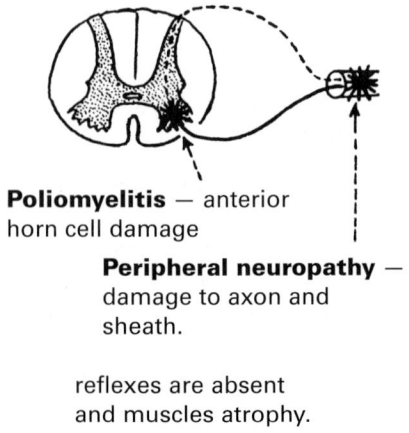

reflexes are absent and muscles atrophy.

MOTOR NEURONE DISEASE

In contrast to these motor disorders, secondary to known diseases, motor neurone disease is of unknown aetiology occurring in adults with a predominant incidence in males.

The basic lesion is a specific progressive degeneration of both cortical and spinal motor neurones with its accompanying pathological effects. There are variations depending on the relative involvement of the upper and lower motor neurone components and the sites of initial damage but there may be considerable overlap.

Historically, 3 main patterns were identified.:

1. In **progressive muscular atrophy**, as the name implies, the main signs are of neurogenic atrophy due to degeneration of the anterior horn cells (LMN).

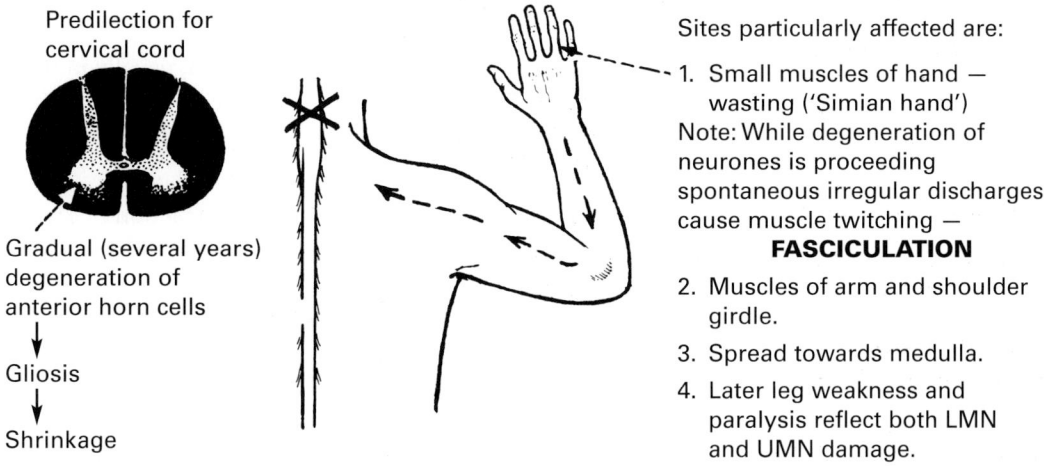

2. In **Amyotrophic lateral sclerosis** there is both UMN and LMN damage: 'lateral sclerosis' indicates the degeneration of the pyramidal tracts.

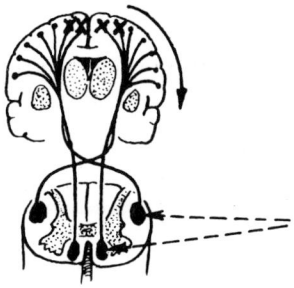

The degeneration affects the cortical motor cells — particularly those supplying the lower limbs but spreading over a few years to involve the neck and head centres. Voluntary movements of the face, jaw and tongue muscles are defective.

Corticospinal tracts showing degeneration and, later, gliosis.

The lesions are very rarely pure UMN type even initially, and with progression, the LMN lesions increase.

3. **Progressive bulbar palsy**

In a few cases, the disease begins with signs of cranial nerve dysfunction — swallowing and facial movements are impaired.

Progress

In motor neurone disease after a long progressive illness, the stage is reached when the bulbar degeneration is severe enough to prevent elimination of secretions from the respiratory tract. Death is usually due to aspiration bronchopneumonia or respiratory failure.

MIXED MOTOR AND SENSORY DISORDERS

SUBACUTE COMBINED DEGENERATION OF CORD

Due specifically to vit B_{12} deficiency. If replacement therapy is begun early enough, there is restoration to normal.

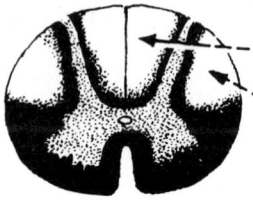

Degenerated tracts		Effects
1. Posterior columns	→	Sensory loss (vibration and proprioception): ataxia
2. Corticospinal tracts	→	Upper motor neurone damage — spastic paralysis

SYRINGOMYELIA

In this condition, a glial-lined cystic space gradually expands within the cord, usually in the cervical region. The pathogenesis is not certain, but it is suggested that the lesion is essentially an expansion of the central canal associated with a mild developmental abnormality of the distal end of the IVth ventricle. Some cases follow spinal trauma.

Effects

Damage to sensory fibres decussating in the cord. Loss of temperature and touch in local segments **(dissociated anaesthesia).**

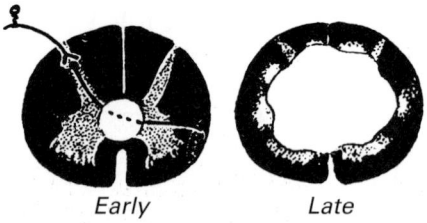

Destruction of grey matter and gradual affection of long tracts. Loss of local reflexes. Severe sensory loss. Spastic paralysis.

FRIEDRICH'S ATAXIA

In this disease, which has a strong familial basis (the FRATAXIN gene on chromosome 9), there is progressive degeneration of sensory (spinocerebellar tracts and posterior columns) and motor tracts. Severe cases begin in childhood and progress to death in a few years. Postural and skeletal deformities complicate the progressive ataxia and paralysis. In some cases there is a cardiomyopathy with arrhythmia.

This disease is mentioned to illustrate the **spinocerebellar degenerations**, a large group of related disorders, usually familial, in which there is neuronal and tract degeneration particularly affecting gait, posture, equilibrium and movement. There is sometimes optic nerve and retinal damage and intellectual disturbance.

SENSORY DISORDERS

In **TABES DORSALIS**, a tertiary manifestation of syphilis in which the lumbar cord is commonly affected, there is degeneration of the posterior nerve roots and columns.

Skin — touch:
Joints and muscles — proprioception

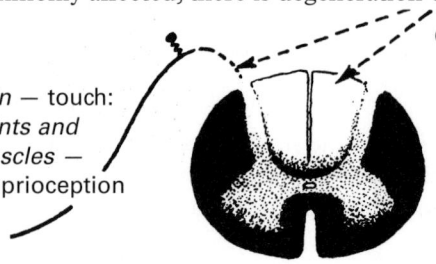

Clinically

Loss of vibration sense and reflexes
Ataxia
Trophic skin ulcers
Severe joint derangement (Charcot p.635)

Additional features

Cranial and sympathetic nerve involvement — disturbance of pupillary reflex

Painful visceral crises

THE PERIPHERAL NERVES

The nerves are a mixture of different types of fibre, myelinated and non-myelinated of varying thickness and length, sub-serving sensory and motor functions. In most disorders, both functions are disturbed, but in the early stages, selective damage to particular fibre types is often seen.

There are numerous disorders which can be classified as follows:

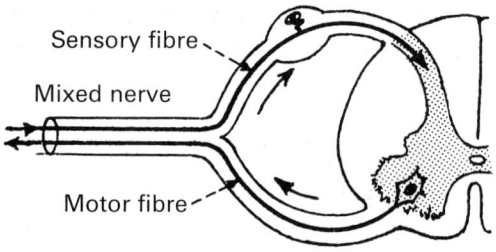

In affection of one or other nerve roots pure motor or sensory disturbance may be seen separately.

(i) Direct damage to peripheral nerve — followed by regeneration or formation of a traumatic neuroma (p. 57).

(ii) The **NEUROPATHIES**
The term neuropathy is preferred to neuritis since most disorders are not essentially inflammatory.

There are two broad groups:

1. ***Parenchymatous***
The axon and its closely associated Schwann cells and myelin sheath are affected primarily; note the myelin is produced and maintained by Schwann cells. Most disorders of this type are due to toxic or metabolic disturbances and affect many nerves — POLYNEUROPATHY.

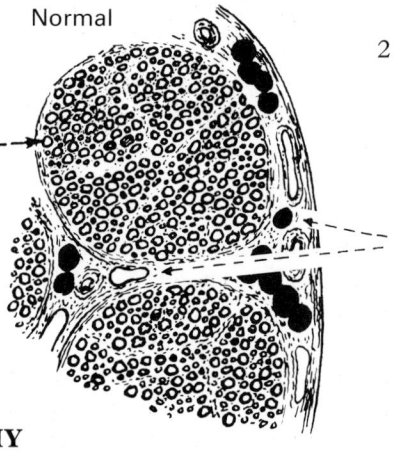

2. ***Interstitial***
The damage is primarily in the blood vessels or supporting tissues (epi-, peri- and endoneurium). In this type, single nerves or several nerves may be affected, depending on the nature of the interstitial damage.

INTERSTITIAL NEUROPATHY

Mononeuropathy

Single nerves are subject to damage by compression. The nerve structures may be damaged directly or more usually as a result of ischaemia.

Examples are the carpal tunnel syndrome in which the median nerve is compressed between the carpal bones and ligaments, and following drunken stupor where abnormal postures have compressed nerves. The cranial nerves within the skull are subject to such distortions leading to degeneration where intracranial pressure is increased.

Prolapsed intervertebral disc (slipped disc) is a common cause of compression damage to nerve roots in the lumbar region particularly.

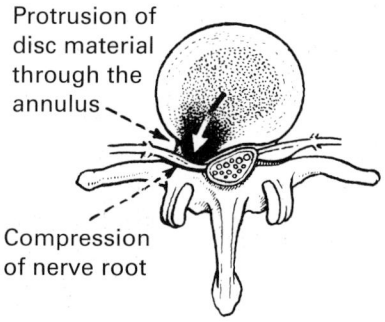

THE NEUROPATHIES

Mononeuritis multiplex

Abnormal function of several nerves is seen. Arteritis is a common cause. Since the vascular lesions are patchy so too is the nerve involvement. The mechanism is essentially ischaemic.

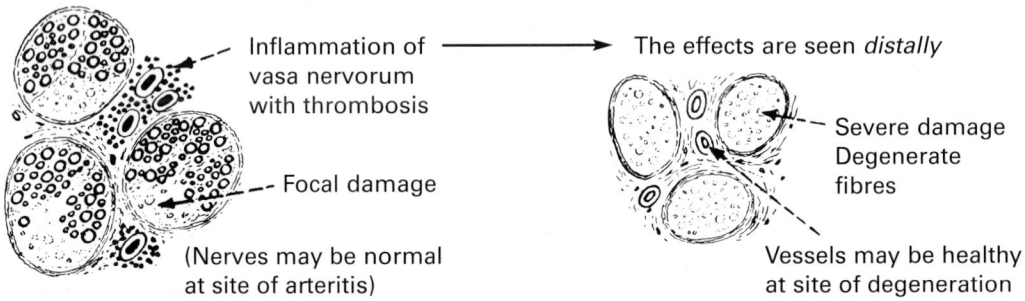

POLYNEUROPATHY

In this, there is extensive and symmetrical disturbance of function, often peripheral in distribution and especially affecting the legs. There are many causes:

Toxic — diphtheria; lead; arsenic; drugs used in medicine.
Deficiency states — particularly vit B complex deficiency causing Beri-Beri.
Metabolic disorders — **diabetes mellitus**, porphyria, metachromatic leukodystrophy, associated with malignant tumours, in uraemia treated by dialysis.

There are two main mechanisms of degeneration.

1. Primary degeneration occurs patchily in Schwann cells; axon degeneration follows slowly. This is the more important mechanism.

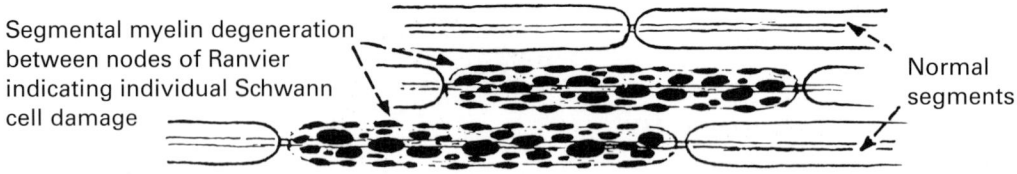

2. Degeneration of the axon with concomitant demyelination. This is closely allied to Wallerian degeneration following nerve transection.

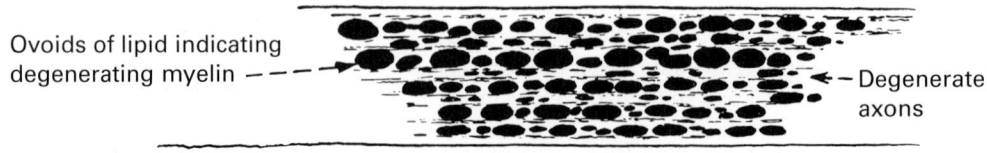

A very common form is a complication of **diabetes mellitus**: there are two distinct mechanisms:

1. A symmetrical polyneuropathy
   — mainly sensory and autonomic
   — metabolic in origin.
2. A focal neuropathy
   — often sensory and motor.
   — vascular in origin due to small vessel disease.

THE NEUROPATHIES

Other forms of neuropathy include:

The Guillain-Barré syndrome.
The onset is acute, often following 7–21 days after a mild non-specific febrile illness. There are peripheral neurological signs with usually a motor (LMN) deficit predominant, beginning in the lumbar nerves and ascending fairly rapidly (ascending paralysis) so that respiratory failure, requiring supportive treatment, is a serious complication.

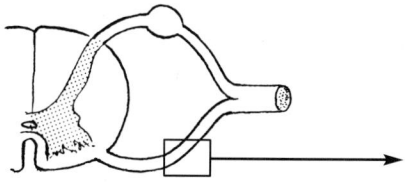

The nerve roots are predominantly affected.

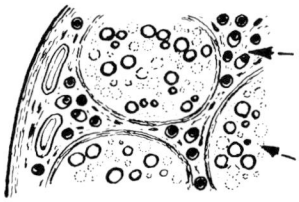

The interstitial tissues are infiltrated with lymphocytes and plasma cells

There is variable axonal and myelin degeneration

The CSF usually contains excessive protein but few cells.

The disease probably has an immunological basis and is allied to acute encephalitis (see p. 580).

Progress: usually recovery is complete.

Bell's palsy
This is a unilateral facial weakness of sudden onset. The cause is not known with certainty, but some cases are associated with draughts and chilling. Reactivation of Herpes Zoster virus may be responsible.

The mechanism is thought to be inflammation with swelling and compression of the facial nerve in its course in the bone adjacent to the internal auditory meatus.

Progress in 75% of cases, there is recovery in about 4–8 weeks.

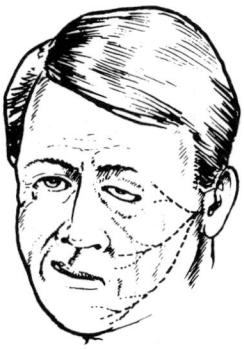

Note drooping and loss of facial expression on paralysed side. Facial muscles pull across the mid line — mouth is distorted.

Leprosy
In the lepromatous form, there is a diffuse neuropathy involving the peripheries (which are at the lower temperature required for proliferation of *M. leprae*).

There is a low grade chronic inflammation of the nerve sheaths associated with fibrosis and nerve fibre degeneration.

HYDROCEPHALUS

In hydrocephalus, the volume of the CSF is increased and the ventricles are dilated. In the majority of cases, there is an increase in intracranial pressure. Three possible theoretical **mechanisms** are considered.

1. **Overproduction of CSF**
   The choroid plexus will secrete more CSF to compensate for any external leak, but overproduction is not a cause of hydrocephalus.
2. **Obstruction to the flow of CSF is the common** mechanism.

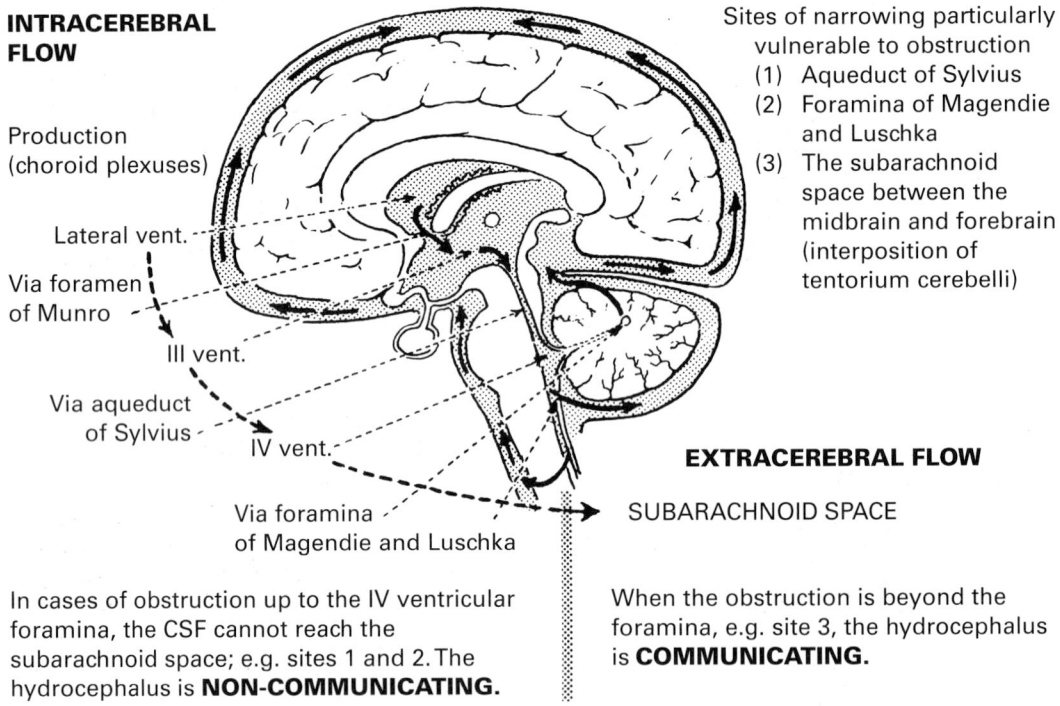

3. **Defective absorption of CSF** is a rare mechanism.

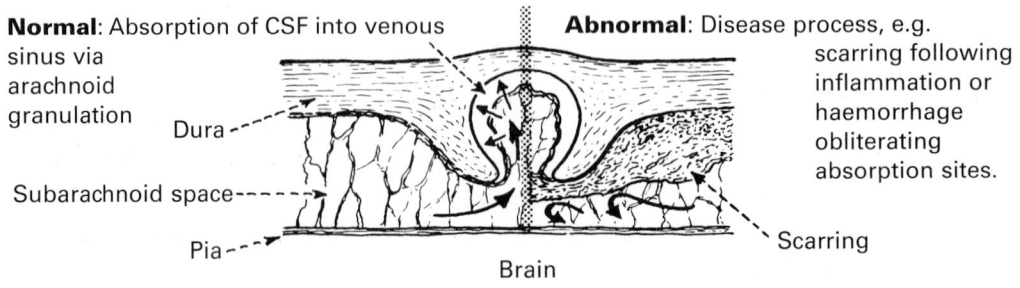

HYDROCEPHALUS

CAUSES

The diseases causing hydrocephalus fall into two groups:

1. **Congenital (developmental) abnormalities**

The common conditions are:

(a) ***The Arnold-Chiari malformation***

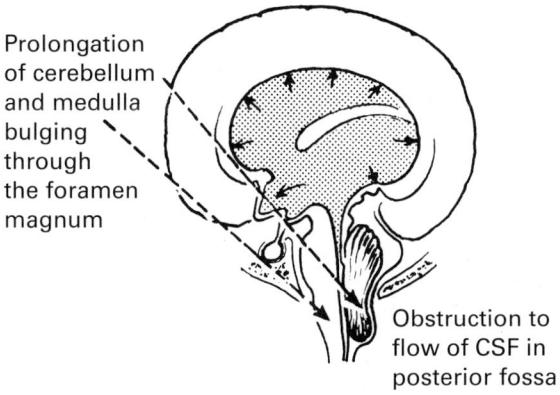

(b) ***Congenital stenosis or atresia of aqueduct of Sylvius***

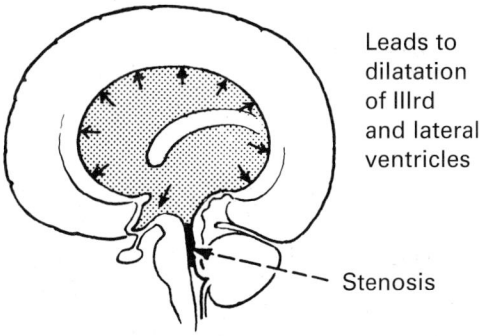

Associated with spina bifida, usually ***meningomyelocele***

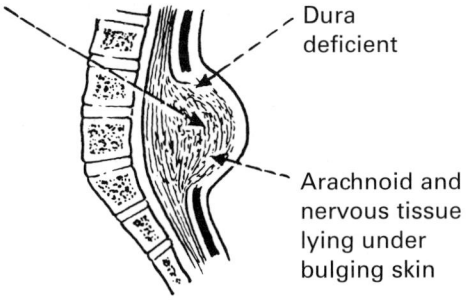

(c) ***Atresia of foramina of Magendie and Luschka***

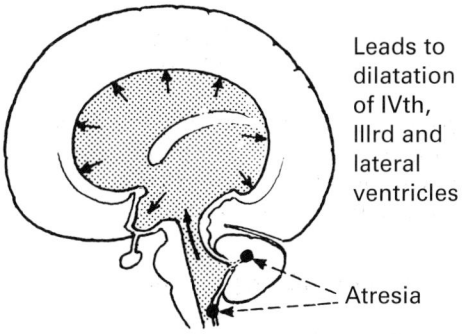

2. **Acquired hydrocephalus**

Of the many possible conditions causing hydrocephalus, the following are most common: (a) cerebral tumour (primary or secondary) and (b) scarring of the meninges following meningitis or subarachnoid haemorrhage.

As already explained, whether any particular disease produces hydrocephalus depends largely on the site affected.

HYDROCEPHALUS

EFFECTS

In **the infant and young child**, the pliable skull expands to accommodate the enlarging brain — but these extreme changes do not occur if an effective shunt is inserted.

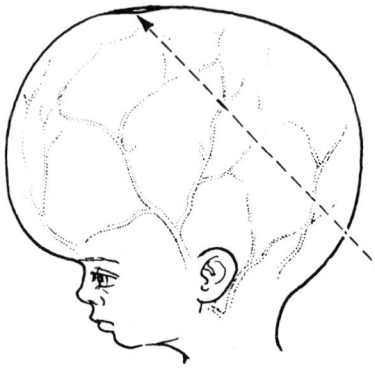

There is great enlargement of the head with prominent scalp veins, and forehead overhanging the eyes. The fontanelle remains open

Clinically mental deficiency is common

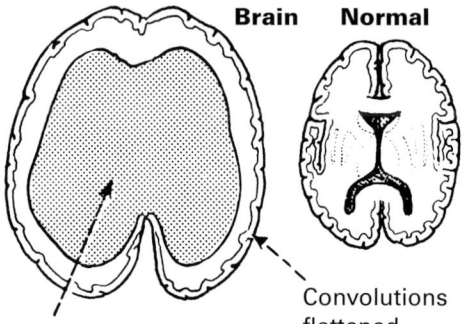

In **the older child and adult**, enlargement of the brain is prevented by the inability of the skull to expand. The main change is dilatation of the ventricles associated with the effects on the brain of increased intracranial pressure.

SPECIAL TYPES OF HYDROCEPHALUS

1 In cases of generalised cerebral atrophy, the ventricular system enlarges to compensate for the loss of cerebral tissue. This also happens locally when cerebral tissue is lost, e.g. following infarction.

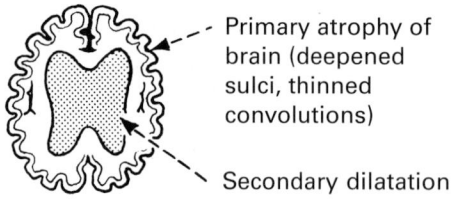

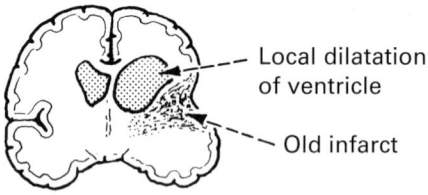

No increase in pressure is involved and the pathological and clinical effects wholly reflect the primary loss of cerebral tissue. The condition is sometimes called **secondary hydrocephalus**.

2. **Normal pressure hydrocephalus**

In this rare condition, progressive mental deterioration (dementia) and disturbances of gait and micturition are associated with ventricular dilatation. Random sampling often shows normal CSF pressures but continuous monitoring shows significant intermittent increases. (Some prefer the title Intermittent Hydrocephalus.) The diagnosis has assumed importance because in some cases CSF shunt procedures have arrested the progress. The aetiology is obscure.

DEVELOPMENTAL ABNORMALITIES

Developmental abnormalities of the brain and cranium are relatively common, varying from virtually complete absence of cerebral substance (anencephaly), with associated failure of formation of the cranial meninges and the skull, to minor local malformations, e.g. meningocele and encephalocele. Often they are associated with congenital defects in other parts of the body.

SPINA BIFIDA

In the lumbosacral and cervical regions particularly, local defects in the development and closure of the neutral tube and vertebral arches result in spina bifida.

(a) **Spina bifida occulta**

Normal skin covering

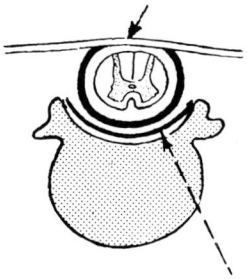

Vertebral arches and dura deficient — may be associated with minor nerve defects — particularly affecting bladder function

(b) **Meningocele**

Skin may be thin at apex

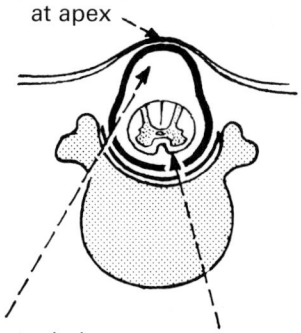

Rounded sac containing CSF

Cord in normal position

(c) **Meningomyelocele**

Skin usually defective

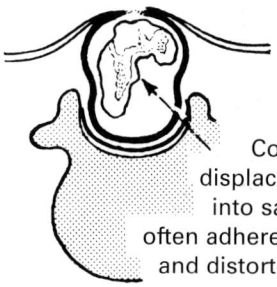

Cord displaced into sac: often adherent and distorted

May be associated with serious nervous deficit — especially in legs, bladder.

Infection through the deficient skin is a serious complication.

There is strong evidence that folic acid deficiency is the cause of these defects.

Diagnosis in utero

α-fetoprotein leaks through the defective skin covering and increased amounts are found in the amniotic fluid. Ultrasonography may also reveal the defect.

Complications

In addition to severe neurological deficits which are aggravated by infection, an important complication even in minor defects is **HYDROCEPHALUS**.

TUMOURS OF THE NERVOUS SYSTEM

The following scheme illustrates the various non-specific clinicopathological effects of a tumour within the skull.

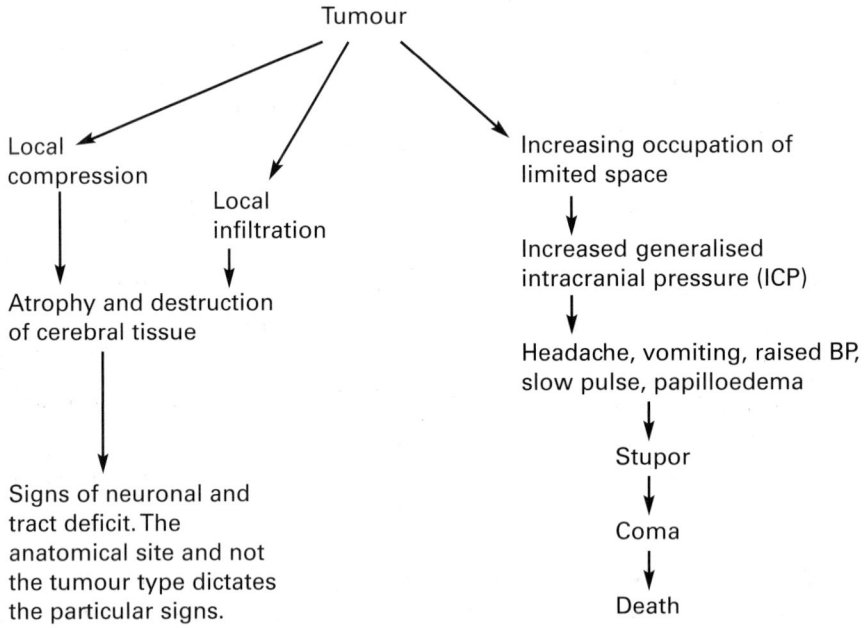

An important factor which materially influences the relative importance of each of these effects is the rate of tumour growth.

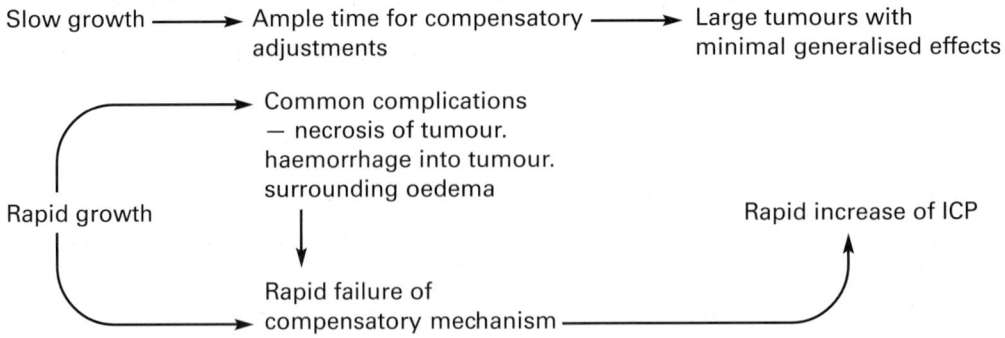

Tumours will be considered in a simplified form under the following broad headings:

1. Secondary neoplasms.
2. Neoplasms of neuroectodermal origin.
3. Neoplasms arising in supporting tissue (mesodermal).
4. Neoplasms and swellings of developmental origin.
5. Neoplasms of nerve sheaths.

SECONDARY BRAIN TUMOURS

In the general population the incidence of metastatic cerebral tumour is much higher than that of primary cerebral neoplasm. The two most common primary sites are lung and breast, but any malignant tumour can metastasise to the brain.

The common presentation is in the form of multiple, well-delineated spherical nodules, randomly distributed

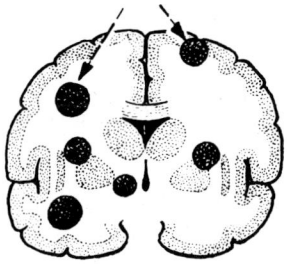

Only occasionally is there a single nodule.

A less common distribution is by permeation of the subarachnoid space — **meningeal carcinomatosis.**

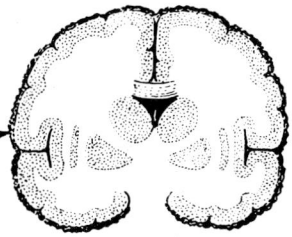

Brain surface covered by a layer of tumour tissue

Carcinoma, leukaemia and lymphoreticular neoplasms may spread in this way (malignant cells may be seen in the CSF).

Secondary tumours may cause serious spinal damage by destroying the integrity of the vertebrae. The prostate and cervix, in addition to lung, breast and kidney, are usual primary sites.

In contrast to tumours causing neurological damage by their physical presence and growth, less commonly *non-metastatic effects of cancer* are seen.

There is a wide range of disorders which are conveniently divided into two groups:

1. Neurological disorders in which the mechanism and association with cancer are known:

Examples	***Mechanism caused by cancer***
Opportunistic infections	Immune depression
Metabolic and hormonal imbalance	Destruction of organs, e.g. liver, kidney Inappropriate secretion
Vascular accidents	Coagulation disorders

2. A group of conditions in which the mechanism is not known. This includes dementia, encephalopathy, cerebellar degeneration, neuropathies and a syndrome mimicking myasthenia gravis (Lambert-Eaton syndrome).

PRIMARY BRAIN TUMOURS

GLIOMAS

Astrocytoma

Derived from astrocytes, these are the commonest primary neurological tumours. They vary in growth rate and differentiation over a wide spectrum. All ages are affected, with a peak at 35 years of age.

Low grade astrocytoma is slow growing and the cells are well differentiated forming many fibres. In childhood, these tumours often occur in the cerebellum but, in adults, the cerebral hemispheres are usually affected.

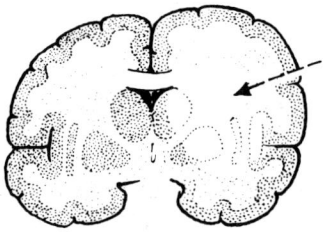

The tumour which has ill-defined margins grows irregularly into the surrounding brain tissues and only latterly causes increased ICP

Note enlargement of hemisphere by ill defined growth.

Because they have ill-defined margins, these tumours are difficult to eradicate and slowly but inexorably grow and eventually cause death.

Transformation to a high grade astrocytoma may occur.

Glioblastoma multiforme is a highly malignant tumour with no well differentiated area and can be regarded as a very poorly differentiated astrocytoma.

The cells are pleomorphic and rapidly growing: proliferation of blood vessels is a striking feature.

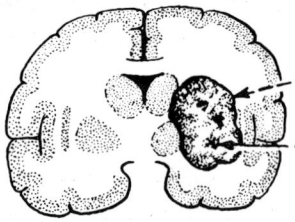

Tumour may look well defined, contrasting with the compressed adjacent cerebral tissue

Necrosis and haemorrhage are common

The prognosis of these patients is very poor.

Oligodendroglioma

These tumours, derived from oligodendroglia, tend to occur in the cerebrum of adults and may present clinically with epilepsy. They usually are slow growing and often show calcification.

Ependymoma

These are also rare and arise from the lining of the ventricles and central spinal cord. They may block the flow of CSF and cause hydrocephalus.

Note: The above gliomas very rarely metastasise outside the nervous system.

TUMOURS OF THE NERVOUS SYSTEM

TUMOURS of NEURONAL TYPE CELLS

Fully differentiated neurones can neither multiply nor give rise to neoplasms. Tumours of this type, derived from primitive nerve precursors (blast cells), are seen in infancy and childhood before completion of differentiation.

They display a basic histological pattern.

Closely aggregated small cells with hyperchromatic round or oval nuclei and scanty cytoplasm

Rosettes, the centres of which are formed by rudimentary nerve fibres, are often seen and represent a step towards differentiation

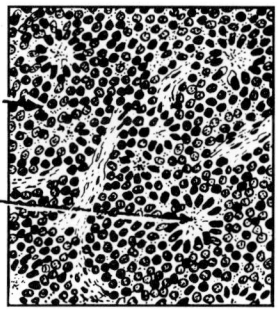

Depending on the site of origin, specific names are given:

Cerebellum:
MEDULLOBLASTOMA

Retina:
RETINOBLASTOMA

Sympathetic ganglia (including adrenal medulla):
NEUROBLASTOMA and GANGLIONEUROMA

Medulloblastoma

This highly malignant tumour arises in and spreads over the surface of the cerebellum, often invading the IVth ventricle. Diffuse tumour nodules may develop on surfaces bathed by CSF.

Retinoblastoma

These tumours, which arise in the retina and cause blindness, spread into the optic nerves. Some cases are clearly seen as a hereditary disease and are bilateral: others arise sporadically due to a genetic mutation after conception and are usually unilateral. The genetic mechanism is now known to be a defective (or missing) tumour suppressor gene [the Retinoblastoma (RB) gene] on chromosome 13.

Neuroblastoma

These tumours occasionally occur in, but more commonly arise from, the precursor cells of the autonomic system; the majority occur in the adrenal medulla. They grow rapidly to become large, soft, haemorrhagic and necrotic retroperitoneal masses soon metastasising to lymph nodes, liver and bones.

Ganglioneuroma

In some cases, neuronal differentiation proceeds, and mature ganglion cells appear and nerve fibres are formed. In some instances, differentiation is complete; such tumours are found in adult life particularly in the mediastinum where they may grow slowly, eventually causing signs due to their size, but never metastasising. With intermediate degrees of differentiation the name ganglioneuroblastoma is used.

TUMOURS OF THE NERVOUS SYSTEM

Meningiomas

These are thought to arise from arachnoid granulations and so are found most commonly adjacent to venous sinuses. They account for 15–20% of intracranial tumours. They are slow growing and essentially 'benign'. A few more aggressive may metastasise.

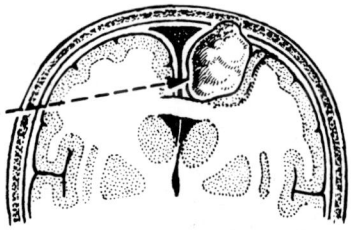

Growth to large size is usually slow so that the compensating mechanisms prevent increased intracranial pressure. Occasional meningiomas arise in the spine.

The histological appearances are variable depending on the relative amounts of cells and collagen, and they mimic in varying degree the arachnoid granulations.

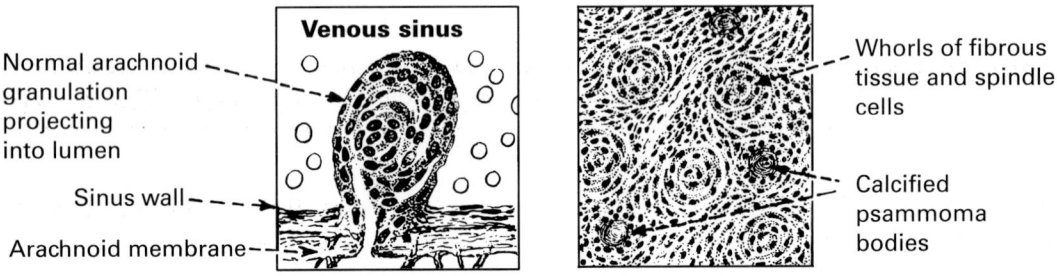

Other mesodermal tumours

True vascular neoplasms are rare, but vascular HAMARTOMAS are fairly common and are a cause of intracranial haemorrhage and epilepsy. These lesions show great variation in site, size and complexity.

Primary microglial and lymphoid tumours are rare; the latter may be intrinsic to the CNS or be metastatic from a primary tumour outside the CNS. Primary lymphomas are an important complication of AIDS.

The incidence of CNS lymphomas is apparently increasing. This may be due to better diagnosis and/or to the more common use of therapeutic immunosuppression.

TUMOURS OF THE NERVOUS SYSTEM

Craniopharyngioma
This is a benign epithelial tumour arising in suprasellar areas. Similar benign cysts also occur.

Germ cell tumours
These occasionally arise in midline structures: they are derived from embryologically misplaced germ cells.

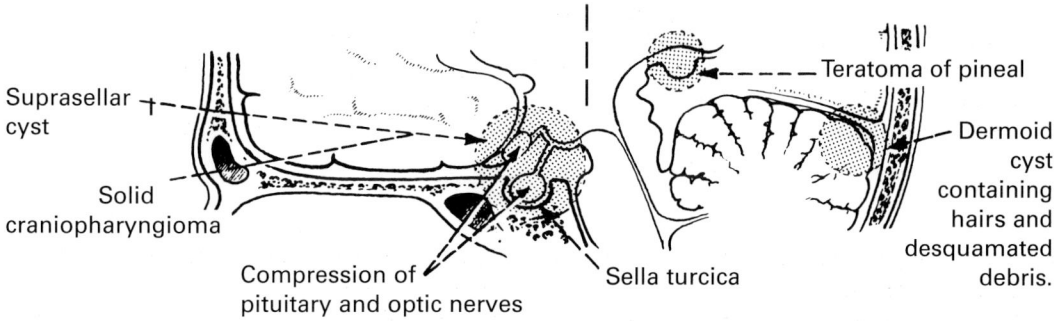

TUMOURS OF PERIPHERAL NERVES

These are essentially collagenous tumours arising in nerve roots within the skull and spine, or in the peripheral nerves. Nomenclature is based on the tissue of origin.

Neurofibroma
Derived from epi- and endoneurium

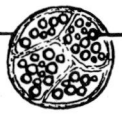

Schwannoma
Derived from Schwann cells intimately surrounding axons.

Spindle cells with wavy nuclei: fine collagen fibres: occasional nerve fibres

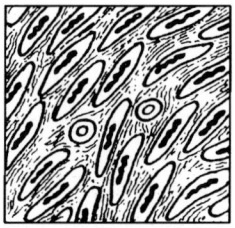

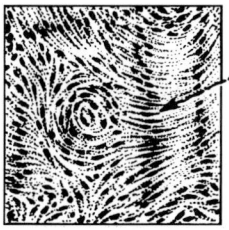

Note nuclear pallisading in addition to whorls and fascicles of collagen

Note: Since neurones do not give rise to these neoplasms, the term neuroma is not used. Traumatic neuroma indicates proliferating nerve endings following injury and is not a true neoplasm (see p. 57).

Nerve sheath tumours may be single or multiple; their effects are due to compression of adjacent nervous tissue and are seen best within the skull or spinal cord.

TUMOURS OF PERIPHERAL NERVES

SCHWANNOMA

Accoustic Neuroma is a good example.

This tumour arises from the VIIIth nerve in the cerebellopontine angle. Although this tumour is benign, it grows around adjacent structures and has an irregular surface so that it may be difficult to remove.

The tumour exerts its effects by compression — distortion of the VIIIth nerve (tinnitus → deafness) and adjacent nerves. Pressure on IVth ventricle → hydrocephalus → increased intracranial pressure.

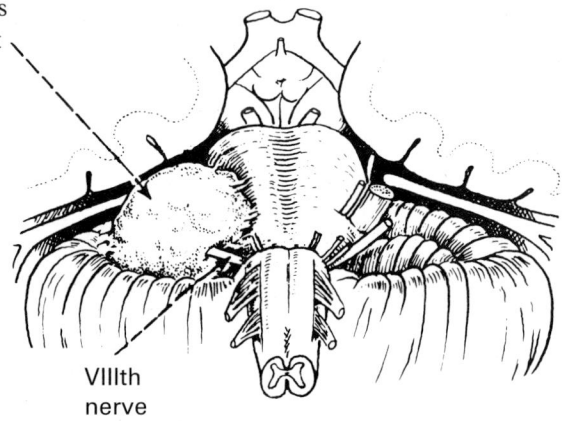

These tumours are rarely multiple as part of neurofibromatosis Type 2 (associated with NF2 gene on chromosome 22).

Neurofibromas

These may be solitary or, in neurofibromatosis, multiple and affect peripheral nerves over a wide area or occupy a single group of nerves. They either form rounded nodules or fusiform swellings and may be cosmetically disfiguring.

These conditions occupy the borderland between neoplasms and hamartomas; very occasionally true neoplasia is superimposed with the development of malignant peripheral nerve sheath tumour.

In **plexiform neurofibroma**, the proliferation slowly proceeds along a group of nerves forming complex thickenings. Growth within the spinal canal causes serious complications.

Pigmentation

The presence of melanin in some of these tumours and the occurrence of skin pigmentation (café au lait spots) in some cases of neurofibromatosis is a reminder of the common neuroectodermal origin of nerve sheath cells and melanocytes.

Aetiology

About half the cases of neurofibromatosis show a family history with an autosomal dominant pedigree. The others are due to sporadic mutations. The defective gene is on chromosome 17 and has tumour suppressor functions. Loss of both copies is associated with malignant transformation.

EPILEPSY

Organic brain disease is a significant factor in only a proportion of epilepsies which are essentially disorders of cerebral function associated with recurrent episodic excessive and abnormal neuronal discharges. The classical signs of generalised convulsions and loss of consciousness are not seen in all epileptics.
Note: The common single seizures associated with febrile illnesses in children are not usually followed by the development of epilepsy.

Incidence: Epilepsy occurs in about 1% of the population.

Mechanism

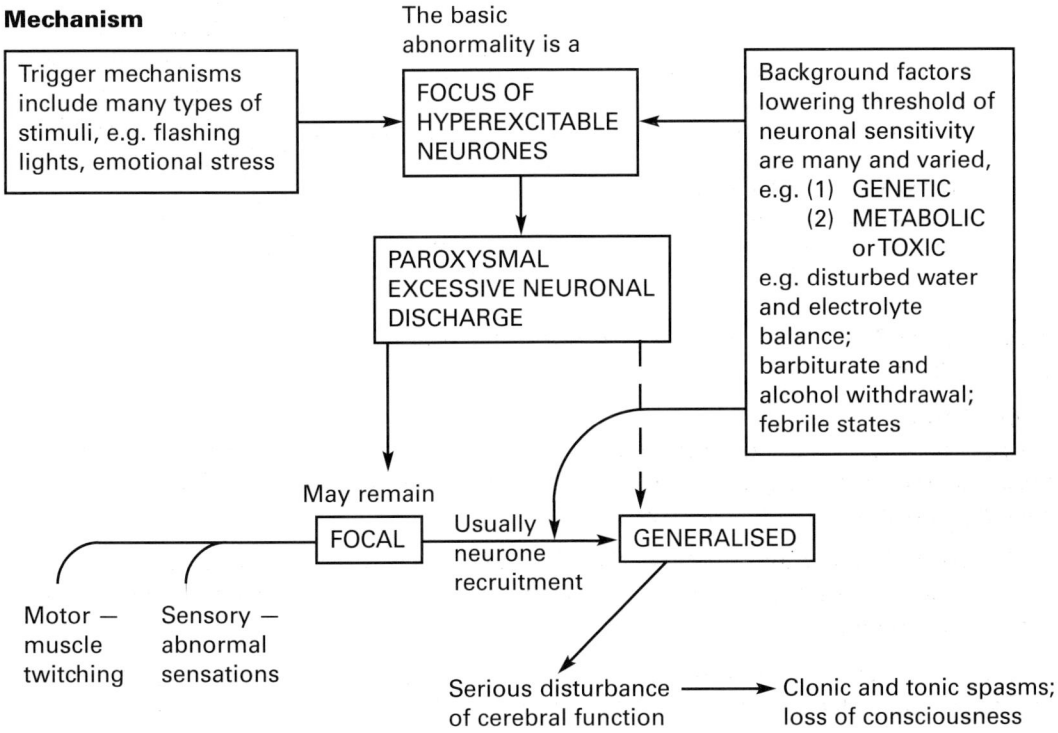

The neurones of the motor cortex, limbic system and the temporal lobe are particularly epileptogenic.

Aetiology

Acquired epilepsy. About 25% of cases are associated with known disease. The hyperexcitable neuronal focus may be due to established brain disease of which congenital abnormalities, post-traumatic scarring and ischaemic change are the most common. Late onset epilepsy may also be due to primary or secondary brain tumours.

Idiopathic epilepsy. In the remaining 75% of cases, although there is no known cause, genetic influences are important. A hyperexcitable focus is often present deep in the brain substance associated with the reticular system.

CEREBROSPINAL FLUID

Although the CSF and extracellular fluid of the central nervous system are essentially similar in composition, changes in the CSF are not reliable indicators of disease within the brain parenchyma.

However, since the CSF reflects conditions in the subarachnoid space, in clinical practice detailed examination and analysis are important and are mandatory in suspected meningitis. The important observations using CSF obtained by lumbar puncture are grouped under headings as follows.

NORMAL	**IN DISEASE**			
	Meningitis		**Virus infection**	**Miscellaneous**
	Pyogenic	*Tuberculous*	*Meningo-encephalitis*	
Pressure 60–180 mm H_2O	↑ Over 200	↑ Over 200	↑High	↓ Below spinal block
Appearance Crystal clear *(for blood staining see below)	Turbid	Opalescent: may be fine fibrin web	Opalescent	–
Cell content 0-4 mononuclears/μl	+ + + >1000 Neutrophils	+ + + Lymphocytes	± + Lymphocytes	–
Biochemistry Protein 0.2–0.4 g/l	↑ 1–10 g/l	↑ 1–3 g/l	↑ 0.5–2 g/l	Very high in spinal block
Glucose 50–80 mg/100 ml (2.8-4.4 mmol/l)	greatly↓ or absent	Low 20–30 mg	Normal	Normal

*When the CSF is blood-stained, it is important to distinguish between contamination due to trauma caused by the tap and true intracranial haemorrhage.

	Contamination	**True haemorrhage**
Supernatant after centrifugation	Clear	Yellow due to bilirubin (red cell degeneration)
Cell count – leucocyte/RBC ratio	Normal	Increased

Microbiology. Identification of organisms is very important.

(1) Deposit and/or fibrin web — stained
- Gram — pyogenic bacteria and fungi
- ZN — tubercle bacilli

(2) Culture: virus isolation

(3) Tests for microbial antigens
- Wassermann reaction for syphilis
- Immunoelectrophoresis for other antigens

CHAPTER 14

MUSCULO-SKELETAL SYSTEM

Skeletal Muscle 606, 607
Atrophy and Hypertrophy 608
Neurogenic Atrophy 608, 609
Myasthenia Gravis 609
Muscle Damage 610
Muscular Dystrophy 611
Inherited Myopathies 612
Acquired Myopathies 613
Muscle Diseases — Diagnosis 614
Post-Viral Fatigue Syndrome 615
Bone 616, 617
Bone Turnover 618
Osteoporosis 619, 620
Osteomalacia and Rickets 621, 622
Bone — Miscellaneous 623–625
Infections of Bone 626, 627
Developmental Abnormalities 628
Cystic Lesions in Bone 629
Tumours in Bone 629–632
Joints 633, 634
Osteoarthritis (OA) 635, 636
Rheumatoid Arthritis (RA) 637, 638
Sero-Negative Arthritis 639
Osteo- and Rheumatoid Arthritis — Comparison .. 640
Infections of Joints 640
Joint and Soft Tissues — Miscellaneous 641
Para-Articular Tissues — Miscellaneous 642
Connective Tissue Diseases 642, 643

SKELETAL MUSCLE

It is useful to consider the anatomy at various levels of magnification.

Naked eye

The muscle consists of bundles of fibres.

External sheath (epimysium)

Tendon

Note: Uniform polygonal shape; nuclei at periphery

Fine collagenous separating membrane (endomysium): no fat within the bundle

Light microscopy (e.g. x 150)

Muscle bundles are seen well in transverse section

Perimysium surrounds bundles

Light microscopy (x 400)

Each muscle fibre is a single specialised cell; within its cytoplasm many myofibrils run in parallel.

Several nuclei immediately underlying sarcolemma

Myofibril

Electron microscopy (e.g. x 15,000)

Z line

I band

A band

H band

Sarcomere

The unique arrangement of the muscle proteins gives characteristic banding.

Loss of banding indicates serious disturbance of intracellular architecture.

MUSCLE CONTRACTION

Within each muscle cell the basic mechanism by which energy is mobilised and released is as follows:

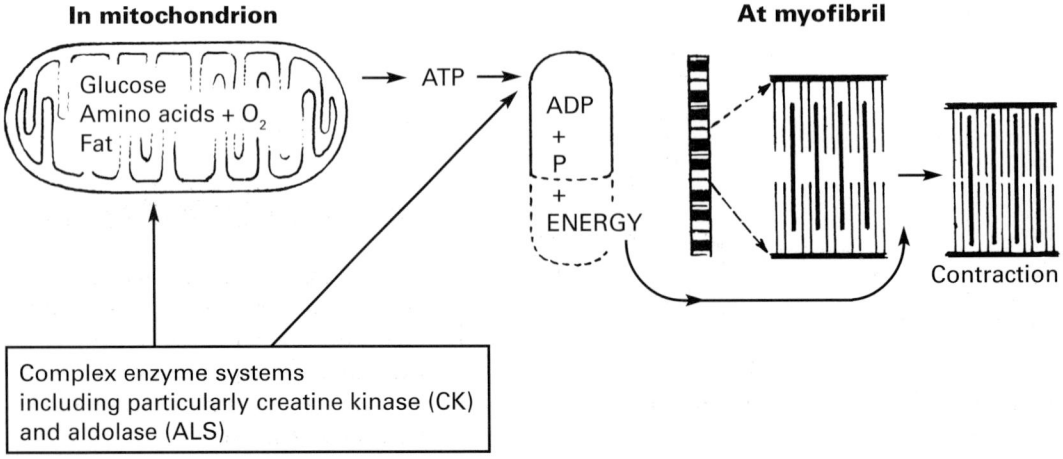

SKELETAL MUSCLE

There are 3 types of muscle fibre, related to differences in functional activity.

	Type of contraction	Location	Myoglobin	Mito-chondria	Metabolism
Type I (red muscle)	SLOW twitch, FATIGUE RESISTANT	POSTURAL MUSCLES	+++	+++	AEROBIC
Type IIa (red muscle)	FAST twitch, FATIGUE RESISTANT	e.g. in LEGS of SPRINTERS	+++	+++	AEROBIC
Type IIb (white muscle)	FAST twitch, FATIGUABLE	ARM MUSCLES	+	+	ANAEROBIC

Note: Most muscles are a mixture of the 3 fibre types, but the proportion varies according to the function of the muscle.

In section, the three fibre types are identified by their ATPase activity.

Normal muscle stained H & E

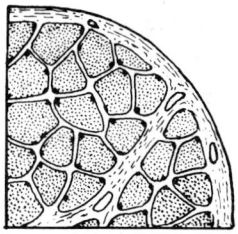

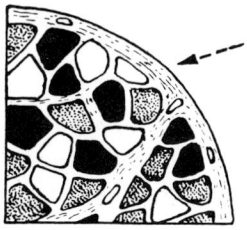

Normal muscle stained for ATPase activity

Type I = black
Type IIa = white
Type IIb = stipple
Note random mosaic pattern.

It is of interest that the muscle fibre function is not intrinsic but is conditioned by its type of nerve supply: any single anterior horn cell innervates fibres of only one type.

MUSCLE INNERVATION

The motor unit consists of:
a single lower motor neurone **(LMN)** —— and the muscle fibres it supplies.

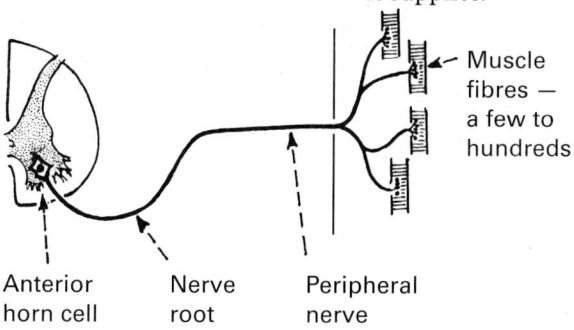

Muscle spindles

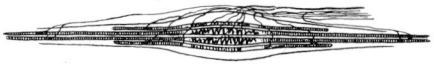

Muscle spindles are bundles of specialised fibres which control and refine muscle contraction and are important for proprioception. They are separately innervated from the surrounding fibres.

ATROPHY AND HYPERTROPHY

Generalised disuse atrophy occurs as a result of prolonged immobilisation in bed. Local atrophy follows immobilisation due to joint disease or after bone fractures.

Hypertrophy of muscle tissue in response to increased work load is well seen in heavy event atheletes. Localised hypertrophy can compensate for damage to adjacent muscular tissues.

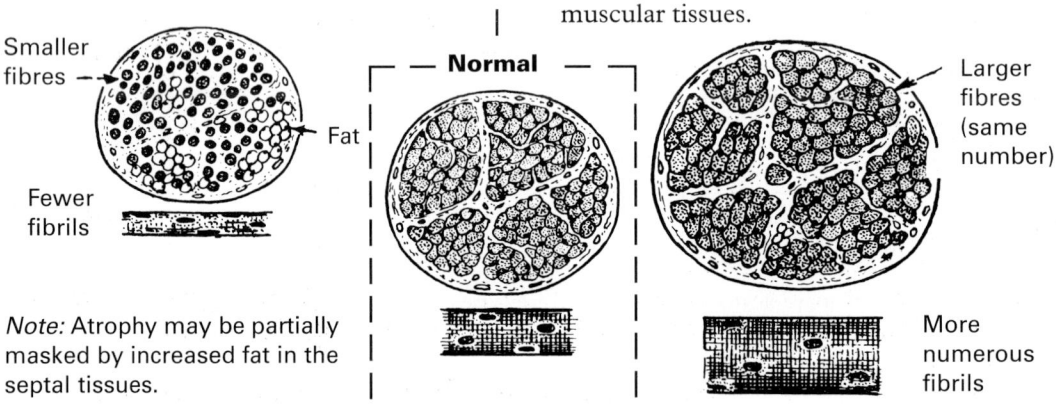

Note: Atrophy may be partially masked by increased fat in the septal tissues.

NEUROGENIC ATROPHY

This is a special form of atrophy seen when the nerve supply is damaged. The distribution of nerve fibres within the muscle is important and is represented diagrammatically in respect of two motor units: A and B.

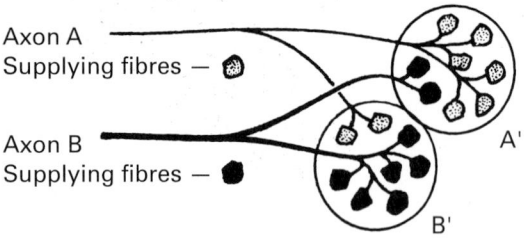

Note that while A and B respectively innervate the majority of fibres in bundles A′ and B′, there is overlap between bundles. Since many axons supply a muscle the overlap is considerable.

Apart from complete traumatic section of a peripheral nerve, it is unusual for all motor fibres to a muscle to be destroyed. Both the basic pattern of innervation and the variations in nerve fibre damage are reflected in the histological appearances in the denervated muscle.

1. Pattern of atrophy

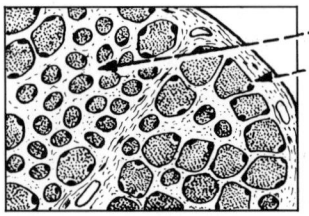

Groups of atrophic denervated fibres with adjacent groups of normal fibres.

Note the overlap — atrophic fibres among normal, and vice versa.

This is the striking basic pattern seen in most diseases of the LMN.

NEUROGENIC ATROPHY

2. **Re-innervation**
   In an area of denervation, the terminal axonal branches of intact neurones sprout and can re-innervate the atrophic fibres. The effects of denervation and re-innervation are shown in a muscle bundle supplied by 2 axons A and B.

Denervation of A

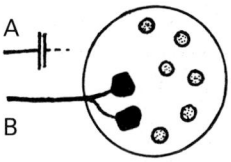

Fibres supplied by A atrophy

Fibres supplied by B remain normal

Re-innervation and **restoration** of fibre size

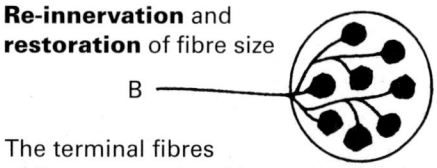

The terminal fibres of B now sprout and innervate the atrophic fibres which are restored to normal size.

This explains

3. **Change in muscle type** which may occur.
   Since the type (fast or slow) of each muscle fibre is conditioned by its nerve supply, the pattern of distribution of fast and slow fibres within a muscle may be changed by re-innervation.
   Thus, although a muscle may be restored to normal in terms of routine histological assessment, slight changes in functional activity may be present.

MYASTHENIA GRAVIS

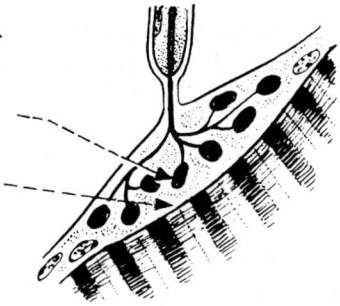

The **MOTOR END-PLATE** is the specialised neuromuscular junction situated at the middle of each muscle fibre. The nervous impulse causes release of **ACETYLCHOLINE** at the specialised nerve endings - depolarisation at this site is the stimulus to contraction. The sarcolemma at this site contains abundant **CHOLINESTERASE**. In MYASTHENIA GRAVIS, the essential disorder is at the motor end-plate where there is a defect in the action of acetylcholine. This rare disease occurs mainly in young females, the important clinical features being muscle weakness and early fatigue of the ocular and head and neck muscles particularly.

Aetiology and mechanism

This is essentially an auto-immune disease (see p. 110).

1. Antibodies to ACETYLCHOLINE RECEPTORS are present in 90% of cases.
2. There is a strong association with THYMIC abnormalities. In young women this is usually *thymic germinal centre hyperplasia*: in middle aged males a *thymoma* (mixed lymphoid or epithelial type) may be present.
3. There is an association with hyperthyroidism (this has an autoimmune basis).

In the affected muscles, aggregates of lymphocytes with occasional single necrotic fibres may be seen.

MUSCLE DAMAGE

(a) **Trauma and ischaemia**

In severe cases where trauma and ischaemia combine to cause necrosis of a considerable mass of muscle, the effects may be serious.

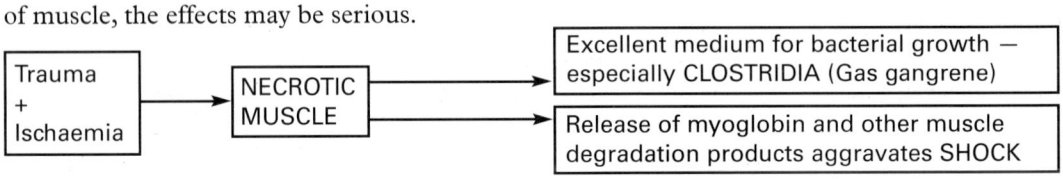

The latter situation is well exemplified in the CRUSH SYNDROME — classically seen in building collapse.

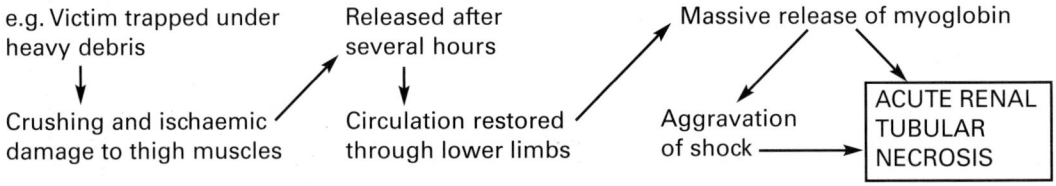

Repair of massive muscle damage

The basic inflammatory response is followed by organisation with removal of the dead muscle.

There are two possible results:

(i) If the gap is not too great, regeneration effects restoration to normal.

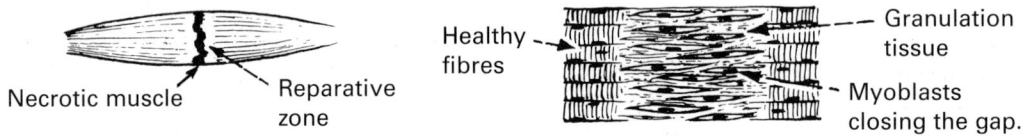

(ii) If the gap is too great, scar tissue prevents the regeneration.

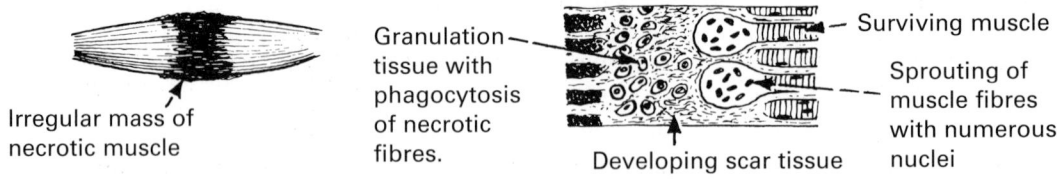

(b) **Inflammation**

In most inflammatory processes, including the common pyogenic infections, the intermuscular fascial planes are involved and muscle damage is negligible and superficial, consisting of degeneration and necrosis of individual fibres.

Abscess formation may follow intramuscular injections.

Viral myositis

A true myositis with focal necrosis of fibres, lymphocyte and macrophage infiltration can be caused by the *Coxsackie group* of viruses. The muscles of the upper thorax are particularly affected.

Parasitic myositis

In trichinosis, the parasitic larvae encyst in the interstitial tissues within muscles. The adjacent muscle fibres become necrotic; focal calcification is often a late sequel.

MUSCULAR DYSTROPHY

Muscular dystrophies are inherited diseases, causing muscle damage and weakness.

Duchenne Muscular Dystrophy

This is the commonest and most serious form.

Clinical features: Muscle weakness in early childhood; typically wheelchair-bound by 12 years of age and death by late teens or early twenties.

Pathology: The main features are

(1) muscle fibre necrosis and

(2) regeneration.

In time, fibres are atrophic and there is fibrosis and fatty replacement.

Biopsy shows:

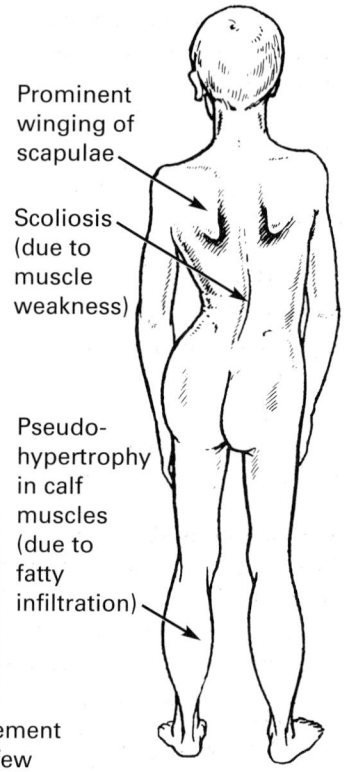

Moderately affected muscle

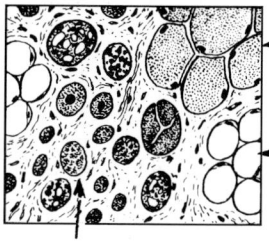

Late stage muscle

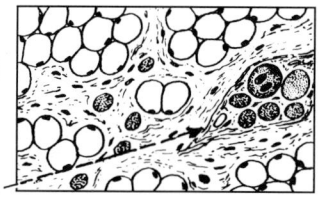

Aetiology: This is an X-linked recessive disease occurring almost exclusively in boys. The dystrophin gene lies on the short arm of chromosome X.

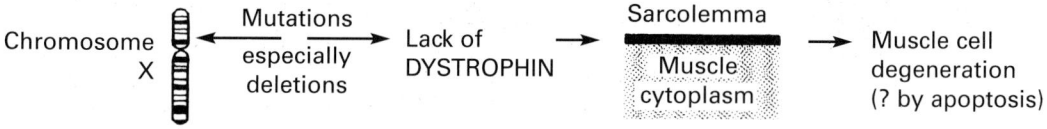

Biopsy in early stages shows a lack of dystrophin using immuno-staining (anti-dystrophin antibodies).

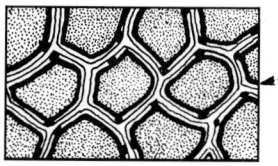

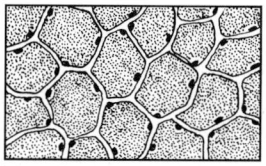

Genetic screening for mutations of the dystrophin gene is now available.

Becker type muscular dystrophy is a milder form caused by mutation in the dystrophin gene resulting in diminished levels of the protein.

Other muscular dystrophies include the facio-scapulohumoral, limb girdle and myotonic dystrophy forms.

INHERITED MYOPATHIES

Specific metabolic defects

An enlarging group of genetic myopathies with specific biochemical or morphological abnormalities is emerging due to the application of modern biochemical, histochemical and morphological (e.g. EM) techniques.

In some, the specific inborn error of metabolism is generalised and includes muscle; in others it is confined to the muscle fibre. Some examples will be given under broad headings:

(1) **Glycogen storage**	(2) **Lipid metabolism**	(3) **Periodic paralysis**
Type 2 (Pompe) — deficiency of acid maltase Type 5 (McArdle) — muscle phosphorylase Type 7 — phosphofructokinase (PEK)	Defect in free fatty acid transport into and utilisation within fibre. (a) carnitine palmityl transferase (CPT) (b) and muscle carnitine deficiency	Associated with hypo- and hyperkalaemia — the muscle defect is a vacuolar degeneration of the sarcolemma

(4) **Morphological abnormalities**

(a) *Mitochondrial*	(b) *Others*	
Large or increased numbers of mitochondria — abnormal oxidative processes	(i) Central core myopathy Central area is abnormal	(iii) Centronuclear myopathy Nucleus in middle of cell
	(ii) Rod body myopathy (nemaline) Rods of tropomysin under sarcolemma	(iv) Disproportion of fibre types I and II

These various myopathies exhibit a wide range in respect of age of onset, clinical presentation and prognosis.

A further rare but interesting autosomal dominant genetic abnormality of muscle is malignant hyperpyrexia. In this condition the administration of general anaesthetic precipitates acute muscle damage. Clinically, there is very high fever, muscle stiffness, cyanosis and acidosis very often resulting in death.

ACQUIRED MYOPATHIES

Inflammatory myopathies — polymyositis and dermatomyositis — are two similar **inflammatory** disorders of muscle.

POLYMYOSITIS — occurs in both sexes and at any age, but especially in middle age. It is characterised by muscle pain and weakness — especially of proximal muscle groups. Progress is variable — deterioration may be rapid or slow.

DERMATOMYOSITIS — has similar muscle changes and also skin lesions often on the face and hands. In adults, dermatomyositis may herald malignancy — often bronchial carcinoma — and there is often evidence of other connective tissue diseases e.g. rheumatoid arthritis.

Pathology:

Muscle fibres show damage varying from atrophy to necrosis and some hypertrophied fibres are seen.

There is lymphocytic infiltrate.

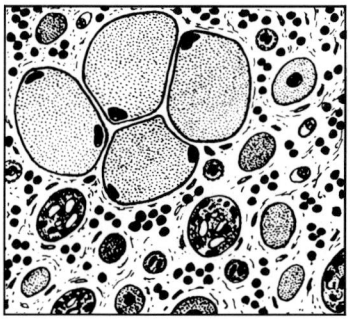

Aetiology

These are both autoimmune diseases although the precise details differ. Polymyositis is a T cell mediated attack on muscle fibres, while dermatomyositis is an immune complex disorder with vascular damage.

CACHECTIC MYOPATHY

In any wasting disease, loss of muscle with weakness is seen.

Primary condition

Chronic infection
Malabsorption
Cancer
Endocrine disorder
Extreme old age

→ Generalised CATABOLISM

↓

The protein of muscle is particularly affected → Loss of muscle bulk; fibres smaller with nuclei closer together; muscle fibre loss — predominantly type II.

Endocrine, toxic and nutritional myopathies

(a) Myopathy is seen in acromegaly, hyperthyroidism, hypothyroidism, hyperaldosteronism (due to hypokalaemia), hyperparathyroidism and in corticosteroid excess.
(b) In alcoholics and a variety of drugs in addition to corticosteroids, e.g. chloroquine, vincristine; and in vitamin D deficiency.

MUSCLE DISEASES – DIAGNOSIS

In clinical practice, although in only a few conditions is curative therapy available, accurate diagnosis of cases of muscular weakness and atrophy is important since there is considerable variation in prognosis and management of these diverse disorders.

A diagnosis is usually reached from a synthesis of the information obtained from investigations under three main headings:

1. **General clinical considerations are fundamental.** Of particular importance are *family history, age of onset, distribution of muscle weakness* and *rate of progress*. To these are added clinical neurological assessment.

2. **Special investigation of neuromuscular electrical activity.** The rate of motor and sensory nerve conduction can be measured electrically.

   The ELECTROMYOGRAM records the activity of groups of muscle fibres and even of individual fibres (usually fine needle electrodes). The broad basic pathological changes already described are reflected in variations of the electrical potential within the muscle during various types of activity.

   These methods are particularly useful in distinguishing primary myopathies, including myotonias, from denervation atrophy.

3. **Laboratory tests**

   (a) *MUSCLE BIOPSY*. The motor unit area of a moderately weak muscle is chosen (end-stage muscle should not be taken). Special precautions must be taken to minimise artifacts. Routine histological examination will usually distinguish the broad groups of disorders and identify the occasional rare myopathy with specific morphological features.

   Histochemical and EM examination and biochemical analysis may identify specific disorders.

   (b) *SERUM ENZYMES*. In the myopathies where actual muscle fibre destruction is proceeding, increased levels of creatine kinase (CK) and aldolase (ALS) are found.

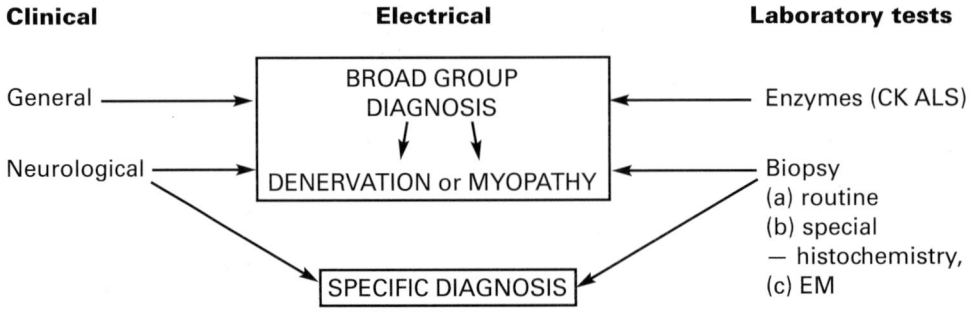

POST-VIRAL FATIGUE SYNDROME

This syndrome has recently come to prominence due to an increased prevalence, both in sporadic cases and in small epidemics. For many years, post-viral depression (e.g. after influenza) and fatigue (e.g. after glandular fever) have been recognised and these symptoms are self-limiting and usually last only a few weeks; the pathological mechanisms are obscure.

The syndrome now so prevalent may be associated with **enterovirus** e.g. coxsackie and other infections and leads to severe functional deficits which are often long-lasting (years). Alternative names for the syndrome are **myalgic encephalomyelitis (ME)** or **chronic fatigue syndrome**.

The clinical signs and symptoms are protean, but the major complaint is extreme fatigue made worse by exercise. For many years the condition was considered to be psychologically induced and was labelled a form of hysteria, but has now been accepted as an organic condition.

The mechanisms however are not yet established with certainty. The flow diagram illustrates the possible mechanisms:

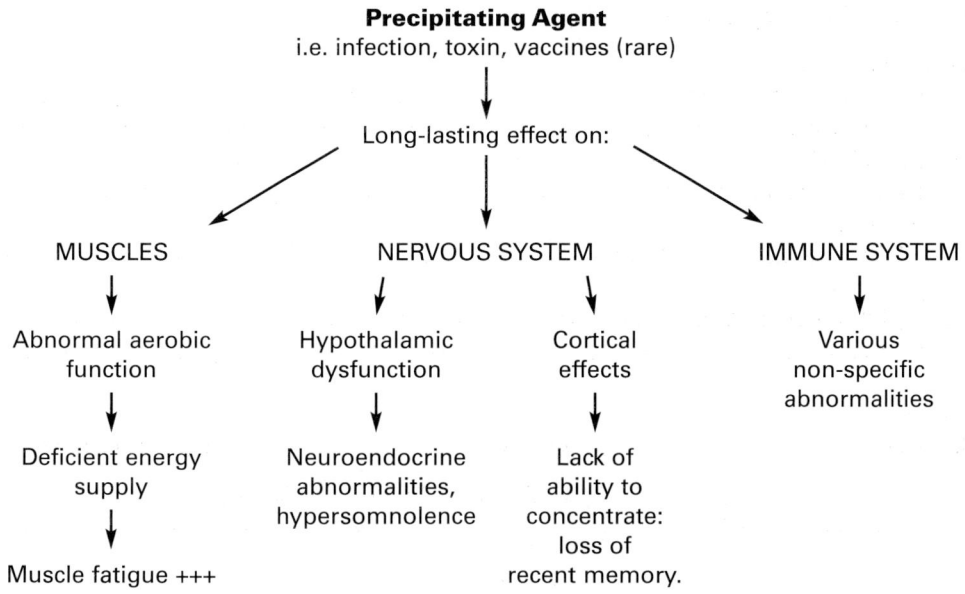

BONE

A bone shows two gross anatomical forms in varying proportions, depending on the particular type of supportive function required of it.

1. **COMPACT BONE**

seen well in long bone shaft, contributes rigidity and forms the dense outer shell (cortex).

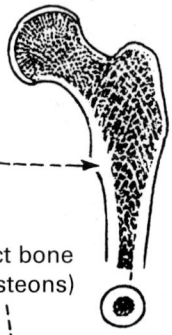

The basic units of compact bone are Haversian systems (osteons) arranged in vertical columns.

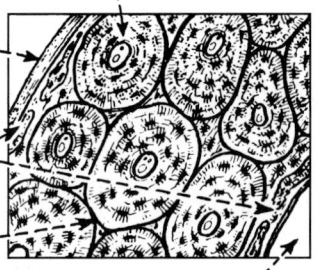

2. **CANCELLOUS BONE**

(along with marrow) occupies the medullary cavities. This arrangement as exemplified in a vertebral body contributes some compressibility and pliability.

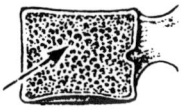

The basic unit of cancellous bone is the trabecula, arranged along lines of stress.

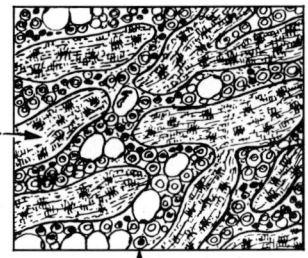

Haemopoietic marrow

In both types of bone, there is a basic **lamellar** structure.

A single Haversian system showing central canal with capillaries, concentric laminae and osteocytes in lacunae.

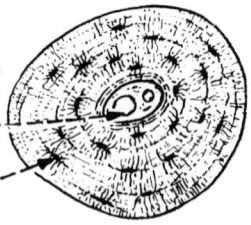

Osteocytes are fairly inactive but communicate through canaliculi in the matrix.

A single trabecula showing:

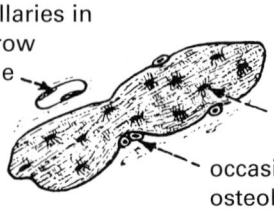

Note: Cancellous bone comprises 20% of bone mass but 80% of bone turnover due to its large surface area.

Bone GROWTH

In **endochondral ossification,** seen at the metaphyseal ends of long bones, the cartilage of the growth plate dies and is invaded by osteoblasts which lay down bone to replace it.

In **membranous ossification,** seen in certain flat bones, the osteoblasts appear in an immature connective tissue matrix. This type is rarely seen in pathological processes.

BONE

WOVEN BONE (non-lamellar), a primitive form laid down in fetal development.

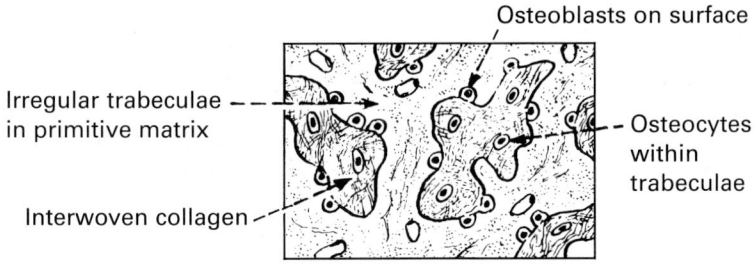

In adult life, this type is seen in bone regeneration and tumours. It may be later replaced by lamellar bone.

BONE and CALCIUM

(a) **Calcification of bone**
Exactly how precipitation of calcium phosphate occurs in osteoid is not well understood. It appears that matrix vesicles are laid down by **osteoblasts** and act as foci for mineralisation. They contain the enzyme **alkaline phosphatase**.

(b) **Bone and calcium homeostasis**
The bony skeleton acts as a reservoir for calcium and responds to the need to maintain plasma levels within a fairly narrow range (9.2–10.4 mg/dl or 2.3–2.6 mmol/l — these figures are for total plasma calcium and are used in clinical practice). This response is controlled mainly by a direct action of parathormone on bone as shown below.

(i) Response to low blood calcium

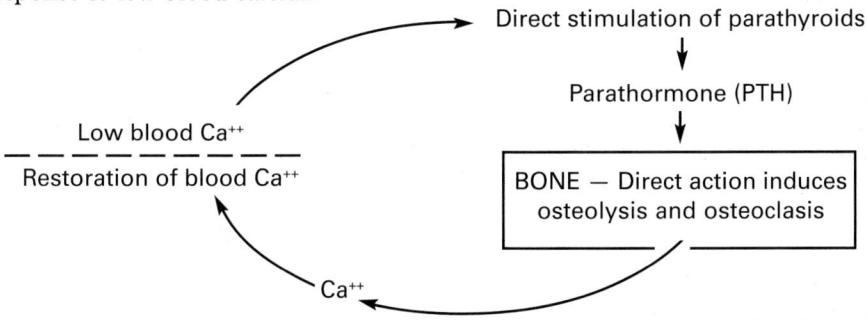

In parathyroid hyperplasia or neoplasia, this process occurs in excess, causing hypercalcaemia and pathological bone resorption. *Note:* PTH also increases calcium absorption from the gut and reabsorption from the kidney.

(ii) When the blood calcium is high, parathormone is not secreted and bone resorption is in abeyance.

Calcitonin antagonises the action of parathormone, but its role in health and disease has not yet been fully assessed. It is probably most important in childhood. The role of vitamin D is discussed on page 622.

BONE TURNOVER

Bone is an active tissue — in the adult 10% turns over each year. The two processes of bone resorption and bone formation are clearly linked — a process known as coupling which is gradually being understood.

In **CANCELLOUS BONE**

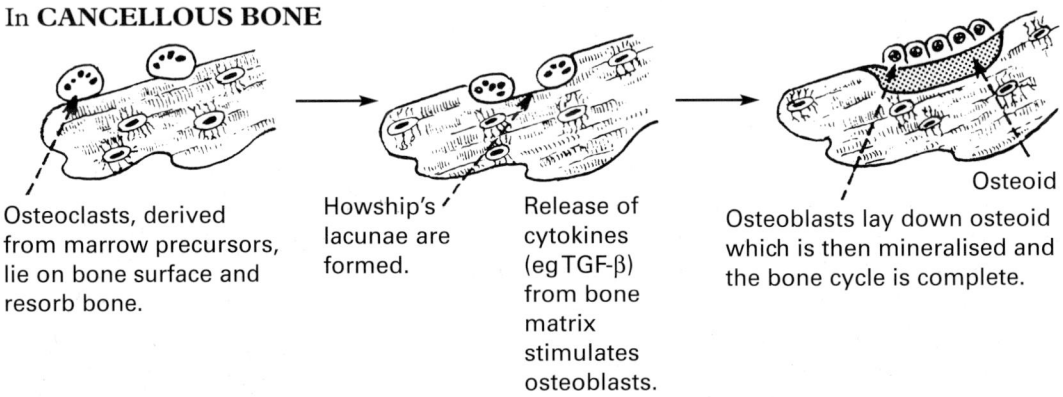

In **CORTICAL BONE**
the same sequence occurs:

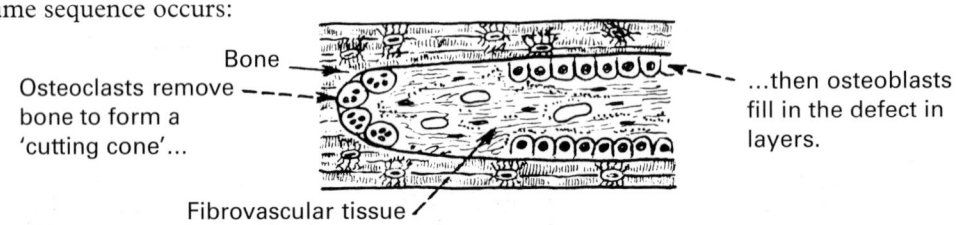

The unit of bone resorption is described as a Basic Multicellular Unit (BMU).

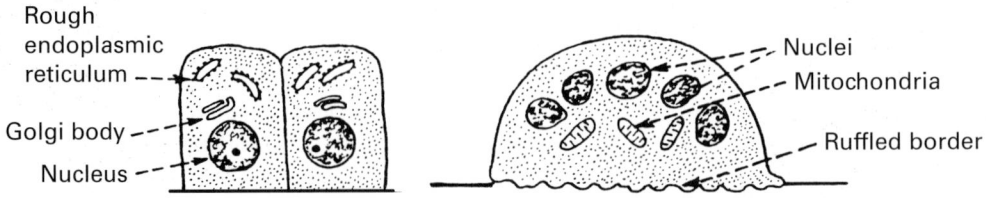

OSTEOBLASTS

— derived from osteoprogenitor cells.
— produce Type I collagen and other proteins.
— secrete alkaline phosphatase — a marker of bone formation.
— stimulated by mechanical stress, androgens, cytokines.

OSTEOCLASTS

— derived from marrow precursors.
— produce acid and enzymes to remove bone.
— produce collagen degradation products e.g. urinary HO Proline — a marker of bone destruction.
— stimulated by cytokines e.g. IL-1 (indirectly by PTH).
— inhibited by oestrogens.

OSTEOPOROSIS

OSTEOPOROSIS is the commonest disorder of bone.
It is defined as a systemic disease characterised by:

(1) low bone mass.
(2) microarchitectural deterioration of bone, with
(3) an increase in bone fragility and susceptibility to fracture.

A patient is said to have osteoporosis if BONE MINERAL DENSITY >2.5 standard deviations below the mean of normal young subjects.

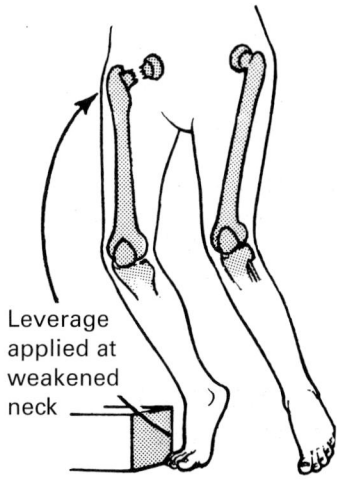

Clinical effects: — osteoporosis is a disease predominantly of post-menopausal females, but men are also affected.

1. Compression (collapse) of vertebral bodies (usually preceded by gradual loss of height and kyphosis); often associated with sudden pain on weight lifting.
2. Fracture of neck of femur or other long bones (especially Colles' fracture of distal radius).

Note: In osteoporosis, the routine serum biochemical tests — particularly the calcium levels — are within the normal range.

Pathology: The changes in the vertebral bodies are illustrative.

Normal

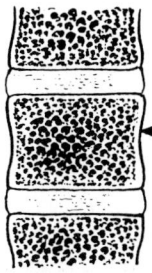

Naked eye and Microscopic appearances

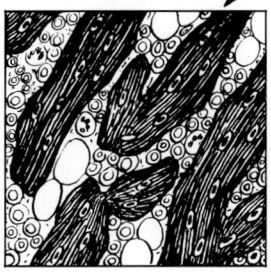

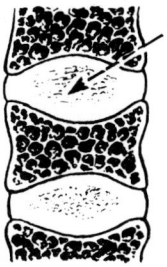

Disc bulging into bone.

Porotic bone: wide honey-comb spaces.

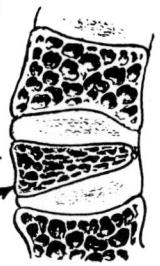

Collapse of vertebral body

Sparse thin trabeculae appear disconnected in 2 dimensions 'Microarchitectural deterioration'.

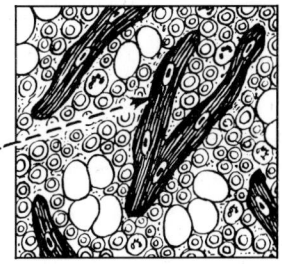

Note: (i) The atrophied trabeculae have a normal calcium content, but because the total trabecular mass is reduced, the total bone calcium is also reduced.
(ii) Bone loss is most marked in cancellous bone with its high turnover, but cortical bone is also affected.

OSTEOPOROSIS

Aetiology

In *normal* bones the dynamic processes of formation and resorption are in balance.

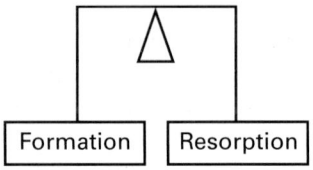

In *osteoporosis* the balance is upset by
(1) diminished formation
(2) increased resorption
(3) both 1 and 2 together

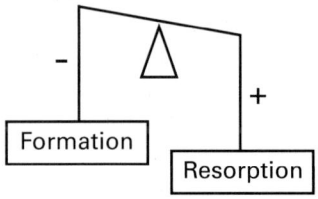

However, bone mass decreases with age in both sexes: in old age, osteoblastic activity falls.

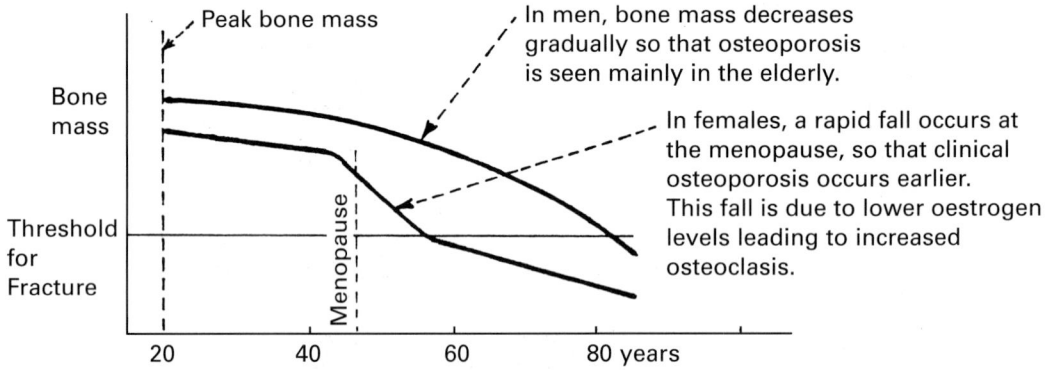

PEAK BONE MASS is important — a high initial figure makes osteoporosis less likely. This depends on factors including:

(a) Genetic predisposition — polymorphisms of vitamin D receptor gene, Type I collagen gene.
(b) Nutrition — especially calcium.
(c) Exercise.

The **aetiology** can be summarised as follows:

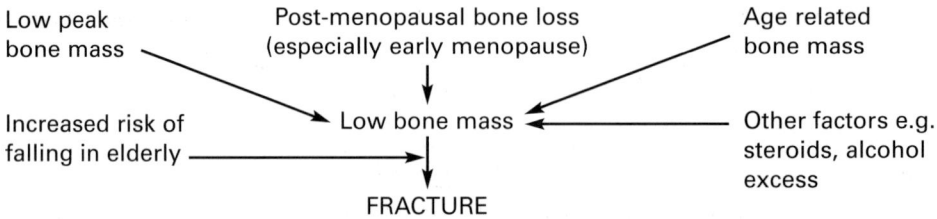

Localised osteoporosis is commonly due to disuse and is seen as a complication of other disorders, e.g. local IMMOBILISATION following fracture; limb paralysis and adjacent to severe joint disease with limitation of movement.

This process can be acute with active osteoclasis, but when function is resumed, normal bone structure is often restored.

OSTEOMALACIA AND RICKETS

Osteomalacia and rickets are disorders of bone in which the essential defect is failure of calcification in newly formed osteoid, caused by vitamin D deficiency in almost all cases.

Osteomalacia occurs in adult life and affects the osteoid which is being continually laid down in the normal remodelling of bone.

Rickets affects the growing child, and serious additional disturbances are seen at the growing ends of long bones. Clinically there is pain, weakness of bones with a tendency to distortion and even fracture. Looser's zones, seen in X-ray, are linear partial fractures of long bones which have failed to calcify.

The mechanisms by which vitamin D deficiency prevents calcification are complex and not completely elucidated. The following simplified diagrams indicate the causes of vitamin D deficiency and its effects on bone.

(a) **Causes of deficiency:**

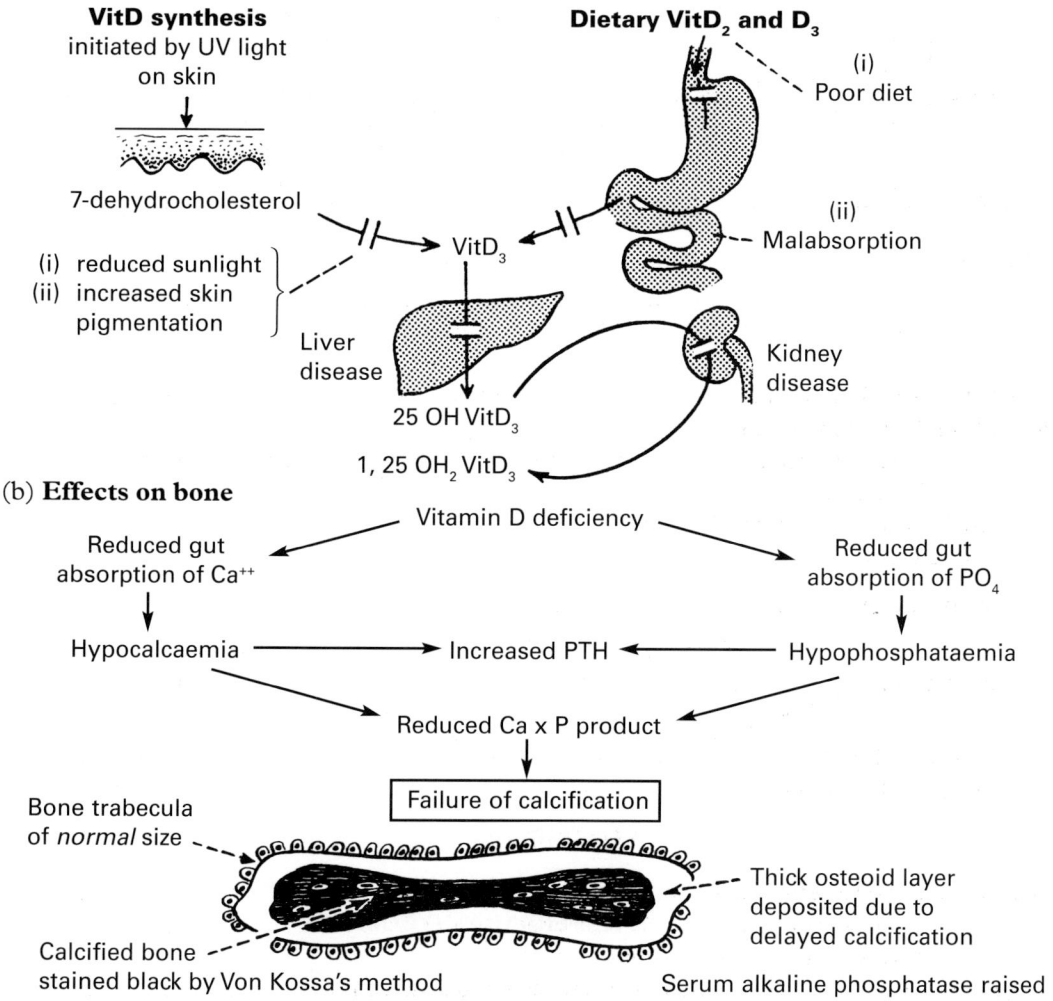

Note: Parathyroid activity tends to restore serum calcium towards normal.

OSTEOMALACIA AND RICKETS

In **rickets** there are important changes at the growing ends of long bones.

Normal

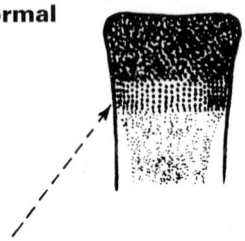

Regularly arranged columns of cartilage cells being replaced by columns of well calcified bone

Rickets

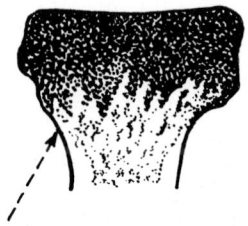

Thickened irregular cartilage — poorly calcified, scanty bone formation

This results in stunting of growth and bowing of the lower limbs.
In females permanent deformities of the pelvis can cause serious difficulty during childbirth

Since osteomalacia can be treated by vitamin D, it is important to distinguish it from osteoporosis: bone biopsy and biochemical tests are useful.

	Osteomalacia	**Osteoporosis**
Biopsy — appearance of trabeculae	Size — normal Thick uncalcified osteoid seams	Thin and small Normal calcification
Osteoblasts	Often increased	Normal numbers
Serum biochemistry		
Alkaline phosphatase	Raised	Normal
Phosphate	Low	Normal
Calcium	May be low	Normal

Osteomalacia and osteoporosis may occur together, especially in the elderly.

Renal osteodystrophy

In any renal disease associated with uraemia, abnormalities of bone occur. The essential factors are failure of kidneys to produce 1,25 DHCC, the active metabolite of vitamin D, and the failure of the kidneys to eliminate phosphate. These lead to important secondary effects:

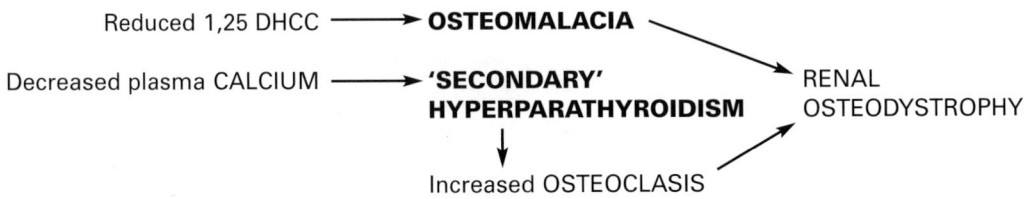

BONE – MISCELLANEOUS

HYPERPARATHYROIDISM

Bone changes may be seen in hyperparathyroidism, especially when severe or long-standing. The essential change is increased bone resorption due to greatly increased osteoclastic activity; usually osteoblastic activity is also increased but the net effect is bone loss.

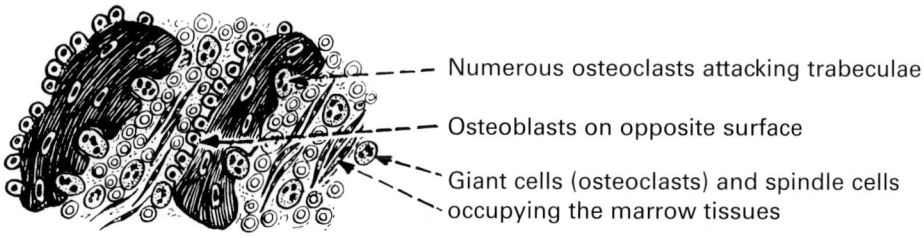

These changes, although generalised, may be locally severe causing cystic spaces — the fully developed disorder is called **osteitis fibrosa cystica.** In some cases giant cell tumour of bone may be mimicked (so-called BROWN TUMOUR of hyperparathyroidism).

HYPERTROPHY OF BONE

In **acromegaly** the enlargement of the jaws, hands and feet is due to subperiosteal osteoblastic proliferation and bone formation under the influence of pituitary growth hormone (soft tissues are also thickened).

Hypertrophic osteoarthropathy (including finger clubbing) affects the digits, distal ends of long bones and the distal joints.

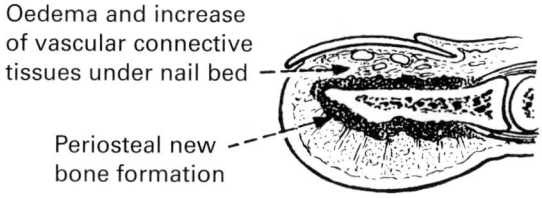

The mechanism is unknown, but the condition is associated with chronic lung disease, lung cancer, cyanotic heart disease and chronic intestinal inflammatory conditions.

Its importance is as an indicator of serious disease elsewhere, and it is of interest that if the primary disease can be cured, the osteoarthropathy may resolve.

BONE – MISCELLANEOUS

FIBROUS DYSPLASIA OF BONE

This disorder may affect a single (monostotic) or several bones (polyostotic). The lesion is of well demarcated fibrous tissue containing small abnormal bone trabeculae. The normal bone is gradually replaced; small cysts may be present. Overexpression of a proto-oncogene is responsible for the polystotic form.

Complications

Fracture or deformity of the weakened bone.

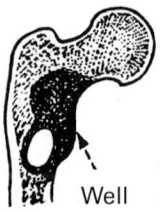

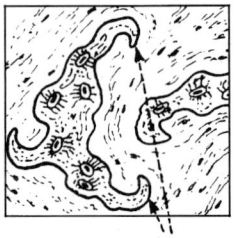

PAGET'S DISEASE OF BONE

This disease of unknown aetiology usually presents after the age of 50 years and affects males predominantly. It is fairly common (3% of autopsies), but only in its more severe forms are there clinical symptoms. The disorder is focal: the bones particularly affected are the pelvis, lower vertebrae, skull and lower limbs. It has been suggested that virus infection (e.g. measles, distemper) of osteoclasts is responsible.

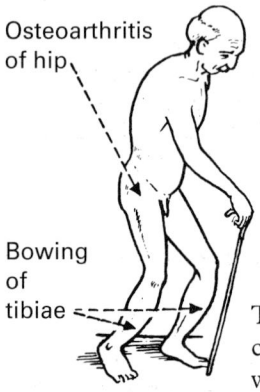

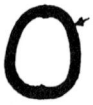

Thickened skull, inner and outer bony tables fused

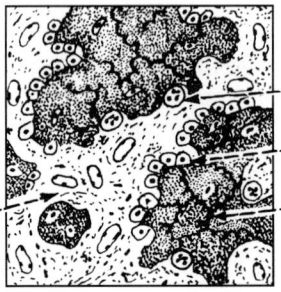

To begin with, there is a localised increase in **osteoclastic** activity causing bone resorption; soon there is a marked **osteoblastic** reaction with bone resorption and deposition proceeding chaotically, so that irregular bone trabeculae with mosaic cement lines are formed. The bone may be thickened, but its structure is defective and weak. Biochemical changes reflect the cellular activity at trabecular level: *Alkaline phosphatase* ↑ (osteoblastic); *urinary hydroxyproline* ↑ (collagen destruction).

The important **complications** are:

1. **Fracture** of weakened bones (including partial long bone fracture and vertebral compression).
2. **Osteoarthritis** of joints due to abnormal stresses caused by bony deformity.
3. An increased risk (×30) of the development of **bone sarcoma**.
4. The increased circulatory load through the vascular stroma may cause high output cardiac failure in patients with compromised cardiac function.

The use of **Calcitonin**, the physiological antagonist of parathormone, and bisphosphonates offer effective therapy in many cases.

BONE – MISCELLANEOUS

AVASCULAR BONE NECROSIS (OSTEONECROSIS)

(a) The usual processes involved in fracture healing have been dealt with (p.63). Due to details of vascular anatomy at particular sites, fractures may be complicated by severance of the blood supply to one of the bone fragments. This results in a high incidence of avascular bone necrosis. Fractures of the femoral neck and scaphoid bone are good examples.

(b) In other cases of osteonecrosis, trauma is not obviously an aetiological factor. In some, but not all of a miscellany of conditions, which includes decompression in those working in increased atmospheric pressure (Caisson disease), alcoholism, Gaucher's disease, sickle cell anaemia and prolonged corticosteroid therapy, local ischaemia may be due to sludging of blood in arteries to bone.
Bone necrosis of this type has important effects when it occurs at an articular surface: serious degenerative arthritis may ensue.

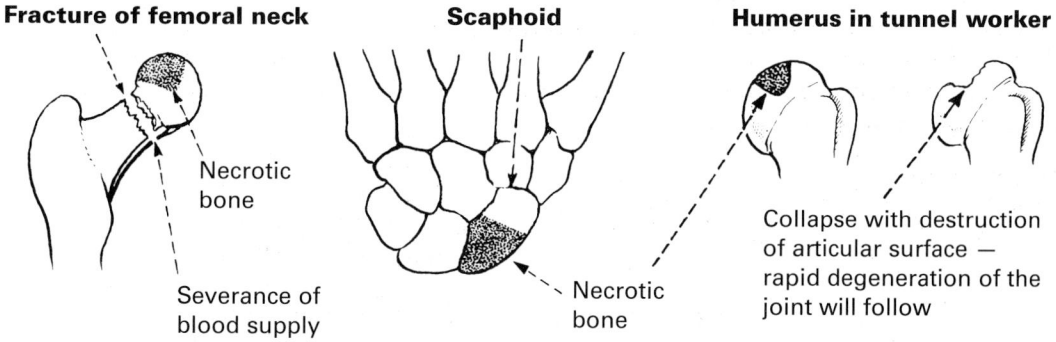

Note: These areas of necrotic bone may be relatively radiodense due to disuse osteoporosis of the adjacent living bone.

(c) In children and adolescents osteonecrosis occurs at several epiphyseal sites for no known cause (repeated minor trauma may be operative in some cases). The general name for this condition is osteochondritis juvenilis, and various eponymous terms are applied depending on the site affected. The commonest is Perthes' disease in which necrosis of one or both femoral heads occurs in children aged 4–10 years: (male: female = 5:1).

SUBPERIOSTEAL HAEMATOMA

In scurvy, the lack of vitamin C is the cause of abnormal collagen synthesis and there is a bleeding tendency due to capillary fragility.

In very young children, large haematomas may form under the periosteum in response to relatively minor trauma. The osteoblasts on the undersurface proceed to form irregular bone and considerable time is required for remodelling to occur. Similar haematomas with ossification may be seen on radiographs of the bones of 'battered babies'.

INFECTIONS OF BONE

The following basic pathological processes occur in all bone infections.

1. Destruction of bone due to necrosis.

NECROSIS

Virulent organisms ± thrombosis of vessels → **Massive**

Too bulky to be removed by natural processes

Bulk of dead bone remains at site and prevents proper repair

← Low grade organisms → ***Single or small groups of osteons or trabeculae***

Dissolution or removal by osteoclasts

2. Reactive and reparative processes.

Fibrosis

New bone formation

Effected by **osteoblastic** activity. This is irregular while infection is still present — later, proper repair with remodelling is completed

As the infection progresses, the balance between the various components changes. In chronic infections, fibrosis and reparative new bone growth may be very striking.

In addition to the usual accompaniments of inflammation, other important complications are: (1) weakening of bone resulting in deformity or fracture and (2) local complications of the inflammation, particularly abscess and sinus formation.

The following bone infections are illustrative:

ACUTE OSTEOMYELITIS

Classically caused by the *Staphylococcus aureus* and affects the growing ends of the metaphyses of long bones in children. Nowadays the incidence has been greatly reduced and the use of antibiotics aborts the development of the disease. The organisms are blood borne and settle in the cancellous bone of the metaphysis. The effects are dramatic and rapidly progressive.

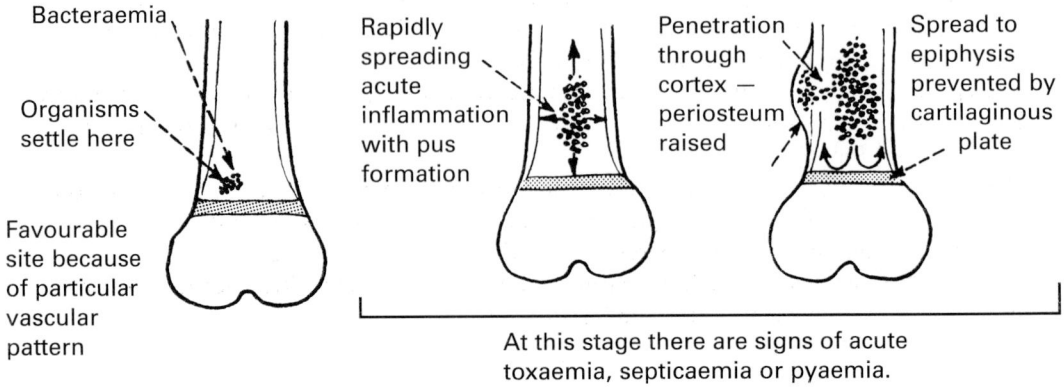

INFECTIONS OF BONE

Acute Osteomyelitis (continued)

Unless treatment is started promptly, the expanding inflammatory process within the rigid bone is seriously complicated.

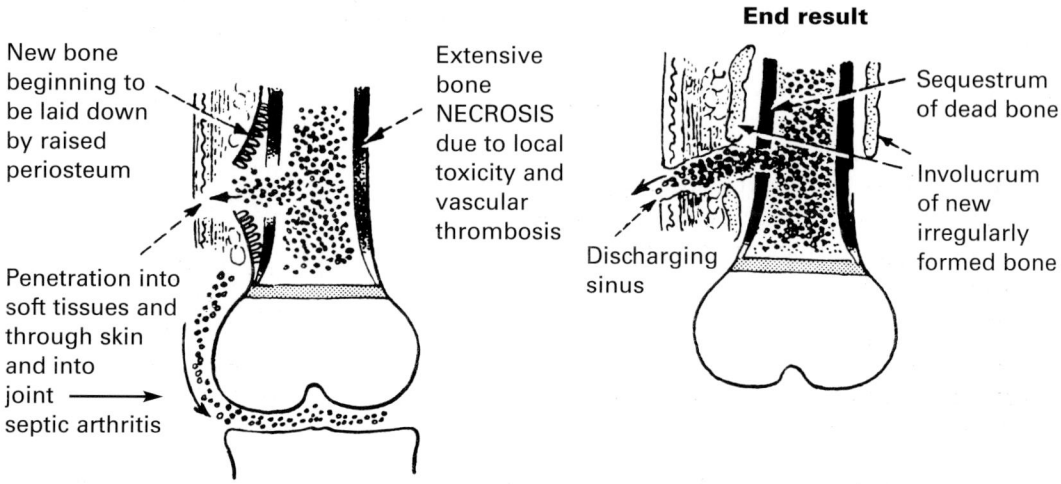

The presence of necrotic bone ensures that the inflammation and sinus discharge continue. With large sequestra, the usual natural methods of removal of dead tissue are inadequate so that surgical treatment is necessary.

At a late chronic stage, in addition to the local disability and disturbance of bone growth, **AMYLOID** disease may supervene and occasionally squamous carcinoma arises in a sinus.

Other pyogenic bacteria can cause osteitis — the salmonella group (esp. *S.typhi*) and brucella, the latter often causing a low grade osteitis of the spine.

With inadequate antibiotic treatment, acute inflammatory processes may be converted into low grade osteitis. Staphylococcal infection of the spine may present in adults in this way.

TUBERCULOSIS

The incidence of bone and joint infection parallels the incidence of the more common pulmonary and intestinal infections. It is therefore low in developed countries but still significant elsewhere, and is associated with HIV infection.

The spine and growing ends of long bones including the epiphyses are commonly affected by blood borne spread and, because of the proximity of joints, tuberculous arthritis is a frequent concomitant.

The basic pathological process is destruction of bone and replacement with tuberculous granulation tissue. Caseous necrosis is common and tracking and spread into adjacent tissues, particularly in relation to spinal tuberculosis, leads to cold abscess formation.

Although the progress is much less rapid than in acute osteomyelitis, without adequate treatment serious damage to bones and joints occurs.

DEVELOPMENTAL ABNORMALITIES

Local abnormalities are fairly common and include cleft palate, spina bifida and many structural variations of limb development. In the majority the aetiology is uncertain: the presence of teratogens (e.g. thalidomide) is suspected in many and, in a few, genetic inheritance has been established.

Generalised abnormalities are rare and usually inherited.

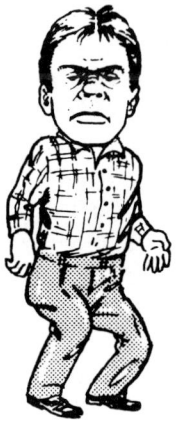

1. **ACHONDROPLASIA** causes a particularly striking dwarfism.
   Short, deformed limbs cause a waddling gait. The bones at the skull base are underdeveloped.
   The basic abnormality is defective, irregular development of cartilage cells, particularly at the growing epiphyseal plate. This results in stunted long bones.
   A mutation of the fibroblast growth factor receptor gene is responsible.

2. In **OSTEOGENESIS IMPERFECTA**, if there is survival beyond infancy, the thin brittle bones fracture easily and a history of multiple fractures with minimal cause is the usual presentation.
   The basic defect is in the osteoblasts which fail to synthesise collagen properly. The defects are due to mutations affecting the Type I collagen genes on chromosomes 7 and 17. The severity of the disorder depends on the type of mutation.

A long bone showing three fractures.

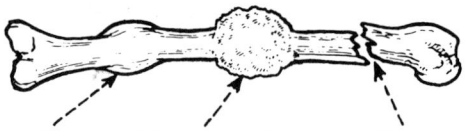

Old, with deformity

More recent, with exuberant callus

Recent, with displacement

Associated conditions due to the same defect are:
(a) very thin sclerae which appear blue
(b) abnormal tooth development due to defective dentine formation.

3. **OSTEOPETROSIS** (Marble bone disease of Albers-Schönberg) is a disorder in which osteoclasts are absent or defective. This results in failure of bone remodelling and abnormal conversion of cartilage to bone. The whole skeleton becomes dense and the bones thickened.
   Complications are: (a) anaemia due to marrow replacement
   (b) fractures
   (c) cranial nerve compression.

Replacement of osteoclasts by marrow transplant has been done with success.

CYSTIC LESIONS IN BONE

True simple cysts in bone are not uncommon. They have an ill defined collagenous capsule and occur in the proximal humeral and femoral metaphyses in children. As they expand, the risk of fracture increases and this is the most usual presenting sign.

Other, cyst-like spaces occur in many bone disorders and even fairly solid non-calcified lesions may appear cystic on radiological examination. Examples of such disorders are cystic degeneration adjacent to osteoarthritic joints, giant cell tumour of bone, aneurysmal bone cyst, hyperparathyroidism, histiocytosis X, localised developmental defects involving fibrous tissue or cartilage and, most commonly, metastatic tumour in bone. Because of the very different prognostic implications, in clinical practice accurate histological diagnosis is essential.

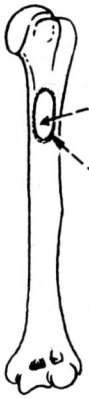

Eosinophilic granuloma (at the benign end of the spectrum of Langerhans histiocytosis) usually presents as single osteolytic radiolucent lesions of bone in children. Vertebral collapse and pathological fractures are sometimes seen. The prognosis is usually good. The histological appearances are typical.

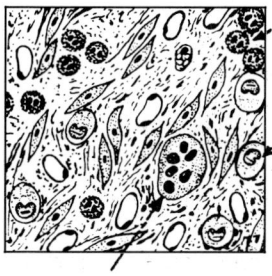

TUMOURS IN BONE

Simple tumours present as proliferations of a variety of tissues, varying from rounded excrescences of cartilage and hard bone (simple exostoses and osteomas) through multiple irregular nodules of cartilage (enchondromas) to areas of replacement of bone by fibrous or myxomatous tissue. In the field of simple bone tumours, the borderland between true neoplasia and developmental defect is ill-defined.
The importance of simple bone tumours is that:

1. They may cause cosmetic and slight functional defects.
2. Pathological fracture may occur.
3. In some conditions (e.g. multiple enchondromatosis and exostoses), there is a tendency to malignant transformation.

TUMOURS IN BONE

OSTEOID OSTEOMA

Although rare, this is worthy of particular mention since it has a striking clinical presentation and a distinctive pathology.

Clinical: Classically, an adolescent complains of well localised, increasingly severe pain in a lower limb long bone. Aspirin gives relief.

Pathological: The essential lesion is a small focus of newly formed irregular trabeculae of osteoid or poorly calcified woven bone in a highly vascular stroma.

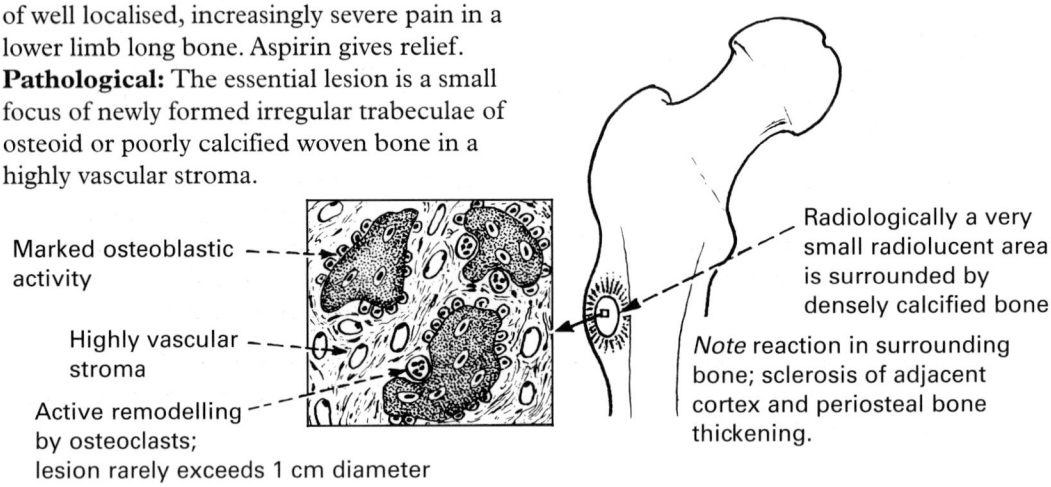

GIANT CELL TUMOUR (osteoclastoma)

This is not a common tumour but presents characteristic histological appearances. The tumour arises in adult life (age 20–40 years), usually at the end of a long bone — especially adjacent to the knee. The basic pathological process is essentially destructive of bone so that the cortex, gradually expanded by the tumour, becomes egg-shell thin and may be ruptured. Pathological fracture is common.

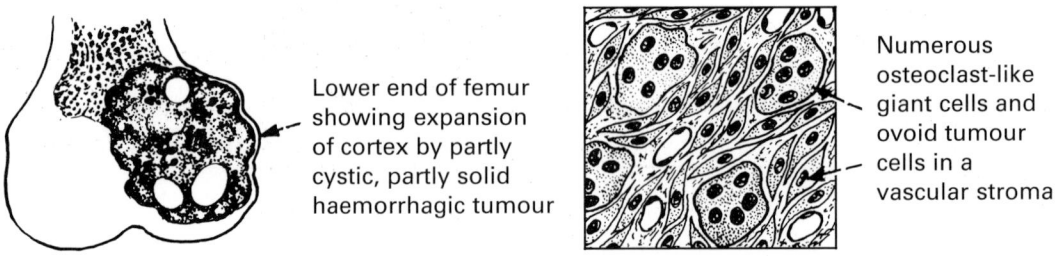

Behaviour: Almost all giant cell tumours are benign. Most are cured by thorough removal: approximately 20% recur: under 5% are malignant or become malignant after radiotherapy and metastasise to the lungs.

TUMOURS IN BONE

MALIGNANT TUMOURS

Primary malignant tumours of bone are not common, but they assume importance because some arise in young people and are highly malignant and in a few, specific pre-existing bone disorders are known precursors, e.g. Paget's disease, multiple enchondromatosis.

Osteosarcoma

This highly malignant tumour is the commonest primary malignant tumour of bone (excluding myelomatosis). It affects two distinct age groups and there is a preponderance of males over females.

Young age group — majority of cases (10–25 years)
The tumour usually arises near the end of a limb long bone (particularly around the knee).

Elderly subjects (over 60 yrs.)
In 50% of this group, Paget's disease is associated. Long bones, vertebrae, pelvis and skull are often affected, and tumours may be multicentric in origin.

The 'classic' tumour in an adolescent will be described: tumour growth begins in the medullary cavity. When the cortex has been destroyed and penetrated there is swelling. Most patients complain of bone pain.

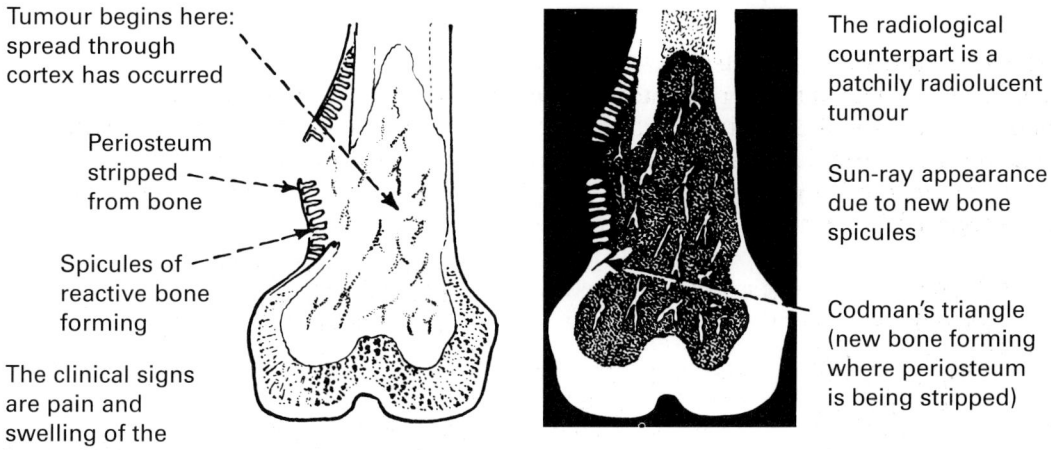

NB at this stage lung metastases may be present.

The tumour arises from primitive cells which retain to a varying extent the ability to form bone. Histologically, varying amounts of osteoid, irregularly woven bone and sometimes islands of primitive cartilage are seen. The tumour cells are pleomorphic and mitotically active. With modern chemotherapy 50–60% of patients survive for 5 years.

TUMOURS IN BONE

Chondrosarcoma.
This shows a much slower growth pattern and affects the age group 40–70 years. Multiple enchondromatosis pre-exists in a number of cases. The tumours arise particularly in the limb girdles and proximal long bones and consist of primitive cartilage. Progressive local destruction is usual. Metastases to the lung are rare.

Ewing's tumour
This rare malignant tumour affects young subjects (age 5–20 years): it arises in long bones, pelvis, ribs and scapulae. The tumour is very aggressive, metastasising early to lungs and other bones.

The tumour cells are small and uniform with pale, open nuclei: the cytoplasm contains glycogen. The histological appearances may mimic lymphoma.

Histogenesis and Aetiology
It is considered to be a primitive neuro-ectodermal tumour and is associated with translocation and fusion of genes typically on chromosomes 11 and 22. With chemotherapy, survival is similar to that of osteosarcoma.

Lymphoid tumours
Lymphoma and myeloma (see p.450) arise in bone, causing osteolysis.

SECONDARY TUMOURS IN BONE
THIS IS THE MOST COMMON TYPE OF TUMOUR IN BONE.
Metastases are usually multiple: occasionally latent renal and thyroid cancers present as single bony metastases with pathological fracture. Tumours which show a predilection for spread to bone are carcinoma of the PROSTATE, BREAST, LUNG, KIDNEY and THYROID particularly. The incidence of bone secondaries ESPECIALLY IN THE SPINE is very high when these tumours become widespread.

The effects of metastatic growth are essentially osteolytic with extensive destruction of bone. In a minority of cases, osteoblastic activity is stimulated by the presence of the tumour so that dense reactive bone is formed. Osteosclerotic secondaries of this type are seen particularly in cancers of the PROSTATE and BREAST.

JOINTS

The diagram illustrates the important components of a **diarthrodial joint.**

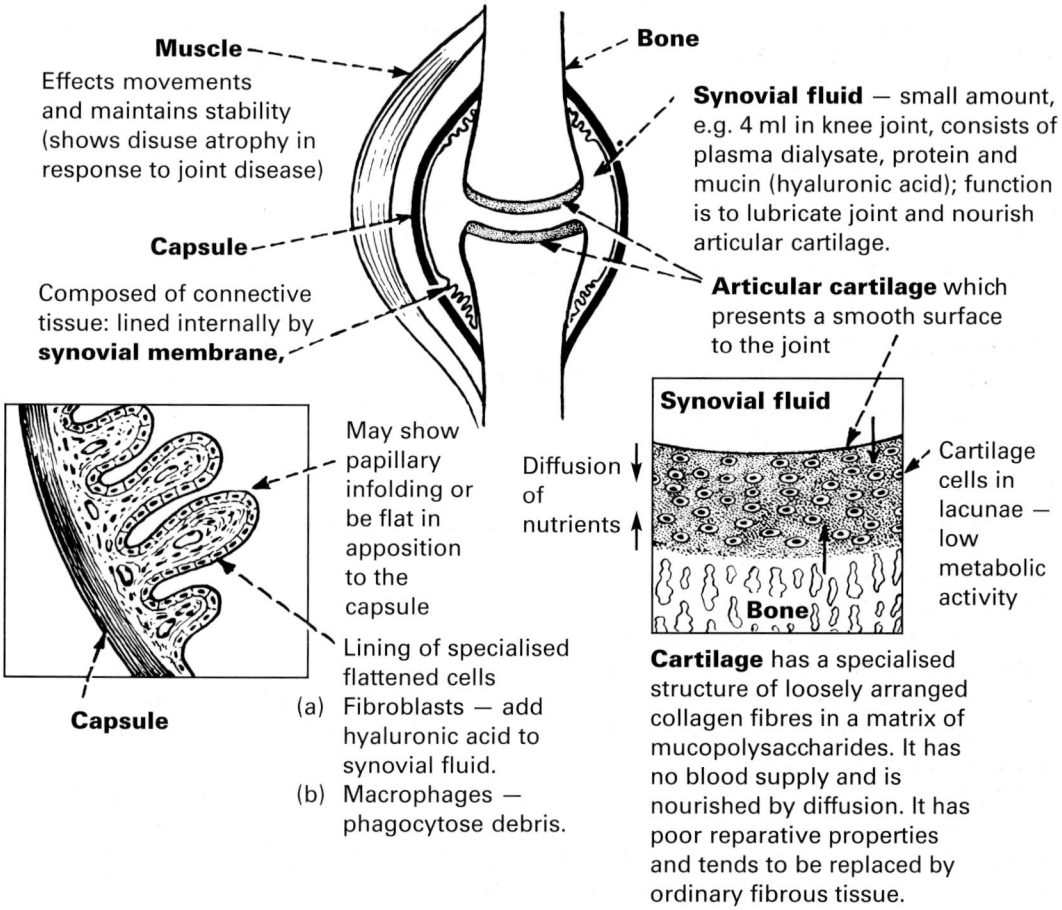

The two most common joint diseases illustrate how individual components of a joint may be initially affected:

Rheumatoid Arthritis essentially an inflammation of **synovial membrane**	**Osteoarthritis** essentially a degeneration of **articular cartilage**

As the diseases progress, other secondary effects are added and may obscure the basic pathology.

JOINT TRAUMA

Trauma is very variable in its severity and effects.

At one end of the scale a single incident of 'sprain or strain' involves only minor soft tissue damage with minimal associated haemorrhage — in these circumstances the healing capacity of joints is rapid and complete.

In contrast, many modern road traffic accidents involve serious damage to joints.

These include:

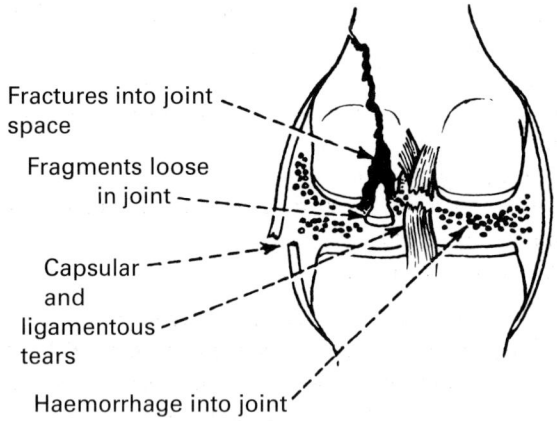

Possible sequels are:

1. The articular surface is permanently deformed (ineffective repair of cartilage).
2. Loose body continues to cause traumatic damage to synovium.
3. Ligaments may not heal or are united by poor scar tissue.
4. Haemorrhagic exudate may not be resorbed — adhesions form within the joint.

With lesser degrees of trauma, particularly if repeated, the synovial membrane shows non-specific reactive changes which include hyperaemia and mild chronic inflammatory cellular infiltrate. There is often a joint **effusion.**

The knee joint is susceptible to a particular type of injury in which one (particularly the medial) of the fibrocartilagenous menisci is torn.

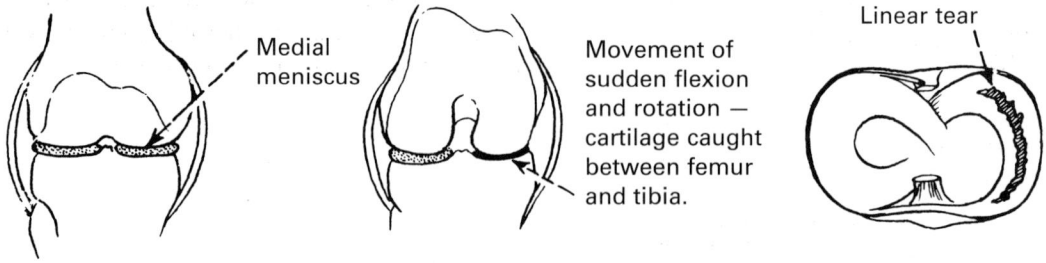

Locking of the joint and effusion are common.

Apart from damage directly attributable to trauma, the most important sequel is that the scene is set within the joint for the more rapid development of **DEGENERATIVE JOINT DISEASE.**

OSTEOARTHRITIS (OA)

OSTEOARTHRITIS (OA)

This is the commonest disorder of joints and, by causing pain and stiffness, is the commonest cause of chronic disability after middle age. The basic pathological progress is degenerative and is similar to that seen in lesser degree in simple ageing. The suffix 'itis' is really inappropriate since any inflammatory changes are secondary.
The disorder is divided into two main groups:

1. In **secondary OA** there is a clear association with some predisposing condition which may be virtually any abnormality of a joint. Of particular importance are:
   (a) alterations to the joint mechanics (e.g. abnormal alignments and angulations); a particularly severe form (Charcot's joint) is seen when the nerve supply to a joint is defective — neuropathic arthropathy.
   (b) abnormality of the articular surfaces (e.g. following injury).
   (c) abnormal stresses on the joint (e.g. the increased weight-bearing demanded by obesity; association with particular occupations and sports).
   (d) previous inflammation e.g. sepsis, rheumatoid arthritis.
2. In **primary OA**, no obvious predisposing cause is evident; there is a presumptive abnormality of chondrocyte metabolism but its essential nature remains obscure. A familial pattern is apparent in some cases — in some, mutation of Type II collagen gene is found.
   In both types of osteoarthritis the basic pathological processes are the same.

Normal

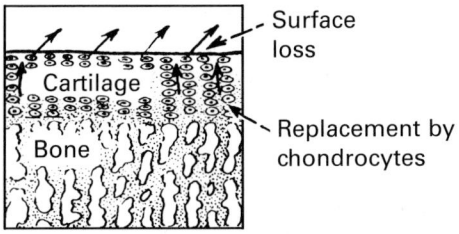

The integrity of the articular cartilagenous surface represents a fine balance between 'wear and tear' losses and replacement by chondrocytes of the specialised matrix.

The earliest change in ageing and OA is in the chemical composition of the matrix which becomes softer. This is followed by progressive characteristic morphological changes.

At site of pressure

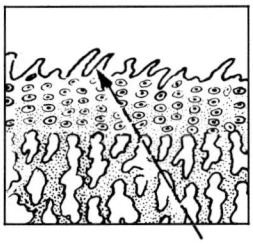

Early OA Flaking and fibrillation of surface

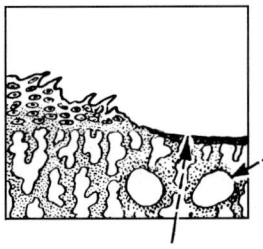

Later OA Loss of cartilage; exposure of bone — becomes hard and polished (eburnated)

OSTEOARTHRITIS (OA)

OSTEOARTHRITIS (continued)

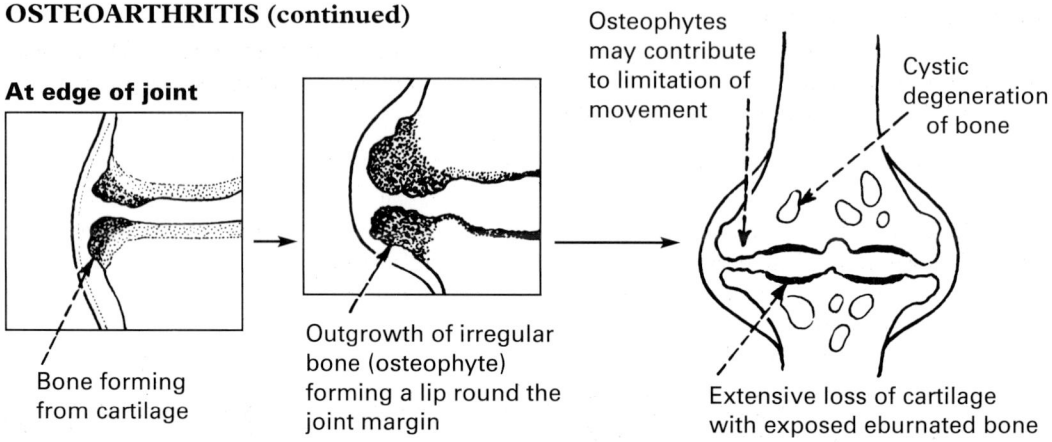

The synovial membrane may show mild, non-specific inflammation and effusion may occur but these changes are secondary.

Distribution: secondary OA often affects a single predisposed joint.

In primary OA, the larger weight bearing joints and the spine in particular are susceptible, but interphalangeal joints bear osteophytic outgrowths (Heberden's nodes). Similar lesions (at the proximal interphalangal joints — Bouchard's nodes) superficially mimic the deformities of rheumatoid arthritis; they are, however, not associated with severe disability and muscle wasting is negligible.

Cervical spondylosis. When osteophytes form around the various intevertebral joints, particularly in the cervical spine, neurological complications ranging from compression of individual nerves to actual spinal cord damage are seen.
Note: OA is a local degenerative disease; there is no associated systemic illness.

GOUT. The arthritis of gout begins as an acute inflammatory process affecting usually a great toe; with repeated attacks, degenerative arthritis supervenes.
Aetiology: the disease is a disorder of purine metabolism. There is hyperuricaemia (serum uric acid >7 mg/dl). Periodically, urate crystals are deposited within the affected joint, at first in the articular cartilage, but later both in the adjacent bone and soft tissues. An acute inflammatory reaction is evoked.

PSEUDO-GOUT. In this condition, crystals of calcium pyrophosphate are deposited in the joint, evoking a similar inflammatory reaction. Larger joints such as the knee tend to be affected; chronic degenerative arthritis often supervenes or co-exists.

RHEUMATOID ARTHRITIS (RA)

Rheumatoid arthritis (RA) is a fairly common systemic disease (1–3% of population in Europe). The main target tissue is the synovial membrane of joints (polyarthritis). The typical clinical course is insidious in its onset and progression. In a minority of cases, the onset is acute and the progress rapid. Frequently there are remissions and exacerbations.

Incidence: female > male 2-3:1

Age of onset: usually 35-55 years, but also in childhood — usually severe.

Typically, the joints of the hands and feet and the knee joints are affected; less commonly there is involvement of the cervical spine and temporomandibular joints.

Pathology: The essential condition is an active chronic inflammation of the synovial membrane.

Early

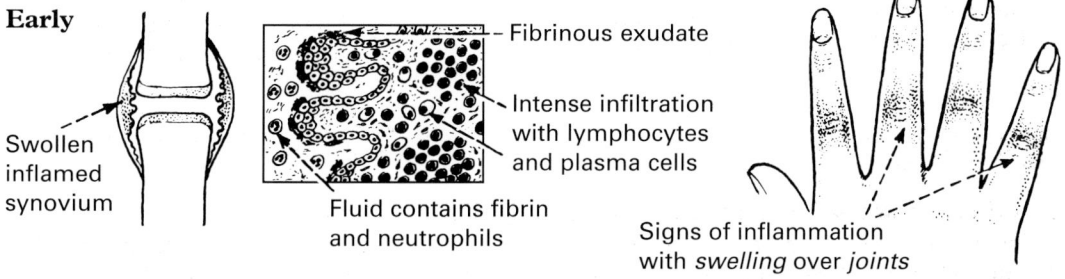

A raised ESR and normochromic anaemia are evidence of the systemic illness.

Intermediate

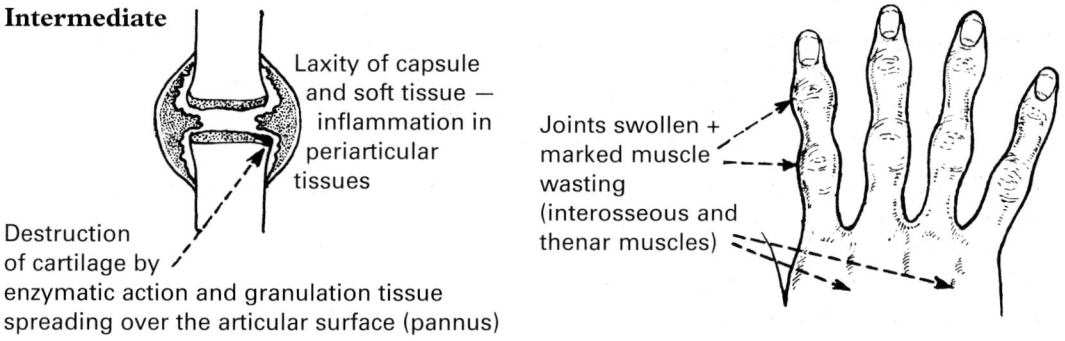

Late

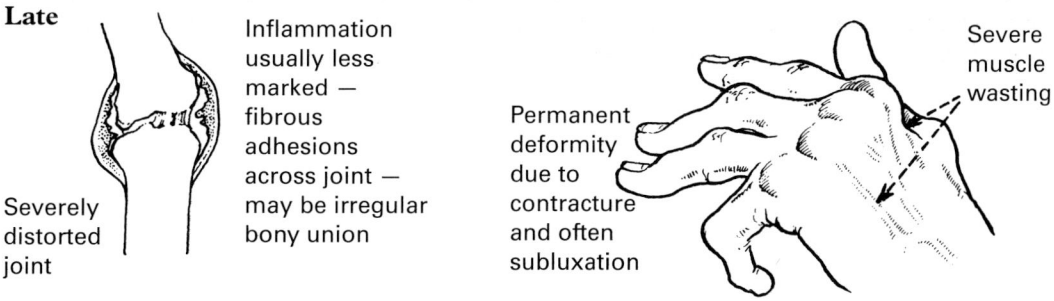

RHEUMATOID ARTHRITIS

The aetiology and mechanisms responsible for the disorder remain unknown. A popular current hypothesis is:

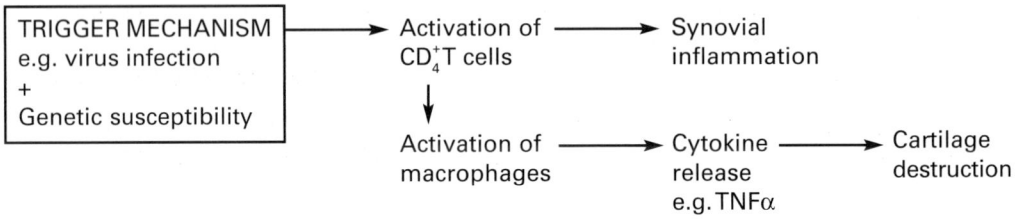

Rheumatoid factors

These are antibodies, mainly of IgM and IgG class, which are directed against the patient's IgG, and may form immune complexes which may contribute to the joint inflammation. Patients in whom these autoantibodies can be found in the serum are described as seropositive. Around 85% of RA patients are seropositive.

The local condition is aggravated by affection of other synovial tissues — particularly tendon sheaths and bursae.

The systemic nature of the disease is illustrated by inflammatory processes affecting the connective tissues at other sites.

1. **Rheumatoid nodules** occur under the skin at pressure points, particularly in the forearms and elbow joints in 1/5 of cases. They range in size up to a few centimeters in diameter. The histological appearance is striking.

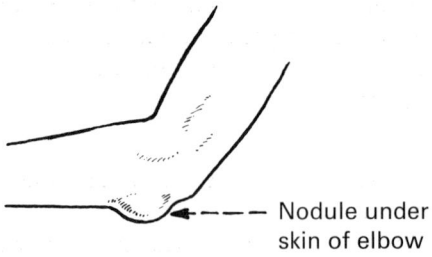

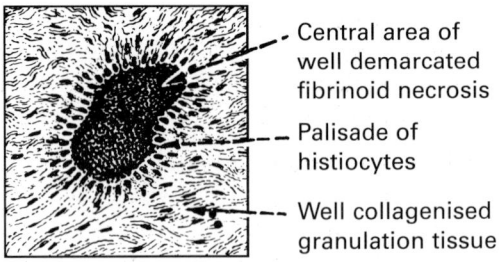

2. The lung may be diffusely affected or, in some cases, lesions similar to rheumatoid nodules are seen. In coal miners, the mixture of coal dust and collagen gives characteristic radiological and pathological appearances — Caplan's nodules.
3. Necrotising arteritis is a serious concomitant in a few cases.
4. A mild interstitial myocarditis, polymyositis or neuritis may be seen in some cases.
5. Lymphoid and splenic reactive enlargements (particularly in juvenile rheumatoid arthritis). Splenomegaly causing hypersplenism — so-called Felty's syndrome.
6. Amyloid disease — may complicate long standing RA.

SERO-NEGATIVE ARTHRITIS

Ankylosing spondylitis (AS) is an arthritis affecting particularly the sacroiliac, costovertebral and vertebral joints, but peripheral arthritis is also seen.

Incidence: .05 per cent of population
male: female; 3:1

Age of onset: Young adults progressive into middle age.
Rheumatoid factor negative

The disorder is, like RA, an active chronic arthritis, but differs in that it may proceed to calcific and osseous ankylosis, so that no movement of the affected joints is possible.

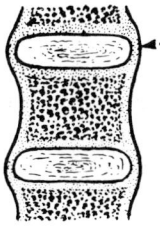

Bony union on the periphery of the intervertebral discs gives the characteristic radiological appearance — bamboo spine.

Aortitis leading to aortic incompetence and uveitis may be seen.

Psoriatic arthritis affects the axial and peripheral joints. Typically the distal inter-phalangeal joints are involved and the adjacent nails are affected.

Reiter's syndrome: This is a syndrome of polyarthritis, urethritis and conjunctivitis following infections e.g. chlamydia, yersinia and salmonella. The detailed mechanisms are unclear.

HLA association. It is of great interest in that ankylosing spondylitis, psoriatic patients with arthritis and Reiter's syndrome all have a close association with HLA-B27 (90% in AS). This suggests that a genetic susceptibility is an important factor predisposing to the arthritis.

No such association with HLA-B27 is evident with RA, which however shows an association with HLA-DR4, twice that of the general population.

Arthritis in acute rheumatic fever

During this stage, arthritis of the knee, ankle and wrist joints is common. The synovial tissues are inflamed and there is an inflammatory cellular infiltrate: the joint fluid contains neutrophils but is sterile. The arthritis is usually self-limiting and without sequelae, in contrast to the cardiac valvular lesions.

OSTEO- AND RHEUMATOID ARTHRITIS – COMPARISON

	OSTEOARTHRITIS	RHEUMATOID ARTHRITIS
Type of disorder	Degenerative	Inflammatory
Site of initial damage	Articular cartilage	Synovial membrane
Age	Late middle age +	3rd decade (any age)
Joints affected	Large weight bearing often single, pre-existing local factors in some cases	Small of hands and feet, multiple
Systemic disease	None ESR – normal Rheumatoid factor – absent	++ ESR ↑ Rheumatoid factor positive Secondary anaemia

INFECTIONS OF JOINTS

1. **Acute infective arthritis**
   (a) Primary pyogenic haematogenous infection is rare nowadays. It remains, however, a serious complication in joints already damaged. *S. aureus* is the common infecting organism. The essential changes are:

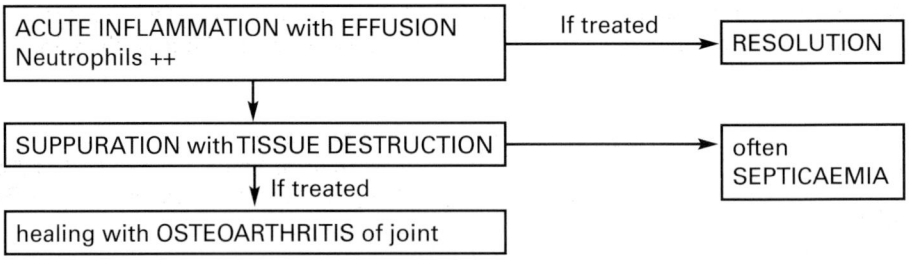

   (b) Arthritis complicating **gonorrhoea** and **brucellosis.**
   In both of these conditions, a polyarthritis may occur in the acute phase and, in a small number, continues as a low grade arthritis. The spine particularly is affected in brucellosis.
2. **Tuberculous arthritis**
   In Western countries the incidence is low: a few cases arise complicating reactivated pulmonary tuberculosis in the elderly. If untreated, there is a low grade chronic inflammation with effusion and progressive destruction of tissues.
   The diagnosis requires culture of joint fluid and/or biopsy when the typical histology of tuberculosis is seen.
3. **Lyme disease** is a polyarthritis due to *Borrelia burgdorferi* transmitted by bites from deer ticks.

JOINT and SOFT TISSUES – MISCELLANEOUS

Pigmented villonodular synovitis (PVNS)
This may affect any synovial tissue, but the knee and hip joints are most commonly affected. There is a strong male predominance (age 20–50). The synovial membrane shows a striking proliferation either in the form of brown pigmented large villi or rounded nodules.

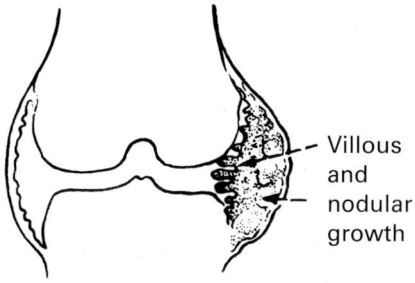

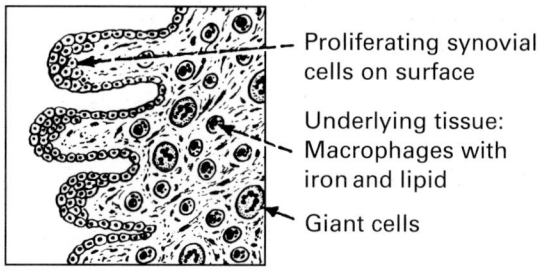

The exact nature of the lesion is not certain. It may be reactive or neoplastic **but to all intents it never metastasises.**

The so-called benign giant cell tumour of tendon sheath is now considered to be a solitary variant of PVNS.

SOFT TISSUE TUMOURS

These are dealt with on pages 123 and 124: 128–130.

Note: The term synovial sarcoma is a misnomer: the tumour does not arise from synovium but from adjacent soft tissues. It is a biphasic tumour (see p. 131).

LOOSE BODIES IN JOINTS

Loose bodies are usually found in diseased or damaged joints and their presence tends to aggravate any existing disease. Clinically, there is often recurrent 'locking' of the joint.

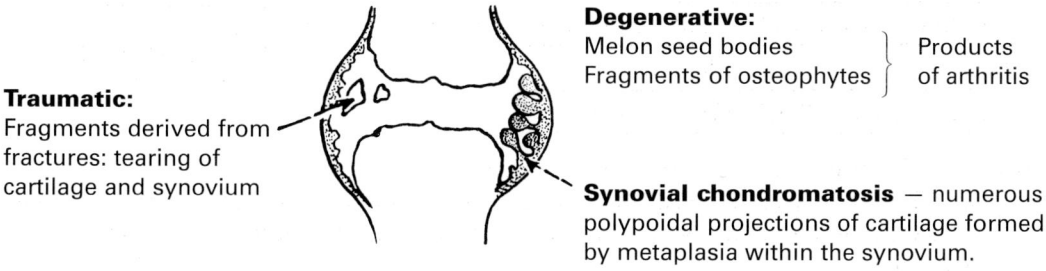

PARA-ARTICULAR TISSUES – MISCELLANEOUS

Bursae
These are synovial-lined spaces usually overlying bony prominences and often connected with adjacent joint spaces. They are subject to traumatic and inflammatory disorders as have been described in joints.

Ganglion
This is a swelling which forms in relation to joint synovium or more usually, tendon sheath. The essential lesion is a myxomatous degeneration of the sheath substance; it is not lined by synovium. Ganglia are classically seen around the wrist.

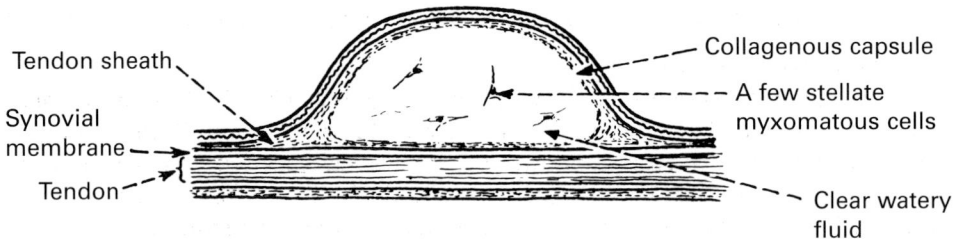

This type of myxomatous cystic degeneration may occur at other less prominent sites, e.g. within the cartilagenous menisci of the knee.

Dupuytren's Contracture. See page 124.

CONNECTIVE TISSUE DISEASES

Some five decades ago, the idea that the collagen component of the connective tissues throughout the body was subject to specific disorders gave rise to the concept of diffuse collagen diseases. Since, in fact, damage to collagen is not usually the primary event, the name was changed to the CONNECTIVE TISSUE DISEASES.

The group includes the 'rheumatic' diseases — rheumatoid arthritis (RA), ankylosing spondylitis (AS) and rheumatic fever; systemic lupus erythematosus (SLE); scleroderma; polyarteritis nodosa (PAN) and dermatomyositis.

Some of these disorders have already been described (RA p. 637; AS p.639; rheumatic fever p.216; PAN p.231; dermatomyositis p. 613).

CONNECTIVE TISSUE DISEASES

Systemic lupus erythematosus (SLE)
This is a rare disease predominantly affecting young women. The clinical progress varies from acute and rapid to insidious and slow. Most frequently the skin, kidneys, joints, serous membranes and endocardium are damaged and, in 20% of cases, the central nervous system. The essential lesion is a vasculitis affecting arterioles, capillaries and venules with fibrinoid necrosis and a variable inflammatory cellular infiltrate. In the kidney the lesion is a glomerulitis (see p.474).

SLE is an autoimmune disorder. Antibodies against many cellular constituents may be found e.g. anti-nuclear, anti-DNA.

Immune complexes activate complement so that low serum levels e.g. of C_3, C_4 are found.

Progressive systemic sclerosis
This is a rare, slowly progressive disease in which there is gradual fibrosis of various organs including the skin (face and hands), gastrointestinal tract, heart and lungs. Raynaud's disease is a common concomitant. The basic abnormality is in the small blood vessels, which show sclerosis with intimal thickening. The change is associated with fibrosis of the surrounding tissues. Auto-antibodies, typically against nuclear components, are often found.

From the description of these various disorders it will be seen that the basic mechanisms are essentially inflammatory and are mediated by autoimmune processes. The inflammatory damage is very variable in its severity, its site of predilection and even its local effects. Multiple factors, of which inherited susceptibility and resistance are important, are involved. The following diagram illustrates the basic mechanisms.

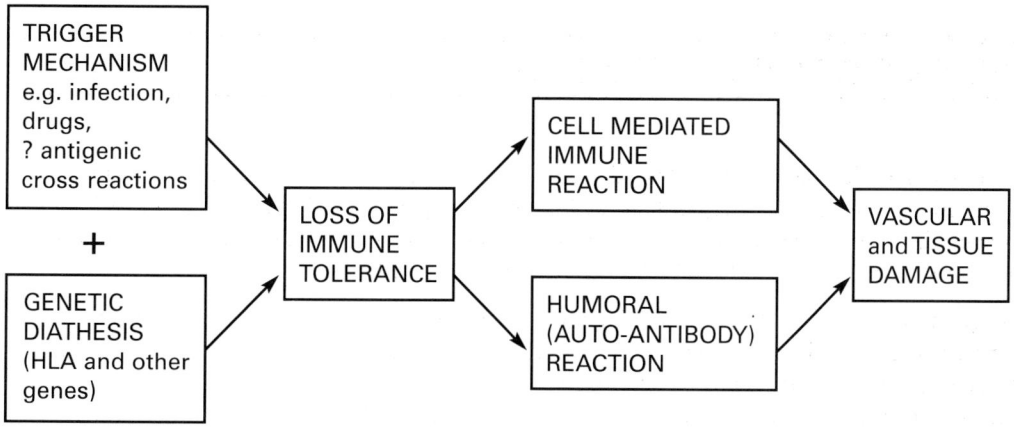

CHAPTER 15

ENDOCRINE SYSTEM

Pituitary Gland 646, 647
Hypopituitarism 648
Pituitary Hyperfunction 649
Thyroid Gland 650–655
Tumours of Thyroid 656
Endocrine Pancreas 657–661
Parathyroid Glands 661, 662
Adrenal Gland 663–667
Multiple Endocrine Neoplasia Syndromes (MENS) 668

PITUITARY GLAND

The endocrine organs form a control system related to the function and metabolism of the organs and peripheral tissues. In this, the pituitary plays a central role.

Anterior pituitary (Adenohypophysis)

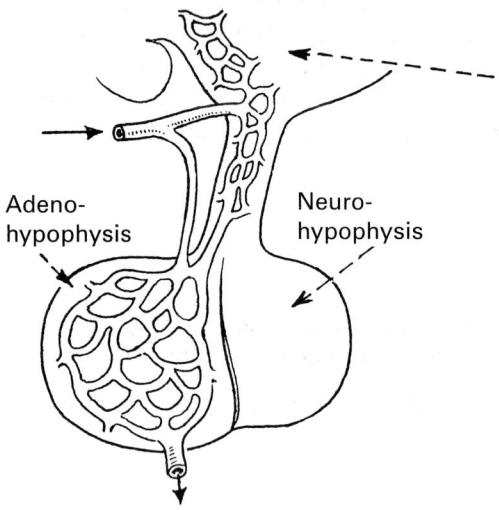

The blood supply to the anterior pituitary is via a portal system which involves the hypothalamus as well as the pituitary, i.e. the direct arterial supply to the pituitary is small.

Histology: Immunostaining has shown that there are 5 types of cell releasing 6 hormones:

Somatotrophs → Growth hormone

Lactotrophs → Prolactin

Thyrotrophs → TSH

Gonadotrophs → FSH and LH

Corticotrophs → ACTH

This modern approach has supplanted the classical histological division into 3 cell types — chromophobes, acidophils and basophils.

CONTROL of ENDOCRINE FUNCTION

A two tier system operates controlling the function of the pituitary and the other endocrines.

1. **Peripheral control.** This can be illustrated by thyroid function. The blood level of the peripheral hormone controls the pituitary secretion of the stimulating hormone.

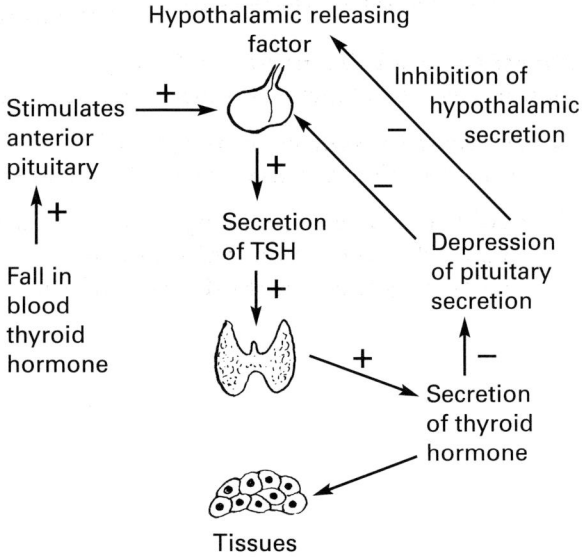

PITUITARY GLAND

Control of endocrine function (continued)

2. **Central control.** In the hypothalamus (median eminence), peptide substances are produced which are transmitted to the anterior pituitary via the portal system of vessels. These peptides act as permissive hormones, allowing release or inhibition of pituitary hormone secretion. Releasing substances have been identified for TSH (TRH), LH/FSH (GnRH), ACTH (CRH), GH (GHRH), Prolactin (PRF). An inhibiting substance, somatostatin, inhibits not only growth hormone and TSH secretion, but also secretion of insulin, glucagon and many other hormones. The action of the hypothalamic centres is controlled by the concentration of hormones in the blood.

Action of anterior pituitary hormones

Growth hormone (GH)

1. Stimulates growth.
2. Acts with insulin and thyroid hormone in controlling protein, fat and carbohydrate metabolism. Promotes nitrogen retention and stimulates protein synthesis.

Note: Some actions of GH are direct — others are mediated by insulin-like growth factors.

Prolactin

Helps to initiate and maintain lactation.

Gonadotrophins

1. Follicular Stimulating Hormone (FSH) — Promotes growth of follicles in ovary; Promotes spermatogenesis

2. Luteinising Hormone (LH) — Induces ovulation; Stimulates testosterone production by testes

Thyroid-stimulating hormone (TSH)

Induces secretion of thyroid hormones and can cause hyperplasia of thyroid epithelium.

Adrenocorticotrophic hormone (ACTH)

Stimulates secretion of glucocorticoids by the adrenal cortex.

Note: ACTH (39 amino acids long) is synthesised as part of a large molecule pro-opiomelanocortin from which a number of other molecules, including melanocyte stimulating hormone (MSH), are derived.

HYPOPITUITARISM

Failure of pituitary secretion may affect one or several hormones. **Causes** include:

(a) Pituitary tumour.
(b) Pituitary surgery/cranial irradiation.
(c) Head injury.
(d) Hypothalamic dysfunction, including craniopharyngioma.
(e) Sheehan's syndrome — is used as an example.

This occurs in women and is due to ischaemic necrosis of the pituitary following post-partum haemorrhage. The normally low pressure in the pituitary portal vascular supply increases the susceptibility of the gland. The results vary with the extent of necrosis and may include the following:

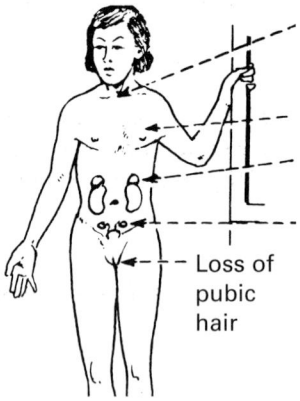

In childhood, growth hormone deficiency is a cause of dwarfism. Skeletal growth is diminished; retarded sexual development; normal intelligence. Hypothalamic GHRH deficiency may be responsible.

Note: Some individuals treated with human growth hormone have developed Creutzfeld-Jacob disease.

In adults, GH deficiency leads to diminished muscle mass, obesity and premature atheroma.

Inflammations of the pituitary gland

Apart from involvement in acute meningitis, inflammation, acute or chronic, is uncommon. Tuberculosis, syphilis and sarcoidosis have been reported.

Lesions of the anterior pituitary generally result in hypofunction or hyperfunction.

POSTERIOR PITUITARY (NEUROHYPOPHYSIS)

This is composed of neural tissue and serves as a store for two hormones produced in the hypothalamus.

1. **Vasopressin (antidiuretic hormone, ADH)**
   By altering the permeability of renal collecting tubules and concentrating the urine, vasopressin helps to control water balance. Diabetes insipidus is the condition which results when it is deficient. Absence of the concentrating mechanism results in the loss of large quantities of fluid. Abnormal thirst and polydypsia result. The condition results from damage (injury, tumour or encephalitis) to the hypothalamus.
2. **Oxytocin**
   This hormone causes contraction of smooth muscle and is often used to aid uterine contraction in labour. It also causes expulsion of milk during lactation.

PITUITARY HYPERFUNCTION

In most cases, this is associated with PITUITARY ADENOMA.
Pituitary adenomas are divided on the basis of size into MACROADENOMAS (>10 mm) and MICROADENOMAS (<10 mm).

Small tumours present only if they produce excess hormones, while larger tumours may cause pressure effects (e.g. on optic chiasma, page 141) or with hypopituitarism due to destruction of normal pituitary. Occasionally haemorrhage into a pituitary adenoma causes raised intracranial pressure (PITUITARY APOPLEXY).

Giantism and acromegaly
These are both the result of excess production of growth hormone by a somatotroph (acidophil) adenoma. Giantism arises in children before the epiphyses have fused; acromegaly arises in adult life.

Giantism
The excess growth hormone induces skeletal growth, the bones retaining their normal shape and relative proportions. Fusion of epiphyses is delayed, but eventually occurs and the features of acromegaly appear. As in acromegaly, there is initially increase in pituitary secretions and there may be sexual precocity.

Acromegaly
The soft tissues increase in thickness. This is followed by periosteal ossification causing thickening of bones.

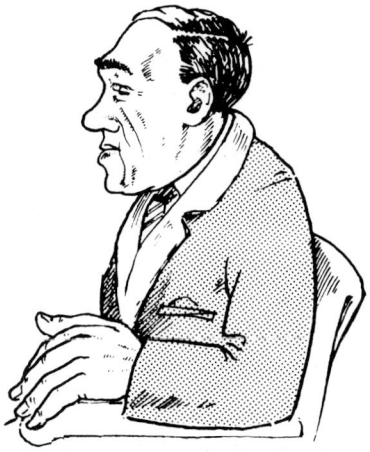

Clinical signs
- Features coarsened: nose enlarged.
- Prognathic (projecting jaw).
- Irregular bone formation — interferes with joint function — leads to osteoarthritis.
- Limbs enlarged.

Pain due to nerve compression is common. Glucose tolerance is diminished and diabetes occurs in 10%. High blood pressure with cardiac hypertrophy and extensive atheroma is common, and the patient may die in cardiac failure.

HYPERPROLACTINAEMIA
Prolactin secreting adenomas are often small. They cause amenorrhoea and infertility in younger women, but are usually asymptomatic in older women and men.

CUSHING's SYNDROME is frequently due to an ACTH secreting adenoma when it is known as Cushing's disease. The effects are described on p.664.

THYROID GLAND

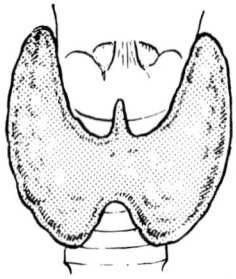

Normal bilobed gland weighs approximately 25 g

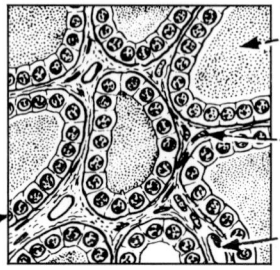

The thyroid gland is under the control of the pituitary thyroid-stimulating hormone (TSH).

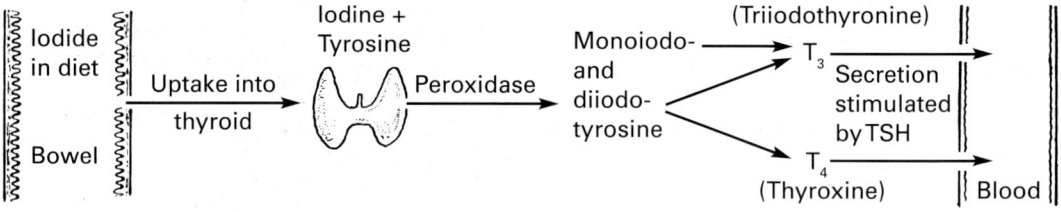

The secretion of TSH is determined by the level of T_3 and T_4 in the blood.

THYROID HYPOFUNCTION

Insufficient thyroid hormone is produced, resulting in myxoedema in adults and cretinism in children.

Adults — MYXOEDEMA

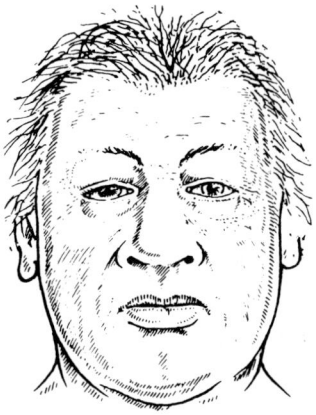

Clinical signs

Basal metabolic rate reduced.
Body temperature falls.
Lethargy and apathy.
Appetite reduced.
Constipation.
Respiratory and heart rates reduced.
Diminished libido.
Lack of ovulation.
Skin thickened, non-pitting oedema due to increase in mucopolysaccharide ground substance.
Hair brittle, dry and falls out.
Blood cholesterol is raised.
TSH secretion is increased.
T_3 and T_4 blood levels low.

THYROID GLAND

Myxoedema (continued)

Causes

1. Autoimmune thyroiditis
   (a) Atrophic form — so-called **primary myxoedema** — the commonest cause of hypothyroidism
   (b) Goitrous form — **Hashimoto's disease.**
2. Severe iodine deficiency.
3. Dyshormonogenesis — inborn errors in the formation of thyroid hormones.
4. Anti-thyroid drugs.
5. Excessive surgical resection of thyroid gland.
6. Treatment with radioiodine.
7. Hypopituitarism → reduced TSH.

Pathological changes in primary myxoedema

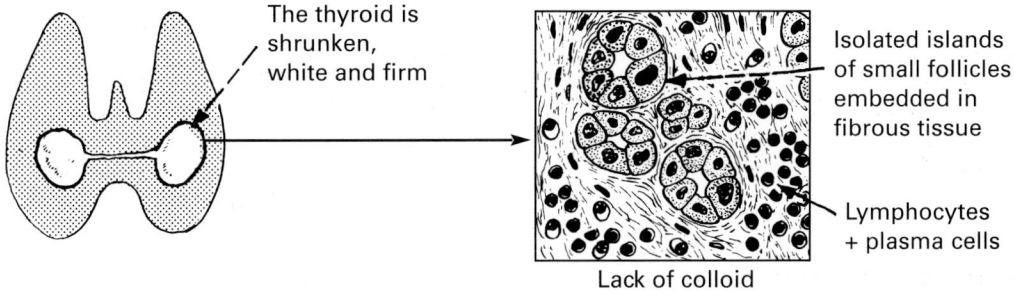

Children — CRETINISM

Infants normal at birth, but abnormality appears within weeks.

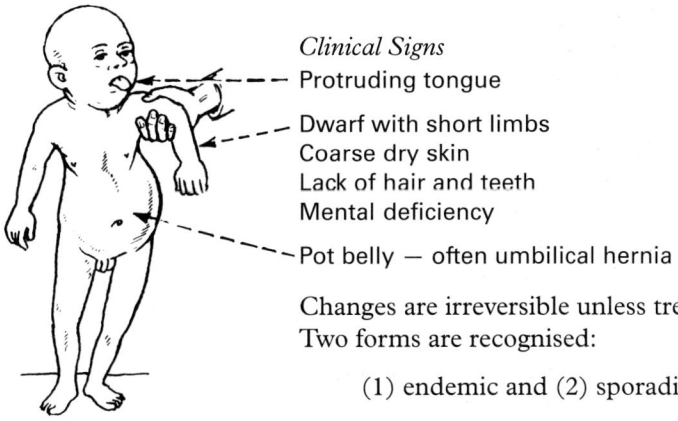

Changes are irreversible unless treatment is given early.
Two forms are recognised:

(1) endemic and (2) sporadic cretinism.

THYROID GLAND

Endemic cretinism

This occurs in districts where goitre is common due to iodine deficiency. It rarely appears until the 3rd generation of a goitrous family and the mother almost always has a goitre. The infantile thyroid is usually enlarged and nodular. Histologically, there are hyperplastic foci containing colloid which compress the intervening tissue. The incidence of this disorder has reduced following addition of iodine to salt.

Sporadic cretinism

This is usually due to congenital hypoplasia or absence of the thyroid. Deaf mutism is often present.

Dyshormonogenesis

In this condition, cretinism is due to a congenital familial recessive enzyme defect leading to inability to complete the formation of thyroid hormone. The thyroid gland is enlarged and shows epithelial hyperplasia. TSH is increased.

THYROID HYPERFUNCTION

Excessive quantities of circulating thyroid hormone (T_3 and T_4) cause thyrotoxicosis. Three types of thyroid lesion can give rise to thyrotoxicosis.

1. Graves' disease (exophthalmic goitre) >80%.
2. Toxic nodular goitre 10%
3. Toxic adenoma <5%.

Graves' Disease (Exophthalmic goitre)

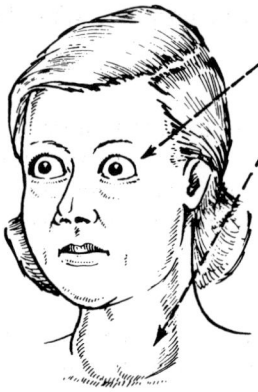

Clinical signs

Exophthalmos
Prominent thyroid.
BMR increased.
Skin warm and sweaty: heat intolerance.
Weakness, hyperkinesia and emotional instability.
Loss of weight.
Glucose tolerance diminished, glycosuria.
Rapid Pulse.
Cardiac arrhythmia, especially atrial fibrillation, and failure in older patients.
TSH low.

THYROID GLAND

Graves' disease

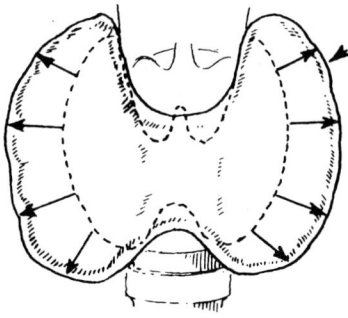

Gland is diffusely enlarged; pale pink in colour

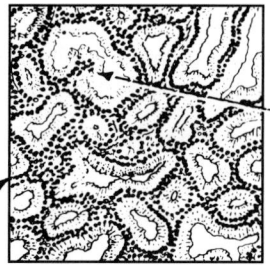

Gland is hyperplastic; numerous closely packed acini of various sizes

Sometimes intra-acinar papilliform growths

Colloid absent

Cells columnar

In some cases there are foci of thyroiditis with lymphocytes and plasma cells.

Other changes: 1. Patches of myxoedema — usually on pre-tibial aspect of legs.
2. Exophthalmos, due to autoimmune damage to the eye muscles.

Aetiology: 1. Usually in females, peak 20–40 years.
2. More common in families showing high incidence of autoimmune disease, e.g. thyroiditis, pernicious anaemia.
3. The stimulation of the thyroid is due to an autoantibody (thyroid stimulating immunoglobulin) which reacts with and activates the surface receptor for TSH on thyroid epithelium. Cyclic AMP is formed and this stimulates hyperplasia of the epithelium and increased formation of thyroid hormone. With the increase in hormone, the blood TSH falls.

Toxic adenoma

Most adenomas are non-active; only a small proportion (1%) give rise to toxic symptoms.

There is usually only one large adenoma present. The histological features are of follicles which may be small or of normal size. Increased production of thyroid hormone by the adenoma, which is autonomous, causes a fall in TSH, and the remainder of the thyroid is inactive.

Toxic nodular goitre

This develops in some cases of non-toxic nodular goitre. Nodules of hyperplasia are interspersed with inactive tissue. The condition is more common over the age of 50. Exophthalmos is absent. Cardiac arrhythmias and failure is common.

THYROID GLAND

Non-toxic goitre

This is a simple enlargement of the thyroid gland, not associated with increased secretion of thyroid hormone.

Two morphological forms are found: (1) parenchymatous and (2) colloid: they are components of a disease spectrum and are separated only on morphological appearances.

1. ***Parenchymatous goitre.*** The gland is enlarged and pale pink. Two phases can be recognised:

   (a) **Diffuse hyperplasia:** The gland consists mainly of small closely packed acini lined by columnar epithelium and containing a small amount of poorly stained colloid. Occasional intra-acinar papilliform epithelial projections may be seen.

   (b) **Nodular hyperplasia:** This is a later stage. Areas of marked hyperplasia cause atrophy of intervening parenchyma. It appears to be related to continuing severity of iodine deficiency.

2. ***Colloid goitre.*** The enlarged gland is translucent and brown due to the large amount of stored colloid.

   This is common in women and appears at puberty or during pregnancy. There are usually no symptoms, but pressure symptoms develop if the thyroid is retrosternal, e.g. pressure on trachea causing stridor, pressure on recurrent laryngeal nerve → hoarseness.

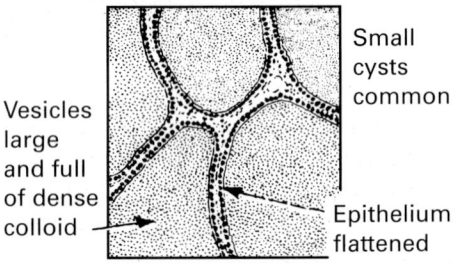

Aetiology. Goitre is endemic in central areas of the world, mountainous regions remote from the sea — Switzerland, Himalayas, Andes, etc. There is a lack of iodine in the soil, hence in the food. Addition of iodine to salt has lowered the prevalence.

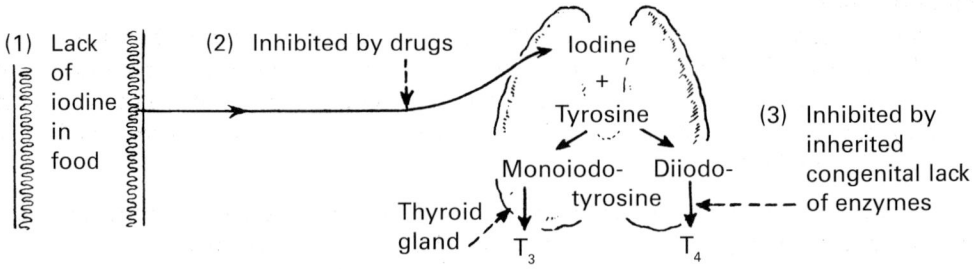

Mechanism of goitre production

Lack of iodine → Deficient production of thyroid hormone → TSH secretion → Enlargement of thyroid to extract maximum amount of iodine from blood

Where the lack of iodine is severe, proliferation is marked (parenchymatous goitre). In colloid goitre, the process is milder.

THYROID GLAND

AUTOIMMUNE THYROIDITIS

This type of disease is associated with the appearance of thyroid antibodies in the blood and inflammatory changes with lymphocytes and plasma cell reaction in the thyroid gland. The degree of pathological change and the clinical effects tend to form a spectrum, but three conditions can be defined.

1. **Hashimoto's thyroiditis (lymphadenoid goitre)**
   This is the most distinctive type of autoimmune thyroid disease, and the changes are widespread.

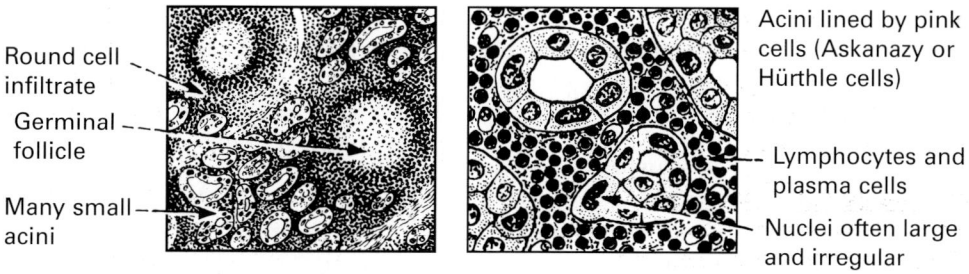

Clinical effects: While the patient may be euthyroid, it is obvious that the balance is precarious. In 50%, the patient, usually a middle-aged female, develops hypothyroidism. Any attempt to reduce the size of the goitre by surgery inevitably causes hypothyroidism.

In a small proportion of cases the patient has thyrotoxicosis in the early stages of the disease. Antibodies to thyroglobulin and to cytoplasmic microsomes of thyroid epithelium are usually present in high concentration.

2. **Primary Myxoedema**
   Antibodies to thyroid hormones and epithelium are found in this disease (p.650) also, but the plasma concentration is lower than in Hashimoto's disease.

3. **Focal thyroiditis**
   This form of autoimmune disease is usually asymptomatic, but again the balance is disturbed and surgical interference may precipitate hypothyroidism. The concentration of antibodies in the plasma is always low. The thyroid in Graves' disease often shows a form of focal thyroiditis and this may account for the occasional occurrence of hypothyroidism as a late complication in that disease.

Patients with autoimmune thyroiditis are apt to have other organ-specific antibodies, e.g. gastric, adrenal etc., and pernicious anaemia and adrenal insufficiency may occur.

4. Graves' disease (p.652).

TUMOURS of THYROID

TUMOURS of the THYROID

Follicular Adenoma

This fairly common tumour is usually single and is encapsulated with compression of the surrounding gland. Very occasionally there is hypersecretion with thyrotoxicosis. Degenerative changes including haemorrhage into the tumour are common.

MALIGNANT TUMOURS are common. Five forms are recognised:

1. ***Papillary carcinoma.*** This is the commonest form affecting particularly young women: the tumours are usually small and may be multiple within the thyroid. They metastasise readily to local lymph nodes and the first clinical sign may be an enlarged cervical lymph node containing metastatic papillary tumour. Remote spread is unusual.

The histological appearances are typical:

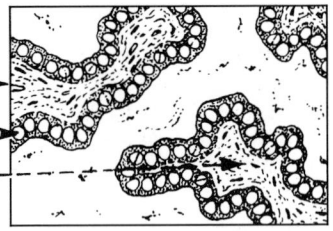

2. ***Follicular carcinoma.*** These tumours have their highest incidence in women over middle age. They present in 2 forms:
   (a) As solitary nodules usually well differentiated: some are well encapsulated and can only be differentiated from adenoma by invasion of the capsule and/or venous venules.
   (b) As a tumour of varying degrees of follicular differentiation, which spreads widely in the thyroid and invades venules.

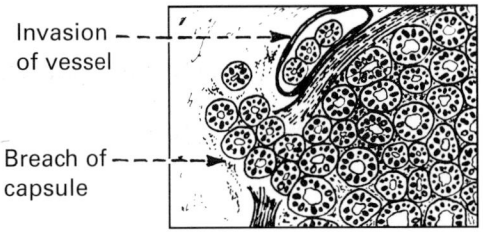

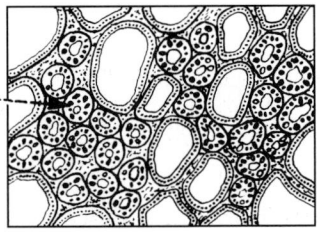

Blood spread particularly to BONES and LUNGS is usual in this type.

3. ***Medullary carcinoma***
   This is a rare tumour arising from the calcitonin-producing cells of the thyroid. Blood calcitonin is high. In addition, there may be production of other hormones resulting in a carcinoid or Cushing's syndrome. There is a familial form in which there are multiple tumours of a number of endocrine organs (MEN II p.668).
4. ***Anaplastic carcinoma***
   This occurs in the elderly and may cause stridor. Distant metastases are common.
5. ***Lymphoma***
   B cell lymphoma occasionally arises in long-standing autoimmune thyroiditis (particularly Hashimoto's disease).

ENDOCRINE PANCREAS

The islets of Langerhans form 1–2% of the pancreatic tissue. Four types of cell make up the islets. The majority are β cells.

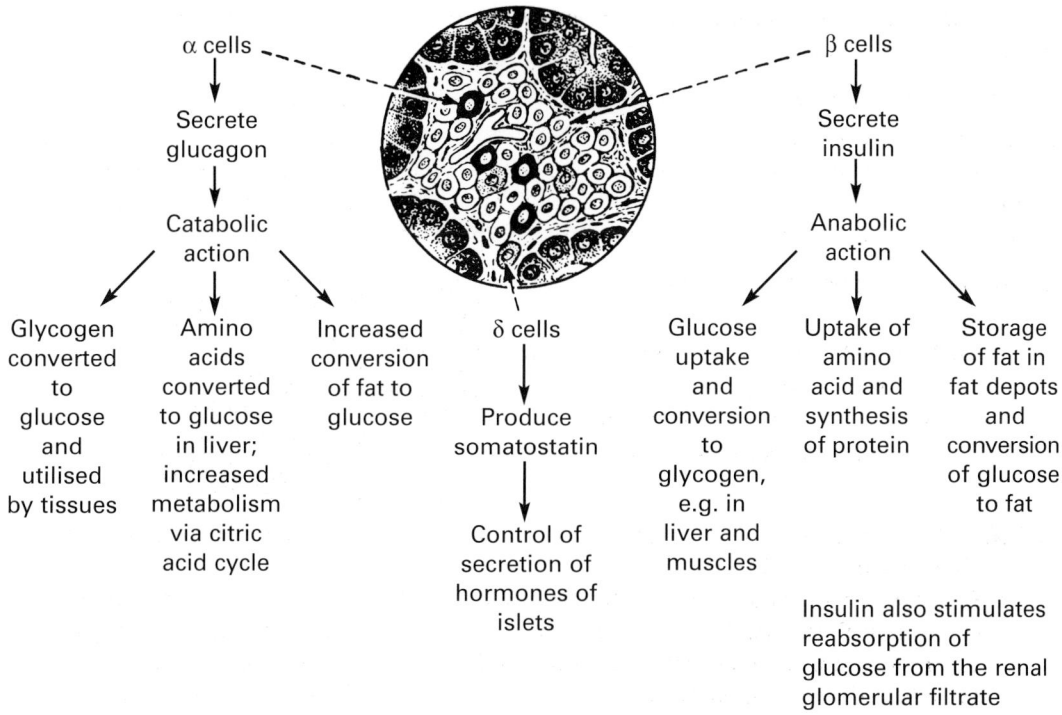

Insulin and glucagon have virtually opposite actions. The action of insulin is also opposed by growth hormone and glucocorticoids.

The fourth type of cell is the pancreatic polypeptide (PP) cell, found in highest concentration in the head of the pancreas.

DIABETES MELLITUS

This condition is due to an absolute or relative lack of insulin activity. In 1997 the American Diabetic Association suggested that the classification of diabetes should be:

Type 1 — immune mediated β cell dysfunction → absolute insulin deficiency.
Type 2 — adult onset due to insulin resistance, relative insulin deficiency or from a secretory defect.
Type 3 — a range of causes including genetic defects of β cell function and diseases of the exocrine pancreas.
Type 4 — gestational diabetes.

ENDOCRINE PANCREAS

BIOCHEMICAL CHANGES AND CLINICAL EFFECTS

The main results of insulin lack are:

1. **Inability to control carbohydrate metabolism, causing:**

Hyperglycaemia → Glycosuria
↓ ↓
Increased plasma osmolarity ← Osmotic diuresis
↓ ↓ ↓
Hypovolaemia → Thirst → Polydipsia
Loss of Na^+ and K^+

2. **Increased fat catabolism**

Leads to:

↓
Excess production of acetyl CoA
→ Conversion to ketone bodies (acetone + hydroxybutyric acid)
→ Ketosis → Acidosis → Acid excreted in combination with Na^+ and K^+
↓
Further electrolyte depletion

3. **Increased catabolism of amino acids** prevents proper protein synthesis and this, together with (1) and (2) above, leads to loss of weight despite polyphagia.

TYPES of DIABETES

Primary forms

TYPE 1 Insulin-Dependent Diabetes (juvenile 'immune-mediated' diabetes)

This form is due to actual destruction of β cells in the islets of Langerhans.

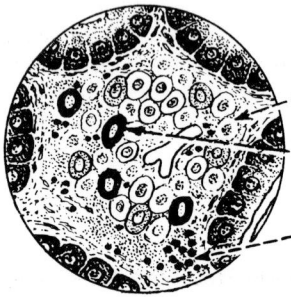

The onset is acute and the peak of incidence is around 13 years. Three factors appear to be of importance in the aetiology

1. There is a familial incidence and in 80% of cases there is an association with Class II HLA antigens (particularly HLA DR3, DR4).
2. The onset of the condition is commonest in autumn and winter.
3. Cell-mediated immunity against islet antigens and humoral antibodies are present in most cases.

This has given rise to a theory of pathogenesis:

GENETIC SUSCEPTIBILITY
– inheritance of particular Class II HLA antigens
+
EXTRINSIC FACTORS
– ? virus infection
– ? foods

↓
Activation of autoimmunity → Damage to β cells → Type 1 diabetes.

Other forms of auto-antibody e.g. gastric, thyroid, adrenal, have been demonstrated. Both sexes are affected and the condition is commoner in lower socio-economic groups.

ENDOCRINE PANCREAS

Types of Diabetes (continued)

Primary forms

TYPE 2 Non-Insulin-Dependent Diabetes (NIDDM)

This is the commonest form of diabetes affecting 5–7% of adults in Western society and 20–35% in certain groups of South Sea Islanders and North American Indians. It is commoner in Asians within Western societies. It is more frequent in females and the incidence increases with age. In contrast to Type 1, the onset is slow and the changes in glucose metabolism mild. (Diet restriction to reduce OBESITY and oral hypoglycaemic drugs usually control the blood sugar.) Clinical presentation is often due to complications, particularly vascular, or the disorder is detected at community screening.

Aetiology

This is a multifactorial disorder involving environmental and genetic factors. The basic mechanism is prolonged INSULIN RESISTANCE in the tissues leading eventually to inadequate secretion of insulin by β cells. The term 'syndrome X' has been applied to the combination of obesity, NIDDM and hyperlipidaemia leading to an increased risk of cardiovascular disease.

The following theory accommodates the known facts:

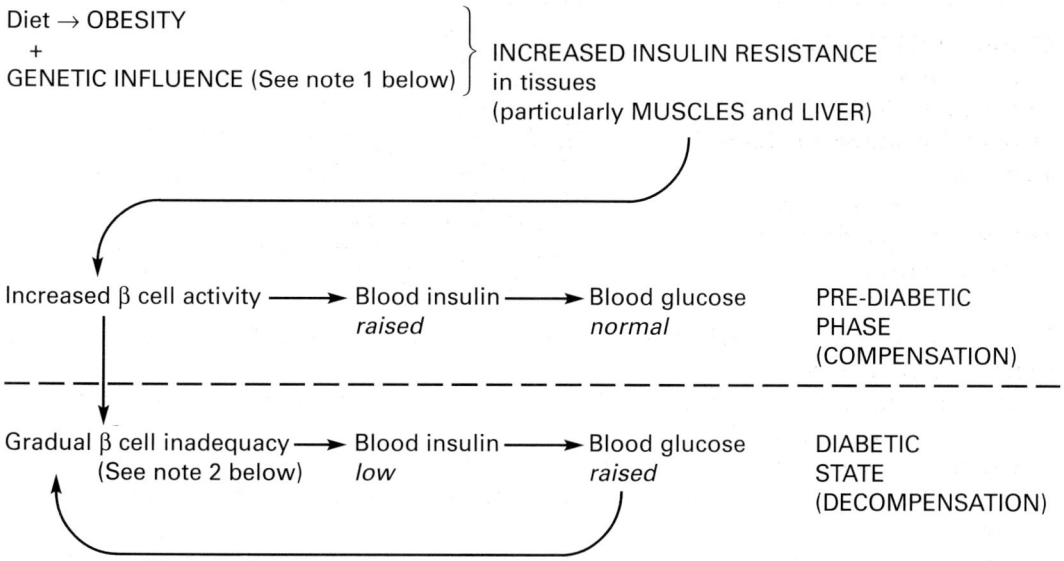

Note 1: The concordance rate for identical twins is over 85% in some studies.
Note 2: β cells secrete islet amyloid protein along with insulin. **Amyloid** is deposited in islets in Type 2 diabetes probably reflecting the prolonged β cell activity.

ENDOCRINE PANCREAS

Types of Diabetes (continued)

***Secondary forms* (Type 3)**

Diabetes may complicate:
1. A number of endocrine diseases (acromegaly, Cushing's syndrome, Conn's syndrome)
2. Metabolic diseases (haemochromatosis, pancreatic calcification)
3. Drug therapy (steroids, thiazide diuretics)
4. Pancreatic inflammation, etc., (chronic pancreatitis, mumps, cystic fibrosis).

Gestational Diabetes (Type 4)
This is associated with glycosuria during pregnancy and the birth of overweight babies. Control of the maternal blood sugar reduces birth weight to normal. Permanent diabetes is apt to develop at a later date.

COMPLICATIONS OF DIABETES

1. **Diabetic Coma.** 2 forms occur:
   (a) **Keto-acidotic coma.** This is common in Type 1 diabetes. Hyperosmolarity, hypovolaemia, acidosis and loss of electrolytes if unchecked lead to coma.
   (b) **Hyperosmolar non-ketotic coma.** This develops slowly in Type 2 diabetes. Hyperglycaemia builds up and produces profound dehydration.

2. **Hypoglycaemic coma.** This occurs when insulin intake is excessive for the amount of food consumed.

3. **Cardiovascular lesions**
   (a) Atheroma develops at an earlier age and with increased severity. Coronary thrombosis is not uncommon.
   (b) Microangiopathy causing occlusion of arterioles and capillaries. These vascular lesions are responsible for many of the clinical lesions e.g. cardiac failure (the commonest cause of death in diabetes) retinopathy, neuropathy, gangrene of limbs, Kimmelstiel-Wilson lesions in the kidney.

4. **Renal failure** is common. It may be due to glomerulosclerosis, but pyelonephritis and renal papillary necrosis are other causes.

5. **Infections.** There is an increased susceptibility to sepsis and fungal infections and to tuberculosis.

6. **Neuropathy.** (a) Peripheral } Possibly due to direct metabolic damage
   (b) Autonomic } ± microvascular occlusion

ENDOCRINE PANCREAS

ISLET CELL TUMOURS

These are uncommon. Most are benign and are asymptomatic unless they secrete excess hormones. 10% are malignant. The clinical effects vary with the hormone produced.

1. Insulin-secreting tumours arising from β cells produce attacks of hypoglycaemia.
2. Gastrin-secreting tumours cause multiple peptic ulcers (Zollinger-Ellison syndrome).
3. Glucagonoma inducing a diabetic condition.
4. Inappropriate hormone secretion, e.g. carcinoid syndrome, Cushing's syndrome, etc.

These tumours may form part of multiple endocrine neoplasia syndromes.

PARATHYROID GLANDS

The parathyroids are four small glands lying posterior to the thyroid gland.

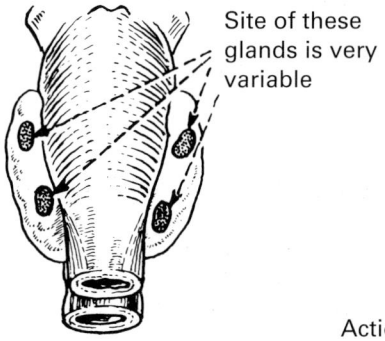

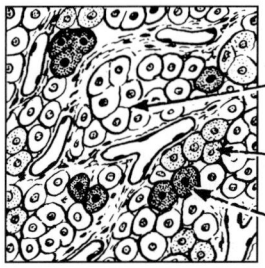

Three types of cell are found:

1. Water clear cells
2. Chief cells

} actively secreting

3. Oxyphil cells – containing numerous mitochondria

Action of parathyroid hormone

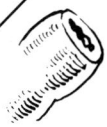

Through vitamin D it regulates absorption of calcium and phosphorus according to blood levels

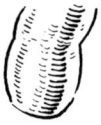

Gut

Increases reabsorption of calcium and excretion of phosphate

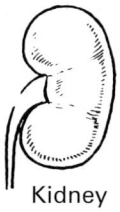

Kidney

Increases mobilisation of calcium and phosphate from bone

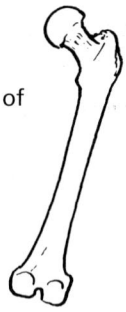

Bone

Maintains relative concentrations of calcium and phosphorus in the blood and helps control acid/base balance

PARATHYROID GLANDS

HYPERFUNCTION (see page 623)
There are 3 forms:

1. **Primary**
   This is due to **adenoma** (>90%), **hyperplasia** (approx. 5%) and **carcinoma** (approx. 2%).
   The **blood calcium** is **raised.**
   The effects are:
   (a) Formation of renal calculi sometimes leading to renal failure.
   (b) Parathyroid bone disease (osteitis fibrosis cystica).
   (c) General muscle weakness.
   (d) Metastatic calcification.

2. **Secondary**
   Parathyroid hyperplasia is a response to the **low blood calcium** from various causes as follows:

   CHRONIC RENAL FAILURE
   Malabsorption syndromes
   Vitamin D deficiency
   } HYPOCALCAEMIA → PARATHYROID HYPERPLASIA

3. **Tertiary**
   In a few cases an autonomous nodule develops in the hyperplastic gland and HYPERCALCAEMIA results.

Note: **Humoral Hypercalcaemia of Malignancy.**
Carcinomas, particularly of the lung and kidney may produce **Parathyroid hormone related peptide** (PTHrP) which causes **hypercalcaemia**. This is not related to parathyroid disease.

HYPOPARATHYROIDISM
This occurs in 3 circumstances:
1. Accidental surgical removal of parathyroids during thyroidectomy
2. Auto-immune disease
3. Congenital deficiency.

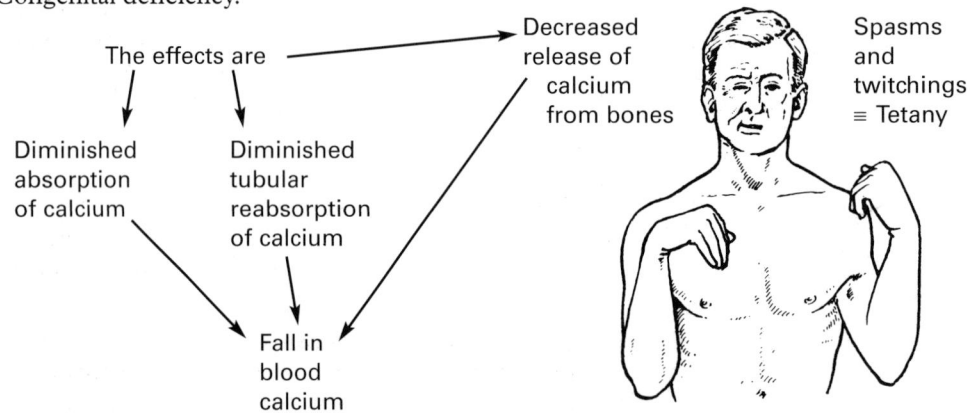

ADRENAL GLAND

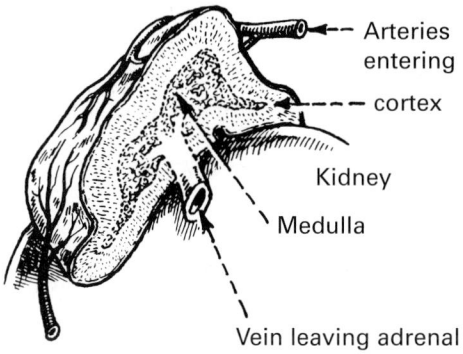

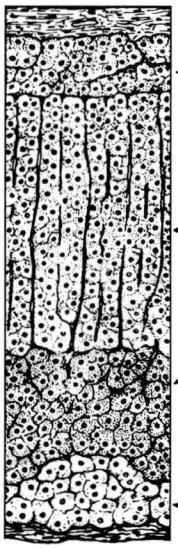

Mineralocorticoids
The main one is aldosterone.
It is involved with the renin-angiotensin system and ADH in the maintenance of blood volume. The mechanism is as follows:

Fall in renal output of Na → Stimulation of juxtaglomerular system
Fall in renal perfusion → Stimulation of juxtaglomerular system

↓

Renin secretion

↓

Angiotensin formed in blood

↓

Aldosterone secretion

→ Increase in renal absorption of sodium → Retention of fluid

→ Increased tubular secretion of K^+

Glucocorticoids
Their actions are:

- Anti-inflammatory action → Prevents migration and activity of neutrophils and macrophages
- Increased gluconeogenesis from protein → Increased protein catabolism + Diminished protein synthesis
- Increased gluconeogenesis from protein → Blood sugar increases → Glycogen deposition in liver
- Cytotoxic effect on lymphocytes → Suppression of immunological response
- Suppress secretion of growth hormone
- Deposition of subcutaneous fat in trunk and face

ADRENAL GLAND

Control Mechanism

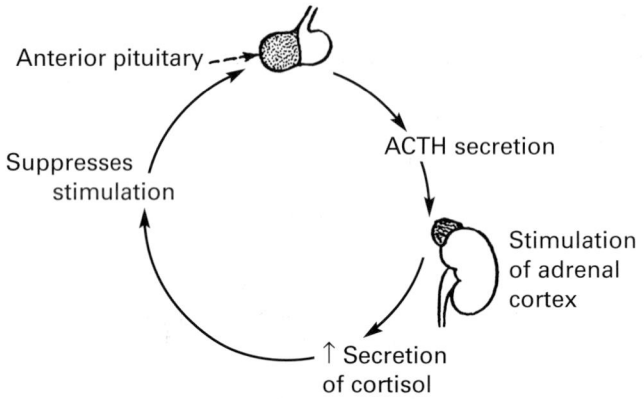

The hypothalamus secretes corticotrophin releasing hormone which stimulates secretion of ACTH.

Sex hormones — androgens and oestrogens — are also produced in small quantities.

HYPERACTIVITY

This manifests itself in three ways:

1. **Cushing's syndrome (hypersecretion of cortisol)**
   This condition is commonest in women, but occurs also in men and rarely in children.

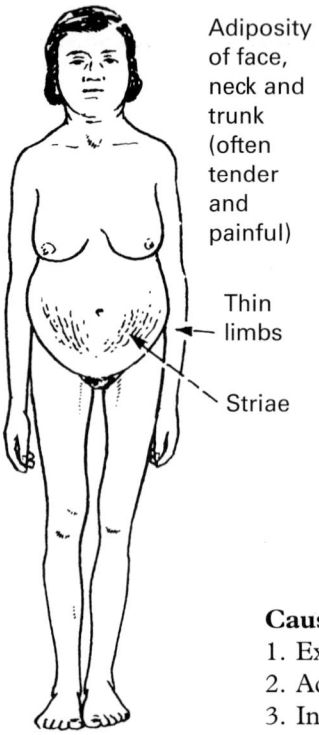

Clinical effects

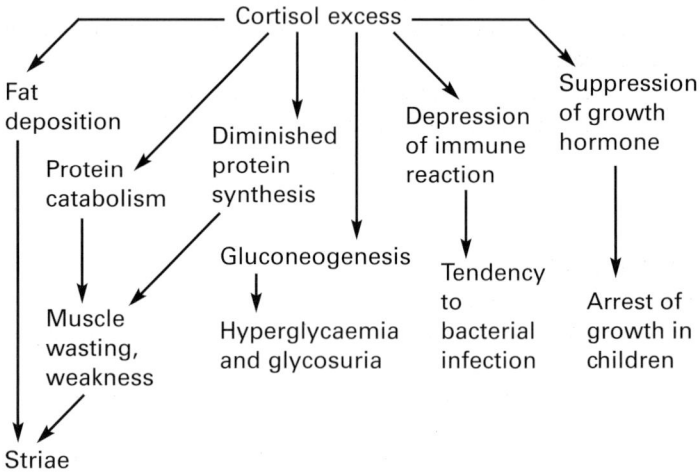

In addition:
1. Osteoporosis → kyphosis
2. Hypertension
3. Degree of virilism common in women.

Causes

1. Excessive secretion of ACTH by pituitary adenoma, 70%.
2. Adenoma of adrenal cortex, occasionally carcinoma, 20%.
3. Inappropriate secretion of ACTH e.g. by bronchial carcinoma, carcinoids, pancreatic tumours.
4. Prolonged administration of glucocorticoids or ACTH as therapy.

ADRENAL GLAND

Hyperactivity (continued)

2. **Primary hyperaldosteronism** (Conn's syndrome).
   This is due to an adenoma (>80%) or hyperplasia of the zona glomerulosa.

Effects

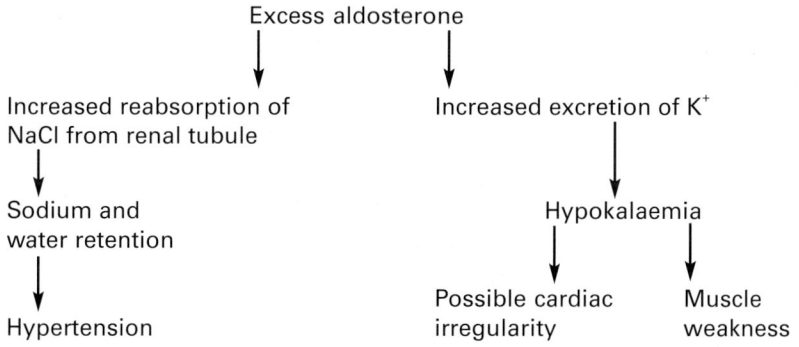

Note: Secondary hyperaldosteronism is a consequence of any high renin state e.g. renal ischaemia.

3. **Excessive sex hormone secretion**
   This can occur occasionally with an adrenal cortical adenoma; usually excessive androgens are secreted.
   (a) In children it causes precocious puberty.
   (b) In female adults — virilism, oligomenorrhoea.

HYPOFUNCTION

Acute adrenal failure

This is usually due to septicaemia, especially due to meningococci.

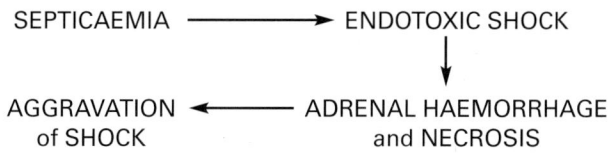

ADRENAL GLAND

Chronic Hypofunction

Inadequate production of MINERALOCORTICOIDS

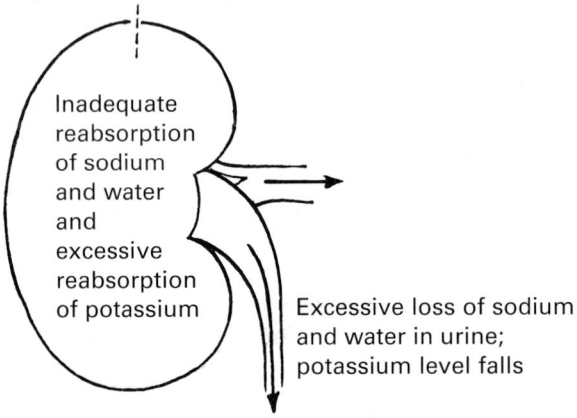

Inadequate production of GLUCOCORTICOIDS

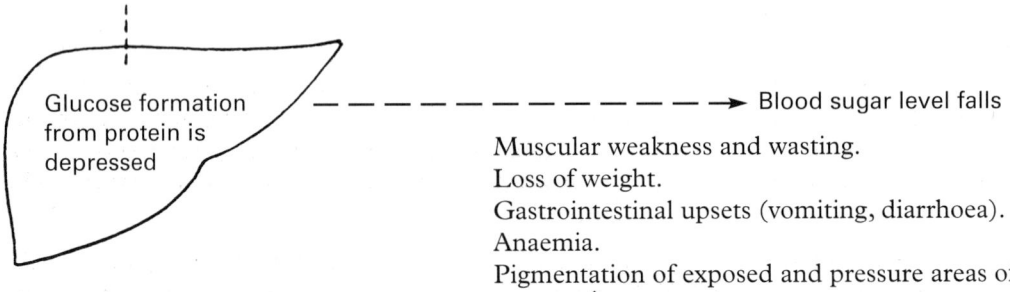

Muscular weakness and wasting.
Loss of weight.
Gastrointestinal upsets (vomiting, diarrhoea).
Anaemia.
Pigmentation of exposed and pressure areas of skin (↑MSH).
Dehydration.
Crises occur especially if acute infection complicates the condition.

Administration of adrenal hormones restores individual to normal.

Note: In adrenal gland failure, a high level of ACTH results. Melanocyte stimulating hormone is derived from the same precursor pro-opiomelanocortin

Causes

1. Addison's disease. This is an autoimmune adrenalitis with humoral or cell mediated damage to the adrenal gland. It is responsible for at least 75% of cases.
2. Tuberculous destruction of adrenals — remains an important cause, especially in developing countries.
3. Pituitary failure.

Other autoimmune diseases affecting other endocrine glands are commonly associated with Addison's disease, e.g. thyroid, parathyroid disease, diabetes.

ADRENAL GLAND

Congenital Adrenocortical Enzyme Defects
These are rare, inherited conditions due to autosomal recessive traits.

Each transformation step in the pathways of steroid formation in the adrenal cortex requires the activity of one or more enzymes. Deficiency of any enzyme will interfere with production of the end product.

21 hydroxylase deficiency
This is the commonest type, and the lack of this enzyme prevents the production of cortisol and aldosterone. The low blood cortisol activates ACTH secretion. Adrenal hyperplasia follows and, although cortisol is not formed, other steroids are produced in excess. The resulting clinical syndrome varies with the severity of the defect, e.g:

1. Symptoms of Addison's disease.

2. Lesser degrees of adrenal failure plus symptoms due to excess of sex steroids.
   (a) Pseudohermaphroditism in females; precocious puberty in males.
   (b) Virilism in female.

3. No signs of adrenal failure but sex disturbance.

Other variations have been described. Some of these syndromes are also seen with adrenocortical tumours.

ADRENAL MEDULLA

This tissue is composed of chromaffin cells producing two catecholamines — adrenaline and noradrenaline. The first stimulates the cardiorespiratory system, increasing blood sugar and general metabolism; the second raises blood pressure. During stress, they act in concert with the adrenocorticosteroids. Excess production may occur with some tumours of the medulla. Three are described:

1. **Phaeochromocytoma.** This tumour is composed of chromaffin cells. Symptoms are due to paroxysmal overproduction of the amines with hypertension, raised metabolic rate and blood sugar. Cerebral haemorrhage may occur. About 10% of phaeochromocytomas are familial, 10% are bilateral and 10% are malignant. It is very difficult to predict behaviour on histological grounds.

   Familial cases may be associated with:
   (a) MEN syndromes.
   (b) Neurofibromatosis.
   (c) Von Hippel Lindau syndrome among others.

2. **Ganglioneuroma:** a benign tumour, composed of well-differentiated ganglion cells (see page 599).

3. **Neuroblastoma:** a very malignant tumour of primitive nerve cells, occurring in children. Catecholamines are occasionally produced by the neurogenic tumours (see page 599).

MULTIPLE ENDOCRINE NEOPLASIA SYNDROMES (MENS)

This is a group of familial conditions (autosomal dominant inheritance) characterised by multiple endocrine tumours.

The main syndromes are:

MEN I — Parathyroid adenoma,
Pancreatic islet cell tumours,
Pituitary adenomas.
This is due to mutation of the MEN I gene on chromosome 11.

MEN IIA — Medullary carcinoma of thyroid,
Phaeochromocytoma,
Parathyroid adenoma or hyperplasia.

MEN IIB — Medullary carcinoma of thyroid (poor prognosis),
Phaeochromocytoma,
Mucosal 'neuromas',
Ganglioneuromas of gut.

These are due to mutations activating the *ret* oncogene on chromosome 10.

Their importance is that family screening may pick up tumours at an early stage, indeed at the stage of hyperplasia which often precedes the development of tumours.

Illustrative family history:

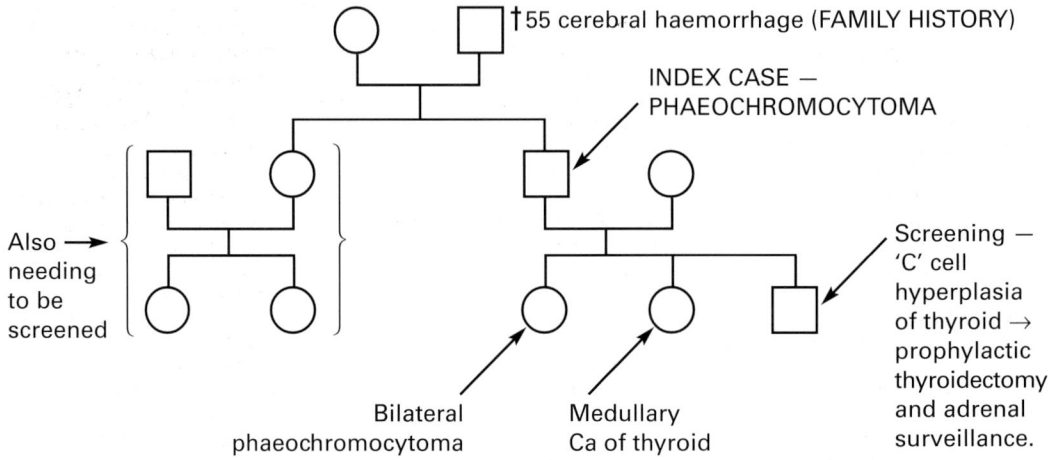

INDEX

Page numbers in **bold type** indicate importance relative to the other page numbers on the same line of the index.

Abetalipoproteinaemia, hereditary, 413
ABO blood groups, **407**, 408
Abscesses, 40–41
  amoebic, 321, **365**
  appendix, 324, 338
  cold, 74, 627
  intracranial, 567, **569**
  liver *see* Liver, abscesses
  lung, 274
  muscle, 610
  peri-apical (teeth), 293
  prostate, 533
  pyaemic, 67
  subphrenic, 324
Acanthocytes, 413
Achalasia of oesophagus, 299
Achlorhydria, 64, 398
Acholuric jaundice, 346, 404
Achondroplasia, 628
Acid phosphatase, prostatic, 142, 537
Acinetobacter infections, 84
Acinic cell carcinoma, 296
Acoustic neuroma, 602
Acquired immune deficiency syndrome *see* AIDS; Human immunodeficiency virus
Acromegaly, 623, **649**
ACTH (adrenocorticotrophic hormone), 647, 648
  Cushing's syndrome, 664
  ectopic secretion, 282
Actinomycosis, 75, 363
Active immunisation, 111
Acute bacterial endocarditis, 224–225
Acute bacterial lymphadenitis, 434
Acute diffuse proliferative glomerulonephritis, 467
Acute leukaemias, 456, 457, 460
Acute pancreatitis, 375–377
Acute phase reactants, 86
Acute post-haemorrhagic anaemias, 389, **401**
Acute pyelonephritis, 479–480, 485
Acute rejection, renal transplants, 492
Acute tubular necrosis, 485, 487–488, 610
  see also Renal tubular necrosis
Addison's disease, 666
Adenoacanthoma, endometrium, 507
Adenocarcinomas, 119, 127
Adenochondroma, 285
Adenoid cystic carcinoma, 296
Adenolymphoma (Warthin's tumour), 295
Adenomas, 118, **121–122**
  bile ducts, 367
  carcinomas from, 143
  colon, 332–333
  Cushing's syndrome, 664
  kidney, 498
  liver cell, 367
  pituitary *see* Pituitary gland, adenomas
Adenomatous polyps, 121, 143
Adenomyosis, 505
Adenosis, breast, 526
Adenosquamous carcinomas, 507, 512
Adhesion molecules, inflammation, 35
Adhesions
  bowel, 324, 338
  pleura, 41
Adrenal gland, 198, 541, 663–667
Adrenocorticotrophic hormone, 647, 648
Adult respiratory distress syndrome, 173, 286
Aflatoxins, 146, 369
African sleeping sickness (trypanosomiasis), 578
Ageing, 15, 546, **564**
Agranulocytosis, 423
AIDS, 106–107
  central nervous system, 564, 575
  haemophilia, 428
Air embolism, 163
Albers-Schönberg disease (osteopetrosis), 628
Alcoholic liver diseases, 353-354, 356, 369
Aldosterone, 166, **663**
  Conn's syndrome, 665
  shock, 175
Aleukaemic leukaemias, 455, 457
Alkaline phosphatase, 618, 624
Allergy, 102
  upper respiratory tract, 252
    hay fever, 90, 103, **251**
α chain disease (Mediterranean lymphoma), 336
α_1-antitrypsin deficiency, 262, 265, **362**
α-fetoprotein
  neural tube defects, 595
  tumours, 142, 368, 540
α-thalassaemias, 416
Aluminium, haemodialysis, 492
Alzheimer's disease, 564, **565**
Amaurotic familial idiocy (Tay-Sach's disease), 583
American Diabetic Association, classification, 657
Amniotic fluid embolism, 163
Amoebic abscesses, 321, **365**
Amoebic dysentery, 321
Amylase, 374, 376
Amyloid (deposition), 22–24
  kidneys, 23, **474**
  myelomatosis, 451
  prion diseases, 576
Amyotrophic lateral sclerosis, 587
Anaemias, 387–420
  see also Haemolytic anaemias
Analgesic nephropathy, 489
Anaphylaxis, 102, 103
Androblastomas (Sertoli-Leydig cell tumours), 521
Aneuploidy, 19, 119, 145
Aneurysms, 234–237
  cardiac, 209
  polyarteritis nodosa, 231
  syphilitic, 77, 237
  thrombus, 159
Angiitis, 232
Angina pectoris, 211
Angiofibroma, nasal, 255
Angiogenesis, chronic inflammation, 42
Angiomas, 132, 246–247
  see also Haemangiomas
Angiosarcoma, 247
Angiotensin, 663

Angiotensin *(continued)*
shock, 175
Anisocytosis, 385, 391
Ankylosing spondylitis, 92, 223, **639**
Ann Arbor staging system, Hodgkin's disease, 453
Anterior pituitary, 646–648
Anterior poliomyelitis, **574**, 586
Anthracosis, 277
Antibodies, 97
AIDS, 106
allergy, 102
complexes with antigens, 98, 104
glomerulonephritis, 467, 469, **473**
complexes with viruses, 83
glomerular basement membrane, 468
haemolytic anaemias, 406
hepatitis viruses, 350, 351
iso-antibodies, 407, 408
syphilis, 77
see also Autoantibodies
Anticoagulants, 161
coumarins, 429
heparin, 431
natural, deficiency, 431
Anti-D antibody (anti-Rh antibody), 408
Antidiuretic hormone, 166
ectopic secretion, 282
shock, 175
see also Vasopressin
Antigens, 90
autoimmune disorders, 108
complexes with antibodies, 98, 104
glomerulonephritis, 467, 469, **473**
hepatitis B virus infection, 350
presentation by phagocytes, 100
Anti-haemophilic globulin (factor VIII), 426, 427, **428**
Antioxidants, 12
Antithrombin deficiency, 431
Antithrombin III, 427
Antitoxins, 71, 98
Anuria, shock, 175
Aortic aneurysms, 235
rupture, 230
Aortic incompetence, 183, 223
Aortic valve disease, 222–223
Aortitis
ankylosing spondylitis, 639
syphilitic, 77
APC gene, 150, 153, 333
Aphthous ulcers, 290
Aplastic anaemias, 390, 417, **419**
Apoferritin, 26, 392
Apolipoprotein E gene, 565
Apoplectic cyst, 557
Apoptosis, 4
gene abnormality in tumours, 151
Appendicitis, 239, 323–324, 338
Argentaffin cells, 337
Arnold-Chiari malformation, 593
Arrhenoblastomas (Sertoli-Leydig cell tumours), 521
Arrhythmias, 207, 226–227
Arteries 190–196, 231–238
Arteriolosclerosis, hypertension, 197
Arteriosclerosis, 190
aneurysms, 237
hypertension, 197
Arterio-venous aneurysms, 236
Arteritis, 231–233
Arthritis
infective, 640
see also Osteoarthritis; Rheumatoid arthritis
Arthus reactions *see* Immune complex reactions
Asbestosis, 279
Ascending cholangitis, 363
Ascending degenerations, spinal cord, 585
Aschoff bodies, 217
Aschoff Rokitansky sinuses, 371
Ascites, 167, **339**
chronic pancreatitis, 379
cirrhosis, 360
tuberculosis, 74
Askanazy cells, 655
Aspergillosis, 84
Aspiration pneumonia, 273
Asthma, 103, **261**
Astrocytes, 547
Astrocytomas, 598
Atelectasis, 286
Atheroma, 191–196
aneurysms, 237
cerebral infarction, 554
coronary arteries, 202
diabetes mellitus, 660
Atopy, 102, 261
Atrial fibrillation, 221, **226**
Atrophic glossitis, 394, 399
Atrophy, 14
heart, 215
muscle, 608–609
neurones, 546
Atypical ductal hyperplasia, breast, 527
Atypical hyperplasia, endometrium, 506
Atypical lobular hyperplasia, breast, 527
Autoantibodies, 109
Autoimmune disorders, 108–110
Addison's disease, 666
coeliac disease, 311
connective tissue diseases, 109, **642–643**
cytotoxic hypersensitivity reactions, 103
diabetes mellitus, 658
Dressler's syndrome, 209
Graves' disease, 653
haemolytic anaemia, 406
idiopathic thrombocytopenic purpura, 426
myopathies, 613
pernicious anaemia, 303, 398
primary biliary cirrhosis, 357
Sjogren's syndrome, 294
thymic hyperplasia, 444
thyroiditis, 651, 655
see also Myasthenia gravis; Rheumatoid arthritis
Autolysis, 9
AV aneurysms (arterio-venous aneurysms), 236
Avascular bone necrosis, 625
Avian tuberculosis, 74

B lymphocytes, 91
deficiency, 105
B_2 microglobulins, HLA antigens, 92
Bacillary dysentery, 320
'Backwash' ileitis, 314
Bacteraemia, 65, **66**
osteomyelitis, 626
Bacteria, 62
central nervous system infections, 567–570
disease mechanisms, 65–77
and influenza, 271
lung abscesses, 274
pyelonephritis, 479
upper respiratory tract infections, 250, 253
Bacterial endocarditis, 66, 67
Bacterial lymphadenitis, acute, 434
Bacterial shock, 168, **172**, 173, 177
acute adrenal failure, 665
Balkan nephritis, 489
Bamboo spine, 639
Barrett's oesophagus, 297
Bartholin's gland, 514
Basal cell carcinoma, 126
Basophils (mast cells), 97, 102, 103
Basophils (pituitary), 646
Battered baby syndrome, 625
bcl-2 gene, 448
Becker type muscular dystrophy, 611
Bell's palsy, 591
Bence-Jones protein, urine, 451
Bends (caisson disease), 163, 625
Benign cystic teratoma, 131

Benign giant cell tumour of tendon sheath, 641
Benign hyperplasia, prostate, 115, 535–536
Benign hypertension, 200–201
  kidney, 475–476
Benign pigmented naevi, 133
Benign tumours, 117, 141
  of connective tissue, 123–124
  epithelial, 120–122
  histology, 118
  malignant transformation, 143
Berger's disease *see* IgA nephropathy
'Berry' aneurysms, 236, 237, 558
β cells, pancreas, 657, 659
β-myosin heavy chain gene, 214
β-pleated sheets, prion protein, 576
β-thalassaemias, 416
Bile, reflux, acute pancreatitis, 377
Bile ducts, 370, 372
  adenoma, 367
Bile salts, gallstones, 373
Bilharzia *see* Schistosomiasis
Biliary cirrhosis, 109, 356–358
Bilirubin, 346
Biopsy
  bone marrow, 386
  kidney, 466
  malignant ulceration, 45
  muscle, 614
Blackwater fever, 412
Bladder
  calculi, 496
  cystitis, 480, **500**
  trabeculae, 535
  tumours, 501
Blind loop syndrome, 396
Blood
  cell counts, 385
  films, 385
  in infections, 86
  leucoerythroblastic picture, 461
  thrombosis, 157-159
  transfusions incompatible, 407
  tumour spread via, 138–139
  see also Leukaemias
Blood groups, 20, 407, 408
Blood pressure
  for cerebral blood supply, 553
  pulmonary and systemic, 181
  shock, 171
  see also Hypertension
Blood-brain barrier, 545
Blue bloaters, 265
Blue naevi, 133
Bone, 616–632
  healing, 58–60
  metastases, 632
    prostate carcinoma, 537, 632
  myelomatosis, 450
  tuberculosis, 73, **627**
  tumours, 629–632
  turnover, 618
Bone marrow
  examination, 386
  failure, 423, *see also* Aplastic anaemias
  haemolytic anaemias, 405
  haemopoiesis, 384
  iron deficiency anaemia, 391
  leukaemias, 455–460
  megaloblastic anaemia, 395
  myelofibrosis, 461
  pernicious anaemia, 398
  thrombocytopenia, 426
  transplantation
    graft *versus* host disease, 112
  see also Anaemias; Stem cells
Boundary zones
  brain infarction, 176, 555
  see also Watershed zones
Bovine spongiform encephalopathy, 81, 576
Bowen's disease, 538
Bradykinin, 38, 337
Brain
  ageing, 564
  AIDS-associated diseases, 106
  contusion, 561
  hydrocephalus, 594
  increased intracranial pressure on, 550
  infarcts *see* Cerebral infarcts
  malaria, 577
  shock, 176
  swelling, 551
  trauma, 560–563
  tumours, 598
BRCA genes, 150, 520, 531
Breast
  benign diseases, 526–528
  carcinomas, 119, 127, **528–531**
    bone metastases, 632
    lymph nodes, 445
    spread, 140
  fibroadenomas, 122, 527
  papilloma, 120
Brenner tumours, 519
Bronchi
  metaplasia, 115
  obstruction, 285, 286
  tumours of glands, 285
  see also Lungs, carcinoma
Bronchiectasis, 266–267
Bronchiolitis, 260, 272
Bronchitis, 260, 262
Bronchopneumonia, 268
  tuberculous, 276
Brown-Kelly-Paterson syndrome, 299, 394
Brucellosis
  arthritis, 640
  osteitis, 627
Budd-Chiari syndrome, 361
Buerger's disease, 232
Bullae, emphysema, 263
Burkitt's lymphoma, 81, 448
  chromosomes, 152
Burns
  haemolysis, 411
  shock, 172
Burr cells, 491
Bursae, 642

CA125 (tumour marker), 520
Caeruloplasmin, Wilson's disease, 362
Caisson disease, 163, 625
Calcification, 9, **25**
  chronic pancreatitis, 379
  Monckeberg arteriosclerosis, 190
Calcitonin, 142, 617, 624
Calcium
  bone, 617
  coagulation system, 427
  parathyroid glands, 661–662
  plasma levels, 617
  vitamin D deficiency, 621
Calcium oxalate, renal calculi, 495
Calculi
  kidney, 495
  salivary, 294
  see also Gallstones
Call-Exner bodies, 521
Callus, 58
Cancer *see* Malignancy
Candida albicans, 84, 290, 297, 514
Capillaries, 178
  granulation tissue, 50
  thrombosis, 160
  tissue fluid circulation, 166
Capillary angioma, 132
Caput medusae, 361
Carcinoembryonic antigen, 142, 335
Carcinogenesis, 145–154
Carcinoid tumours, 337, 367
Carcinoma in situ
  breast, 528–529
  see also Intraepithelial neoplasia
Carcinomas, 125–127
  see also named sites
Carcinomatosis, meningeal, 597
Carcinosarcoma, 131
Cardiogenic shock, 168, 173
Cardiomyopathy, 213–214
Cardiovascular diseases, 156–248
Caries, dental, 293

Carpal tunnel syndrome, 589
Carriers
  hepatitis viruses, 349, 351
  inherited disorders, 20
  staphylococcus aureus, 68
  typhoid, 319
Caseation, 8, 9, 43, 72
Casoni test, 366
Casts, urine, 464
Cat scratch fever, 434
Catecholamines, 667
  blood pressure, 198
Cavernous angioma, 132, 367
$CD4^+$ T lymphocytes, 93
  counts in AIDS, **106**, 111
$CD8^+$ T lymphocytes, 93
Cell cycle, 3
Cell-mediated hypersensitivity reactions, 104
Cell-mediated immunity, 91, **93–94**
Cells, 2–15
Cellulitis, 46
Central nervous system, 544–588, 592–601, 603–604
Centromeres, 16
Cerebellum, tonsillar hernia, 550
Cerebral atrophy, hydrocephalus, 594
Cerebral haemorrhage, 557
Cerebral infarcts, 165, **554–556**
  multi-infarct dementia, 564, **566**
Cerebral malaria, 412, **577**
Cerebral oedema, 551, 563
Cerebral perfusion pressure, 553
Cerebrospinal fluid, 544, 545, **604**
  absorption defect, 592
  meningitis, 569–572
  obstruction, 592
    from increased intracranial pressure, 552
  subarachnoid haemorrhage, 558
Cerebrovascular disease, 553–559
Cervical spondylosis, 636
Cervicitis, 510
Cervix, 510–513
  carcinoma, 512–513
    human papilloma virus, 81, 513
  cytology screening, 511
  intraepithelial neoplasia, 144, 511
  squamous cell carcinoma, 125
CFTR gene, 380
Charcot-Leyden crystals, 261
Charcot's joint, 635
Chemotaxis, 36, 424
Chickenpox, 80
Chlamydia trachomatis, 434, 510, 514, 535
Chloramphenicol, aplastic anaemia, 419
Chlorinated hydrocarbons, on liver, 344, 345
Cholangiocarcinoma, 369
Cholangiolitis, bacterial shock, 177
Cholangitis
  ascending, 363
  primary sclerosing, 357
Cholecystitis, 371
Cholera, 316
Cholestasis, intrahepatic, 346
Cholesterol, 195
  gallstones, 370, 373
Chondromas, 118, 123, 629
Chondrosarcoma, 632
Choreas, 216, 581
Choriocarcinoma, 523, 525, 539
Chorionic gonadotrophin, 142, 525, 540
Christmas factor, 427, **428**
Chromaffin cells, 667
Chromatolysis, motor neurones, 56
^{51}Chromium, red cell life span, 403
Chromosomes, 16
  abnormalities, 19–20
  ageing, 15
  damage, 2
  oncogenesis, 152
  Philadelphia, 458
  radiation on, 148
Chronic fatigue syndrome, 615
Chronic granulomatous disease, 424
Chronic obstructive pulmonary disease, 262–265
Chronic renal failure, 477–478
CIN (cervical intraepithelial neoplasia), 144, 511
Cirrhosis, 355–357
  hepatocellular carcinoma, 368
  liver failure, 358
  splenomegaly, 439
  see also Biliary cirrhosis
Cirsoid aneurysms (arterio-venous aneurysms), 236
Clearance tests, 464
Clonal evolution, 145
Clonal selection, plasma cells, 97
Clonorchiasis, 366, 369
Clostridium, 70, 71, 322
Coagulation system, 161, **425–431**
Coagulative necrosis, 5, **6**
Coal miners, pneumoconiosis, 277
Co-carcinogens, 147
Coeliac disease, 310
Cold abscesses, 74, 627
Cold agglutination disease, 406
Cold sores, 80, 290
Colitis, ischaemic, 326
  see also Ulcerative colitis
Collagen diseases (connective tissue diseases), 109, **642–643**
Collagenase, 52
Collapse, lungs, 286
Colliquative necrosis, 5, 7
Colloid goitre, 654
Colon
  carcinoma, 127, 143, 333, **334–335**
    ulcerative colitis, 143, 314
Comedocarcinoma, 528
Commensal organisms, 62, 64
Common bile duct, gallstones, 372
Common cold, 251
Communicating hydrocephalus, 592
Complement system, 98,99
  chemotactic agents, 36
  glomerulonephritis, 471, 473
Complex acini, liver, 343
Complex sclerosing lesions, breast, 527
Compound fractures, 59
  skull, 567
Compound naevi, 133
Conducting system, heart, 227
Condylomata acuminata, 515, 538
Congenital heart disease, 228
Congenital syphilis, 77
Congestive cardiomyopathy, 213
Congo red staining, 22
Coning, medulla oblongata, 550
Connective tissue diseases, 109, **642–643**
Conn's syndrome, 199, 665
Constrictive pericarditis, 230
Contact dermatitis, 104
Continuous ambulatory peritoneal dialysis, complications, 492
Contraceptives, oral, 504
  see also Intra-uterine devices
Contre-coup injury, 561
Contusion, brain, 561
Copper, Wilson's disease, 362
Copper binding protein, primary biliary cirrhosis, 357
Cor pulmonale, 187–188
Coronary arteries, ischaemic heart disease, 202–204
Coronaviruses, 250
Cortical necrosis, kidneys, 485
Coryza (common cold), 251
Coumarin anticoagulants, 429
Councilman bodies, 347
Coxsackie virus infections, 229, 290, 610
Craniopharyngiomas, 601
Creatinine clearance test, 464
Cretinism, 651–652
Creutzfeldt-Jakob disease (CJD), 81, 564, **576**